Pharmacology, Characterizations, Toxicity, and Herb-Drug Interactions of Herbs in Traditional Medicine

Olubunmi Atolani
University of Ilorin, Nigeria

Learnmore Kambizi
Cape Peninsula University of Technology, South Africa

M.T. Bakare-Odunola
University of Ilorin, Nigeria

IGI Global
Scientific Publishing
Publishing Tomorrow's Research Today

Vice President of Editorial	Melissa Wagner
Director of Acquisitions	Mikaela Felty
Director of Book Development	Jocelynn Hessler
Production Manager	Mike Brehm
Cover Design	Jose Rosado

Published in the United States of America by
IGI Global Scientific Publishing
701 East Chocolate Avenue
Hershey, PA, 17033, USA
Tel: 717-533-8845 | Fax: 717-533-7115
Website: https://www.igi-global.com E-mail: cust@igi-global.com

Library of Congress Cataloging-in-Publication Data

LCCN: 2025038284 (CIP Data Pending)
ISBN13: 979-8-3373-5876-5
Isbn13Softcover: 979-8-3373-5877-2
EISBN13: 979-8-3373-5878-9

British Cataloguing in Publication Data
A Cataloguing in Publication record for this book is available from the British Library.

Table of Contents

Detailed Table of Contents

Nrf2 is a key transcription factor regulating genes for antioxidant defense, inflammation control, and detoxification, protecting cells from oxidative stress. Natural Nrf2 activators like sulforaphane, curcumin, and quercetin enhance cellular resilience and show promise in treating neurodegenerative, cardiovascular, and metabolic diseases. Conversely, Nrf2 inhibitors such as halofuginone and bardoxolone methyl are used in oncology to suppress tumour-promoting overactivation. Indigenous medicinal plants—especially turmeric (Curcuma longa) and moringa (Moringa oleifera)—are rich in phytochemicals that modulate Nrf2, offering a natural strategy for chronic disease prevention. However, African plants remain underexplored, and clinical trials on natural modulators are limited, with gaps in dosage, efficacy, and safety data. Despite these limitations, the chapter highlights the therapeutic potential of indigenous plants in modulating Nrf2 pathways and recommends intensified research and clinical validation.

Environmental pollution remains a global health issue linked to numerous diseases, primarily through the generation of reactive oxygen species (ROS) that induce lipid peroxidation, protein and DNA damage, and cellular dysfunction. This review examines the therapeutic potential of medicinal ethnobotanicals in mitigating

Piper betle L. is widely recognized for its diverse medicinal properties, including antimicrobial activity, therapeutic efficacy in dermatological disorders, analgesic effects, and its beneficial role in managing respiratory disorders. The plant contains a variety of bioactive chemical constituents, such as hydroxychavicol, chavibetol, chavibetol acetate, caryophyllene, allyl pyrocatechol diacetate, camphene, chavibetol methyl ether, eugenol, α-pinene, β-pinene, limonene, sabinene, 1,8-cineol, and allyl pyrocatechol monoacetate. These compounds exhibit notable pharmacological activities, contributing to the potential as stimulants with properties such as antiplatelet, anti-inflammatory, immunomodulatory, gastroprotective, and antidiabetic activities. This review aims to provide a comprehensive overview of the phytochemical constituents and pharmacological properties of Piper betle L., with particular emphasis on its antimicrobial, antioxidant, antidiabetic, anticancer, and anti-gout potential.

This chapter discusses the critical need for scientific validation of complex traditional herbal formulations, particularly those widely used in Africa, which frequently lack established efficacy, safety, and consistency. It offers a comprehensive framework that integrates advanced chemical profiling and biological assays. Various spectroscopic and hyphenated techniques used for characterization of herbal medicines are discussed, as well as common assays used for validating herbal formulations' medicinal properties. The use of spectroscopy for standardization, quality control, and safety assessment of herbal formulations is also covered. The chapter demonstrates how bridging indigenous knowledge with modern evidence-based healthcare can help researchers, regulators, and healthcare providers realize the full potential of the world's botanical heritage in disease treatment.

Herbal medicine involves the use of medicinal plants for treatment of diseases in developing and developed countries. Plants have been used for medical purposes in human history and it's still widely practiced today. Herbal remedies have active constituent/ingredient which is known to have curative effects on the body. They are used as treatment and relief for various diseases such as diabetes, low sperm count, anemia as well as cancer. Herbal remedies in Nigeria have become popular and are majorly classified into monoherbal and polyherbal remedies. The use of herbal remedies tends to affect humanity both positively and negatively. Some positive importance reported includes high level of effectiveness of the herb, cheap and readily availabile with numerous health benefits and vitality. The disadvantages however are the observed side effects, high percentage of alcohol content, and lack of dosage regulation of the herbs.

Inflammation in the body might be viewed as a cascade (driven by the immune, vascular, and signaling systems) whenever the body is affected by some foreign agents. This cascade boils and terminates at activated repair mechanisms when the host detects the offending stimulus. The persistence of states of drug resistance and toxicological effects in the human body stimulates the search for new therapeutic agents that can combat inflammation and analgesia. Ethnopharmacological research of plants with traditional uses as anti-inflammatory and analgesic agents demonstrates an extensive variety of bioactive constituents that have been utilized traditionally by various tribal communities to alleviate pain and restrain the inflammatory processes. Phytochemical analysis of these ethnomedicinal herbs has revealed that be contain secondary metabolites such as curcumin, ursolic acid, escin, withaferin A, etc., often showing the ability to inhibit important inflammatory mediators, viz., cyclooxygenase-2 (COX-2), nuclear factor-κB (NF-κB), and pro-inflammatory cytokines, e.g., TNF-α and IL-1β.

Cancer remains the second leading cause of death globally, with classical therapies limited by selectivity, toxicity, and resistance. This review examines polyphenol-rich preparations and their multi-target interactions in cancer cells. Polyphenols (flavonoids, phenolic acids, stilbenes, lignans) simultaneously modulate multiple targets, addressing key cancer hallmarks: sustained proliferative signaling, apoptosis evasion, replicative immortality, and angiogenesis. Key pathways include PI3K/Akt/mTOR, MAPK, RAS, and p53. Notable compounds like curcumin, resveratrol, quercetin, and EGCG induce apoptosis, inhibit angiogenesis, arrest cell cycle, and modulate epigenetics. Despite encouraging preclinical evidence, clinical translation faces challenges from low bioavailability, rapid metabolism, and conflicting data. Strategies include stable derivatives, nano-encapsulation, personalized medicine, and combination with established drugs. Polyphenolic compounds emerge as promising multi-target anticancer agents with low toxicity. Further research on bioavailability and trials is needed.

Parkinson's disease (PD) is a progressive neurodegenerative disorder involving α-synuclein aggregation in the substantia nigra and the loss of dopaminergic neurons. Its pathophysiology involves oxidative stress, mitochondrial dysfunction, impaired neurotransmission, and neuroinflammation. The existing treatments, including levodopa, dopamine agonists, and monoamine oxidase B inhibitors, are symptomatic but fail to halt disease progression or side effects, and therefore, neuroprotective strategies are needed. Zingiber officinale (ginger) contains phenolic compounds (6-gingerol, 6-shogaol, zingerone, and paradol) with antioxidant, anti-inflammatory, and anti-apoptotic properties. Preclinical studies show the neuroprotection of ginger by scavenging reactive oxygen species, enhancing defenses, inhibiting mediators, and controlling signaling cascades. Although clinical trials in PD are lacking, cognitive

Preface

INTRODUCTION

Traditional medicine continues to occupy a central place in healthcare systems across the world, particularly in regions where medicinal plants remain deeply embedded in cultural heritage and everyday health practices. In recent decades, renewed scientific interest has brought herbal medicine to the forefront of pharmacological, toxicological, and clinical research, creating a vital bridge between indigenous knowledge and modern biomedical science. It is within this context that we present this edited reference book, *Pharmacology, Characterizations, Toxicity, and Herb–Drug Interactions of Herbs in Traditional Medicine.*

This volume is published in commemoration of the 10th anniversary of the African Centre for Herbal Research, Ilorin (ACHRI). Over the past decade, ACHRI has served as a hub for multidisciplinary research, capacity building, and scientific validation of traditional herbal remedies. This book stands as both a celebration of that milestone and a scholarly contribution that reflects the Centre's commitment to advancing evidence-based herbal medicine.

The chapters in this book collectively highlight the multifaceted applications of herbal remedies across diverse cultures, with particular emphasis on general human health, skin conditions, oral discomfort, and dental hygiene. Through comprehensive reviews and experimental studies, contributors examine the antimicrobial, anti-inflammatory, analgesic, and other bioactive properties of a wide range of medicinal plants. Equal attention is given to toxicological evaluations and safety considerations, recognizing that efficacy must be accompanied by responsible and informed use.

This reference work provides in-depth profiles of over twenty medicinal herbs, detailing their traditional uses, pharmacological activities, chemical composition, and spectroscopic characterization, alongside documented toxicities. Cutting-edge scientific findings, including studies on herbal formulations and cosmetic preparations, further underscore the relevance of herbal medicine in contemporary healthcare.

Beyond its scientific rigor, this volume situates herbal medicine within its rich historical and cultural context, acknowledging the folklore and indigenous knowledge systems that have sustained these practices for generations. By doing so, it reinforces the value of traditional medicine not only as a therapeutic resource but also as a repository of cultural identity and biodiversity.

This book is intended as a comprehensive resource for researchers exploring the pharmacological potential of medicinal plants, healthcare professionals seeking to responsibly integrate traditional medicine into practice, and students and enthusiasts interested in the botanical foundations of human health. Natural products scientists, biochemists, pharmacologists, pharmaceutical scientists, agriculturists, food technologists, ethnobotanists, herbal practitioners, and allied professionals will find this volume both informative and enriching.

As Editors, we are grateful to all contributing authors for their scholarly dedication and to ACHRI for fostering a decade of impactful research. We hope this book will inspire further investigation, promote safe and effective use of herbal remedies, and strengthen the dialogue between traditional knowledge and modern science for the benefit of global health.

ORGANIZATION OF THE BOOK

Chapter 1 explores the central role of nuclear factor erythroid 2–related factor 2 (Nrf2) as a master regulator of antioxidant defense, inflammation control, and cellular detoxification. The chapter critically examines both natural activators and inhibitors of Nrf2, highlighting their therapeutic relevance in chronic diseases such as neurodegenerative, cardiovascular, metabolic disorders, and cancer. Particular emphasis is placed on indigenous medicinal plants, including turmeric (*Curcuma longa*) and moringa (*Moringa oleifera*), which are rich in phytochemicals capable of modulating Nrf2 signaling pathways. While underscoring the promise of these botanicals for disease prevention and management, the chapter also draws attention to significant gaps in clinical validation, especially regarding African medicinal plants, dosage optimization, efficacy, and long-term safety. It ultimately calls for intensified translational and clinical research to harness the full therapeutic potential of natural Nrf2 modulators.

Chapter 2 addresses the growing global health burden posed by environmental pollution and its strong association with oxidative stress–mediated diseases. This chapter provides a mechanistic review of how medicinal ethnobotanicals mitigate pollution-induced oxidative damage through their antioxidant and cytoprotective properties. Drawing on in vitro and in vivo evidence, it highlights the roles of phytochemicals such as flavonoids, phenolic acids, alkaloids, and terpenoids in scavenging reactive oxygen species and modulating redox-sensitive signaling pathways. The chapter convincingly demonstrates how these plant-derived compounds restore cellular and tissue homeostasis, positioning ethnobotanicals as promising therapeutic agents in counteracting the adverse health effects of environmental pollutants.

Chapter 3 offers a comprehensive and critical examination of traditional herbal anxiolytics within the emerging discipline of neurophytomedicine. It situates anxiety disorders within their neurobiological and global health contexts, while acknowledging the limitations of conventional pharmacotherapies. The chapter evaluates botanicals historically used for anxiety relief, focusing on key phytochemical classes and their interactions with GABAergic, serotonergic, and hypothalamic–pituitary–adrenal pathways. By addressing challenges such as standardization, placebo effects, and ethical sourcing, the chapter lays the groundwork for future innovations, including pharmacogenomic approaches, artificial intelligence–driven phytochemical discovery, and the integration of validated botanicals into mainstream psychiatric care.

Chapter 4 presents an in-depth appraisal of *Piper betle* L., a medicinal plant renowned for its extensive pharmacological versatility. The chapter systematically details the phytochemical composition of the plant, highlighting bioactive constituents such as hydroxychavicol, eugenol, chavibetol, and various terpenes that underpin its biological activities. Emphasis is placed on its antimicrobial, antioxidant, anti-inflammatory, antidiabetic, anticancer, and anti-gout potentials, as well as its traditional and contemporary therapeutic applications in dermatological, respiratory, and metabolic disorders. This chapter reinforces the scientific basis for the continued medicinal relevance of *Piper betle* and underscores its promise as a source of lead compounds for drug development.

Chapter 5 focuses on the scientific evaluation of complex herbal formulations, emphasizing the urgent need for standardization, quality control, and safety validation, particularly for widely used African traditional medicines. The chapter outlines an integrative framework combining advanced spectroscopic techniques with biological assays to characterize chemical composition and therapeutic efficacy. It discusses the role of spectroscopy and hyphenated analytical methods in ensuring consistency, detecting adulteration, and assessing safety. By bridging indigenous knowledge systems with modern evidence-based methodologies, this chapter provides a practical roadmap for researchers, regulators, and healthcare professionals seeking to translate traditional formulations into validated therapeutic products.

Chapter 6 critically examines the widespread use of herbal remedies in Nigeria, framing them as both beneficial and potentially harmful depending on their preparation, regulation, and use. The chapter explores the classification of Nigerian herbal remedies into monoherbal and polyherbal formulations and highlights their reported effectiveness, affordability, and accessibility. At the same time, it addresses pressing concerns related to adverse effects, high alcohol content, lack of dosage standardization, and regulatory oversight. By presenting a balanced perspective, this chapter emphasizes the need for informed use, scientific evaluation, and policy-driven regulation to maximize benefits while minimizing risks.

Chapter 7 delves into the ethnopharmacology and toxicological profiles of medicinal plants traditionally used as anti-inflammatory and analgesic agents. It contextualizes inflammation as a complex biological cascade and highlights the growing demand for safer, more effective alternatives to conventional drugs. The chapter reviews ethnomedicinal herbs rich in bioactive secondary metabolites such as curcumin, ursolic acid, escin, and withaferin A, which target key inflammatory mediators including COX-2, NF-κB, and pro-inflammatory cytokines. By integrating traditional knowledge with modern pharmacological insights, this chapter underscores the therapeutic promise of ethnomedicinal plants while stressing the importance of toxicity evaluation and dose optimization.

Chapter 8 examines polyphenol-rich formulations and their multi-target interactions with molecular pathways involved in cancer development and progression. The chapter highlights the ability of polyphenols to simultaneously modulate multiple cancer hallmarks through pathways such as PI3K/Akt/mTOR, MAPK, RAS, and p53. Key compounds, including curcumin, resveratrol, quercetin, and epigallocatechin gallate, are discussed for their roles in inducing apoptosis, inhibiting angiogenesis, regulating epigenetics, and arresting the cell cycle. While acknowledging the strong preclinical evidence supporting these compounds, the chapter critically discusses challenges related to bioavailability and clinical translation, proposing innovative strategies such as nano-encapsulation and combination therapies.

Chapter 9 highlights the neuroprotective potential of ginger (*Zingiber officinale*) in the context of Parkinson's disease. The chapter outlines the complex pathophysiology of the disease and the limitations of existing symptomatic treatments. It then examines the bioactive constituents of ginger, including gingerols, shogaols, and zingerone, emphasizing their antioxidant, anti-inflammatory, and anti-apoptotic properties. Preclinical evidence supporting ginger's neuroprotective effects is reviewed, alongside emerging data on cognitive benefits and safety. The chapter positions ginger as a promising adjunctive therapy while emphasizing the need for rigorous clinical trials to substantiate its role in neurodegenerative disease management.

Chapter 10 provides a comprehensive appraisal of *Adansonia digitata* (baobab), a culturally significant and pharmacologically rich African tree species. The chapter synthesizes ethnomedicinal uses of its various parts with phytochemical and pharmacological evidence supporting its antioxidant, anti-inflammatory, antimicrobial, and antidiabetic activities. With growing applications in nutraceuticals, cosmetics, and herbal formulations, baobab is presented as an underutilized yet highly valuable botanical resource. The chapter underscores its potential contribution to natural product drug discovery, food security, and public health innovation.

Chapter 11 concludes the volume by exploring the intersection of folklore medicine, environmental science, and modern pharmacology in multitarget disease mitigation. The chapter emphasizes ecochemical interface studies, demonstrating how environmental factors influence plant chemistry and therapeutic efficacy. Through case studies and interdisciplinary approaches, it illustrates how traditional knowledge, when combined with contemporary tools such as systems biology and artificial intelligence, can unlock novel therapeutic pathways. The chapter calls for ethically grounded, eco-centric research frameworks that support sustainable drug discovery and personalized medicine, reinforcing the future relevance of plant-based therapeutics in global healthcare.

Chapter 12 explores Tropical herbs are rich in bioactive phytochemicals with untapped cosmeceutical potential. Constituents such as flavonoids, terpenoids, saponins, alkaloids, tannins, and phenolics provide antioxidant, antimicrobial, anti-inflammatory, and rejuvenating effects. These structures enable free radical scavenging, UV protection, collagen stabilization, and modulation of inflammation, supporting uses in hair growth, skin lightening, nail strengthening, and odor control. Evidence spans in vitro assays (coffeeberry, tea tree, garlic), in vivo studies (calendula, bergamot, ginseng), and clinical trials (soy, aloe, rosehip) showing benefits in wound healing, hydration, tone, and acne reduction. Yet, most tropical herbs lack standardized formulations, toxicity profiling, and large-scale validation. Systematic exploration and commercialization could foster innovation, biodiversity conservation, and sustainable development in the global cosmeceutical industry.

CONCLUSION

As this edited reference book draws to a close, it becomes evident that traditional medicine—when examined through rigorous scientific lenses—offers far more than historical or cultural relevance; it represents a dynamic and evolving frontier in modern healthcare. The chapters assembled in this volume collectively demonstrate that medicinal herbs and herbal formulations possess measurable pharmacological activities, complex chemical architectures, and clinically relevant therapeutic potentials.

The contributions herein reflect a deliberate balance between tradition and innovation. Indigenous knowledge systems, particularly those rooted in African ethnomedicine, are thoughtfully integrated with contemporary advances in pharmacology, spectroscopy, molecular biology, and clinical science. By addressing mechanisms of action, safety profiles, and multi-target disease modulation, this book reinforces the necessity of evidence-based validation for herbal remedies, especially in the face of increasing global reliance on natural products for health maintenance and disease management.

Importantly, this volume does not shy away from the challenges confronting herbal medicine research. Issues such as variability in plant chemistry, lack of dosage standardization, regulatory gaps, and limited clinical trials are critically examined, underscoring the need for coordinated multidisciplinary efforts. At the same time, the promising roles of emerging technologies—including systems biology, artificial intelligence, and advanced analytical platforms—highlight new pathways for transforming traditional remedies into standardized, safe, and effective therapeutic options.

Published in commemoration of the 10th anniversary of the African Centre for Herbal Research, Ilorin (ACHRI), this book stands as both a scholarly milestone and a forward-looking call to action. It is our hope that this work will inspire further research, foster cross-sector collaborations, inform policy and regulation, and encourage responsible integration of validated herbal medicines into mainstream healthcare systems.

As Editors, we trust that this volume will serve as a valuable and enduring resource for researchers, clinicians, educators, students, and practitioners alike. More importantly, we hope it will contribute to preserving botanical heritage, advancing scientific understanding, and improving global health outcomes through the thoughtful and ethical use of medicinal plants.

Chapter 1
Nrf2 Modulators and the Prospects of Indigenous Medicinal Plants

Abisola Aminat Afolabi
http://orcid.org/0009-0003-1011-2110
Bowen University, Nigeria

Emmanuel Henry Ezenabor
http://orcid.org/0009-0009-0231-7734
Bowen University, Nigeria

Godwin Ayebaitari Berena
Bowen University, Nigeria

ABSTRACT

Nrf2 is a key transcription factor regulating genes for antioxidant defense, inflammation control, and detoxification, protecting cells from oxidative stress. Natural Nrf2 activators like sulforaphane, curcumin, and quercetin enhance cellular resilience and show promise in treating neurodegenerative, cardiovascular, and metabolic diseases. Conversely, Nrf2 inhibitors such as halofuginone and bardoxolone methyl are used in oncology to suppress tumour-promoting overactivation. Indigenous medicinal plants—especially turmeric (Curcuma longa) and moringa (Moringa oleifera)—are rich in phytochemicals that modulate Nrf2, offering a natural strategy for chronic disease prevention. However, African plants remain underexplored, and clinical trials on natural modulators are limited, with gaps in dosage, efficacy, and safety data. Despite these limitations, the chapter highlights the therapeutic potential of indigenous plants in modulating Nrf2 pathways and recommends intensified research and clinical validation.

DOI: 10.4018/979-8-3373-5876-5.ch001

1.0 INTRODUCTION

Non-communicable diseases, encompassing cardiovascular diseases, cancers, diabetes, chronic respiratory illnesses, and neurodegenerative disorders, now account for approximately 74% of all deaths globally, translating to over 41 million lives lost annually (Shitaw et al., 2025; VanderJagt et al., 2022). Persistent inflammation and oxidative stress are now widely accepted as driving forces in the pathogenesis and progression of these diseases (VanderJagt et al., 2022).

Despite their often slow and insidious progression, NCDs have collectively surpassed communicable diseases as the principal cause of death, disability, and economic burden in the 21st century (Oso et al., 2023). Recent projections estimate that this global burden will intensify by an additional 17% over the next decade, disproportionately impacting low and middle-income countries (LMICs) (Wang et al., 2020). These regions, particularly Africa, are projected to experience a 27% rise in NCD-related mortality, driven by urbanization, lifestyle changes, and persistent challenges to health system capacity (Wang et al., 2020). In 2020, up to 80% of NCD deaths in LMICs occurred before age 70, illustrating the premature and devastating nature of the epidemic (Oso et al., 2023; VanderJagt et al., 2022).

Nigeria, home to over 219 million people in 2022, now faces a dual disease burden, with NCDs representing about 27–30% of all deaths (over 600,000 annually) (WHO Regional Office for Africa, 2023; Oso et al., 2023). As shown in Table 1, additional statistical data on the occurrence of major NCDs in Nigeria are provided.

Across the spectrum of NCDs in Nigeria, major risk factors include hypertension (prevalence above 31%), obesity, tobacco use, physical inactivity, unhealthy diets, and excessive alcohol consumption. See more details in Table 1.

The concentration of NCDs among economically disadvantaged and rural populations is accentuated by out-of-pocket health costs, late presentations, and inaccessible preventive care, driving further impoverishment and social inequities (Oso et al., 2023).

Table 1. Major NCDs and occurrence in Nigeria (2020–2025)

Disease	Occurrence	Key Findings	References
Cardiovascular Disease	10–27%	Leading NCD cause; high DALYs	Ojo et al., 2024; Ogah et al., 2023
Diabetes (all forms)	4.1 – 5.8%	South-south zone highest (8.5%)	Olamoyegun et al., 2024; Esan et al., 2024.
Cancer (incidence)	100,000/ year	High case-fatality (delayed diagnoses)	Olayeriju et al., 2021

continued on following page

Table 1. Continued

Disease	Occurrence	Key Findings	References
COPD/asthma	6.9–13%	Asthma is high in urban youth	Oso, A. (2023)
Hypertension	31.2%	Poor awareness and control	Adeloye et al., 2021; Ojo et al., 2024
Obesity	14.3%	Rapidly rising, urban-centric	Adeloye et al., 2021; Chukwuonye et al., 2022.
Physical inactivity	52–75%	Greatest among urban dwellers	Adeloye et al., 2021.
Tobacco use	5.6%	Higher than the global average (especially for men)	WHO Tobacco Country Profile (2023)

These statistics generally highlight the fast-moving epidemiological transition currently taking place in Nigeria.

There are two interconnected processes in nearly all major NCDs: oxidative stress and chronic low-grade inflammation (Nediani et al., 2024).

Oxidative stress is essentially an imbalance between the generation of reactive oxygen species (ROS) and the cellular antioxidant defences, leading to molecular and cellular damage, affecting proteins, lipids, and DNA alike (Ezema et al., 2024; Grant et al., 2021). In obesity-driven metabolic syndrome, for instance, adipose tissue becomes infiltrated with immune cells, which generate inflammatory cytokines and ROS, perpetuating insulin resistance and endothelial dysfunction (Hosseinkhani et al., 2021).

Conversely, inflammation, while initially essential for wound repair and pathogen defence, becomes pathogenic when it remains unresolved. Chronic, non-resolving inflammation sustains cellular damage, promotes fibrosis, and is now recognized as a foundational process in atherosclerosis, cancer progression, and neurodegenerative diseases such as Alzheimer's and Parkinson's (Nediani et al., 2024; Shitaw et al., 2025; Lastra et al., 2020).

Notably, ROS themselves act as signalling molecules that activate pro-inflammatory transcription factors such as NF-κB, thereby compounding tissue damage and establishing a self-perpetuating vicious cycle (Saha et al., 2024; Nediani et al., 2024).

Clinical and experimental studies repeatedly demonstrate that the oxidative-inflammatory axis not only initiates NCDs but also amplifies their progression and complications, whether endothelial dysfunction in heart disease, β-cell failure in diabetes, mutagenesis in cancer, or dopaminergic neuron loss in Parkinson's disease (Nediani et al., 2024; Wang et al., 2021).

Nigeria is one of the most biodiverse countries in Africa, having thousands of plant species, with hundreds used in traditional medicine (Abdulazeez et al., 2024). Newer phytochemical investigations between 2020 to 2025 have further validated that Nigerian medicinal plants harbour rich arrays of bioactive compounds, including flavonoids, alkaloids, polyphenols, terpenoids, lignans, glycosides, and saponins, which underpin their therapeutic effects (Wang et al., 2021; Popoola et al., 2021; Olayeriju et al., 2021). Furthermore, these constituents exhibit potent antioxidant and anti-inflammatory activity, with some mimicking or surpassing the effects of known pharmaceuticals in laboratory models (Martínez-Rizo et al., 2024; VanderJagt et al., 2022; Popoola et al., 2021).

Over the years, research has affirmed that many Nigerian medicinal plants directly modulate oxidative stress and inflammatory pathways central to NCD pathophysiology (VanderJagt et al., 2022; Popoola et al., 2021). Emerging survey support antioxidant and antinflammatory properties (Nwozo et al., 2023; Ogbonnaya et al., 2024; VanderJagt et al., 2022). These findings span in vitro, in vivo, and computational studies, and increasingly validate traditional ethnomedicinal knowledge.

This chapter discusses research published from 2020 to 2025, focusing on the regulation of Nrf2, recent progress in identifying and characterizing Nigerian medicinal plants as natural Nrf2 modulators, identified gaps, and recommendations for future studies and clinical validation.

1.1 NUCLEAR FACTOR ERYTHROID 2-RELATED FACTOR 2 (NRF2)

Nuclear factor erythroid 2-related factor 2 (Nrf2) is a transcription factor that regulates redox balance, metabolism, and protein homeostasis, while modulating several genes associated with iron synthesis, storage, or transit, hence playing crucial roles in both ferroptosis and renal disorders. The protein products of its target genes exhibit diverse cytoprotective effects, encompassing antioxidant, anti-inflammatory, metabolic, and drug-metabolizing activities, as well as contributing to the maintenance of protein homeostasis (Dinkova-Kostova & Copple, 2023).

NRF2, in conjunction with KEAP1 and antioxidant response elements (AREs), is involved in the KEAP1/NRF2/ARE signalling pathway, which governs the cytoprotective functions of the cell (Wadowski et al., 2024). It is also a transcription factor responsible for managing mitochondrial function, inflammation, and various cytoprotective actions like metabolism of xenobiotics and drugs (Gjorgieva et al., 2023; Islam et al., 2023). Because of this, it is considered to be the main agent in maintaining redox balance at both the cellular level and tissue level, as it is responsible for regulating about 200 genes (Gjorgieva et al., 2023; Pouremamali et al., 2022).

1.1.1 Nrf2 Structure

Nrf2 belongs to the cap 'n' collar (CNC) subfamily of basic leucine zipper (bZIP) transcription factors together with NF-E2 p45-related factors 1 and 3 (Nrf1 and Nrf3), NF-E2 p45, and transcriptional repressors BTB Domain and CNC homolog 1 and 2 (Bach1 and Bach2) (Ngo et al., 2022). Structural studies of the protein have shown the presence of seven highly conserved functional domains (Neh1–Neh7) which are referred to as the Nrf2-ECH homology (Neh) domains (Wadowski et al., 2024; Ngo et al., 2022).

a. Neh1 has a leucine zipper domain that allows it to interact with DNA and small MAF (*v-Maf* avian musculoskeletal fibrosarcoma oncogene homolog) proteins.
b. The Neh2 domain interacts with the negative KEAP1 regulator through specific DLG and ETG motifs and plays an important role in NRF2 degradation.
c. Neh3 – Neh5 domains participate in NRF2 transactivation. The Neh3 domain enables transcription activation of genes containing the ARE motif.
d. The Neh4 and Neh5 domains cooperatively bind to the cAMP response element-binding (CREB) protein (CBP), which allows them to perform a co-activating function for numerous transcription factors.
e. The Neh6 and Neh7 domains' activity relates to post-translational regulation of NRF2. The Neh6 domain next to Neh2 is crucial in the degradation of NRF2.
f. The Neh7 domain can interact with the retinoic X receptor α, resulting in NRF2 repression.

Figure 1. Domain structure of Nrf2, showing the functional domains of Nrf2 and Keap1, which regulate the antioxidant response. Nrf2 contains seven conserved Neh domains (Ngo et al., 2022)

1.1.2 Nrf2 Biochemical Regulation

Nrf2 is a ubiquitous transcription factor that orchestrates the cellular response to oxidative, electrophilic, and metabolic stress by transactivating a suite of antioxidant and detoxification genes (over 500 known targets, including HO-1, NQO1, GCLC, and GSTs) (Dodson et al., 2022; Xiao et al., 2024; Kumar et al., 2024).

The stability and nuclear localization of Nrf2 are tightly regulated by its repressor, Kelch-like ECH-associated protein 1 (Keap1) (Sykiotis et al., 2021).

In the absence of stress, NRF2 is a transient and unstable protein. Its levels are mainly regulated by Kelch-like ECH-associated protein 1 (KEAP1), which serves as an E3 ubiquitin ligase substrate adaptor, directing NRF2 for ubiquitination and subsequent degradation by the proteasome (Dinkova-Kostova & Copple, 2023). And upon exposure to oxidative or electrophilic stress, critical cysteine residues on Keap1 are modified, disrupting Keap1-Nrf2 binding, allowing Nrf2 to escape degradation, translocate to the nucleus, and drive the transcription of cytoprotective genes through binding to antioxidant response elements (AREs) in target promoters (Lastra et al., 2020; Panieri et al., 2020).

Additionally, KEAP1 functions as a sensor for various internal and external electrophiles and oxidants due to its multiple highly reactive cysteine residues. When these residues undergo chemical alterations, KEAP1's ability to target NRF2 for degradation is hindered, which leads to the accumulation of Nrf2 and the upregulation of several cytoprotective proteins. Both NRF2 and KEAP1 are susceptible to post-translational modifications and can interact with other proteins that affect their respective functions (Kopacz et al., 2020; Matzinger et al., 2020).

The primary mechanisms regulating NRF2 operate through post-transcriptional KEAP1-dependent regulation, post-transcriptional KEAP1-independent regulation, and transcriptional regulation.

Nrf2 regulation is multi-layered:

a. Canonical (Keap1-Dependent): In normal situation, a Keap1 holds onto Nrf2 inside the cell and help tag it for destruction by the cell's waste-disposal system, so Nrf2 doesn't become active (Table 2). This leads to a rapid Nrf2 turnover (half-life <20 min), keeping its basal levels low (Tamaru et al., 2024; Zhang et al., 2025). Stress-induced Keap1 cysteine modification leads to Nrf2 stabilization and activation. Nrf2 then heterodimerizes with sMaf proteins and binds AREs, activating downstream genes (Yang et al., 2022; Mukherjee et al., 2023; Tamaru et al., 2024).
b. Non-canonical (Keap1-Independent): Involvement of β-TrCP and GSK-3-mediated phosphorylation, interactions with p62/SQSTM1 (in autophagy-linked pathways), and regulation by other signalling pathways such as Notch, NF-κB, and PI3K/Akt (Dodson et al., 2022; Xiao et al., 2024; Kumar et al., 2024). Alternative regulators such as p62/SQSTM1, p21, DPP3, WTX, and PALB2 compete for Keap1 binding, leading to its autophagic degradation and further Nrf2 activation. GSK-3β can phosphorylate Nrf2's Neh6 degron, leading to β-

TrCP-mediated degradation (Keap1-independent) (Yang et al., 2022; Adeniran & Akindele, 2024; Park et al., 2023).

c. Post-translational Modifications: Phosphorylation and acetylation affect Nrf2's stability, localization, and activity (Dodson et al., 2022; Lastra et al., 2020). MicroRNAs (miR-144, miR-28, miR-152-3p, miR-380-5p) further modulate Nrf2 by targeting its mRNA for degradation or enhancing translation, providing an additional layer of post-transcriptional regulation (Gray et al., 2022; Yang et al., 2022).

Figure 2. Nrf2 regulation pathway. The Kelch-like ECH-associated protein 1 (KEAP1)–nuclear factor erythroid 2-related factor 2 (Nrf2) system (Saha et al., 2020)

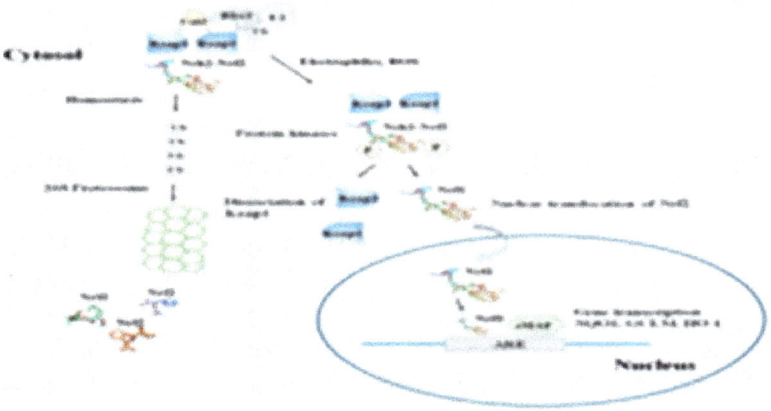

1.1.3 Nrf2 Signal Integration and Crosstalk

Nrf2 does not act in isolation; rather, it cross-regulates and is regulated by the PI3K/Akt, MAPK (ERK, p38, JNK), and AMPK pathways. Activation of PI3K/Akt and MAPK often leads to phosphorylation of Nrf2, enhancing its dissociation from Keap1 and nuclear accumulation. AMPK, as an energy sensor, can also influence Nrf2 nuclear translocation in energy-depleted states, as shown in See Table 2.

Table 2. Mechanisms of Nrf2 modulation

Regulatory Mechanism	Molecular Players	Outcome for Nrf2	References
Keap1-dependent degradation	Keap1, Cul3, Rbx1	Ubiquitination and degradation	Tamaru et al., 2024; Yang et al., 2022
Keap1 cysteine modification	ROS, Electrophiles	Nrf2 stabilization	Zhang et al., 2025
p62-mediated autophagy	p62/SQSTM1	Keap1 degradation	Yang et al., 2022; Tamaru et al., 2024
GSK-3/β-TrCP pathway	GSK-3β, β-TrCP	Keap1-independent degradation	Tamaru et al., 2024
MicroRNA modulation	miR-144, miR-28	Nrf2 mRNA repression or depression	Yang et al., 2022; Gray et al., 2022
Kinase signalling	PI3K/Akt, MAPK, AMPK	Nrf2 phosphorylation and activation	Adeniran & Akindele, 2024

1.2 PHYSIOLOGICAL AND PATHOLOGICAL ROLES OF NRF2

Nrf2 is indispensable for redox homeostasis, regulation of inflammatory tone, and cellular resilience to toxic challenges. Mouse knockout studies show increased susceptibility to oxidative damage and chemical carcinogens. In humans, diminished Nrf2 activity is associated with worsened outcomes in metabolic syndrome, diabetes, and neurodegenerative disorders, while appropriate activation confers cytoprotection and resilience (Dodson et al., 2022; Kumar et al., 2024; Fasipe & Laher, 2023).

However, persistent Nrf2 activation in cancer cells can promote tumour growth, chemoresistance, and metabolic reprogramming, emphasizing the "double-edged sword" nature of the pathway (Sykiotis et al., 2021). Therefore, successful therapeutic targeting requires contextual understanding of Nrf2 regulation.

1.2.1 Oxidative Stress, Inflammation, and Diseases

Chronic oxidative stress and low-grade inflammation, partly through NF-κB activation, are established mediators of NCD onset and progression, including cardiovascular diseases, diabetes, obesity, neurodegeneration, and cancer (VanderJagt et al., 2022).

As the primary transcription factor promoting antioxidant defence, Nrf2 regulates genes encoding phase II detoxifying enzymes (e.g., HO-1, NQO1, glutathione S-transferases), phase III transporters, components involved in glutathione biosynthesis, and iron sequestration proteins (Dodson et al., 2022; Yagishita et al., 2020).

Enhancement of Nrf2 activity has been shown to:

a. Reduce inflammatory cytokine production and oxidative injury;
b. Diminish lipid peroxidation and DNA damage;
c. Preserve mitochondrial function and cellular homeostasis;
d. Protect β-cells in the pancreas and vascular endothelium in models of metabolic and cardiovascular disease (Dodson et al., 2022; Kumar et al., 2024; Fasipe & Laher, 2023).

Conversely, insufficient or dysregulated Nrf2 activity contributes to enhanced susceptibility to metabolic dysfunction, endothelial injury, and organ fibrosis, highlighting its centrality in preventing and mitigating NCDs (Kumar et al., 2024; Lastra et al., 2020).

1.2.2 The Role of Nrf2 in Non-Communicable Disease (NCD) Prevention and Therapy

Nrf2 controls the transcription of over 200 cytoprotective genes, including those encoding antioxidant enzymes (HO-1, SOD, GPx), phase II detoxification enzymes (GST, NQO1, UGT), proteins involved in GSH biosynthesis, xenobiotic transporters, and more (Tee et al., 2025; Adeniran & Akindele, 2024; Zhang et al., 2025).

This orchestration is central to redox homeostasis, inflammation control, and protection against tissue damage.

a. Neurodegenerative Diseases: Defective Nrf2 signalling is implicated in Alzheimer's, Parkinson's, Huntington's, and ALS. In these neurodegenerative conditions, Nrf2 deficiency exacerbates ROS, impairs antioxidant defences, and promotes oxidative neuronal injury, inflammation, and protein misfolding. Preclinical studies demonstrate that pharmacological activation of Nrf2 (with curcumin, sulforaphane, resveratrol, naringenin) can attenuate neuroinflammation, improve mitochondrial function, and reduce behavioural deficits in rodent models (Adeniran & Akindele, 2024; Park et al., 2023; Yang et al., 2022; Tee et al., 2025).
b. Metabolic and Cardiovascular Disorders: Nrf2 activation protects against diabetic complications (nephropathy, neuropathy, cardiomyopathy), atherosclerosis, and hypertension by mitigating oxidative stress, improving endothelial function, and inhibiting inflammatory cytokines(Wadowski et al., 2024; Gu et al., 2025; Moratilla-Rivera et al., 2023).
c. Cancer: Nrf2's dual roles are highlighted in cancer, acute activation prevents genotoxicity, while chronic/constitutive activation (often due to KEAP1 or

NFE2L2 mutations) enables metabolic reprogramming, therapy resistance, and tumour progression (Tee et al., 2025). Thus, Nrf2 modulators must be contextually targeted.

d. Pulmonary and Hepatic Disorders: Nrf2 attenuates acute lung injury, COPD, idiopathic pulmonary fibrosis, and drug-induced liver injury by modulating inflammation, promoting detoxification, and regulating cellular regeneration (Zhang et al., 2025). Recent studies also show that traditional herbal compounds activating Nrf2 can confer significant hepatoprotection in animal models.

1.3 ETHNOBOTANICAL SURVEY OF NIGERIA'S INDIGENOUS MEDICINAL PLANTS

The traditional herbal medicine in Nigeria is a deeply rooted practice, reflecting generations of indigenous knowledge, biodiversity, and local therapeutic needs. Recent ethnobotanical surveys and biochemical screening studies have begun systematically evaluating the pharmacological properties of key medicinal plants, many of which are already integrated into local healthcare for the management of fevers, metabolic ailments, infectious diseases, and chronic inflammatory conditions (Olawale et al., 2022; Idaguko & Adeniyi, 2023).

Among these, several species have been prioritized for their high antioxidant content, traditional use in NCD-relevant conditions, and emerging biomolecular evidence of Nrf2 pathway modulation. Table 3 summarizes the most studied plants in this context, their ethnopharmacological uses, and relevant bioactivity findings.

The data presented in table 3 were drawn from studies conducted between 2020 to 2025, involving sample sizes ranging from 30 to over 200 plant specimens. Geographic coverage spans multiple Nigerian regions, including Osun, Kaduna, Cross River, and Enugu States, ensuring ethnobotanical diversity across major ecological zones. Validation methods includes in vitro assays (e.g., antioxidant enzyme activity, Nrf2 nuclear translocation), in vivo models (e.g., rodent studies for anti-inflammatory and metabolic effects), and in silico docking to predict compound interactions with Keap1-Nrf2 targets. These approaches collectively support the reliability of the findings and their translational relevance.

1.3.1 Mechanistic Basis of Traditional Use

Across Nigeria's diverse ethnolinguistic groups, medicinal plants are routinely used to manage fevers, metabolic disorders, infectious diseases, and inflammatory conditions. While theses use was historically justified through empirical observation, modern biochemical screening has revealed that many of these species contain:

a. Polyphenols and flavonoids that neutralize ROS (Nwozo et al., 2023; Attahiru, 2025).
b. Terpenoids and alkaloids with antimicrobial or anti-inflammatory activity (Attahiru & Attahiru, 2025).
c. Saponins and tannins that modulate metabolic and immune pathways (Attahiru, 2025; Nwozo et al., 2023).

Table 3. Nigerian medicinal plants, ethnobotanical relevance, plant parts used, and traditional application

Common Name	Botanical Name	Traditional Use	Part of the Plant Used	References
Bitter leaf	*Vernonia amygdalina*	Malaria, diabetes, gastrointestinal disorders	Leaves	Oseghale et al., 2024; Lawal et al., 2022; Tauchen et al., 2023
Scent leaf	*Ocimum gratissimum*	Respiratory infections, fever, malaria, dysentery	Leaves	Lawal et al., 2022; Oseghale et al., 2024; Oyelakin et al., 2020
Neem	*Azadirachta indica*	Malaria, infections, skin ailments	Leaves, bark, seeds	Lawal et al., 2022; Tauchen et al., 2023
Moringa	*Moringa oleifera*	Diabetes, hypertension, anemia, nutrition	Leaves, Seeds	Okorie et al., 2023; Lawal et al., 2022
Bitter kola	*Garcinia kola*	Cough, cold, infections, longevity	Seeds (Kernels)	Tauchen et al., 2023; Lawal et al., 2022; Chijindu et al., 2020
Miracle leaf/ Leaf of life	*Bryophyllum pinnatum*	Epilepsy, longevity, wound healing	Leaves	Lawal et al., 2022; Chijindu et al., 2020
African snakeroot	*Rauvolfia vomitoria*	Hypertension, malaria, gastrointestinal issues	Roots and leaves	Lawal et al., 2022
Bush banana/ Finger root	*Uvaria chamae*	Snakebite, respiratory, and reproductive issues	Roots and leaves	Okosodo and Sarada, 2021; Lawal et al., 2022
Goat weed	*Ageratum conyzoides*	Fever, wounds, respiratory ailments	Leaves	Lawal et al., 2022;
Caesar weed	*Urena lobata*	Snake bites, cough, reproductive health	Leaves	Lawal et al., 2022
Giant milkweed	*Calotropis procera*	Skin diseases and diabetes	Leaves	Okosodo and Sarada, 2021; Lawal et al., 2022
Negro pepper	*Xylopia aethiopica*	Bone dislocation, respiratory, and fertility	Leaves and fruits	Ihinmikaiye and Akinjagunla, 2020
Mango	*Mangifera indica*	Antimalarial, fever, diabetes	Leaves, bark	Lawal et al., 2022; Chijindu et al., 2020

continued on following page

Table 3. Continued

Common Name	Botanical Name	Traditional Use	Part of the Plant Used	References
Alligator pepper	*Aframomum melegueta*	Digestion. Anti-epilepsy	Seeds and rhizomes	Ihinmikaiye and Akinjagunla, 2020; Okosodo and Sarada, 2021
Garlic	*Allium sativum*		Bulbs (cloves)	Lawal et al., 2022; Oyelakin et al., 202

Xylopia aethiopica demonstrates the strongest and most consistent Nrf2 activation, supported by both in vitro and in vivo evidence, making it a top candidate for further clinical development. Its high fold-change, multi-pathway engagement, and rich phytochemical profile give it a clear edge over other species studied.

These plants are not only culturally significant but have now been biochemically profiled for their antioxidant, anti-inflammatory, and Nrf2-modulating activities (VanderJagt et al., 2022).

1.4 AN OVERVIEW OF RECENT RESEARCH ON NRF2 MODULATION BY NIGERIAN INDIGENOUS MEDICINAL PLANTS

Nrf2 has emerged as a master regulator of antioxidant response, orchestrating gene expression vital for cellular protection against oxidative stress and inflammation (Ayustaningwarno et al., 2024).

Traditional medicinal systems across Nigeria have long utilized indigenous plants, both for their direct therapeutic value and enhancement of the body's defence mechanisms. Among the most recognized of these are ginger (*Zingiber officinale*) and bitter leaf (*Vernonia amygdalina*) (Table 8), which are widely consumed as teas or aqueous extracts. Recent research, including contributions by Adeyemi et al. (2024) and Elebiyo et al. (2022), has placed particular emphasis on defining the molecular mechanisms by which these plants modulate the Nrf2 pathway, their antioxidant and anti-inflammatory properties (Ayustaningwarno et al., 2024; Adeyemi et al., 2024; Rotimi et al., 2024).

Growing evidence from in vitro cell-based assays, phytochemical analysis, and computational studies has shed light on several Nigerian medicinal plants, identifying them as potent modulators of the Nrf2 signalling pathway. As shown in Table 4, a summary of how extracts from *Erythrina senegalensis*, *Sclerocarya birrea*, *Boswellia dalzielli*, *Pseudocedrela kotschyi*, *Sterculia setigera*, *Sarcocephalus esculentus*, and *Xylopia aethiopica* demonstrated significant activation of Nrf2 was highlighted (VanderJagt et al., 2022).

Table 4. Nigerian indigenous medicinal plants with Nrf2-modulating activity

Plant and part used	Nrf2 Activation (Fold Increase)	NF-κB Inhibition (%)	Major Observed Effects	References
Boswellia dalzielli (Leaves)	7.4	-	Strong Nrf2 activation, anti-inflammatory, antioxidant	D'Amico et al., 2022; VanderJagt et al., 2022
Xylopia aethiopica (Leaves)	7.7	-	Nrf2 activation, cytokine suppression, pain reduction	Boakye et al., 2022; VanderJagt et al., 2022
Sclerocarya birrea (Bark)	-	77.5	Nrf2 activation, antioxidant, anti-inflammatory	Olas et al., 2025
Sarcocephalus esculentus (Bark)	-	91.8	Highest NF-κB inhibition, antioxidant, cytoprotective	VanderJagt et al., 2022
Erythrina senegalensis (Leaves)	-	81.4	Nrf2 activation, wound healing, hepatoprotection	VanderJagt et al., 2022
Sterculia setigera (Bark)	-	75.5	Antioxidant, anti-apoptotic, neuroprotection	Kantati et al., 2024

1.4.1 Antioxidant and Anti-inflammatory Activities

Extracts of these plants showed strong radical-scavenging capacity by TRAP and FRAP assays, correlating with their inhibition of NF-κB activation and Nrf2 upregulation, as shown in Table 5 (VanderJagt et al., 2022).

Table 5. Biochemical activities of selected Nigerian medicinal plants

Genes/Protein	Functions	Health Implications
HO-1 (heme oxygenase-1)	Antioxidant, anti-inflammatory	Cytoprotection, anti-inflammation
NQO1(quinine oxidoreductase)	Detoxification, antioxidant	Redox regulation, chemoprevention
GSTs (glutathione S-transferases)	Detoxification, antioxidant	Cancer prevention, metabolic stability
GCLC/GCLM (glutamate-cysteine ligase)	Glutathione synthesis	GSH homeostasis, ROS neutralization

continued on following page

Table 5. Continued

Genes/Protein	Functions	Health Implications
SOD, CAT, PRDXs	ROS or RNS scavenging, peroxidase action	Reduce cell or tissue injury
FTL/FTH (ferritin subunits)	Iron sequestration, metabolism	Limit ROS generation, decrease ferroptosis
Proteasome subunits, SQSTM1/p62	Protein degradation, autophagy	Remove damaged proteins, prevent toxicity

1.5 NRF2 MODULATORS

Nrf2 modulators refer to compounds, which may be either naturally occurring or synthesised, that regulate the Nrf2 pathway by either enhancing or suppressing it to impact cellular defence mechanisms (Wang et al., 2021). These modulators can either activate or inhibit Nrf2 activity, thereby affecting its protective functions.

The modulation of Nrf2 can yield either beneficial or detrimental outcomes, depending on the specific context and the associated disease or condition. Nrf2 modulators are primarily classified into two categories based on whether they boost or inhibit Nrf2 activity (Dinkova-Kostova & Copple, 2023). Modulation of Nrf2 can either be direct or indirect, as shown in Table 6.

1.5.1 Types of Nrf2 modulators

Nrf2 modulators play a dual role in health and disease, with their effects depending on cellular context, especially between normal and cancerous cells. This duality is central to understanding their therapeutic potentials and risk. They are broadly categorized into two groups:

a. Nrf2 activators
b. Nrf2 inhibitors

1.5.2 Nrf2 activators

Nrf2 activators are used to augment antioxidant defences and provide protection against oxidative stress in conditions such as neurodegenerative diseases, cardiovascular disorders, diabetes, and liver and kidney diseases (Ngo et al., 2022). These activators can be derived from natural sources or be synthetically produced. Some examples of natural Nrf2 activators include Epigallocatechin-3-gallate (EGCG), curcumin, resveratrol, and quercetin. While certain synthetic Nrf2 activators include dimethyl fumarate (Tecfidera), diroximel fumarate (Vumerity), and omaveloxolone (Skyclarys).

a. Curcumin, also known as diferuloylmethane, is a well-researched polyphenolic compound derived from *Curcuma longa*, known for its anti-inflammatory, antioxidant, and anticancer effects, primarily functioning as an Nrf2 activator (Table 6). Its activation mechanisms involve demethylation of the Nrf2 promoter region and facilitation of Nrf2's nuclear translocation, along with interference with KEAP1 by interacting with its cysteine thiols to prevent Nrf2 degradation. It influences the expression of various Nrf2-dependent proteins, including HO-1, NQO1, GST, GR, AR, and phase-II detoxifying and antioxidant enzymes (Panieri et al., 2020; Chen et al., 2024; Tascioglu et al., 2021). It is also important to note that curcumin has low bioavailability and poor pharmacokinetic properties, which limit its therapeutic application (Panieri et al., 2020).
b. Epigallocatechin-3-gallate (EGCG) is a polyphenol predominantly found in green tea extract. Chemically, EGCG is an ester formed from epigallocatechin and gallic acid (3,4,5-trihydroxybenzoic acid), categorised as a catechin. It is primarily recognised as an Nrf2 activator. It promotes the nuclear translocation of Nrf2, leading to increased expression of its target genes, especially phase-II detoxifying enzymes, thus exerting anti-inflammatory and antioxidative effects (Saha et al., 2020; Panieri et al., 2020; Chen et al., 2024). Its mechanism of action involves oxidising or modifying cysteine residues in KEAP1, encouraging the dissociation of Nrf2 from the complex. Research between 2020 to 2025 has shown that low doses activate Nrf2, while higher doses may inhibit it (Panieri et al., 2020).
c. Resveratrol (3,5,4-trihydroxystilbene) is a polyphenol that activates Nrf2. It exhibits anticancer, antioxidant, anti-inflammatory, and antidiabetic properties and plays a significant role in regulating various signalling pathways (Table 7) related to cellular growth, division, angiogenesis, invasion, metastasis, and apoptosis (Pouremamali et al., 2022).
d. Quercetin (3,3′,4′,5,7-pentahydroxyflavone), a flavonoid found in fruits and vegetables that also activates Nrf2. It activates Nrf2 through sustained phosphorylation by PKC, promotes its nuclear translocation, and enhances the expression and activity of phase-II detoxifying enzymes. Quercetin interacts directly with KEAP1, inhibiting its capacity to bind to Nrf2 (Table 7) (Suraweera et al., 2020; Saha et al., 2020).

1.5.3 Nrf2 inhibitors

Nrf2 inhibitors are compounds that hinder or reduce the activity of the Nrf2 transcription factor (Lv et al., 2024). They are primarily used in cancer treatment, where excessive Nrf2 activity may enable tumour cells to survive and resist chemotherapy. Some natural Nrf2 inhibitors include luteolin, apigenin, and berberine, while synthetic Nrf2 inhibitors include halofuginone and bardoxolone-methyl. Currently, the number of identified Nrf2 inhibitors is relatively limited (Dinkova-Kostova & Copple, 2023).

a. Luteolin, a polyphenolic flavonoid, is present in *Vernonia amygdalina*, commonly known as bitter leaf, and is recognised as an Nrf2 inhibitor. This compound exhibits a range of beneficial activities, including antibacterial, anti-inflammatory, antioxidant, anticancer, and cytoprotective effects, and has been demonstrated to inhibit cell proliferation and the promotion of the cell cycle (Pouremamali et al., 2022). Its mechanism of action leads to reduced levels of NRF2 mRNA and protein, as well as hindrance of Nrf2's binding to AREs and depletion of GSH (Bukowski et al., 2020; Sanchez-Ortega et al., 2021; Ghareghomi et al., 2022).
b. Apigenin, another bioflavonoid, also demonstrates Nrf2 inhibitory effects and can be found in various plants native to Nigeria, such as *Newbouldia laevis* (traditionally used for diabetes), *Stachytarpheta jamaicensis*, *Vernonia amygdalina*, and *Ocimum gratissimum*. This compound is noted for its antioxidant, anti-inflammatory, anticancer, and antiviral properties (Pouremamali et al., 2022). Apigenin reduces NRF2 levels at both the mRNA and protein levels by downregulating the PI3K/Akt pathway and impeding its translocation to the nucleus (Sánchez-Ortega et al., 2021; Ghareghomi et al., 2023). Its inhibitory effects are not dependent on KEAP1.
c. Berberine, an isoquinoline alkaloid, is found in the plant *Annickia chlorantha*, which is utilised in traditional medicine throughout Nigeria for various health issues. Its properties indicate its potential in addressing neurodegenerative, metabolic, and cardiovascular conditions as well as in cancer prevention, treatment, and drug sensitisation (Ashrafizadeh et al., 2020; Och et al., 2020; Xiong et al., 2022). Berberine influences Nrf2 activity through mechanisms such as KEAP1 suppression, modulation of Nrf2 nuclear translocation, alteration of Nrf2 mRNA expression, and interaction with upstream mediators of Nrf2 (Xiong et al., 2022).

1.5.4 Nrf2 modulation occurs under two primary circumstances:

a. Overactivation (Upregulation): This takes place in cancer, wherein Nrf2 aids cancer cell survival and chemotherapy resistance. Consequently, Nrf2 inhibitors are being investigated to diminish its activity.
b. Underactivation (Downregulation): This is evident in chronic non-cancer diseases such as neurodegenerative, respiratory, cardiovascular, kidney, and liver diseases. In these instances, NRF2 activators are utilised to enhance the body's defensive responses.

The significance of modulating Nrf2 in the context of non-communicable diseases (NCDs) lies in the fact that these chronic, non-infectious conditions constitute a leading source of mortality and disability for the population at large (Wang et al., 2020). The increasing prevalence of NCDs correlates with demographic shifts, urbanisation, and lifestyle changes (Wang et al., 2020). Targeting Nrf2 presents opportunities to:

a. Restore antioxidant defence mechanisms.
b. Mitigate oxidative stress and inflammation.
c. Safeguard cells and tissues from harm.
d. Slow down disease progression in ailments such as Alzheimer's, asthma, heart failure, and liver or kidney disorders.

Table 6. Recent experimental evidence on phytochemistry and Nrf2 modulation (in vitro and in vivo)

Plant Name	Bioactive Compounds	Nrf2 Modulation	Study Type	NCD Relevance	Mechanism of Action	References
Curcuma longa	Curcumin	Direct activator	In vitro	Anti-inflammatory, anti-diabetic	Keap1 cysteine covalent modification	VanderJagt et al., 2022
Moringa oleifera	Isothiocyanates, flavonoids	Indirect activator	In vivo	Antioxidant, anti-diabetic	Enhances Nrf2 nuclear translocation	Elebiyo et al., 2022
Vernonia amygdalina	Sesquiterpene lactones	activator	In vitro	Anti-cancer, anti-inflammatory	Indirect oxidative stress signalling	Olamoyegun et al., 2024
Monodora myristica	Eugenol, flavonoids	activator	In vivo	Cardioprotective, anti-inflammatory	ROS scavenging and Nrf2 induction	Elebiyo et al., 2022
Ocimum gratissimum	Eugenol, thymol	activator	In vitro	Antioxidant, antimicrobial	Enhances antioxidant enzyme expression	Olamoyegun et al., 2024
Piper guineense	Piperine	Direct activator	In vitro	Anti-obesity, anti-diabetic	Modulates Keap1-Nrf2 interaction, Enhances Nrf2 nuclear translocation	Elebiyo et al., 2022
Azadirachta indica	Azadirachtin, nimbolide	activator	In silico	Anti-cancer, hepatoprotective	Induces phase II detox enzymes	VanderJagt et al., 2022

1.5.5 Limitations of Current In Vitro and In Vivo Studies

Despite their value, existing studies on Nrf2 modulators especially those from plant sources face several challenges:

1. Lack of Clinical Translation: many studies stop at the preclinical stage, with few progressing to human trials. In vitro models often use immortalized cell lines that don't fully mimic human physiology. In vivo studies, typically in rodents, may not accurately predict human responses due to species differences (Ford et al., 2021).

2. Non-Physiological Conditions: In vitro studies often use synthetic media that lack the complexity of real biological environments, leading to misleading results. For example, some Nrf2 activators like brusatol show strong effects in vitro but also cause cytotoxicity, which is reduced in more realistic serum-based models (Wadowski et al., 2024).
3. Limited Mechanistic Insight: Some studies report Nrf2 activation without fully explaining the molecular pathways involved (e.g., Keap1 binding, oxidative stress signalling). This hinders the development of targeted therapies or combination treatments.

1.5.6 Risks of Chronic Nrf2 Activation

Persistent Nrf2 activation, while protective in acute stress, can become harmful when sustained over time. Chronic upregulation of Nrf2 has been associated with enhanced tumour cell survival, metabolic reprogramming, and resistance to chemotherapy, particularly in cancers such as lung, liver, and pancreatic tumors (Ungvari et al., 2025).

Cancer cells often hijack the Nrf2 pathway to escape apoptosis and detoxify anticancer agents, making them harder to eliminate. This contributes to poor treatment outcomes and tumour recurrence, especially when Nrf2 is constitutively activated due to mutations in Keap1 or Nrf2 itself.

Beyond cancer, prolonged Nrf2 activation may impair immune responses, promote tissue fibrosis, and disrupt redox homeostasis. These effects have been observed in models of chronic kidney disease, liver fibrosis, and autoimmune conditions, where excessive antioxidant signalling blunts necessary inflammatory responses (Baird & Yamamoto, 2020).

Therefore, therapeutic use of Nrf2 modulators, especially from natural sources must be carefully dosed, time-limited, and validated for safety. This is particularly important for plant-based compounds with multiple active constituents, as their long-term effects on systemic redox balance and immune modulation remain underexplored (Wadowski et al., 2024; Ford et al., 2021).

1.6 PHYTOCHEMISTRY AND NRF2 MODULATION

The antioxidant and anti-inflammatory efficacy of these Nigerian plants is attributed to diverse phytochemicals.

These compounds function through electrophilic modification of Keap1 cysteine residues, enhancement of Nrf2 nuclear translocation, and modulation of intracellular redox-sensitive signalling pathways (Jiménez-Cabrera et al., 2020; Boakye et al., 2022; Egbujor et al., 2022)

Table 7. Principal Nrf2 target genes, their functions, and health implications

Compound	Phytochemical Class	Experiment Type	Nrf2 Activity Impact	References
Quercetin	Flavonoid	Cell-based, animal model	↑ Nrf2, HO-1, SOD, GPx, CAT	Park et al., 2023; Moratilla-Rivera et al., 2023
Curcumin	Polyphenol	Cell-based, animal/clinical	Nrf2 translocation, HO-1, NQO1	Park et al., 2023;
Naringenin	Flavonoid	In vitro / in vivo (PD)	↑ Nrf2, HO-1, GCL, GSH	Yang et al., 2022
Resveratrol	Stilbene	Mouse, clinical samples	↓ Aβ (AD), ↑ HO-1/ NQO1	Wadowski et al., 2024; Yang et al., 2022
Baicalin	Flavone glucuronide	Animal model	Hepatoprotection via Nrf2	Zhang et al., 2025
Chlorogenic acid	Polyphenol	Animal model	Hepatoprotective, Nrf2-dependent	Zhang et al., 2025

Key: ↑ - indicates upregulation; ↓ - indicates downregulation

Nrf2 regulates the transcription of antioxidant and cytoprotective genes, including HO-1, NQO1, and glutathione-related enzymes, as shown in Table 8. Research has established the role of Nrf2, its modulators, mechanisms of action, and supporting evidence from preclinical studies. Significant advances in research over the last five years highlight the following.

a. In vitro and In vivo Efficiency: Multiple studies demonstrate that aqueous and ethanolic extracts from Nigerian plants not only provide strong radical scavenging activity but also significant upregulation of Nrf2 and downstream cytoprotective genes in cell-based and preclinical animal models, as shown in Table 6 (VanderJagt et al., 2022)
b. Correlative Antioxidant Metrics: There is a strong correlation between measured antioxidant capacities (in TRAP or FRAP assays) and the degree of NF-κB inhibition/Nrf2 activation, suggesting efficacy in redox modulation aligns with in vivo anti-inflammatory effects (VanderJagt et al., 2022)
c. Multi-Target Bioactivity: Beyond Nrf2, several plant-derived compounds also inhibit inflammatory signalling (e.g., NF-κB and MAPKs), contributing dual antioxidant and anti-inflammatory action (Boakye et al., 2022; Jayakumar et al., 2022).

d. Computational Pharmacology: Docking and in silico studies have identified specific bioactive plant metabolites (such as rutin, chlorogenic acid, and vitexin) with high affinity for disease-related molecular targets, including those downstream of Nrf2, in diabetes and metabolic diseases (Olawale et al., 2022). **Hea**

Table 8. Key current research findings and corresponding references

Research Focus	Key Findings	Plant(s) Involved	Reference
Nrf2 Activation via Infusions	Upregulation of Nrf2, suppression of NF-κB, improved organ function	Ginger (*Zingiber officinale*), Bitter leaf (Vernonia amygdalina)	Adeyemi et al., 2024; Elebiyo et al., 2022
Synergistic Antioxidant Effects	Combined extracts show enhanced Nrf2 activation and radical scavenging	Ginger + Bitter leaf	Adeyemi et al., 2024
Bioactive Compound Identification	Gingerols, sesquiterpenes, and flavonoids linked to Nrf2 modulation	Ginger, Bitter leaf	Elebiyo et al., 2022
Benchmark Comparability	Nrf2 activation comparable to sulforaphane	*Boswellia dalzielli, Xylopia aethiopica*	VanderJagt et al., 2022
Computational Pharmacology	Rutin, chlorogenic acid, and vitexin bind Nrf2 targets	Multiple Nigerian plants	Olawale et al., 2022
Neuroprotection via Nrf2	Reduced apoptosis, improved cognition in rodents	*Sterculia setigera*	Kantati et al., 2024
Lipid Profile Improvement	Reduced oxidative stress, improved lipid metabolism	*Sclerocarya birrea*	Olas et al., 2025
Anti-diabetic and Hepatoprotective	Limonoids and triterpenes linked to Nrf2 activation	*Pseudocedrela kotschyi*	Alhassan et al., 2021; Olawale et al., 2022

1.7 IDENTIFIED KNOWLEDGE GAPS

Despite the increasing proof of the therapeutic significance of Nrf2 modulation, several critical gaps still exist.

a. Clinical validation deficiency: The strongest evidence thus far resides at the in vitro and animal-model stages. Clinical trials validating efficacy, demonstrating optimal dosing, and establishing robust safety profiles for plant-derived Nrf2 modulators from Nigeria are notably lacking (Dodson et al., 2022; Lastra et al., 2020; Fasipe & Laher, 2023).

b. Safety and toxicity data: while traditional use supports presumed safety, robust dose-response and toxicity studies are sparse. Some extracts reveal dose-related cytotoxicity in cell-based assays, and concern remains about the cumulative effect of pyrrolizidine alkaloids and other potentially mutagenic plant constituents at pharmacological doses (VanderJagt et al., 2022; Kantati et al., 2024).
c. Mechanistic Under exploration: detailed analyses dissecting the specific molecular mechanisms, active phytocompounds responsible for Nrf2 activation, and potential off-target effects (such as chronic Nrf2 overactivation promoting chemoresistance or metabolic dysregulation) are underrepresented in current literature (Boakye et al., 2022; Egbujor et al., 2022).
d. Synergistic and polypharmacological interactions: most plant extracts are complex mixtures, with potential synergistic or antagonistic interactions among their bioactive constituents. Comprehensive understanding of these interactions remains underdeveloped despite their probable importance for both efficacy and safety (VanderJagt et al., 2022).
e. Interaction with conventional pharmaceuticals: potential interference with drug absorption, metabolism, or action due to co-administration of traditional plant medicine with pharmaceutical agents is a further gap seldom addressed in clinical or pharmacovigilance studies, bearing direct relevance for Nigerian healthcare users (VanderJagt et al., 2022).

1.8 RECOMMENDATIONS FOR INTENSIFIED RESEARCH AND VALIDATION

a. Safety Profiling and Risk Assessment: Conduct comprehensive dose–response and chronic toxicity studies in vivo, especially for high-bioactivity extracts. Screen for hepatotoxicity, nephrotoxicity, mutagenicity, and possible drug interactions.
b. Dose, Route, and Formulation Optimisation: Leverage nanotechnology, encapsulation, and other novel formulation methods to overcome solubility and bioavailability challenges. Conduct pharmacokinetic analyses in both animal models and humans.
c. Mechanistic Dissection and Biomarker Integration: Isolate and characterise the bioactive phytocompounds using modern analytic technologies (e.g., high-resolution mass spectrometry, NMR) that most effectively activate Nrf2, and use validated biomarkers (such as HO-1, NQO1, GCLC induction) (Table 7) in both preclinical and early-phase trials.

d. Policy, Regulation, and Health Systems Integration: Support harmonised policy development for herbal medicines, combining traditional intellectual property knowledge with contemporary regulation, ensuring both cultural preservation and patient safety.

1.9 CONCLUSION

Nrf2 serves as a fundamental cellular defence system, safeguarding the body against damage and disease. It protects cells by activating potent antioxidant and detoxification systems. Nrf2 modulators, particularly those from natural origins, present considerable potential for addressing chronic and non-communicable diseases by improving cellular defences. However, the limited number of clinical trials and the ambiguity regarding safe dosages impede their optimal therapeutic application.

Nrf2 modulation represents a central axis for the prevention and treatment of various non-communicable diseases. This book chapter describes extensively the molecular regulation of Nrf2, its cross-pathway interactions, and the accumulating preclinical and ethnobotanical evidence positioning indigenous medicinal plants as a promising source of Nrf2 modulators

Recent research convincingly underscores the growing potential of Nigerian indigenous medicinal plants as sources of natural Nrf2 modulators, particularly in the context of NCD prevention and management. Evidence from 2020–2025 research demonstrates antioxidant, anti-inflammatory, and cytoprotective effects mediated via activation of the Nrf2 pathway.

To leverage this unique therapeutic opportunity, Nigeria must intensify multidisciplinary research efforts, invest in modern phyto-medical and toxicological infrastructure, and promote regulatory harmonisation. This approach will not only enrich the scientific basis for integrating traditional plant medicine into the national health system but also address the escalating NCD crisis with cost-effective, accessible, and culturally rooted solutions.

Table 9. Summary of key findings of top candidate plant and compounds

Plant Species	Part Used	Key Compounds
Erythrina senegalensi	Leaves	flavonoids, alkaloids, phenolic acids
Xylopia aethiopica	Leaves	Diterpenes, flavonoids, essential oils
Boswellia dalzielli	Leaves and bark	Boswellic acids, terpenoids, phenolics.
Sclerocarya birrea	Bark	Flavonoids, saponins, phenolic comounds.

Actionable Recommendations

a. Clinical Translation: Conduct phase I/II clinical trials to prioritize top-performing plants for safety and efficacy testing in NCD contexts. Enhancement of bio-availability can be used for formulation technologies (e.g., nanoemulsions, liposomes) to improve compound absorption and stability.
b. Policy and Infrastructure: establishing a national Nrf2 phytomedicine research consortium can facilitate collaboration among universities, traditional medicine practitioners, and biotech firms. Invest in toxicological and pharmacokinetic labs will enable in-country validation of herbal products to meet international standards.

REFERENCES

Abdulazeez, M. A., Jasim, H. A., Popoola, T. D., Benson, S. O., Manosroi, J., Sallau, A. B., Tabari, M. A., & Fatokun, A. A. (2024). Nigerian medicinal plants with potential anticancer activity—A review. *Exploration of Targeted Anti-tumor Therapy*, *5*(6), 1393–1434. DOI: 10.37349/etat.2024.00282 PMID: 39764419

Adeloye, D., Owolabi, E. O., Ojji, D. B., Auta, A., Dewan, M. T., Olanrewaju, T. O., Ogah, O. S., Omoyele, C., Ezeigwe, N., Mpazanje, R. G., Gadanya, M. A., Agogo, E., Alemu, W., Adebiyi, A. O., & Harhay, M. O. (2021). Prevalence, awareness, treatment, and control of hypertension in Nigeria in 1995 and 2020: A systematic analysis of current evidence. *Journal of Clinical Hypertension*, *23*(5), 963–977. DOI: 10.1111/jch.14220 PMID: 33600078

Adeniran, L. A., & Akindele, O. (2024). Ethnobotanical survey of medicinal plants used by the indigenous people of Ilorin, North Central, Nigeria. *Medicine India*, *3*, 21–32. DOI: 10.25259/MEDINDIA_26_2023

Adeyemi, S. O., Rotimi, D. E., Fatinukun, H. D., Adeogun, V. O., Evbuomwan, I. O., Adebayo, O. L., & Akanji, M. A. (2024). Antioxidant and inflammatory-modulating properties of ginger and bitter leaf teas. *International Journal of Environmental Health Research*, *34*(12), 4122–4136. DOI: 10.1080/09603123.2024.2338894 PMID: 38591815

Alhassan, A. M., Ahmed, Q. U., Malami, I., & Zakaria, Z. A. (2021). Pseudocedrela kotschyi: A review of ethnomedicinal uses, pharmacology, and phytochemistry. *Pharmaceutical Biology*, *59*(1), 953–961. DOI: 10.1080/13880209.2021.1950776 PMID: 34283002

Ashrafizadeh, M., Fekri, H. S., Ahmadi, Z., Farkhondeh, T., & Samarghandian, S. (2020). Therapeutic and biological activities of berberine: The involvement of the Nrf2 signalling pathway. *Journal of Cellular Biochemistry*, *121*(2), 1575–1585. DOI: 10.1002/jcb.29392 PMID: 31609017

Attahiru, A. (2025). Bioactive compounds and therapeutic prospects of Nigerian medicinal plants. *International Journal of African Health and Medical Research*, *9*(5), 45–60.

Ayustaningwarno, F., Anjani, G., Ayu, A. M., & Fogliano, V. (2024). A critical review of Ginger's (*Zingiber officinale*) antioxidant, anti-inflammatory, and immunomodulatory activities. *Frontiers in Nutrition*, *11*, 1364836. DOI: 10.3389/fnut.2024.1364836 PMID: 38903613

Baird, L., & Yamamoto, M. (2020). The molecular mechanisms regulating the KEAP1–NRF2 pathway. Molecular and Cellular Biology, 40(13), Bioltif, Y. E., Sase, T. J., and Nehemiah, T. O. (2020). Phytochemical screening and review of the pharmacological importance of Erythrina senegalensis. *International Journal of Trend in Scientific Research and Development*, *4*(3), 292–296.

Boakye, Y. D., Osafo, N., Oppong-Kyekyeku, J., Abotsi, W. K. M., Boakye-Gyasi, E., Heiss, E., & Agyare, C. (2022). Regulation of Nrf2 and NF-κB activities may contribute to the anti-inflammatory mechanism of xylopic acid. *Inflammopharmacology*, *30*(5), 1835–1841. DOI: 10.1007/s10787-022-00950-y PMID: 35260973

Bukowski, K., Kciuk, M., & Kontek, R. (2020). Mechanisms of multidrug resistance in cancer chemotherapy. *International Journal of Molecular Sciences*, *21*(9), 3233. DOI: 10.3390/ijms21093233 PMID: 32370233

Chen, T., Xiao, Z., Liu, X., Wang, T., Wang, Y., Ye, F., Su, J., Yao, X., Xiong, L., & Yang, D. H. (2024). Natural products for combating multidrug resistance in cancer. *Pharmacological Research*, *202*, 107099. DOI: 10.1016/j.phrs.2024.107099 PMID: 38342327

Chijindu, P. C. I., Okpoma, M. O., & Atubi, O. (2020). Ethnobotanical survey of medicinal plants used in Erhuwaren community in Ughelli South Local Government Area of Delta State. *Unilag Journal of Medicine. Science and Technology*, *8*(1), 176–206.

Chukwuonye, I. I., Ohagwu, K. A., Ogah, O. S., John, C., Oviasu, E., Anyabolu, E. N., Ezeani, I. U., Iloh, G. U. P., Chukwuonye, M. E., Raphael, C. O., Onwuchekwa, U., Okafor, U. H., Oladele, C., Obi, E. C., Okwuonu, C. G., Iheji, O., Nwabuko, O. C., Nnoli, M. A., & Okpechi, G. (2022). Prevalence of overweight and obesity in Nigeria: Systematic review and meta-analysis of population-based studies. *PLOS Global Public Health*, *2*(6), e0000515. DOI: 10.1371/journal.pgph.0000515 PMID: 36962450

D'Amico, R., Fusco, R., Cordaro, M., Interdonato, L., Crupi, R., Gugliandolo, E., Di Paola, D., Peritore, A. F., Siracusa, R., Impellizzeri, D., Cuzzocrea, S., & Di Paola, R. (2022). Modulation of NrF-2 pathway contributes to the therapeutic effects of Boswellia serrata gum resin extract in a model of experimental autoimmune myocarditis. *Antioxidants*, *11*(11), 2129. DOI: 10.3390/antiox11112129 PMID: 36358503

Dinkova-Kostova, A. T., & Copple, I. M. (2023). Advances and challenges in therapeutic targeting of NRF2. *Trends in Pharmacological Sciences*, *44*(3), 137–149. DOI: 10.1016/j.tips.2022.12.003 PMID: 36628798

Dodson, M., Shakya, A., Anandhan, A., Chen, J., Garcia, J. G., & Zhang, D. D. (2022). NRF2 and diabetes: The good, the bad, and the complex. *Diabetes*, *71*(12), 2463–2476. DOI: 10.2337/db22-0623 PMID: 36409792

Egbujor, M. C., Buttari, B., Profumo, E., Telkoparan-Akillilar, P., & Saso, L. (2022). An overview of Nrf2-activating compounds bearing α, β-unsaturated moiety and their antioxidant effects. *International Journal of Molecular Sciences*, *23*(15), 8466. DOI: 10.3390/ijms23158466 PMID: 35955599

Elebiyo, T. C., Olori, O. O., Rotimi, D. E., Al-Megrin, W. A. I., De Waard, M., Alkhuriji, A. F., Batiha, G. E.-S., Adeyanju, A. A., & Adeyemi, O. S. (2022). Chemical fingerprinting, comparative in vitro antioxidant properties, and biochemical effects of ginger and bitterleaf infusion. *Biomedicine and Pharmacotherapy*, *155*, 113788. DOI: 10.1016/j.biopha.2022.113788 PMID: 36271566

Elebiyo, T. C., Rotimi, D., Evbuomwan, I. O., Maimako, R. F., Iyobhebhe, M., Ojo, O. A., Oluba, O. M., & Adeyemi, O. S. (2022). Reassessing vascular endothelial growth factor (VEGF) in anti-angiogenic cancer therapy. *Cancer Treatment and Research Communications*, *32*, 100620. DOI: 10.1016/j.ctarc.2022.100620 PMID: 35964475

Esan, C. O., Ratcliffe, C., Talabi, J. Y., Diaz-Martinez, R., & Enujiugha, V. N. (2024). Factors that influence the management of type 2 diabetes mellitus among adults in Nigeria: A systematic review and meta-analysis. *IPS Journal of Public Health*, *4*(2), 118–142. DOI: 10.54117/ijph.v4i2.29

Ezema, B. O., Eze, C. N., Ayoka, T. O., & Nnadi, C. O. (2024). Antioxidant-enzyme Interaction in Non-communicable Diseases. *Journal of Exploratory Research in Pharmacology*, *9*(4), 262–275. DOI: 10.14218/JERP.2024.00020

Fasipe, B., & Laher, I. (2023). Nrf2 modulates the benefits of evening exercise in type 2 diabetes. *Sports Medicine and Health Science*, *5*(4), 251–258. DOI: 10.1016/j.smhs.2023.09.001 PMID: 38314046

Ford, B. M., Taylor, A. M. W., & McIntosh, J. M. (2021). In vitro–in vivo hybrid approaches for studying modulation of the NRF2 pathway. *Frontiers in Animal Science (Online)*, *8*, 674355. DOI: 10.3389/fanim.2021.674355

Ghareghomi, S., Habibi-Rezaei, M., Arese, M., Saso, L., & Moosavi-Movahedi, A. A. (2022). Nrf2 modulation in breast cancer. *Biomedicines*, *10*(10), 2668. DOI: 10.3390/biomedicines10102668 PMID: 36289931

Ghareghomi, S., Moosavi-Movahedi, F., Saso, L., Habibi-Rezaei, M., Khatibi, A., Hong, J., & Moosavi-Movahedi, A. A. (2023). Modulation of Nrf2/HO-1 by natural compounds in lung cancer. *Antioxidants, 12*(3), 735. DOI: 10.3390/antiox12030735 PMID: 36978983

Gjorgieva Ackova, D., Maksimova, V., Smilkov, K., Buttari, B., Arese, M., & Saso, L. (2023). Alkaloids as natural NRF2 inhibitors: Chemoprevention and cytotoxic action in cancer. *Pharmaceuticals (Basel, Switzerland), 16*(6), 850. DOI: 10.3390/ph16060850 PMID: 37375797

Grant, R., & Seyedsadjadi, N. (2021). The Potential Benefit of Monitoring Oxidative Stress and Inflammation in the Prevention of Non-Communicable Diseases (NCDs).

Gray, N. E., Farina, M., Tucchi, P., & Saso, L. (2022). The Role of the NRF2 Pathway in Maintaining and Improving Cognitive Function. *Biomedicines, 10*(8), 2043. DOI: 10.3390/biomedicines10082043 PMID: 36009590

Gu, H., Liu, J., Jiang, J., Ma, H., Wu, S., Sun, L., & Yao, L. (2025). The role of Nrf2 signalling pathway in diabetic cardiomyopathy: From pathogenesis to traditional Chinese medicine interventions. *Frontiers in Cardiovascular Medicine, 12*, 1492499. DOI: 10.3389/fcvm.2025.1492499 PMID: 40727576

Hosseinkhani, F., Heinken, A., Thiele, I., Lindenburg, P. W., Harms, A. C., & Hankemeier, T. (2021). The contribution of gut bacterial metabolites in the human immune signalling pathway of non-communicable diseases. *Gut Microbes, 13*(1), 1882927. DOI: 10.1080/19490976.2021.1882927 PMID: 33590776

Idaguko, C. A., & Adeniyi, M. J. (2023). Indigenous Antidiabetic Medicinal Plants Used in Nigeria: A Review. *Asian Plant Research Journal, 11*(6), 81–97. DOI: 10.9734/aprj/2023/v11i6234

Ihinmikaiye, S. O., and Akinjagunla, A. D. (2020). Ethnobotanical survey of medicinal plants used by the indigenous people of Bayelsa State, Nigeria. *International Journal of Engineering Applied Sciences and Technology.*

Islam, M. A., Medha, M. M., Nahar, A. U., Al Fahad, M. A., Siraj, M. A., & Seidel, V. (2023). Cancer protective role of selected dietary polyphenols via modulating Keap1/Nrf2/ARE And interconnected signalling pathways. *Nutrition and Cancer, 75*(4), 1065–1102. DOI: 10.1080/01635581.2023.2183546 PMID: 37078744

Jayakumar, T., Huang, C. J., Yen, T. L., Hsia, C. W., Sheu, J. R., Bhavan, P. S., Huang, W.-C., Hsieh, C.-Y., & Hsia, C. H. (2022). Activation of Nrf2 by Esculetin mitigates inflammatory responses through suppression of NF-κB signalling Cascade in RAW 264.7 cells. *Molecules (Basel, Switzerland)*, *27*(16), 5143. DOI: 10.3390/molecules27165143 PMID: 36014382

Jiménez-Cabrera, T., Bautista, M., Velázquez-González, C., Jaramillo-Morales, O. A., Guerrero-Solano, J. A., Urrutia-Hernández, T. A., & De la O-Arciniega, M. (2020). Promising antioxidant activity of Erythrina genus: An alternative treatment for inflammatory pain? *International Journal of Molecular Sciences*, *22*(1), 248. DOI: 10.3390/ijms22010248 PMID: 33383701

Kantati, Y. T., Kodjo, M. K., Lefranc, B., Basille-Dugay, M., Hupin, S., Schmitz, I., Leprince, J., Gbeassor, M., & Vaudry, D. (2024). Neuroprotective effect of Sterculia setigera leaves hydroethanolic extract. *Journal of Molecular Neuroscience*, *74*(2), 44. DOI: 10.1007/s12031-024-02222-6 PMID: 38630337

Kopacz, A., Kloska, D., Forman, H. J., Jozkowicz, A., & Grochot-Przeczek, A. (2020). Beyond repression of Nrf2: An update on Keap1. *Free Radical Biology & Medicine*, *157*, 63–74. DOI: 10.1016/j.freeradbiomed.2020.03.023 PMID: 32234331

Kumar, A. V., Selvaraj, D., Garg, V. K., Buttar, H. S., Kashyap, D., and Wilson, D. W. (2024). The impact of Nrf2 Signalling Pathway in Redox Regulation, Inflammation Attenuation, and Management of Metabolic Syndrome: A Systematic Review. *Biochemical Mechanisms for Metabolic Syndrome*, 223-241.

Lastra, D., Fernández-Ginés, R., Manda, G., and Cuadrado, A. (2020). Perspectives on the clinical development of NRF2-targeting drugs. *Reactive Oxygen Species: Network Pharmacology and Therapeutic Applications*, 93-141.

Lawal, I. O., Rafiu, B. O., Ale, J. E., Majebi, O. E., & Aremu, A. O. (2022). Ethnobotanical survey of local flora used for medicinal purposes among indigenous people in five areas in Lagos State, Nigeria. *Plants*, *11*(5), 633. DOI: 10.3390/plants11050633 PMID: 35270103

Lv, B., Xing, S., Wang, Z., Zhang, A., Wang, Q., Bian, Y., Pei, Y., Sun, H., & Chen, Y. (2024). NRF2 inhibitors: Recent progress, future design and therapeutic potential. *European Journal of Medicinal Chemistry*, *279*, 116822. DOI: 10.1016/j.ejmech.2024.116822 PMID: 39241669

Martínez-Rizo, A. B., Fosado-Rodríguez, R., Torres-Romero, J. C., Lara-Riegos, J. C., Ramírez-Camacho, M. A., Herrera, A. L. A., & Arana-Argáez, V. E. (2024). Models in vivo and in vitro for the study of acute and chronic inflammatory activity: A comprehensive review. *International Immunopharmacology*, *135*, 112292. DOI: 10.1016/j.intimp.2024.112292 PMID: 38788446

Matzinger, M., Fischhuber, K., Pölöske, D., Mechtler, K., & Heiss, E. H. (2020). AMPK leads to phosphorylation of the transcription factor Nrf2, tuning transactivation of selected target genes. *Redox Biology*, *29*, 101393. DOI: 10.1016/j.redox.2019.101393 PMID: 31805502

Moratilla-Rivera, I., Sánchez, M., Valdés-González, J. A., & Gómez-Serranillos, M. P. (2023). Natural Products as Modulators of Nrf2 Signalling Pathway in Neuroprotection. *International Journal of Molecular Sciences*, *24*(4), 3748. DOI: 10.3390/ijms24043748 PMID: 36835155

Mukherjee, A. G., & Gopalakrishnan, A. V. (2023). The mechanistic insights of the antioxidant Keap1-Nrf2 pathway in oncogenesis: A deadly scenario. *Medical Oncology (Northwood, London, England)*, *40*(9), 248. DOI: 10.1007/s12032-023-02124-4 PMID: 37480500

Nediani, C., Ruzzolini, J., & Dinu, M. (2024). Oxidative stress and inflammation as targets for novel preventive and therapeutic approaches in non-communicable diseases III. *Antioxidants*, *13*(11), 1404. DOI: 10.3390/antiox13111404 PMID: 39594546

Ngo, V., & Duennwald, M. L. (2022). Nrf2 and oxidative stress: A general overview of mechanisms and implications in human disease. *Antioxidants*, *11*(12), 2345. DOI: 10.3390/antiox11122345 PMID: 36552553

Nwozo, O. S., Effiong, E. M., Aja, P. M., & Awuchi, C. G. (2023). Antioxidant, phytochemical, and therapeutic properties of medicinal plants: A review. *International Journal of Food Properties*, *26*(1), 359–388. DOI: 10.1080/10942912.2022.2157425

Och, A., Podgórski, R., & Nowak, R. (2020). Biological activity of berberine—A summary update. *Toxins*, *12*(11), 713. DOI: 10.3390/toxins12110713 PMID: 33198257

Ogah, O. S., Orimolade, O. A., & Jinadu, T. O. (2023). Cardiovascular diseases in Nigeria: Current status, threats, and opportunities. *Circulation*, *148*(19), 1441–1444. DOI: 10.1161/CIRCULATIONAHA.123.063671 PMID: 37931020

Ogbonnaya, F. C., Amah, G. H., Ogunbiyi, B. T., Ukangwa, N. A., Adewole, O. A., Akani, E. O., & Oladele, L. O. (2024). Antinutrients Properties and Antioxidant Activity of Some Nigerian Leafy Vegetable Plants. *Tropical Journal of Natural Product Research*, *8*(11).

Ojo, A. E., Ojji, D. B., Grobbee, D. E., Huffman, M. D., & Peters, S. A. (2024). The burden of cardiovascular disease attributable to hypertension in Nigeria: A modelling study using summary-level data. *Global Heart, 19*(1), 50. DOI: 10.5334/gh.1332 PMID: 38863890

Okorie, P. N., Onuoha, C. C., & Adebayo, R. A. (2023). Moringa oleifera in traditional healthcare practice in Nigeria: An ethnobotanical review. *Frontiers in Pharmacology, 14*, 1132456.

Okosodo, E. F., & Sarada, P. M. (2021). Ethno botanical survey and sustainable use of medicinal plant species for the treatment of tropical diseases, Yewa North Southwestern Nigeria. *European Journal of Research Development and Sustainability, 2*(9), 134–149.

Olamoyegun, M. A., Alare, K., Afolabi, S. A., Aderinto, N., & Adeyemi, T. (2024). A systematic review and meta-analysis of the prevalence and risk factors of type 2 diabetes mellitus in Nigeria. *Clinical Diabetes and Endocrinology, 10*(1), 43. DOI: 10.1186/s40842-024-00209-1 PMID: 39639395

Olas, B., Adebayo, O., & Rotimi, D. (2025). Polyphenolic-rich extracts of Sclerocarya birrea improve oxidative stress and lipid metabolism in diabetic rats. *Phytomedicine, 123*, 155678.

Olawale, F., Olofinsan, K., Iwaloye, O., & Ologuntere, T. E. (2022). Phytochemicals from Nigerian medicinal plants modulate therapeutically-relevant diabetes targets: Insight from computational direction. *Advances in Traditional Medicine, 22*(4), 723–737. DOI: 10.1007/s13596-021-00598-z

Olayeriju, O. S., Elekofehinti, O. O., Olaleye, M. T., & Akindahunsi, A. A. (2021). Activation of NRF2/HO-1 Pathway by aqueous methanolic leaf extract of Triclisia gilletii and selected identified compounds in Triclisia gilletii, modulates crystal binding genes (CD44/OPN) in Ethane-1, 2-diol-induced nephrolithic rats. *Phytomedicine Plus : International Journal of Phytotherapy and Phytopharmacology, 1*(4), 100066. DOI: 10.1016/j.phyplu.2021.100066

Oseghale, I. D., Lawal, O. P., Ubebe, D. O., Orjiewulu, V. C., Igunma, A. A., Odey, O. P., Ajibola, D. T., Chima, D. I., Tuador, N. K., & Ani, C. P. (2024). Ethnomedicinal and phytopharmacological aspects of Vernonia amygdalina (bitter leaf) utilised as a traditional medicinal herb. *Asian Journal of Research in Biochemistry, 14*(6), 41–57. DOI: 10.9734/ajrb/2024/v14i6326

Oso, A. (2023). Non-communicable Diseases: An Emerging Epidemic in Nigeria. *Tropical Journal of Nephrology, 18*(1 and 2), 31-37.

Oyelakin, A. O., Olubode, T. P., & Olawale, B. R. (2020). Ethnobotanical survey and phytochemical analysis of selected medicinal plants used in treating digestive disorders. *Journal of Medicinal Plants Studies*, *8*(2), 38–42.

Panieri, E., Buha, A., Telkoparan-Akillilar, P., Cevik, D., Kouretas, D., Veskoukis, A., Skaperda, Z., Tsatsakis, A., Wallace, D., Suzen, S., & Saso, L. (2020). Potential applications of NRF2 modulators in cancer therapy. *Antioxidants*, *9*(3), 193. DOI: 10.3390/antiox9030193 PMID: 32106613

Park, J. S., Rustamov, N., & Roh, Y. S. (2023). The roles of NRF2-regulated oxidative stress and mitochondrial quality control in chronic liver diseases. *Antioxidants*, *12*(11), 1928. DOI: 10.3390/antiox12111928 PMID: 38001781

Popoola, T. D., Guetchueng, S. T., Ritchie, K. J., Awodele, O., Dempster, N. M., Akinloye, O., Sarker, S. D., & Fatokun, A. A. (2021). Potent Nrf2-inducing, antioxidant, and anti-inflammatory effects and identification of constituents validate the anti-cancer use of Uvaria chamae and Olax subscorpioidea. *BMC Complementary Medicine and Therapies*, *21*(1), 234. DOI: 10.1186/s12906-021-03404-0 PMID: 34537049

Pouremamali, F., Pouremamali, A., Dadashpour, M., Soozangar, N., & Jeddi, F. (2022). An update of Nrf2 activators and inhibitors in cancer prevention/promotion. *Cell Communication and Signaling : CCS*, *20*(1), 100. DOI: 10.1186/s12964-022-00906-3 PMID: 35773670

Rotimi, D. E., Ben-Goru, G. M., Evbuomwan, I. O., Elebiyo, T. C., Alorabi, M., Farasani, A., Batiha, G. E., & Adeyemi, O. S. (2024). *Zingiber officinale* and Vernonia amygdalina infusions improve redox status in rat brain. *Metabolic Brain Disease*, *39*(3), 721–732.

Saha, S., Buttari, B., Panieri, E., Profumo, E., & Saso, L. (2020). An overview of Nrf2 signalling pathway and its role in inflammation. *Molecules (Basel, Switzerland)*, *25*(22), 5474. DOI: 10.3390/molecules25225474 PMID: 33238435

Saha, S., Buttari, B., & Saso, L. (2024). Modulation of oxidative stress and inflammation via the NRF2 signalling pathway. *Frontiers in Pharmacology*, *15*, 1483289. DOI: 10.3389/fphar.2024.1483289 PMID: 39359243

Sanchez-Ortega, M., Carrera, A. C., & Garrido, A. (2021). Role of NRF2 in lung cancer. *Cells*, *10*(8), 1879. DOI: 10.3390/cells10081879 PMID: 34440648

Shitaw, E. E., AlAhmad, M., & Sivaprasadarao, A. (2025). Inter-Organelle Crosstalk in Oxidative Distress: A Unified TRPM2-NOX2 Mediated Vicious Cycle Involving Ca2+, Zn2+, and ROS Amplification. *Antioxidants, 14*(7), 776. DOI: 10.3390/antiox14070776 PMID: 40722879

Suraweera, L., Rupasinghe, T., Dellaire, H. P. V., & Xu, G. (2020). Regulation of Nrf2/ARE pathway by Dietary flavonoids: A friend or foe for Cancer Management? *Antioxid (Basel), 9*(10), 973. DOI: 10.3390/antiox9100973 PMID: 33050575

Sykiotis, G. P. (2021). Keap1/Nrf2 signalling pathway. *Antioxidants, 10*(6), 828. DOI: 10.3390/antiox10060828 PMID: 34067331

Tamaru, E., Kokubu, D., Ushida, Y., & Itoh, K. (2024). Nrf2 induction potency of plant-derived compounds determined using an antioxidant response element luciferase reporter and conventional NAD(P)H-quinone acceptor oxidoreductase 1 activity assay. *BMC Research Notes, 17*(1), 373. DOI: 10.1186/s13104-024-07038-6 PMID: 39707451

Tascioglu Aliyev, A., Panieri, E., Stepanić, V., Gurer-Orhan, H., & Saso, L. (2021). Involvement of NRF2 in breast cancer and possible therapeutical role of polyphenols and melatonin. *Molecules (Basel, Switzerland), 26*(7), 1853. DOI: 10.3390/molecules26071853 PMID: 33805996

Tauchen, J., Frankova, A., Manourova, A., Valterova, I., Lojka, B., & Leuner, O. (2023). Garcinia kola: A critical review on chemistry and pharmacology of an important West African medicinal plant. *Phytochemistry Reviews, 22*(5), 1305–1351. DOI: 10.1007/s11101-023-09869-w PMID: 37359709

Tee, T. X., Kee, L. T., Chai, T. T., Yam, H. C., Reza, H. M., Wong, F. C., Law, J. X., & Tan, S.-A. (2025). Plant-derived Nrf2 activators to enhance liver antioxidative and regenerative potentials. *Revista Brasileira de Farmacognosia, 35*(1), 61–77. DOI: 10.1007/s43450-024-00609-5

Ungvari, Z., Menyhart, O., Lehoczki, A., Fekete, M., Fazekas-Pongor, V., Ocana, A., Varga, P., & Győrffy, B. (2025). NRF2 pathway activation predicts poor prognosis in lung cancer: A cautionary note on antioxidant interventions. *GeroScience*. Advance online publication. DOI: 10.1007/s11357-025-01736-0 PMID: 40537696

VanderJagt, D., Hunsaker, L., Otimenyin, S. O., & Uguru, M. O. (2022). The anti-inflammatory activities of twelve Nigerian medicinal plants: Inhibition of NfkB, activation of Nrf2, and antioxidant content. *African Journal of Biochemistry Research, 16*(1), 1–10.

Wadowski, P., Juszczak, M., & Woźniak, K. (2024). NRF2 modulators of plant origin and their ability to overcome multidrug resistance in cancers. *International Journal of Molecular Sciences*, *25*(21), 11500. DOI: 10.3390/ijms252111500 PMID: 39519053

Wang, J., Xiao, M., Wang, J., Wang, S., Zhang, J., Guo, Y., Tang, Y., & Gu, J. (2021). NRF2-related epigenetic modifications in cardiac and vascular complications of diabetes mellitus. *Frontiers in Endocrinology*, *12*, 598005. DOI: 10.3389/fendo.2021.598005 PMID: 34248833

Wang, Y., & Wang, J. (2020). Modelling and prediction of global non-communicable diseases. *BMC Public Health*, *20*(1), 822. DOI: 10.1186/s12889-020-08890-4 PMID: 32487173

World Health Organisation, Regional Office for Africa. (2023, August). Nigeria – Country Disease Outlook. WHO Regional Office for Africa.

Xiao, J. L., Liu, H. Y., Sun, C. C., & Tang, C. F. (2024). Regulation of Keap1-Nrf2 signalling in health and diseases. *Molecular Biology Reports*, *51*(1), 809. DOI: 10.1007/s11033-024-09771-4 PMID: 39001962

Xiong, R. G., Huang, S. Y., Wu, S. X., Zhou, D. D., Yang, Z. J., Saimaiti, A., Zhao, C.-N., Shang, A., Zhang, Y.-J., Gan, R.-Y., & Li, H. B. (2022). Anticancer effects and mechanisms of berberine from medicinal herbs: An update review. *Molecules (Basel, Switzerland)*, *27*(14), 4523. DOI: 10.3390/molecules27144523 PMID: 35889396

Yagishita, Y., Gatbonton-Schwager, T. N., McCallum, M. L., & Kensler, T. W. (2020). Current landscape of NRF2 biomarkers in clinical trials. *Antioxidants*, *9*(8), 716. DOI: 10.3390/antiox9080716 PMID: 32784785

Yang, R., Zhang, J., Li, J., Qin, R., Chen, J., Wang, R., Goltzman, D., & Miao, D. (2022). Inhibition of Nrf2 degradation alleviates age-related osteoporosis induced by 1,25-Dihydroxyvitamin D deficiency. *Free Radical Biology & Medicine*, *178*, 246–261. DOI: 10.1016/j.freeradbiomed.2021.12.010 PMID: 34890768

Zhang, X., Qian, J. W., Wei, B. T., & Zhang, B. (2025). Flavonoids as Modulators of Nrf2 Signalling Pathway in Alleviating Cisplatin-Induced Organ Toxicity. *Yangtze Medicine*, *9*(1), 52–77. DOI: 10.4236/ym.2025.91006

Chapter 2

Medicinal Ethnobotanicals in Mitigating Pollution-Induced Oxidative Damage With Mechanisms and Therapeutic Potential:

Mechanistic Basis of Plant Antioxidant Defense

Temidayo Daniel Adeniyi
http://orcid.org/0000-0002-8482-9136
University of Ilorin, Nigeria

Emmanuel Tolulope Adegoke
http://orcid.org/0009-0005-6856-4958
University of Ilorin, Nigeria

Akinpelu Moronkeji
http://orcid.org/0000-0001-5186-8676
Osun State University, Osogbo, Nigeria

Oluwadarasimi Osundara
http://orcid.org/0009-0007-1052-1503
University of Ilorin, Nigeria

Godwin Olawoyin Adunmo
http://orcid.org/0000-0001-7938-8092
University of Ilorin, Nigeria

Hanifat Abake Olaitan
http://orcid.org/0009-0006-5507-3129
University of Ilorin, Nigeria

Gbadebo Maroof Oyeniyi
http://orcid.org/0009-0007-0034-7177
University of Ilorin, Nigeria

DOI: 10.4018/979-8-3373-5876-5.ch002

ABSTRACT

Environmental pollution remains a global health issue linked to numerous diseases, primarily through the generation of reactive oxygen species (ROS) that induce lipid peroxidation, protein and DNA damage, and cellular dysfunction. This review examines the therapeutic potential of medicinal ethnobotanicals in mitigating pollution-induced oxidative stress, with a focus on their molecular mechanisms and therapeutic potentials. Ethnobotanicals, rich in bioactive phytochemicals such as flavonoids, phenolic acids, alkaloids, and terpenoids, exhibit potent antioxidant and cytoprotective properties. Their protective effects are largely mediated through the enhancement of endogenous antioxidant systems and modulation of redox-sensitive signalling pathways. Evidence from both in vivo and in vitro studies highlights the efficacy of selected ethnobotanicals in reducing oxidative biomarkers and restoring tissue homeostasis, particularly in mammalian systems. This review highlights the potential of ethnobotanicals as promising agents in mitigating the health effects of environmental pollutants.

1.0 INTRODUCTION

Environmental pollution has emerged as a critical global health and ecological challenge in the 21st century, with significant impacts on human well-being and ecosystems. Various types of pollution, including air, water, soil, and noise, are linked to numerous health issues such as respiratory diseases, cardiovascular problems, cancer, and neurological disorders (Adigun & Odeleye, 2025). The primary causes of pollution include rapid industrialisation, urbanisation, unsustainable agricultural practices, and poor waste management. Despite global attention, the long-term consequences of environmental degradation persist, particularly in developing countries where awareness and regulations are lacking (Ukaogo et al., 2020).

Air pollution, primarily composed of particulate matter (PM), ozone (O_3), nitrogen oxides (NOx), sulfur dioxide (SO_2), and carbon monoxide (CO), poses significant health risks (Moronkeji and Akinbo 2024). These pollutants, mainly emitted from energy production, industry, traffic, and agriculture, affect multiple organ systems, leading to cardiovascular, respiratory, and neurological diseases (Sigsgaard & Hoffmann, 2024). Exposure to air pollution is a major contributor to morbidity and premature mortality globally. Specific health impacts include chronic obstructive pulmonary disease (COPD), asthma, lung cancer, and central nervous system dysfunctions. The growing concern over air pollution's health effects necessitates a multidisciplinary approach involving public awareness, scientific expertise, and sustainable solutions (Manisalidis et al., 2020). Soil pollution, resulting from industrial activities, agricultural practices, and improper waste disposal, poses significant threats to ecosystems and human health (Adeniyi et al., 2023; Koushal et al., 2025). Key pollutants include heavy metals, pesticides, and micro/nanoplastics, which reduce soil fertility, contaminate food crops, and contribute to water pollution (Adeniyi et al, 2017). These contaminants can bioaccumulate in plants and enter the food chain, leading to various health implications, particularly neurodegenerative disease (Adeniyi et al., 2019). Heavy metals like cadmium, lead, copper, and zinc, along with pesticides, have adverse effects on agricultural ecosystems and human health. The toxicity of these pollutants is influenced by their bioavailability in soil and plant uptake mechanisms (Alengebawy et al., 2021; Adeniyi et al., 2024a)

1.1 The Burden Of Oxidative Stress And Its Link To Pollution

Environmental pollution, particularly air pollution, is a major contributor to adverse health effects through the induction of oxidative stress (Itziou et al., 2024). Fine particulate matter ($PM_{2.5}$) and ozone are key pollutants that generate ROS in biological systems, triggering inflammatory responses and cellular damage. This oxidative stress impacts multiple organ systems, including respiratory, cardiovascular, and central nervous (Moronkeji and Akinbo 2024; Wang et al., 2025).

Particulate matter (PM) in the air can trigger the generation of ROS in biological systems, leading to oxidative stress and inflammation, which can damage cellular biomolecules, including lipids, proteins, and DNA, contributing to various chronic diseases affecting the respiratory, cardiovascular, and nervous systems. PM's toxicity is largely attributed to its metal and polycyclic aromatic hydrocarbon (PAH) components, which activate the Nrf2 pathway as a protective mechanism (Pardo et al., 2020; Wang et al., 2025).

1.2 The Rise Of Interest In Ethnobotanical Medicine

Medicinal plants have been integral to traditional medicine for millennia, with approximately 80% of people relying on herbal remedies as their primary health solution (Popoola et al., 2021). These plants possess rich phytochemical profiles, particularly antioxidants like phenolic compounds and flavonoids, which play crucial roles in combating oxidative stress and inflammation (Figure 1) (Said & Ibrahim, 2024). Recent research has explored the therapeutic potential of medicinal plants in addressing modern health challenges, including air pollution-induced inflammation and anxiety. Studies have focused on plants such as *Passiflora incarnata* and *Withania somnifera*, investigating their mechanisms in modulating cytokines, NF-κB signalling, and neurophysiological regulation (Rathore et al., 2025). Herbal remedies have gained popularity as accessible and culturally acceptable healthcare options, particularly in low- and middle-income countries. These plant-based interventions show promise in managing various health conditions, including diabetes, by enhancing insulin sensitivity and reducing glucose absorption (Emmanuel, 2025). Herbal medicines also demonstrate potential in combating particulate matter-induced health effects through their antioxidant and anti-inflammatory properties (Intharuksa et al., 2024). The growing interest in natural remedies is driven by concerns over synthetic drug side effects and a shift towards holistic health approaches (Fouche, 2025). Plant-derived compounds, especially polyphenols, exhibit strong antioxidant properties that may help treat neurodegenerative diseases by scavenging free radicals and reducing oxidative stress (Chandran & Abrahamse, 2020).

1.3 Oxidative Stress and Environmental Pollution

Oxidative stress is a pathological condition characterised by an imbalance between the generation of ROS and the capacity of the biological system to neutralise these reactive intermediates through antioxidant defences (Kıran et al., 2023). Under physiological conditions, ROS, including superoxide anion (O_2•$^-$), hydrogen peroxide (H_2O_2), and hydroxyl radical (•OH), are generated as natural byproducts of cellular metabolism, particularly within the mitochondria during oxidative phosphorylation (Napolitano et al., 2021). In moderate concentrations, ROS serve essential roles in cellular signalling, immune defence, and apoptosis regulation. However, excessive accumulation due to internal dysfunction or external exposure leads to oxidative damage to cellular biomolecules (Martinvalet and Walch, 2022). At the biochemical level, oxidative stress involves the activation of redox-sensitive transcription factors such as nuclear factor kappa B (NF-κB), activator protein 1 (AP-1), and nuclear factor erythroid 2–related factor 2 (Nrf2), which modulate inflammatory responses and the expression of antioxidant enzymes. ROS-induced lipid peroxidation leads to the formation of secondary cytotoxic products like malondialdehyde (MDA) and 4-hydroxynonenal (4-HNE), which further propagate cellular injury. DNA oxidation results in mutagenic lesions compromising genomic integrity (Gambhir et al., 2022). Antioxidant defences are categorised into enzymatic and non-enzymatic systems. Key enzymatic antioxidants include superoxide dismutase (SOD), which converts superoxide into hydrogen peroxide; catalase and glutathione peroxidase (GPx), which reduce hydrogen peroxide into water (Bandodkar et al., 2025). Non-enzymatic antioxidants include reduced glutathione (GSH), vitamins C and E, flavonoids, and other polyphenolic compounds derived from dietary or botanical sources (Abdulfatah, 2022; Adeniyi et al., 2024b). A well-coordinated interaction between these systems is essential to maintain redox homeostasis and prevent oxidative injury. When disrupted by environmental insults such as air pollutants, heavy metals, or industrial toxins, oxidative stress is chronic and contributes to the pathogenesis of cardiovascular, neurodegenerative, pulmonary, and metabolic diseases (Ehsanifar et al., 2021; Akinpelu & Akinbo, 2024).

1.3.1 Heavy Metals, Particulate Matter, Hydrocarbons as major environmental pollutants

Environmental pollutants are primary external sources of oxidative stress, with many of them possessing redox-active properties or interfering with cellular antioxidant defences. Among the most significant contributors are heavy metals, particulate matter, and hydrocarbons, all of which have been shown to induce ROS formation leading to oxidative damage in biological systems (Adeniyi et al., 2023; Moronkeji et al. 2024a). Heavy metals such as lead (Pb), cadmium (Cd), mercury (Hg), and arsenic (As) are toxic environmental contaminants that persist in air, soil, and water (Adeniyi et al., 2024a; Angon et al., 2025).

1.3.2 Heavy metals, Particulate matter (PM) and Polycyclic aromatic hydrocarbons (PAHs)

Heavy metals disrupt redox homeostasis by directly generating ROS or by depleting intracellular antioxidants (Jomova et al. 2025). Heavy metals like Cd can displace essential metals from antioxidant enzymes, reducing their activity, while Pb interferes with mitochondrial electron transport, resulting in excessive ROS formation (Sun et al., 2022). Arsenic exposure is also associated with oxidative DNA damage and lipid peroxidation, contributing to carcinogenesis and cardiovascular dysfunction (Balali-Mood et al., 2021). Particulate matter like ($PM_{2\cdot5}$) and ultrafine particles ($PM_{0\cdot1}$), are airborne pollutants derived from combustion engines or industrial emissions, and are capable of penetrating deep into the respiratory tract, where they stimulate inflammation and oxidative stress through multiple mechanisms (Moronkeji and Akinbo 2024; Park et al. 2021) PM contains redox-active substances such as transition metals and polycyclic aromatic hydrocarbons (PAHs) that catalyse the formation of superoxide and hydroxyl radicals (Vimukthi et al., 2025). Chronic exposure to PM has been linked to respiratory illnesses, cardiovascular diseases, and neurodegenerative disorders through persistent oxidative injury and mitochondrial dysfunction (Sierra-Vargas et al., 2023). Polycyclic aromatic hydrocarbons (PAHs) are organic pollutants produced by the incomplete combustion of organic materials like coal, oil, and wood. PAHs such as benzo[a]pyrene can undergo enzymatic metabolism in the body, forming electrophilic intermediates and quinones that generate ROS and form DNA adducts (Ammar et al., 2021). These processes lead to oxidative stress, mutagenesis, and inflammatory responses. Occupational and environmental exposures to PAHs are associated with increased risks of lung cancer, atherosclerosis, and impaired reproductive function (Montano et al., 2025). The interaction of these pollutants with biological systems often activates redox-sensitive signalling pathways such as NF-κB and MAPK, amplifying inflammation and further ROS production. Moreover, the combined exposure to multiple pollutants can produce synergistic toxic effects, heightening the extent of oxidative damage (Gambhir et al., 2022).

Figure 1. Medicinal ethnobotanicals in the mitigation of pollution-induced oxidative damage

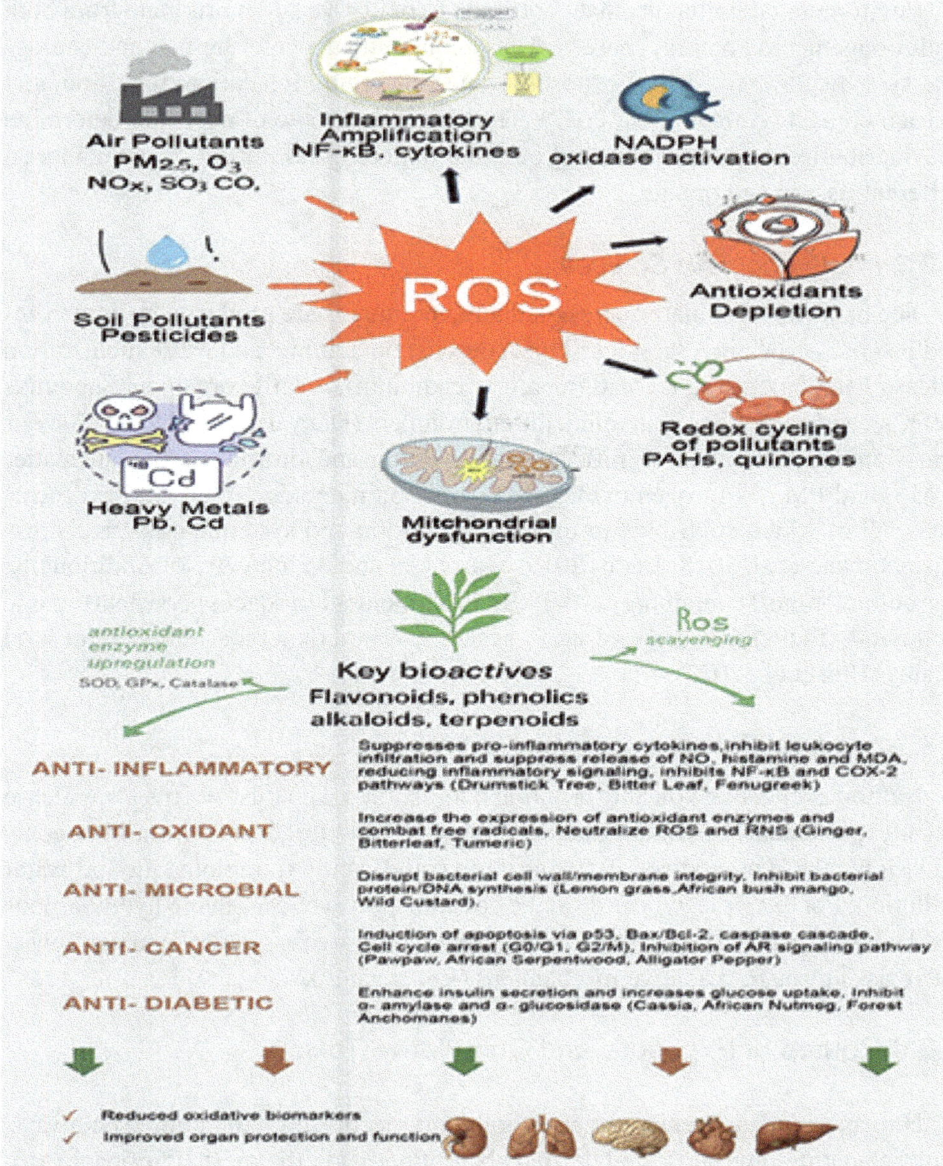

1.3.3 Sources and Routes of Exposure

Environmental pollutants that contribute to oxidative stress originate from both anthropogenic and natural sources. These contaminants enter human and ecological systems through various exposure routes, including inhalation, ingestion, and dermal contact (Anetor et al., 2022). The source and route of exposure determine the distribution, accumulation, and eventual toxicological impact of pollutants on different tissues and organs.

1.3.3.1 Anthropogenic Sources

The majority of oxidative stress-inducing pollutants are produced by human activities. Industrial processes, fossil fuel combustion, mining, and waste incineration release heavy metals (e.g., lead, mercury, cadmium), volatile organic compounds (VOCs), and particulate matter into the environment (Danyal et al., 2023). Vehicular emissions are particularly significant sources of fine and ultrafine particulate matter ($PM_{2 \cdot 5}$ and $PM_{0 \cdot 1}$), nitrogen oxides (NO_X), carbon monoxide (CO), and hydrocarbons, all of which contribute to urban air pollution and systemic oxidative stress (Brinchmann et al. 2018; Kadir, 2019; Moronkeji and Akinbo 2024). Additionally, agricultural runoff containing pesticides and herbicides introduces persistent organic pollutants (POPs) into soil and water systems, where they bioaccumulate in food chains (Hua et al., 2022).

1.3.3.2 Natural Sources

Natural events like volcanic eruptions, forest fires, and dust storms also release harmful pollutants into the environment. Although less frequent than anthropogenic emissions, these natural sources contribute significantly to regional air and water pollution. For example, wildfire smoke contains polycyclic aromatic hydrocarbons (PAHs), fine particulates, and oxidising gases that pose respiratory and cardiovascular risks through oxidative mechanisms (Lei et al., 2024).

1.3.4 Routes of Exposure and Cumulative Toxicity

Human exposure to environmental pollutants occurs through multiple pathways, with inhalation, ingestion, and dermal absorption being the most significant (Moronkeji and Akinbo, 2024; Adeniyi et al., 2024a).Among these, inhalation represents the most direct and prevalent route, particularly for airborne pollutants. Fine and ultrafine particles can bypass the upper respiratory defences, penetrate deep into the alveolar spaces, and enter systemic circulation, leading to the initiation of oxidative stress and provoking systemic inflammation through the activation of redox-sensitive signaling pathways (Ali et al., 2022). Ingestion of heavy metals, pesticides, and microplastics often present in polluted water, crops, and animal products can result in chronic internal exposure. Over time, these toxicants may bioaccumulate in vital organs like the liver, testes, kidneys, and nervous system, contributing to widespread oxidative damage and metabolic disturbances (Moini and Ferdowsi, 2023; Adeniyi et al., 2023; Adeniyi et al., 2024a; Adeniyi et al., 2024b; Adeniyi et al., 2024c). Dermal absorption also represents a relevant exposure route, especially in occupational or cosmetic contexts. Harmful substances, including pesticides, industrial chemicals, and certain additives in personal care products, can breach the skin barrier, cause localised oxidative injury and contribute to systemic toxicity when absorbed into circulation (Morlock & Zoller, 2025). In reality, individuals are seldom exposed to a single pollutant or route. Rather, cumulative and combined exposures are the norm, involving simultaneous contact with diverse pollutants across multiple pathways. This complex exposure scenario leads to the amplification of oxidative burden and complicates the prediction of toxicological outcomes with risks particularly heightened in vulnerable populations, including children, pregnant women, the elderly, and individuals with underlying health conditions (Mao et al., 2024).

1.4 Mechanisms of Pollutant-Induced ROS Generation

Pollutants induce oxidative stress primarily through the excessive generation of ROS, either by direct redox activity or by disrupting intracellular pathways that regulate redox balance. These mechanisms vary by pollutant class but converge on common cellular and molecular pathways that amplify oxidative damage and trigger pathophysiological responses.

1.4.1 Mitochondrial Dysfunction

One of the primary mechanisms by which pollutants induce ROS is through the disruption of mitochondrial electron transport chains.Heavy metals such as cadmium, lead, and arsenic interfere with mitochondrial complexes I and III, causing electron leakage and the partial reduction of oxygen to form superoxide radicals (Liu et al., 2022). Similarly, $PM_{2.5}$ and nanoparticles localise to mitochondria and impair oxidative phosphorylation, promoting mitochondrial ROS production and the opening of mitochondrial permeability transition pores (Chen et al., 2021).

1.4.2 Activation of NADPH Oxidase (NOX)

Enzymes Environmental stimuli such as diesel exhaust particles, ozone, and PAHs activate membrane-bound NADPH oxidases, especially NOX1, NOX2, and

NOX4, which catalyse the reduction of oxygen to superoxide ($O_2\bullet^-$) (Zhou et al., 2023). This NOX-dependent ROS generation is prominent in pulmonary epithelial and endothelial cells and plays a central role in pollutant-induced vascular inflammation and oxidative lung injury.

1.4.3 Redox-Cycling of Pollutant Components

Certain organic pollutants, particularly PAHs and quinones, undergo metabolic redox cycling, which is a process by which they alternate between oxidised and reduced forms, continuously generating superoxide and hydrogen peroxide in the presence of oxygen (Sarkar et al., 2020). These intermediates, produced via cytochrome P450 enzymes (e.g., CYP1A1, CYP1B1), also form DNA adducts, compounding genotoxicity and oxidative stress.

1.4.5 Transition Metal Catalysis (Fenton and Haber-Weiss Reactions)

Redox-active transition metals such as iron (Fe^{2+}) and copper (Cu^{+}), often bound to particulates or present in industrial pollutants, catalyse the Fenton and Haber-Weiss reactions. In these processes, hydrogen peroxide is converted into highly reactive hydroxyl radicals (•OH), which indiscriminately damage cellular macromolecules (Zhang et al., 2021). This catalytic activity significantly contributes to oxidative tissue injury following pollutant exposure.

1.4.6 Antioxidant Depletion and Inflammatory Amplification

Pollutants not only induce excessive production of ROS but also impair cellular antioxidant defence mechanisms. Toxic metals such as arsenic and cadmium inhibit key antioxidant enzymes like SOD, GPx and Catalase while also depleting GSH, thereby increasing cellular susceptibility to oxidative insults (Rahman et al., 2021). Simultaneously, pollutants including ozone and ultrafine particles activate macrophages and neutrophils, which generate ROS through respiratory bursts and release pro-inflammatory cytokines. This dual process of antioxidant depletion and immune cell activation perpetuates oxidative stress and establishes a chronic inflammatory cycle, ultimately driving tissue injury (Cascio, 2022). Table 1.0 shows the mechanisms of action of ethnobotanicals and their effects on organs and tissues.

1.5 Overview of Ethnobotanicals in Traditional Medicine

Ethnobotanicals refer to plants and their derivatives used by various ethnic and indigenous communities for healing, spiritual, or nutritional purposes (Mekonnen et al., 2022). They are integral to traditional medicine systems such as Ayurveda, Traditional Chinese Medicine, and African Traditional Medicine (Yuan et al., 2016). Ethnobotanical plants have been integral to traditional medicine systems globally, with approximately 80% of the global population relying on plant-based remedies for primary healthcare. Studies have documented over 6,000 plant species utilised globally for therapeutic, ceremonial, and dietary purposes (Hossain et al., 2022). These plants represent an essential reservoir of bioactive compounds with pharmacological potential and continue to serve as foundational resources for both modern pharmaceuticals and traditional medicine systems (Popoola et al., 2021).

Table 1. Mechanisms of action of ethnobotanical agents and their effects on tissue and organ systems

Notable Ethnobotanicals	Mechanism of Action	Target Tissues/ Organs	Observed Effects	References
Anti-inflammatory				
Fenugreek *(Trigonella foenum-graecum)*	Stimulates insulin secretion, delays gastric emptying; inhibits NF-κB and COX-2 pathways; antioxidant activity via flavonoids and saponins	Pancreas, GI tract, liver, adipose tissue	Improved glucose tolerance, reduced inflammation, and lipid-lowering effect	(Arya et al., 2023)
Jungle Geranium *(Ixora coccinea)*	Lowers the production of pro-inflammatory mediators by blocking inflammatory pathways like cyclooxygenase (COX) and lipoxygenase (LOX).	Skin, GI tract, Joint.	Lessen inflammation-related discomfort, redness, and oedema in the skin and joints.	(Bharathy et al., 2024)
West African black pepper *(Piper guineense)*	Piperine disrupts bacterial cell wall, inhibits prostaglandin synthesis, modulates TRPV1 pain receptors	GI tract, respiratory system, joints, nervous system	Relief of pain, treatment of respiratory infections, reduced microbial load	(Alagbe et al., 2021), (Akbar et al., 2025), (Deniz et al., 2024)

continued on following page

Table 1. Continued

Notable Ethnobotanicals	Mechanism of Action	Target Tissues/ Organs	Observed Effects	References
Scent Leaf *(Ocimum gratissimum)*	Inhibits NF-κB, a crucial transcription factor that controls inflammatory cytokines. Additionally, they alter JNK, STAT-3, AP-1, and NFAT expression, which helps to lessen inflammatory reactions.	Lungs, GI tract.	Efficient in treating gastritis, colitis, and bronchitis.	(Gholijani et al., 2016; Pereira et al., 2023)
African Basil (*Ocimum canum*)	Exerts anti-inflammatory effects through interactions with carbonic anhydrase family proteins and important enzymes in the arachidonic pathway, such as COX-1 and COX-2.	Lungs and joints.	Effective for asthma, arthritis, and musculoskeletal discomfort.	(Beltrán-Noboa et al., 2022)
African star apple (*Chrysophyllum albidum*)	Rich in flavonoids and proanthocyanidins that scavenge ROS; inhibits α-amylase and α-glucosidase enzymes; suppresses pro-inflammatory cytokines.	Pancreas, liver, kidney, cardiovascular system	Reduced oxidative stress, improved glycemic control, prevention of organ damage	(Imaga et al., 2023), (Hamzah, 2024), (Oyetayo et al., 2021), (Owolabi & Okubor, 2024)
Wild Custard Apple (*Annona senegalensis*).	Inhibits leukocyte infiltration and suppresses the release of NO, histamine and MDA, reducing inflammatory signalling	Skin, GI tract	Reduced inflammatory cytokines, Reduced edema, Accelerated healing of inflammation	(Togbenou et al., 2020)
False Sesame (*Ceratotheca sesamoides*)	Downregulates pro-inflammatory cytokines and reduces prostaglandin synthesis; flavonoids inhibit COX activity.	Skin, joints, mucous membranes	Relief of inflammatory symptoms and analgesic effects Improved joint mobility	(Osuagwu & Idika, 2021)
Guinea Pepper (*Xylopia aetheopica*)	Modulate inflammatory mediators (histamine, serotonin, bradykinin) and the arachidonate pathway. Suppresses ICAM-1 expression, decreases pro-inflammatory cytokines (IL-6 and TNF-α).	Skin, liver, GIT	Relief of pain and inflammation	(Osafo et al., 2018)

continued on following page

Table 1. Continued

Notable Ethnobotanicals	Mechanism of Action	Target Tissues/ Organs	Observed Effects	References
Hyptis suaveolens *Cassia alata,* *Cajanus cajan* *Morinda lucida*	NF-κB and COX-2 inhibition Suppression of pro-inflammatory cytokines (TNF-α, IL-1β, IL-6) Inhibition of prostaglandin synthesis	Joints, brain, liver, lungs, GI tract	Reduced tissue oedema, neutrophil infiltration, and histological evidence of inflammation	(Patel & Bhutani, 2014; Yada et al., 2021), (Ayertey et al., 2020)
Hog plum *(Spondias mombin)*	Contains vitamin C and carotenoids; enhances glutathione levels; disrupts microbial membranes	Liver, GI tract, skin, immune system	Improved liver function, prevention of gastrointestinal infections, and reduced inflammation	(Santos et al., 2023), (Ogunro et al., 2023), (Adetuyi et al., 2025).
Crinum glaucum, *Enantia chlorantha,* *Struchium sparganophora,* *Spathodea campanulata,* *Tithonia diversifolia,* *Laggera pterodonta*	Attenuates the expression of proteins iNOS and COX-2. Inhibits the interactivity between Nrf2 and Keap1 protein	Gastrointestinal tract	Increases free radical scavenging potential.	(Coolborn et al., 2015; Tagne et al., 2018)
Antioxidant				
Bitter Leaf *(Vernonia amygdalina)*	Supports the antioxidant qualities of the plant by lessening oxidative stress and scavenging free radicals.	Liver and pancreas.	Prevents hepatotoxicity and the consequences of diabetes.	(Ekaluo et al., 2015)
Drumstick Tree *(Moringa oleifera).*	Increases the expression of antioxidant enzymes and combats free radicals.	Liver, kidneys, and heart	Protects against kidney damage, hypertension, and oxidative damage.	(Vongsak et al., 2015; Chi et al., 2023).
Loranthus micranthus, *Pavetta crassipes*	Scavenging of free radicals Neutralisation of ROS and RNS.	Heart, Lungs, Liver	Increased cellular protection, improved immune system and slowed down ageing of cells.	(Hlophe & Bassey, 2023) (Esievo et al., 2023)
Spider Plant (*Chlorophytum comosum*) False Sesame *(Ceratotheca sesamoides)*	Enhances antioxidant enzymes such as SOD and catalase, reduces oxidative stress markers.	Blood, liver tissue	Reduced oxidative biomarkers, enhanced antioxidant enzymes Neutralisation of ROS, antioxidant protection	(Ibrahim & Fasakin, 2022) (Osuagwu & Idika, 2021)

continued on following page

Table 1. Continued

Notable Ethnobotanicals	Mechanism of Action	Target Tissues/ Organs	Observed Effects	References
Turmeric (*Curcuma longa*) Ginger (*zingiber officinale*)	It neutralizes ROS/RNS directly and also upregulate antioxidant enzymes such as glutathione peroxidase, superoxide dismutase, and catalase. It activates Nrf2 by releasing it from Keap1, enabling its nuclear translocation and Subsequent upregulation of genes that code for antioxidant proteins and phase II detoxification enzymes It contains (6)-gingerol, which protects cells from oxidative stress	Liver, joints, GIT	Improved digestion, protection of liver function, antioxidant and immune boosting	(Burapan et al., 2020; Lakitaningsih et al., 2019) Sindhoora & Bhattacharjee, 2020; Unuofin et al., 2021)
Lemon grass *(Cymbopogon citratus)*	Represses the expression of TNF-α and TGF-β and upregulates IL-10 and Nrf-2 levels	Liver and Kidneys	Modulates TNF-α, TGF-β, Nrf-2 and IL-10 in the liver and kidneys	Adeniyi et al 2024d Moronkeji et., 2024b
Antioxidant, Cardioprotective, Antimicrobial				
Bush buckthorn *(Ziziphus spp. or Rhamnus spp., depending on context)*	Rich in anthraquinones and flavonoids; induces apoptosis in abnormal cells; modulates gut microbiota.	Cardiovascular system, GI tract, skin	Enhanced cardiovascular protection, improved digestion, antimicrobial protection	(Oruka & Achuba, 2023), (Sinan et al., 2021)
Anticancer				
African Serpentwood *(Rauvolfia vomitoria).*	Generation of ROS, modification of the mitochondrial membrane potential, and caspase activation.	Colon, prostate, and brain.	Beneficial for neurological and gastrointestinal malignancies.	(Adico, 2024)

continued on following page

Table 1. Continued

Notable Ethnobotanicals	Mechanism of Action	Target Tissues/ Organs	Observed Effects	References
Alligator Pepper *(Aframomum melegueta).*	The anti-cancer properties of AM and its components include altering cell signalling pathways, which include suppressing tumour development, inducing apoptosis, and inhibiting NF-κB.	Colon, breast, and prostate.	Investigated in malignancies of the gastrointestinal tract and hormones.	(Almatroudi et al., 2019)
Diospyros mespiliformis, Bryophyllum pinnatum, Byrsocarpus coccineus	Induces p53-dependent apoptosis of colorectal cancer cells	Colon	It induces apoptosis in HCT-116 colon cancer cells	(Mukherjee et al., 2025)
Pawpaw (*Carica papaya*)	Papain and chymopapain degrade parasite proteins; induces apoptosis via caspase activation; boost wound collagen deposition.	Skin, GI tract, liver, reproductive organs	Accelerated wound healing, reduced tumour cell proliferation, anti-helminthic effects	(Ayodipupo Babalola et al., 2024), (Usmani et al., 2023), (Kong et al., 2021), (Masooma et al., 2024)
Abrus precatorius Azadirachta indica Khaya grandifoliola	Induction of apoptosis (via p53, Bax/Bcl-2, caspase cascade) Cell cycle arrest (G0/G1, G2/M) Anti-angiogenic & anti-proliferative effects, Inhibition of AR signalling pathway	Breast, colon, prostate,	Tumour size reduction, inhibited proliferation, DNA fragmentation in cancer cells	(Ismail et al., 2019)
		Antimicrobial		
Christmas Bush *(Alchornea cordifolia).*	Suppress the production of microbial cell walls and DNA replication, targeting bacteria and protozoa.	Urinary tract, GI tract, and skin.	Traditional use for malaria, dysentery, and urinary tract infections.	(Ajayi et al., 2020)
Ganoderma colossum Berlina grandiflora	Disruption of bacterial cell wall/membrane Inhibition of protein/ DNA synthesis, Interference with quorum sensing	Skin, GI tract, respiratory system	Reduced bacterial load; healing of infected wounds; inhibition of *H. pylori* and enteropathogens	(Zhu et al., 2011; Karunarathna et al., 2024)

continued on following page

Table 1. Continued

Notable Ethnobotanicals	Mechanism of Action	Target Tissues/ Organs	Observed Effects	References
Wild Custard *Apple (Annona senegalensis)*	Disrupts microbial cell wall integrity and inhibits bacteria and fungi growth.	Skin, microbial pathogens	Inhibition of *S. aureus and Candida strains* Decreased infection severity	(Nwafor & Igboeli, 2021)
Lemon grass (*Cymbopogon citratus*) African Bush Mango (Irvingia gabonensis	Inhibit glucosyltransferase activity and disrupt biofilm formation. Contains saponins, flavonoids, and alkaloids which contribute to antimicrobial activity	Respiratory tract, skin	Reduces fever and antimicrobial activity	(Ortega Ramirez et al., 2020; Olanrewaju et al., 2018)
Antidiabetic				
Cassia siamea	α-amylase and α-glucosidase inhibition,	Pancreatic enzymes	Controlled blood glucose level	(Tanty & Herlina, 2018)
African nutmeg (Monodora myristica) African Bush Mango (Irvingia gabonensis	By inhibition of α-amylase and α-glucosidase Fat absorption by amylase and lipase inhibition	GIT, liver	Pain relief, improved liver function. Weight reduction, improved lipid profile.	(Awojide et al., 2023).
Forest Anchomanes *(Anchomanes difformis)*	Enhances insulin secretion and increases glucose uptake; modulates glucose-metabolising enzymes such as α-amylase inhibition	Pancreas, blood glucose pathway	Lower blood glucose levels, improved insulin sensitivity.	(Onukak et al.,2020)
Antihyperlipidemic				
African Oil Bean Tree *(Pentaclethra macrophylla)*	Inhibits HMG-CoA reductase pathways, lowers triglycerides and LDL; suppresses inflammatory markers such as TNF-α and COX-2	Liver, plasma	Reduced LDL, lowered triglycerides	(Ezeani & Okafor, 2019)

continued on following page

Table 1. Continued

Notable Ethnobotanicals	Mechanism of Action	Target Tissues/ Organs	Observed Effects	References
Allium sativum, Picralima nitida	Increasing lecithin-cholesterol acyl transferase (LCAT) activity	Adipose tissues, liver	Improves lipid profiles by decreasing triglycerides, total cholesterol, and LDL-cholesterol	(Siddiqui et al., 2020)
Allium sativum	Reversibly inhibits platelet aggregation	Blood vessels	Reduced clot formation, improved vascular flow,	(Hiyasat et al., 2009)

1.5.2 Indigenous Knowledge Systems and Herbal Pharmacopoeias

Ethnobotanical knowledge, passed down through generations, plays a crucial role in traditional medicine and modern drug discovery. Indigenous communities globally rely on plant-based remedies for primary healthcare, with over 6,000 species used for medicinal purposes (Hossain et al., 2022). This knowledge encompasses plant identification, preparation methods, dosage, and therapeutic indications (Srinivas & Singh, 2023). Integrating traditional wisdom with advanced scientific techniques, such as multi-omics approaches and bioinformatics tools, enhances natural product discovery and drug development (Chele et al., 2025). Ethnopharmacology bridges the gap between traditional knowledge and modern medicine, offering a valuable source for drug discovery (Zargaran, 2024). Many contemporary pharmaceuticals, including aspirin and artemisinin, have ethnobotanical roots (Chele et al., 2025).

1.5.3 Safety, Availability, and Sustainability

Ethnobotanicals are increasingly popular as natural alternatives to synthetic drugs, but their safety requires scientific validation (Fouche, 2025). While often perceived as safer, issues of toxicity and herb-drug interactions remain concerns (Mensah et al., 2019). Sustainable harvesting practices are crucial for preserving medicinal plant biodiversity and ecological balance (Alum, 2025). The widespread availability and minimal processing of these plants make them cost-effective, particularly in developing countries where traditional medicine is prevalent (Fouche, 2025; Mensah et al., 2019). However, overexploitation threatens many medicinal plant species and their ecosystems. To address these challenges, a holistic approach integrating scientific research, policy formulation, and community engagement is necessary (Alum, 2025).

2.1 COMPARATIVE EVALUATION OF PLANT EXTRACTS IN MITIGATING OXIDATIVE STRESS

Plant-derived extracts are becoming more and more well-known for their antioxidant properties in reducing oxidative stress, which is linked to several pathological illnesses such as cancer, cardiovascular disease, and dementia. These bioactive substances provide a variety of benefits, including anti-ageing and anti-inflammatory qualities (Salehi et al., 2020). However, a number of important factors, including dosage and exposure time, affect how effective they are. When evaluating antioxidant capability, the extraction process and the detection methods employed are also very important (Pisoschi et al., 2016).

Plant-derived bioactives have shown potential in controlling neurodegenerative illnesses through diverse pathways such as decreasing oxidative stress, neuroinflammation, and protein aggregation (Shoaib et al., 2023). Although these substances may have therapeutic uses, it's crucial to remember that certain bioactive compounds may have pro-oxidant effects in specific situations. Thus, the use of antioxidants produced from plants for disease prevention and health promotion requires careful consideration (Salehi et al., 2020).

2.1.1 Dose-response relationships

The dual nature of phytochemicals as pro-oxidants and antioxidants depends on their concentration and the surrounding environment. They efficiently scavenge free radicals and strengthen antioxidant defences at low dosages. However, they may have pro-oxidant effects at high concentrations, which could result in cell damage and oxidative stress (Rajashekar, 2023). Plant extracts' antioxidant effects frequently follow a concentration-dependent pattern, as represented by sigmoidal dose-response curves (Furger et al., 2022). As concentration rises, some polyphenols show bidirectional activity, changing from pro-oxidant to antioxidant effects (or vice versa) (Nowak et al., 2022). The presence of redox metals, pH, and the production of benzoquinones are some of the factors affecting this dual behaviour. Although phytochemicals' pro-oxidant hazards are typically outweighed by their antioxidant benefits, it is important to carefully examine their concentration-dependent effects when developing oxidative stress management techniques (Castañeda-Arriaga et al., 2018). Antioxidants such as N-acetylcysteine, polyphenols, and vitamin C can activate redox pathways, resulting in cytoprotective responses at low dosages but potentially detrimental at high concentrations (Tyuryaeva & Lyublinskaya, 2023). This biphasic relationship has been shown in several phytochemicals, including phytoestrogens, resveratrol, and sulforaphane, especially in cell culture research concentrating on tumour and non-cancerous cell growth (Jodynis-Liebert & Kujawska, 2020).

2.1.2 Tissue-Specific and Exposure-Dependent Effects of Phytochemicals

The antioxidant effects of phytochemicals are tissue-specific and influenced by the duration of exposure. In the brain, polyphenols such as hesperidin exhibit neuroprotective effects by lowering oxidative stress, preserving neurotransmitter levels, and crossing the blood–brain barrier (Khan & Parvez, 2015; Miranda et al., 2018). Dietary phytochemicals modulate the Nrf2/ARE signalling pathway, which is a key regulator of antioxidant enzymes, thereby protecting against oxidative stress-mediated diseases, including diabetes, cancer, and neurodegenerative disorders (Thiruvengadam et al., 2021). In the liver, phytochemicals maintain membrane integrity and enhance detoxifying enzymes, while flavonoid-rich extracts reduce inflammation-induced oxidative stress in the lungs (Forni et al., 2019).

The therapeutic outcome also depends on the duration of exposure. Short-term administration of aspalathin-enriched green rooibos extract (28 days) altered glutathione redox balance and antioxidant gene expression in rats (Van der Merwe et al., 2015). Extracts from *Azadirachta indica, Khaya senegalensis, Anogeissus leiocarpus,* and *Tamarindus indica* produced reversible toxicity upon acute exposure but caused more severe hepatic and renal damage with prolonged use (Tauheed et al., 2021). Conversely, *Citrus aurantium* extract demonstrated hepatoprotective effects against CCl4-induced injury in both acute (3-day) and chronic (28-day) models by enhancing antioxidant enzymes and reducing lipid peroxidation (Kim et al., 2016). Similarly, 28-day treatment with Phoenix dactylifera fruit extract reduced aluminium chloride-induced neurotoxicity in rats, improving antioxidant levels and neurobehavioral outcomes in a dose-dependent manner (Olufunmilayo et al., 2025).

2.1.3 Synergistic and Combinatorial Roles of Phytochemicals in Therapy

Plant-derived antioxidants can act synergistically with conventional therapies to enhance efficacy while reducing toxicity. Combinations of phenolic or terpenoid compounds with chemotherapeutic agents such as cisplatin or doxorubicin not only mitigate adverse effects but also sensitise resistant cancer cells (Wagner & Efferth, 2017; Negrette-Guzmán, 2019). These effects are mediated through modulation of oxidative stress pathways, including inhibition of NF-κB and HIF-1α, which are linked to chemoresistance (Haddad et al., 2000). Additionally, redox-active substances that elevate ROS production and weaken antioxidant defences selectively induce cancer cell death without harming normal cells (Akladios et al., 2015). Beyond oncology, combinations of antioxidants like vitamins C and E, glutathione, and N-acetylcysteine (NAC) can enhance total antioxidant capacity, improve glutathione levels, and reduce oxidative stress markers, including ROS, nitrites, and lipid peroxidation (Muñoz-Sánchez et al., 2023).

2. 2 BIOAVAILABILITY AND METABOLIC STABILITY

Phytochemicals exhibit considerable therapeutic potential, but their efficiency is frequently hampered by poor bioavailability, fast metabolism, and low systemic concentrations (Hu et al., 2023; Rassu et al., 2023). Several strategies have been devised to overcome these challenges. These include encapsulation techniques, chemical alterations, and nanoformulations utilising micelles, liposomes, and nanoparticles as carriers (Singh et al., 2019). Curcumin, a natural compound with different pharmacological effects, suffers from poor bioavailability due to its low solubility and fast metabolism. In order to improve its therapeutic potential, a number of strategies have been established. Nanoformulations enhance the solubility and absorption of curcumin and include lipid-based carriers, nanoparticles, and microparticles (Mahran et al., 2017). Furthermore, prodrug use and co-administration with other medications have demonstrated promise, especially when paired with nanotechnologies (Rassu et al., 2023). Co-administration of piperine, which is present in black pepper, dramatically increases the bioavailability of curcumin by up to 20 times. Piperine accomplishes this via generating hydrogen-bonded complexes with curcumin and attaching to enzymes involved in curcumin metabolism, such as CYP3A4 and UDP-glucuronosyltransferase (Patil et al., 2016). By overcoming curcumin's drawbacks, these pharmacological approaches hope to improve its therapeutic potential for a range of uses, such as the prevention of cancer and the management of inflammatory diseases (Mahran et al., 2017).

Additionally, food matrix composition and processing methods are important factors in increasing the bioavailability of phytochemicals (Hu et al., 2023). It is anticipated that these developments in delivery systems would expand the use of phytochemicals in meals, supplements, and medications, perhaps enhancing their therapeutic effectiveness in a range of ailments, such as cancer and neurological illnesses (Rassu et al., 2023).

2.3 THERAPEUTIC POTENTIAL AND PHARMACOLOGICAL PROMISE

Medicinal plants hold considerable promise in addressing pollution-induced oxidative damage and its related health complications. Herbal extracts have been used for centuries in traditional medicine to treat various health conditions, valued for their cost-effectiveness, clinical success, and fewer side effects compared to synthetic drugs. Recently, the pharmaceutical industry has increasingly incorporated phytochemicals from medicinal plants into modern therapies (Bencharif-Betina et al., 2023). Medicinal plants are rich in bioactive secondary metabolites such as steroids, alkaloids, phenolics, glycosides, and flavonoids, which exhibit a wide range of beneficial biological activities, including antimicrobial, anti-inflammatory, anticancer, and antioxidant effects (Dar et al., 2023). They also play a role in managing diabetes mellitus by regulating hyperglycemia associated with pancreatic beta-cell dysfunction (Yeshi et al., 2022) and offer natural protection against oxidative stress (Zhao et al., 2025). Notably, high-altitude species produce elevated levels of flavonoids and phenolic compounds, enhancing their antioxidative potential (Ashraf et al., 2024). In addition to their therapeutic applications, medicinal and aromatic plants have shown promise in environmental management and pollution mitigation. However, exposure to heavy metal pollutants can disrupt their biosynthetic pathways, reducing their pharmacological efficacy (Asiminicesei et al., 2024).

2.4 TRANSLATIONAL RELEVANCE

Translational research in medicinal plants aims to bridge laboratory discoveries and clinical applications, supporting the development of affordable and effective therapies. Techniques such as micropropagation scale the cultivation of medicinal plants to meet therapeutic demand (Moraes et al., 2021). Tools such as transcriptomics aid in exploring functional genes and biosynthetic pathways (Guo et al., 2021), while studies on essential oils highlight the ethnopharmacological relevance of indigenous herbs (Pirintsos et al., 2020). Promising results from in vitro studies to clinical trials support the anti-diabetic potential of certain medicinal plants (Omale et al., 2023). However, translating these findings to clinical use requires careful consideration of bioavailability and mechanisms of action (Sadgrove & Jones, 2019). Many phytochemicals, including boswellic acids, curcumin, quercetin, and resveratrol, show in vivo efficacy despite plasma concentrations below their in vitro IC50 values, suggesting a need to reassess conventional pharmacokinetic models (Abdel-Tawab, 2021). Tissue-level analysis and combination therapies may provide better insights into herbal efficacy. In Nigeria, ongoing efforts aim to advance translational herbal medicine to improve healthcare access and medicinal security (Ilomuanya & Adegun, 2023). While plant-based diets benefit metabolic health, their effects on mental and cognitive function remain unclear, potentially influenced by diet, specific nutrients, or broader lifestyle factors.

2.5 PATENTABILITY AND DRUG DEVELOPMENT

Patents remain integral in advancing drug discovery and protecting pharmaceutical innovations, covering novel compounds, processes, and medicinal plant applications (Imran, 2025). Plant-derived natural products are increasingly recognised for their patent potential, with reports indicating that 75% of assessed remedies were eligible for protection (Périne et al., 2022). Rosemary-based products, for instance, have shown significant patent activity in China for pharmaceutical and cosmetic uses (Boukhari & Fatimi, 2023). Natural compounds such as *Annona muricata* and *Cannabis sativa* demonstrate anti-tumour effects through apoptosis and antioxidant mechanisms, while *Moringa oleifera* and *Curcuma longa* exhibit strong antidiabetic activity, offering safer alternatives to conventional therapies (Salehi et al., 2020). These therapeutic potentials are supported by modern approaches such as bioactivity-guided fractionation, high-throughput screening, and advanced structural analysis, which enhance druggability assessment and patent opportunities (Najmi et al., 2022; Chaachouay & Zidane, 2024). Despite this progress, challenges remain in formulation, quality control, safety, and regulatory compliance. Global regulatory agencies are increasingly working to integrate herbal medicines into formal approval frameworks, while emerging technologies applying ADMET (Absorption, Distribution, Metabolism, Excretion, and Toxicity) principles are reshaping natural product drug discovery (Hossain et al., 2022). These advances reinforce the importance of safeguarding plant-based innovations to address future global health needs.

3.1 CHALLENGES IN STANDARDISATION AND VALIDATION OF HERBAL AND TRADITIONAL MEDICINE

Standardising and validating herbal medicine remains difficult due to variability in plant materials, preparation methods, and the absence of universally accepted quality control protocols.Factors such as geography, harvesting time, and processing influence drug consistency, while the complex, multi-constituent composition of herbal remedies complicates pharmacopoeial assessments (Busia, 2024; Hussain et al., 2024; Indrayanto, 2024). Limited scientific data on efficacy and safety further hinders integration into mainstream healthcare (Yadav et al., 2023). The growing demand for herbal therapies, particularly for lifestyle diseases, highlights the need for advanced analytical methods aligned with international guidelines (Paul & Kumar, 2023).

3.2 REGULATORY AND SAFETY CONCERNS

In Nigeria, the regulation of herbal medicine is challenged by cultural reliance on traditional healers, limited enforcement, and safety issues. Despite the WHO's call for integration of traditional medicine into healthcare systems, many products remain unregulated and sold by unlicensed practitioners, raising risks of adulteration and poor compliance (Eruaga et al., 2024; Modibbo et al., 2024; Awodele et al., 2014). While NAFDAC provides oversight, gaps in regulation persist, necessitating stronger frameworks to ensure quality and safety (Eruaga, 2024).

3.3 NEED FOR INTEGRATIVE RESEARCH AND CLINICAL TRIALS

Although 70–80% of Africans depend on herbal medicine, its integration into healthcare is limited by inadequate standardisation, lack of validation, and stigma (Salau et al., 2024; Ayuba et al., 2024). In Nigeria, new university curricula now include Complementary and Alternative Medicine, yet insufficient clinical, pharmacological, and toxicological studies remain a barrier. Collaborative research, standardised dosages, and international endorsement are essential for evidence-based use (Ilomuanya, 2023; Salau et al., 2024). Effective integration also requires cooperation among healers, healthcare providers, and policymakers to build inclusive systems that improve health outcomes (Ayuba et al., 2024).

3.4 ROLES OF LOCAL COMMUNITIES AND KNOWLEDGE PRESERVATION

Local communities are central to preserving indigenous knowledge and sustaining biodiversity, as traditional medicine often relies on cultural practices that encourage sustainable plant use (Xie, 2022; Ajewole, 2024). In Nigeria, this knowledge forms the basis of rural healthcare. However, integrating these practices into modern healthcare must balance respect for indigenous heritage with regulatory safeguards to ensure safety (Akunna et al., 2023; Eruaga et al., 2024).

4.0 CONCLUSION

Herbal medicine is widely used in Nigeria and other developing regions largely due to cultural acceptability and affordability. However, it faces challenges of standardisation, regulation, and stigma, further limiting its integration into formal healthcare. While global organisations like the WHO support evidence-based use through research and regulatory initiatives, strengthening scientific validation, plant conservation, and collaboration between traditional and modern healthcare is essential for safe integration and sustainable innovation.

REFERENCES

Abdel-Tawab, M. (2021). Considerations to Be Taken When Carrying Out Medicinal Plant Research—What We Learn from an Insight into the IC50 Values, Bioavailability and Clinical Efficacy of Exemplary Anti-Inflammatory Herbal Components. *Pharmaceuticals (Basel, Switzerland)*, *14*(5), 437. DOI: 10.3390/ph14050437 PMID: 34066427

Abdulfatah, H. F. (2022). Non-enzymatic antioxidants in stressed plants: A review. *Journal of university of Anbar for Pure science*, 16, 25-37. https://www.academia.edu/download/103370295/article_176435_425a95431c7afdc7f9ac1e18d8493a9b.pdf

Adeniyi, T., Moronkeji, A., Oluwatunase, G., Adekomi, A., & Adunmo, G. (2024a). Mercury-induced oxidative stress and neuropathologic changes in the prefrontal cortex of Wistar rats. *Nigerian Journal of Neuroscience*, *15*(4), 97–104. DOI: 10.47081/njn2024.15.4/001

Adeniyi, T. D., Achukwu, P. U., & Abubakar, A. A. (2017). Frequency of electronics waste generated heavy metals in urban waterways. *International Journal of Human Capital in Urban Management*, *2*(2), 89–100.

Adeniyi, T. D., Achukwu, P. U., Abubakar, A. A., & Adedayo, D. A. (2019). Heavy metals obtained from waterways induced neurodegeneration in the prefrontal cortex of Wistar rats. *European Journal of Anatomy : Official Journal of the Spanish Society of Anatomy*, *23*(1), 65–76.

Adeniyi, T. D., Moronkeji, A., Ajala, I. O., Oyeleke, A., Moronkeji, A. I., Falana, F., & Ngeri, B. (2024d). Mitigation of Diclofenac-Induced Hepatorenal Toxicity by Methanolic Extract of Cymbopogon citratus. *Nigerian Journal of Physiological Sciences; Official Publication of the Physiological Society of Nigeria*, *39*, 241–249. PMID: 40156783

Adeniyi, T. D., Moronkeji, A., & Ekundina, V. O. (2023). Histological evaluation of the liver, kidney, and tests of adult male Wistar rats exposed to heavy metals-contaminated waterways. *Medical Laboratory Journal*, *17*(5), 4–8. DOI: 10.61186/mlj.17.5.4

Adeniyi, T. D., Moronkeji, A., & Eyovwerhuvwu, D. E. (2024b). Effects of Pyrethroid Exposure on Testicular Histopathology and Biochemistry in Adult Male Wistar Rats: Evaluation of Ascorbic Acid and Alpha-Tocopherol Administration. *Journal of Advanced Pharmacy Research*, *8*(1), 29–37. DOI: 10.21608/aprh.2023.234710.1235

Adetuyi, A. R., Salawu, S. O., Akinmoladun, A. C., & Akindahunsi, A. A. (2025). Protective effect of Spondias mombin leaf extracts against aluminum chloride-induced brain oxidative stress, inflammation and apoptosis in rats. *Future Journal of Pharmaceutical Sciences* 2025 11:1, 11(1), 1–15. DOI: 10.1186/s43094-025-00803-9

Adico, M. D. (2024). In vitro activities and mechanisms of action of anti-cancer molecules from African medicinal plants: A systematic review. *American Journal of Cancer Research*, *14*(3), 1376–1401. DOI: 10.62347/AUHB5811 PMID: 38590420

Adigun, O. J., & Odeleye, D. A. (2025). The Devastating Consequences of Environmental Pollution on Human Health. *British Journal of Multidisciplinary and Advanced Studies*, *6*(1), 37–46. DOI: 10.37745/bjmas.2022.04230

Ajayi, O. F., Olasunkanmi, O. O., Agunbiade, M. O., Alayande, K. A., Aiyegoro, O. A., & Akinpelu, D. A. (2020). Study on antimicrobial and antioxidant potentials of Alchornea cordifolia (Linn.): An in vitro assessment. *Transactions of the Royal Society of South Africa*, *75*(3), 266–281. DOI: 10.1080/0035919X.2020.1830868

Ajewole, S. (2024). The Role of Medicinal Plants in Nigerian Traditional Medicine. *ScienceOpen Preprints*. DOI: 10.14293/PR2199.001210.v1

Akbar, S., Cogburn, H., Meyer, A., & Sheridan, D. 2, S. N., Juliani, H. R., Kotwal, S., Simon, J. E., Rafferty, B., Priano, C., Fernández Romero, J., & Koroch, A. (2025). Antioxidant, Antibacterial, and Antiviral Activity of Commercial Products of Piper guineense and Piper borbonense. *Journal of Medicinally Active Plants*, 14(1). DOI: 10.7275/JMAP.2940

Akladios, F. N., Andrew, S. D., & Parkinson, C. J. (2015). Selective induction of oxidative stress in cancer cells via synergistic combinations of agents targeting redox homeostasis. *Bioorganic & Medicinal Chemistry*, *23*(13), 3097–3104. DOI: 10.1016/j.bmc.2015.05.006 PMID: 26022081

Akunna, G. G., Lucyann, C., & Saalu, L. C. (2023). Rooted in Tradition, Thriving in the Present: The Future and Sustainability of Herbal Medicine in Nigeria's Healthcare Landscape. *Journal of Innovations in Medical Research*. DOI: 10.56397/JIMR/2023.11.05

Alagbe, O. A., Alagbe, G. O., Adekunle, E. A., Ayodele, O. O., Olorode, E. M., Oyediran, R. I., Oloyede, E. O., Oluwaloni, F. O., & Oyeleye, A. O. (2021). Ethnomedicinal Uses and Therapeutic Activities of Piper Guineense: A Review. *Journal of Applied Science & Environmental Management*, *25*(6), 927–937. DOI: 10.4314/jasem.v25i6.6

Alengebawy, A., Abdelkhalek, S. T., Qureshi, S. R., & Wang, M.-Q. (2021). Heavy Metals and Pesticides Toxicity in Agricultural Soil and Plants: Ecological Risks and Human Health Implications. *Toxics*, *9*(3), 42. DOI: 10.3390/toxics9030042 PMID: 33668829

Ali, M. U., Lin, S., Yousaf, B., Abbas, Q., Munir, M. A. M., Rashid, A., Zheng, C., Kuang, X., & Wong, M. H. (2022). Pollution characteristics, mechanism of toxicity and health effects of the ultrafine particles in the indoor environment: Current status and future perspectives. *Critical Reviews in Environmental Science and Technology*, *52*(3), 436–473. https://drive.google.com/file/d/12bQHQmViB4EjE3p-1ieaS_wEWQcLuZvb/view. DOI: 10.1080/10643389.2020.1831359

Almatroudi, A., Alsahli, M. A., Alrumaihi, F., Allemailem, K. S., & Rahmani, A. H. (2019). Ginger: A Novel Strategy to Battle Cancer through Modulating Cell Signalling Pathways: A Review. *Current Pharmaceutical Biotechnology*, *20*(1), 5–16. DOI: 10.2174/1389201020666190119142331 PMID: 30659535

Alum, E. U. (2025). Sustainable harvesting of medicinal plants: Balancing therapeutic benefits with environmental conservation. *Agroecology and Sustainable Food Systems*, *49*(3), 380–385. DOI: 10.1080/21683565.2024.2421948

Ammar, R. B., Al Saeedi, F. J., Ahmed, E. A., & Rajendran, P. (2021). Benzo (a) Pyrene Induced ROS-Mediated Lung Cancer. In *Handbook of Oxidative Stress in Cancer: Mechanistic Aspects* (pp. 1–14). Springer Singapore. DOI: 10.1007/978-981-15-4501-6_37-1

Anetor, G. O., Nwobi, N. L., Igharo, G. O., Sonuga, O. O., & Anetor, J. I. (2022). Environmental pollutants and oxidative stress in terrestrial and aquatic organisms: Examination of the total picture and implications for human health. *Frontiers in Physiology*, *13*, 931386. DOI: 10.3389/fphys.2022.931386 PMID: 35936919

Angon, P. B., Islam, M. S., Kc, S., Das, A., Anjum, N., Poudel, A., & Suchi, S. A. (2025, July 16). 2024. 'Sources, Effects and Present Perspectives of Heavy Metals Contamination: Soil, Plants and Human Food Chain'. *Heliyon*, *10*(7), e28357. https://www.sciencedirect.com/science/article/pii/S2405844024043883. DOI: 10.1016/j.heliyon.2024.e28357 PMID: 38590838

Arya, P., Kumari, N., Ahmad Wani, S., & Kumar, P. (2023). Trigonella foenum graecum. *Herbs, Spices and Their Roles in Nutraceuticals and Functional Foods*, 133–148. DOI: 10.1016/B978-0-323-90794-1.00001-6

Ashraf, M. V., Khan, S., Misri, S., Gaira, K. S., Rawat, S., Rawat, B., Khan, M. A. H., Shah, A. A., Asgher, M., & Ahmad, S. (2024). High-Altitude Medicinal Plants as Promising Source of Phytochemical Antioxidants to Combat Lifestyle-Associated Oxidative Stress-Induced Disorders. *Pharmaceuticals (Basel, Switzerland)*, *17*(8), 975. DOI: 10.3390/ph17080975 PMID: 39204080

Asiminicesei, D.-M., Fertu, D. I., & Gavrilescu, M. (2024). Impact of Heavy Metal Pollution in the Environment on the Metabolic Profile of Medicinal Plants and Their Therapeutic Potential. *Plants*, *13*(6), 913. DOI: 10.3390/plants13060913 PMID: 38592933

Aude Périne, M. N. A., Kevin, E., Saurelle, M., Vanessa Charlotte, S. L., Martin, N. N., Jeanne Mauricette, M. M., Chimène, B., & Nga, N. (2022). Evaluation of the Patentability of Medicines based on plants produced in Cameroon: Case of Yaounde. *International Journal of Drug Regulatory Affairs*, *10*(3), 19–24. DOI: 10.22270/ijdra.v10i3.547

Awodele, O., Amagon, K. I., Wannang, N. N., & Aguiyi, J. C. (2014). Traditional medicine policy and regulation in Nigeria: An index of herbal medicine safety. *Current Drug Safety*, *9*(1), 16–22. DOI: 10.2174/15748863086661311261554 34 PMID: 24274707

Awojide, S. H., Akinlade, B., Oyewole, K. A., Adeyemo, A. G., Adeniyi, E. O., Fadunmade, O. E., & Anifowose, A. J. (2023). Synergistic and antagonistic medicinal activities of essential oil of Monodora myristica. *CTU Journal of Innovation and Sustainable Development*, *15*(3), 1–11. DOI: 10.22144/ctujoisd.2023.046

Ayertey, F., Ofori-Attah, E., Antwi, S., Amoa-Bosompem, M., Djameh, G., Lartey, N. L., Ohashi, M., Kusi, K. A., Appiah, A. A., Appiah-Opong, R., & Okine, L. K. (2020). Anti-inflammatory activity and mechanism of action of ethanolic leaf extract of Morinda lucida Benth. *Journal of Traditional and Complementary Medicine*, *11*(3), 249–258. DOI: 10.1016/j.jtcme.2020.07.001 PMID: 34012871

Ayodipupo Babalola, B., Ifeolu Akinwande, A., Otunba, A. A., Ebenezer Adebami, G., Babalola, O., & Nwuofo, C. (2024). Therapeutic benefits of Carica papaya: A review on its pharmacological activities and characterization of papain. In Arabian Journal of Chemistry (Vol. 17, Issue 1). Elsevier B.V. DOI: 10.1016/j.arabjc.2023.105369

Ayuba, D., Fadele, P., Ogaya, J. B., Olayinka, K. E., Sharma, S. N., & Lucero-Prisno, D. E. I.III. (2024). Understanding the root of healing and beyond: Exploring the way forward for Alternative Medicine in Nigeria. *Bhutan Sorig Journal*, *1*(1), 42–47. DOI: 10.47811/bsj.0004050304

Balali-Mood, M., Naseri, K., Tahergorabi, Z., Khazdair, M. R., & Sadeghi, M. (2021). Toxic mechanisms of five heavy metals: Mercury, lead, chromium, cadmium, and arsenic. *Frontiers in Pharmacology*, *12*, 643972. DOI: 10.3389/fphar.2021.643972 PMID: 33927623

Bandodkar, V. V., Moger, V. S., & Baliga, P. (2025). Antioxidant Defense Mechanisms: Enzymatic and non-enzymatic. In The Role of Reactive Oxygen Species in Human Health and Disease (pp. 43-80). IGI Global Scientific Publishing.

Beltrán-Noboa, A., Proaño-Ojeda, J., Guevara, M., Gallo, B., Berrueta, L. A., Giampieri, F., Perez-Castillo, Y., Battino, M., Álvarez-Suarez, J. M., & Tejera, E. (2022). Metabolomic profile and computational analysis for the identification of the potential anti-inflammatory mechanisms of action of the traditional medicinal plants Ocimum basilicum and Ocimum tenuiflorum. *Food and Chemical Toxicology*, *164*, 113039. DOI: 10.1016/j.fct.2022.113039 PMID: 35461962

Bencharif-Betina, S., Benhamed, N., Benabdallah, A., Bendif, H., Benslama, A., Negro, C., Plavan, G., Abd-Elkader, O. H., & De Bellis, L. (2023). A Multi-Approach Study of Phytochemicals and Their Effects on Oxidative Stress and Enzymatic Activity of Essential Oil and Crude Extracts of Rosmarinus officinalis. *Separations*, *10*(7), 394. DOI: 10.3390/separations10070394

Bharathy, P., Thanikachalam, P. V., Shoban, A. N., & Himayavendhan, H. V. (2024). Floral Fusion: Unravelling the Potent Blend of Ixora coccinea and Rhododendron arboreum for Health and Safety Benefits. *Cureus*. Advance online publication. DOI: 10.7759/cureus.70038 PMID: 39449919

Brinchmann, B. C., Skuland, T., Rambøl, M. H., Szoke, K., Brinchmann, J. E., Gutleb, A. C., Moschini, E., Kubátová, A., Kukowski, K., Le Ferrec, E., Lagadic-Gossmann, D., Schwarze, P. E., Låg, M., Refsnes, M., Øvrevik, J., & Holme, J. A. (2018). 'Lipophilic Components of Diesel Exhaust Particles Induce Pro-Inflammatory Responses in Human Endothelial Cells through AhR Dependent Pathway(S)'. *Particle and Fibre Toxicology*, *15*(1), 1–17. DOI: 10.1186/s12989-018-0257-1 PMID: 29298690

Burapan, S., Kim, M., Paisooksantivatana, Y., Eser, B. E., & Han, J. (2020). Thai curcuma species: Antioxidant and bioactive compounds. *Foods*, *9*(9), 1219. DOI: 10.3390/foods9091219 PMID: 32887356

Busia, K. (2024). Herbal Medicine Dosage Standardisation. *Journal of Herbal Medicine*, *46*, 100889. DOI: 10.1016/j.hermed.2024.100889

Castañeda-Arriaga, R., Pérez-González, A., Reina, M., Alvarez-Idaboy, J. R., & Galano, A. (2018). Comprehensive Investigation of the Antioxidant and Pro-oxidant Effects of Phenolic Compounds: A Double-Edged Sword in the Context of Oxidative Stress? *The Journal of Physical Chemistry B*, *122*(23), 6198–6214. DOI: 10.1021/acs.jpcb.8b03500 PMID: 29771524

Chaachouay, N., & Zidane, L. (2024). Plant-Derived Natural Products: A Source for Drug Discovery and Development. *Drugs and Drug Candidates*, *3*(1), 184–207. DOI: 10.3390/ddc3010011

Chandran, R., & Abrahamse, H. (2020). Identifying Plant-Based Natural Medicine against Oxidative Stress and Neurodegenerative Disorders. *Oxidative Medicine and Cellular Longevity*, *2020*, 1–9. DOI: 10.1155/2020/8648742 PMID: 33014278

Chele, K. H., Piater, L. A., van der Hooft, J. J. J., & Tugizimana, F. (2025). Bridging Ethnobotanical Knowledge and Multi-Omics Approaches for Plant-Derived Natural Product Discovery. *Metabolites*, *15*(6), 362. DOI: 10.3390/metabo15060362 PMID: 40559386

Chen, R., Zhang, Y., & Liu, Y. (2021). Airborne particulate matter induces mitochondrial damage and oxidative stress in lung epithelial cells. *Toxicology Letters*, *347*, 26–35. DOI: 10.1016/j.toxlet.2021.04.005

Chi , A., Noubissi, P. A., Pop, O. L., Mure an, C. I., Fokam Tagne, M. A., Kamgang, R., Fodor, A., Sitar-Tăut, A. V., Cozma, A., Oră an, O. H., Heghe , S. C., Vulturar, R., & Suharoschi, R. (2023). Bioactive Compounds in Moringa oleifera: Mechanisms of Action, Focus on Their Anti-Inflammatory Properties. *Plants*, *13*(1), 20. DOI: 10.3390/plants13010020 PMID: 38202328

Coolborn, A., Bolatito, B., Omolara, A., & Adetuyi, F. (2015). Phytochemical and Antioxidant Effect of Spathodea campanulata leaf Extracts. *International Journal of Biochemistry Research & Review*, *7*(3), 148–159. DOI: 10.9734/IJBCRR/2015/16371

Danyal, Y., Mahmood, K., Ullah, S., Rahim, A., Raheem, G., Khan, A. H., & Ullah, A. (2023). Phytoremediation of industrial effluents assisted by plant growth promoting bacteria. *Environmental Science and Pollution Research International*, *30*(3), 5296–5311. DOI: 10.1007/s11356-022-23967-w PMID: 36402881

Dar, R. A., Shahnawaz, M., Ahanger, M. A., & Majid, I. U. (2023). Exploring the Diverse Bioactive Compounds from Medicinal Plants: A Review. *The Journal of Phytopharmacology*, *12*(3), 189–195. DOI: 10.31254/phyto.2023.12307

Deniz, S., Kamsu, G. T., & Ndebia, E. J. (2024). A Comprehensive Review of the Ethnobotanical Uses, Pharmacological, and Toxicological Profiles of Piper capense L.f. (Piperaceae). *Drugs and Drug Candidates, 3*(3), 598–614. DOI: 10.3390/ddc3030034

Ehsanifar, M., Banihashemian, S., & Ehsanifar, M. (2021). Exposure to air pollution nanoparticles: Oxidative stress and neuroinfl ammation. *Journal of Biomedical Research & Environmental Sciences, 2*(10), 964–976. DOI: 10.37871/jbres1339

Ekaluo, U. B., Ikpeme, E. V., Ekerette, E. E., & Chukwu, C. I. (2015). In vitro Antioxidant and Free Radical Activity of Some Nigerian Medicinal Plants: Bitter Leaf (Vernonia amygdalina L.) and Guava (Psidium guajava Del.). *Research Journal of Medicinal Plant, 9*(5), 215–226. DOI: 10.3923/rjmp.2015.215.226

El Boukhari, R., & Fatimi, A. (2023). A Review of the Patentability of Rosemary-Derived Drugs and Bioactive Compounds. *Drugs and Drug Candidates, 2*(1), 172–188. DOI: 10.3390/ddc2010011

Emmanuel K., M. (2025). Diabetes and Herbal Medicine: Understanding Plant-Based Dietary Interventions. *Research invention journal of biological and applied sciences*, 5(1), 5–9. DOI: 10.59298/RIJBAS/2025/5159

Eruaga, M. A., Itua, E. O., & Bature, J. T. (2024). Exploring herbal medicine regulation in Nigeria: Balancing traditional practices with modern standards. *GSC Advanced Research and Reviews,* 18(3), 083-090 DOI: 10.30574/gscarr.2024.18.3.0094

Esievo, K. B., Gegele, I. B., Aliyu, A., Fidelis, S. A., Fatokun, O. T., & Ibrahim, J. A. (2023). Evaluation of Phenolic Content, Anti-oxidant and modulation of blood indices of Pavetta crassipes. *Plant Science Today, 172-174*. Advance online publication. DOI: 10.14719/pst.2453

Ezeani, A., & Okafor, P. (2019). Lipid-lowering potentials of Pentaclethra macrophylla seed fermentation. *African Journal of Food Science, 13*(7), 166–172.

Forni, C., Facchiano, F., Bartoli, M., Pieretti, S., Facchiano, A., D'Arcangelo, D., Norelli, S., Valle, G., Nisini, R., Beninati, S., Tabolacci, C., & Jadeja, R. N. (2019). Beneficial Role of Phytochemicals on Oxidative Stress and Age-Related Diseases. *BioMed Research International, 2019*, 1–16. DOI: 10.1155/2019/8748253 PMID: 31080832

Fouche, G. (2025). *Exploring medicinal plants as natural remedies through scientific investigation*. ScienceBank., DOI: 10.61340/EMPNR

Furger, C., Gironde, C., Rigal, M., Dufour, C., & Guillemet, D. (2022). Cell-Based Antioxidant Properties and Synergistic Effects of Natural Plant and Algal Extracts Pre and Post Intestinal Barrier Transport. *Antioxidants*, *11*(3), 565. DOI: 10.3390/antiox11030565 PMID: 35326215

Gambhir, L., Tyagi, G., Bhardwaj, R., Kapoor, N., & Sharma, G. (2022). Status: Role of Nrf2, a Master Regulator of Cellular Redox. *Reactive oxygen species*, 181. https://www.intechopen.com/chapters/80024

Gholijani, N., Gharagozloo, M., Farjadian, S., & Amirghofran, Z. (2016). Modulatory effects of thymol and carvacrol on inflammatory transcription factors in lipopolysaccharide-treated macrophages. *Journal of Immunotoxicology*, *13*(2), 157–164. DOI: 10.3109/1547691X.2015.1029145 PMID: 25812626

Guo, J., Huang, Z., Sun, J., Cui, X., & Liu, Y. (2021). Research Progress and Future Development Trends in Medicinal Plant Transcriptomics. *Frontiers in Plant Science*, *12*, 691838. Advance online publication. DOI: 10.3389/fpls.2021.691838 PMID: 34394145

Haddad, J. J., Olver, R. E., & Land, S. C. (2000). Antioxidant/pro-oxidant equilibrium regulates HIF-1α and NF-κB redox sensitivity: Evidence for inhibition by glutathione oxidation in alveolar epithelial cells. *The Journal of Biological Chemistry*, *275*(28), 21130–21139. DOI: 10.1074/jbc.M000737200 PMID: 10801793

Hamzah, U. (2024). Nature's healing touch: investigating the anti-inflammatory and analgesic potential of methanol extracts from chrysophyllum albidum stem bark in formalin-induced paw edema in albino rats. American *Journal of Biomedical Science & Pharmaceutical Innovation*, 4(01), 08–14. DOI: 10.37547/AJBSPI/VOLUME04ISSUE01-02

Hiyasat, B., Sabha, D., Grötzinger, K., Kempfert, J., Rauwald, J. W., Mohr, F. W., & Dhein, S. (2009). Antiplatelet activity of Allium ursinum and Allium sativum. *Pharmacology*, *83*(4), 197–204. DOI: 10.1159/000196811 PMID: 19174616

Hlophe, S., & Bassey, K. (2023). Phytochemical Profiling, and Antioxidant Potentials of South African and Nigerian Loranthus micranthus Linn.: The African Mistletoe Exposé. *Plants*, *12*(10), 2016. DOI: 10.3390/plants12102016 PMID: 37653933

Hossain, C. M., Gera, M., & Ali, K. A. (2022). Current Status and Challenges of Herbal Drug Development and Regulatory Aspect: A Global Perspective. *Asian Journal of Pharmaceutical and Clinical Research*, •••, 31–41. DOI: 10.22159/ajpcr.2022.v15i12.46134

Hu, Y., Lin, Q., Zhao, H., Li, X., Sang, S., McClements, D. J., Long, J., Jin, Z., Wang, J., & Qiu, C. (2023). Bioaccessibility and bioavailability of phytochemicals: Influencing factors, improvements, and evaluations. *Food Hydrocolloids*, *135*, 108165. DOI: 10.1016/j.foodhyd.2022.108165

Hua, Y., Yuan, Y., Qin, Y., Zhang, C., Wang, X., Feng, S., & Lu, Y. (2022). Advances in the agro-environment migration of organic chemical pollutants and their biotransformation in crops. *Agronomy (Basel)*, *12*(12), 3009. https://www.mdpi.com/2073-4395/12/12/3009. DOI: 10.3390/agronomy12123009

Hussain, S., Garcia, M. C., Jamal, A., Hernández, F. D. C., Fasil, M., Shahabas, M. A. K., Baboo, C. R. V., & Sirajudheen, M. K. (2024). A Review on Standardization of Traditional Herbal Formulations. *International Journal of Pharmaceutical Research and Applications*, *09*(05), 116–123. DOI: 10.35629/4494-0905116123

Ibrahim, M. T., & Fasakin, A. F. (2022). Antioxidant properties of Chlorophytum comosum leaf extracts. *Journal of Phytomedicine*, *18*(2), 77–85.

Ilomuanya, M., & Adegun, A. (2023). Translational Herbal Medicines Availability: A Necessity to Ensure Medicine Security in Nigeria. *The Nigerian Journal of Pharmacy : the Official Organ of the Pharmaceutical Society of Nigeria*, *57*(1), 512–524. DOI: 10.51412/psnnjp.2023.12

Ilomuanya, M. O., & Adegun, A. (2023). Translational Herbal Medicines Availability: A Necessity to Ensure Medicine Security in Nigeria. *The Nigerian Journal of Pharmacy : the Official Organ of the Pharmaceutical Society of Nigeria*, *57*(1), 512–524. DOI: 10.51412/psnnjp.2023.12

Imaga, N. A., Iheagwam, F. N., Urua, E., & Ebigwai, E. A. (2023). Nutritional, Phytochemical, and Biological Activities of Chrysophyllum albidum Fruit Extracts from Lagos. *TheScientificWorldJournal*, *2023*(1), 8701848. DOI: 10.1155/2023/8701848

Imran, M. (2025). Patent: An Important Tool for Promoting Drug Discovery and Improving Public Health. *Asian Journal of Pharmaceutics*, *19*(01). Advance online publication. DOI: 10.22377/ajp.v19i01.6059

Indrayanto, G. (2024). *Regulation and standardization of herbal drugs: Current status, limitation, challenges and future prospects*. Elsevier BV., DOI: 10.1016/bs.podrm.2023.11.003

Intharuksa, A., Arunotayanun, W., Takuathung, M. N., Boongla, Y., Chaichit, S., Khamnuan, S., & Prasansuklab, A. (2024). Therapeutic Potential of Herbal Medicines in Combating Particulate Matter (PM)-Induced Health Effects: Insights from Recent Studies. *Antioxidants*, *14*(1), 23. DOI: 10.3390/antiox14010023 PMID: 39857357

Ismail, N., Wan-Ibrahim, W., Mohd-Salleh, S., Yajid, A., Wong, M., & Hashim, M. M. (2019). Methanolic extract of Abrus precatorius promotes breast cancer MDA-MB-231 cell death by inducing cell cycle arrest at G0/G1 and upregulating Bax. *Asian Pacific Journal of Tropical Biomedicine*, *9*(6), 249. DOI: 10.4103/2221-1691.260397

Itziou, A., Balis, V., Lakioti, E., Karayannis, V., & Tsanaktsidis, C. (2024). Environmental Pollution and Oxidative Stress: Health Effects During Pregnancy: A Review. *Applied Sciences (Basel, Switzerland)*, *14*(21), 9884. DOI: 10.3390/app14219884

Janet Olufunmilayo, O., Olugbenga Ayodeji, A., & James Oluwabusayo, A. (2025). Neurobehavioural Changes and Oxidative Damage due to Aluminium Chloride-Induced Neurotoxicity in Adult Female Wistar Rats: Phoenix Dactylifera L. Fruit to the Rescue. *Brain Science Advances*, *11*(2), BSA.2024.9050012. Advance online publication. DOI: 10.26599/BSA.2024.9050012

Jodynis-Liebert, J., & Kujawska, M. (2020). Biphasic Dose-Response Induced by Phytochemicals: Experimental Evidence. *Journal of Clinical Medicine*, *9*(3), 718. DOI: 10.3390/jcm9030718 PMID: 32155852

Jomova, K., Alomar, S. Y., Nepovimova, E., Kuca, K., & Valko, M. (2025). Heavy metals: Toxicity and human health effects. *Archives of Toxicology*, *99*(1), 153–209. DOI: 10.1007/s00204-024-03903-2 PMID: 39567405

Kadir, A. (2019). Near-roadway air pollution: evaluation of fine particulate matter ($PM_{2.5}$) and ultrafine particulate matter ($PM_{0.1}$) in Interior Alaska (Doctoral dissertation). https://scholarworks.alaska.edu/bitstream/handle/11122/10507/Kadir_A_2019.pdf?sequence=1

Karunarathna, S. C., Ediriweera, A., Prasannath, K., Mingfei, Y., & Hapuarachchi, K. K. (2024). Exploring the health benefits of Ganoderma: Bioactive compounds and mechanisms of action; immunomodulatory, and anti-tumour activities. *New Zealand Journal of Botany*. Advance online publication. DOI: 10.1080/0028825X.2024.2375996

Khan, M. H. A., & Parvez, S. (2015). Hesperidin ameliorates heavy metal induced toxicity mediated by oxidative stress in brain of Wistar rats. *Journal of Trace Elements in Medicine and Biology*, *31*, 53–60. DOI: 10.1016/j.jtemb.2015.03.002 PMID: 26004892

Kim, T.-W., Lee, D.-R., Choi, B.-K., Kang, H.-K., Jung, J.-Y., Lim, S.-W., Yang, S. H., & Suh, J.-W. (2016). Hepatoprotective effects of polymethoxyflavones against acute and chronic carbon tetrachloride intoxication. *Food and Chemical Toxicology*, *91*, 91–99. DOI: 10.1016/j.fct.2016.03.004 PMID: 26980244

Kıran, T. R., Otlu, O., & Karabulut, A. B. (2023). Oxidative stress and antioxidants in health and disease. *Journal of Laboratory Medicine*, *47*(1), 1–11. DOI: 10.1515/labmed-2022-0108

Kong, Y. R., Jong, Y. X., Balakrishnan, M., Bok, Z. K., Weng, J. K. K., Tay, K. C., Goh, B. H., Ong, Y. S., Chan, K. G., Lee, L. H., & Khaw, K. Y. (2021). Beneficial Role of Carica papaya Extracts and Phytochemicals on Oxidative Stress and Related Diseases: A Mini Review. *Biology (Basel)*, *10*(4), 287. DOI: 10.3390/biology10040287 PMID: 33916114

Koushal, S., Arya, D., Anbarasan, S., Haloi, D. M. R., Rahman, T., Singh, V., & Deekshithulu, N. V. G. (2025). Soil Pollution: Sources, Effects, and Mitigation Strategies. *Asian Journal of Soil Science and Plant Nutrition*, *11*(1), 280–290. DOI: 10.9734/ajsspn/2025/v11i1480

Lei, Y., Lei, T. H., Lu, C., Zhang, X., & Wang, F. (2024). Wildfire smoke: Health effects, mechanisms, and mitigation. *Environmental Science & Technology*, *58*(48), 21097–21119. DOI: 10.1021/acs.est.4c06653 PMID: 39516728

Liu, J., Wang, Q., & Li, Y. (2022). Mitochondrial oxidative stress and pollutant-induced toxicity: Mechanistic insights. *Redox Biology*, *54*, 102389. DOI: 10.1016/j.redox.2022.102389 PMID: 35792437

Lukitaningsih, E., Rohman, A., & Rafi, M., AF, N., & Windarsih, A. (. (2019). In vivo antioxidant activities of Curcuma longa and Curcuma xanthorrhiza: A review. *Food Research*, *4*(1), 13–19. DOI: 10.26656/fr.2017.4(1).172

Mahran, R. I., Hagras, M. M., Sun, D., & Brenner, D. E. (2017). Bringing Curcumin to the Clinic in Cancer Prevention: A Review of Strategies to Enhance Bioavailability and Efficacy. *The AAPS Journal*, *19*(1), 54–81. DOI: 10.1208/s12248-016-0003-2 PMID: 27783266

Manisalidis, I., Stavropoulou, E., Stavropoulos, A., & Bezirtzoglou, E. (2020). Environmental and Health Impacts of Air Pollution: A Review. *Frontiers in Public Health*, *8*, 14. Advance online publication. DOI: 10.3389/fpubh.2020.00014 PMID: 32154200

Mao, X., Liu, Y., Wei, Y., Li, X., Liu, Y., Su, G., Wang, X., Jia, J., & Yan, B. (2024). Threats of per- and poly-fluoroalkyl pollutants to susceptible populations. *The Science of the Total Environment*, *921*, 171188. DOI: 10.1016/j.scitotenv.2024.171188 PMID: 38395163

Martinvalet, D., & Walch, M. (2022). The role of reactive oxygen species in protective immunity. *Frontiers in Immunology*, *12*, 832946. https://www.frontiersin.org/journals/immunology/articles/10.3389/fimmu.2021.832946/pdf. DOI: 10.3389/fimmu.2021.832946 PMID: 35145515

Masooma, Q., Qaiser, A., Ali, D. S., & Manzoor, D. S. (2024). Prospects of Carica papaya in the treatment of human viral infections: A comprehensive and a systematic review. *Heliyon*, *10*(21), e39635. DOI: 10.1016/j.heliyon.2024.e39635 PMID: 39553635

Mekonnen, A. B., Mohammed, A. S., & Tefera, A. K. (2022, September 19). Ethnobotanical Study of Traditional Medicinal Plants Used to Treat Human and Animal Diseases in Sedie Muja District, South Gondar, Ethiopia. *Evidence-Based Complementary and Alternative Medicine : eCAM*, *7328613*, 1–22. Advance online publication. DOI: 10.1155/2022/7328613 PMID: 36193157

Mensah, M. L., Komlaga, G., Forkuo, A. D., Firempong, C., Anning, A. K., & Dickson, R. A. (2019). Toxicity and safety implications of herbal medicines. Herbal medicine, 63, 1-17.

Miranda, A. R., Albrecht, C., Cortez, M. V., & Soria, E. A. (2018). Pharmacology and Toxicology of Polyphenols with Potential As Neurotropic Agents in Non-communicable Diseases. *Current Drug Targets*, *19*(2), 97–110. DOI: 10.2174/1389450117666161220152336 PMID: 28000547

Modibbo, M. R., Ibrahim, H., Sulaiman, M. Y., & Zakir, B. (2024). Maganin Gargajiya: Assessing the Benefits, Challenges, and Evidence of Traditional Medicine in Nigeria. *Cureus*. Advance online publication. DOI: 10.7759/cureus.71425 PMID: 39411369

Moini, J., & Ferdowsi, K. (2023). Environmental Pollutants and Nutrition. In Handbook of Nutritional Disorders (pp. 428-444). CRC Press. DOI: 10.1201/9781003453376-38

Montano, L., Baldini, G. M., Piscopo, M., Liguori, G., Lombardi, R., Ricciardi, M., Esposito, G., Pinto, G., Fontanarosa, C., Spinelli, M., Palmieri, I., Sofia, D., Brogna, C., Carati, C., Esposito, M., Gallo, P., Amoresano, A., & Motta, O. (2025). Polycyclic Aromatic Hydrocarbons (PAHs) in the Environment: Occupational Exposure, Health Risks and Fertility Implications. *Toxics*, *13*(3), 151. https://www.mdpi.com/2305-6304/13/3/151. DOI: 10.3390/toxics13030151 PMID: 40137477

Moraes, R. M., Cerdeira, A. L., & Lourenço, M. V. (2021). Using Micropropagation to Develop Medicinal Plants into Crops. *Molecules (Basel, Switzerland)*, *26*(6), 1752. DOI: 10.3390/molecules26061752 PMID: 33800970

Morlock, G. E., & Zoller, L. (2025). Fast unmasking toxicity of safe personal care products. *Journal of Chromatography. A, 1752*, 465886. DOI: 10.1016/j.chroma.2025.465886 PMID: 40252263

Moronkeji, A., Adeniyi, T., Oyeleke, A., Igunbor, C., Ayeni, J., Adelabi, T., & Moronkeji, A. (2024b). Cymbopogon citratus: A modulator of TNF-A and IL-10 in NSAID-induced hepatorenal toxicity in adult Wistar rats. *Bulletin of Pharmaceutical Sciences Assiut University, 47*(2), 1251–1262. DOI: 10.21608/bfsa.2024.297319.2162

Moronkeji, A., & Akinbo, F. O. (2024). 'Genotoxic Response and Histological Alterations in Rat Lungs Exposed to Gasoline Generator Exhaust'. *Sultan Qaboos University Journal for Science [SQUJS]* 29(1): 15–27. https://journals.squ.edu.om/index.php/squjs/article/view/5780

Moronkeji, A., Temidayo, A., Benita, A., & Latifat, O. (2024a). 'Methanolic Leaf Extract of Vernonia Amygdalina Mitigates Cadmium-Induced Oxidative Stress in the Liver and Kidney of Adult Male Wistar Rats'. *Egyptian Journal of Basic and Applied Sciences, 11*(1), 469–478. DOI: 10.1080/2314808X.2024.2360364

Mukherjee, S., Banik, S. K., Chakraborty, S., Das, T., Choudhury, M. D., & Tripathi, A. (2025). Bryophyllum pinnatum Induces p53-Dependent Apoptosis of Colorectal Cancer Cells via Increased Intracellular ROS and G2/M Cell-Cycle Arrest In Vitro and Validated in Silico by Molecular Docking. *Cell Biology International, 49*(5), 534–554. DOI: 10.1002/cbin.70004

Muñoz-Sánchez, G., Godínez-Méndez, L. A., Fafutis-Morris, M., & Delgado-Rizo, V. (2023). Effect of Antioxidant Supplementation on NET Formation Induced by LPS In Vitro; the Roles of Vitamins E and C, Glutathione, and N-acetyl Cysteine. *International Journal of Molecular Sciences, 24*(17), 13162. DOI: 10.3390/ijms241713162 PMID: 37685966

Najmi, A., Javed, S. A., Al Bratty, M., & Alhazmi, H. A. (2022). Modern Approaches in the Discovery and Development of Plant-Based Natural Products and Their Analogues as Potential Therapeutic Agents. *Molecules (Basel, Switzerland), 27*(2), 349. DOI: 10.3390/molecules27020349 PMID: 35056662

Napolitano, G., Fasciolo, G., & Venditti, P. (2021). Mitochondrial management of reactive oxygen species. *Antioxidants, 10*(11), 1824. https://www.mdpi.com/2076-3921/10/11/1824. DOI: 10.3390/antiox10111824 PMID: 34829696

Negrette-Guzmán, M. (2019). Combinations of the antioxidants sulforaphane or curcumin and the conventional antineoplastics cisplatin or doxorubicin as prospects for anticancer chemotherapy. *European Journal of Pharmacology, 859*, 172513. DOI: 10.1016/j.ejphar.2019.172513 PMID: 31260654

Nowak, M., Tryniszewski, W., Sarniak, A., Wlodarczyk, A., Nowak, P. J., & Nowak, D. (2022). Concentration Dependence of Anti- and Pro-Oxidant Activity of Polyphenols as Evaluated with a Light-Emitting Fe2+-Egta-H2O2 System. *Molecules (Basel, Switzerland)*, *27*(11), 3453. DOI: 10.3390/molecules27113453 PMID: 35684391

Nwafor, N., & Igboeli, L. (2021). Antimicrobial activity of Annona senegalensis fruit extract against pathogenic microbes. *Scientific African*, *13*, e00988.

Ogunro, O. B., Oyeyinka, B. O., Gyebi, G. A., & Batiha, G. E. S. (2023). Nutritional benefits, ethnomedicinal uses, phytochemistry, pharmacological properties and toxicity of Spondias mombin Linn: A comprehensive review. *The Journal of Pharmacy and Pharmacology*, *75*(2), 162–226. DOI: 10.1093/jpp/rgac086 PMID: 36632807

Olanrewaju, I. O., Mordi, R. C., & Echeme, J. O. (2018). Antibacterial, antifungal and anti-tubercular activities of chloroform fraction of the leaf extract of Irvingia gabonensis (African bush mango). *Anti-Infective Agents*, *18*(2), 109–114. DOI: 10.2174/2211352517666181122125411

Omale, S., Amagon, K. I., Johnson, T. O., Bremner, S. K., & Gould, G. W. (2023). A systematic analysis of anti-diabetic medicinal plants from cells to clinical trials. *PeerJ*, *11*, e14639. DOI: 10.7717/peerj.14639 PMID: 36627919

Onukak, A. C., Musa, I., & Abdullahi, Z. (2020). Hypoglycemic potential of Anchomanes difformis rhizome extract in diabetic rats. *Journal of Ethnopharmacology*, *260*, 112921.

Ortega-Ramirez, L. A., Gutiérrez-Pacheco, M. M., Vargas-Arispuro, I., González-Aguilar, G. A., Martínez-Téllez, M. A., & Ayala-Zavala, J. F. (2020). Inhibition of Glucosyltransferase Activity and Glucan Production as an Antibiofilm Mechanism of Lemongrass Essential Oil against Escherichia coli O157:H7. *Antibiotics (Basel, Switzerland)*, *9*(3), 102. DOI: 10.3390/antibiotics9030102 PMID: 32121319

Oruka, O., & Achuba, F. I. (2023). In vitro Antioxidant and Anti-Inflammatory Activities of Aqueous Leaf Extract of Alchornea cordifolia. *Journal of Applied Science & Environmental Management*, *27*(2), 299–304. DOI: 10.4314/jasem.v27i2.16

Osafo, N., Obiri, D. D., Antwi, A. O., & Yeboah, O. K. (2018). The acute anti-inflammatory action of xylopic acid isolated from Xylopia aethiopica. *Journal of Basic and Clinical Physiology and Pharmacology*, *29*(6), 659–669. DOI: 10.1515/jbcpp-2018-0019 PMID: 30052517

Osuagwu, G. G., & Idika, G. C. (2021). Anti-inflammatory and antioxidant activity of Ceratotheca sesamoides leaf infusion in Wistar rats. *Nigerian Journal of Natural Products and Medicine*, *25*(1), 54–62.

Owolabi, T., & Okubor, P. (2024). Anti-Ulcer and Antioxidant Activities of Chrysophyllum albidum G. Don. Seeds Cotyledons. *Jurnal Farmasi Dan Ilmu Kefarmasian Indonesia, 11*(2), 260–268. DOI: 10.20473/jfiki.v11i22024.260-268

Oyetayo, F. L., Akomolafe, S. F., & Balogun, G. B. (2021). Effects of Chrysophyllum albidum fruit pulp on haemodynamic parameters, pro-inflammatory markers, antioxidant parameters and critical biomolecules associated with hypertension–in vivo. *Inflammopharmacology, 29*(3), 825–839. DOI: 10.1007/s10787-021-00830-x PMID: 34120250

Pardo, M., Qiu, X., Zimmermann, R., & Rudich, Y. (2020). Particulate Matter Toxicity Is Nrf2 and Mitochondria Dependent: The Roles of Metals and Polycyclic Aromatic Hydrocarbons. *Chemical Research in Toxicology, 33*(5), 1110–1120. DOI: 10.1021/acs.chemrestox.0c00007 PMID: 32302097

Park, S. Y., An, K. S., Lee, B., Kang, J. H., Jung, H. J., Kim, M. W., Ryu, H. Y., Shim, K. S., Nam, K. T., Yoon, Y. S., & Oh, S. H. (2021). Establishment of particulate matter-induced lung injury model in mouse. *Laboratory Animal Research, 37*(1), 20. DOI: 10.1186/s42826-021-00097-x PMID: 34330339

Patel, N. K., & Bhutani, K. K. (2014). Pinostrobin and Cajanus lactone isolated from Cajanus cajan (L.) leaves inhibits TNF-α and IL-1β production: In vitro and in vivo experimentation. *Phytomedicine, 21*(7), 946–953. DOI: 10.1016/j.phymed.2014.02.011 PMID: 24680612

Patil, V. M., Das, S., & Balasubramanian, K. (2016). Quantum Chemical and Docking Insights into Bioavailability Enhancement of Curcumin by Piperine in Pepper. *The Journal of Physical Chemistry A, 120*(20), 3643–3653. DOI: 10.1021/acs.jpca.6b01434 PMID: 27111639

Paul, T. K., & Kumar, K. J. (2023). *Standardization of Herbal Medicines for Lifestyle Diseases.*, DOI: 10.1007/978-981-99-7703-1_27

Pereira, R. B., Rahali, F. Z., Nehme, R., Falleh, H., Ben Jemaa, M., Sellami, I. H., Ksouri, R., Bouhallab, S., Ceciliani, F., Abdennebi-Najar, L., & Pereira, D. M. (2023). Anti-inflammatory activity of essential oils from Tunisian aromatic and medicinal plants and their major constituents in THP-1 macrophages. *Food Research International, 167*, 112678. DOI: 10.1016/j.foodres.2023.112678 PMID: 37087210

Pirintsos, S. A., Bariotakis, M., Kampa, M., Sourvinos, G., Lionis, C., & Castanas, E. (2020). The Therapeutic Potential of the Essential Oil of Thymbra capitata (L.) Cav., Origanum dictamnus L. and Salvia fruticosa Mill. And a Case of Plant-Based Pharmaceutical Development. *Frontiers in Pharmacology, 11*, 522213. Advance online publication. DOI: 10.3389/fphar.2020.522213 PMID: 33390932

Pisoschi, A. M., Pop, A., Cimpeanu, C., & Predoi, G. (2016). Antioxidant Capacity Determination in Plants and Plant-Derived Products: A Review. *Oxidative Medicine and Cellular Longevity, 9130976*(1), 9130976. Advance online publication. DOI: 10.1155/2016/9130976 PMID: 28044094

Olugbenga Kayode Popoola, Kayode Damilola Adekeye, Eunice Damilola Akinbinu, Lanre Tope Adekeye, Michael Bolaji Afolayan, Emmanuel Ayomide Bakare, & Oluwatobi Emmanuel Akande. (2021). Ethnobotanical plants and their tradomedicinal values: A review. *World Journal of Biology Pharmacy and Health Sciences,* 5(1), 066–088. DOI: 10.30574/wjbphs.2021.5.1.0108

Rahman, M. S., Kabir, H., & Islam, M. R. (2021). Heavy metal exposure and oxidative damage: A review of mechanisms. *Toxics*, *9*(9), 218. DOI: 10.3390/toxics9090218 PMID: 34564369

Rajashekar, C. B. (2023). Dual Role of Plant Phenolic Compounds as Antioxidants and Prooxidants. *American Journal of Plant Sciences*, *14*(01), 15–28. DOI: 10.4236/ajps.2023.141002

Rassu, G., Sorrenti, M., Catenacci, L., Pavan, B., Ferraro, L., Gavini, E., Bonferoni, M. C., Giunchedi, P., & Dalpiaz, A. (2023). Conjugation, Prodrug, and Co-Administration Strategies in Support of Nanotechnologies to Improve the Therapeutic Efficacy of Phytochemicals in the Central Nervous System. *Pharmaceutics*, *15*(6), 1578. DOI: 10.3390/pharmaceutics15061578 PMID: 37376027

Rathore, T., Upadhyay, E., & Jain, A. K. (2025). Therapeutic Role of Medicinal Plants in Combating Air Pollution-Induced Inflammation and Anxiety. *International Journal of Environmental Sciences*, *11*(10s), 635–649. DOI: 10.64252/y86v7b35

Sadgrove, N. J., & Jones, G. L. (2019). From Petri Dish to Patient: Bioavailability Estimation and Mechanism of Action for Antimicrobial and Immunomodulatory Natural Products. *Frontiers in Microbiology*, *10*, 2470. Advance online publication. DOI: 10.3389/fmicb.2019.02470 PMID: 31736910

Said, M., & Ibrahim, M. M. (2024). Antioxidants and Phytochemical Profiles in Medicinal Plants: Unraveling Molecular Mechanisms. *Scholars International Journal of Biochemistry*, *7*(07), 106–117. DOI: 10.36348/sijb.2024.v07i07.003

Salau, A. K., Shehu, S., & Bakare-Odunola, M. T. (2024). Navigating the Challenges of Integrating African Herbal Medicines: A Path to Universal Acceptance. *Fountain Journal of National Ad Applied Sciences*, *13*(1). Advance online publication. DOI: 10.53704/fujnas.v13i1.474

Salehi, B., Azzini, E., Zucca, P., Maria Varoni, E., & Anil Kumar, V., N., Dini, L., Panzarini, E., Rajkovic, J., Valere Tsouh Fokou, P., Peluso, I., Prakash Mishra, A., Nigam, M., El Rayess, Y., El Beyrouthy, M., N. Setzer, W., Polito, L., Iriti, M., Sureda, A., Magdalena Quetglas-Llabrés, M., … Sharifi-Rad, J. (. (2020). Plant-Derived Bioactives and Oxidative Stress-Related Disorders: A Key Trend towards Healthy Aging and Longevity Promotion. *Applied Sciences (Basel, Switzerland)*, *10*(3), 947. DOI: 10.3390/app10030947

Santos, É. M., Ataide, J. A., Coco, J. C., Fava, A. L. M., Silvério, L. A. L., Sueiro, A. C., Silva, J. R. A., Lopes, A. M., Paiva-Santos, A. C., & Mazzola, P. G. (2023). Spondias sp: Shedding Light on Its Vast Pharmaceutical Potential. *Molecules (Basel, Switzerland)*, *28*(4), 1862. DOI: 10.3390/molecules28041862 PMID: 36838849

Sarkar, A., Roy, D., & Ghosh, S. (2020). PAHs and oxidative stress: Metabolic activation and redox cycling in human toxicity. *Molecular and Cellular Biochemistry*, *469*, 21–34. DOI: 10.1007/s11010-020-03813-z

Shoaib, S., Ansari, M. A., Al Fatease, A., Safhi, A. Y., Hani, U., Jahan, R., Alomary, M. N., Ansari, M. N., Ahmed, N., Wahab, S., Ahmad, W., Yusuf, N., & Islam, N. (2023). Plant-Derived Bioactive Compounds in the Management of Neurodegenerative Disorders: Challenges, Future Directions and Molecular Mechanisms Involved in Neuroprotection. *Pharmaceutics*, *15*(3), 749. DOI: 10.3390/pharmaceutics15030749 PMID: 36986610

Siddiqui, N. A., Taj, F. B., Ishaque, I., Shahid, A., & Ayaz, A. (2020). Role of simvastatin and allium sativum on lipid profile in diabetic dyslipidemic patients: A comparative study. *The Professional Medical Journal*, *27*(02), 353–358. DOI: 10.29309/TPMJ/2020.27.02.3974

Sierra-Vargas, M. P., Montero-Vargas, J. M., Debray-Garcia, Y., Vizuet-de-Rueda, J. C., Loaeza-Roman, A., & Teran, L. M. (2023). Oxidative stress and air pollution: Its impact on chronic respiratory diseases. *International Journal of Molecular Sciences*, *24*(1), 853. https://www.mdpi.com/1422-0067/24/1/853. DOI: 10.3390/ijms24010853 PMID: 36614301

Sigsgaard, T., & Hoffmann, B. (2024). Assessing the health burden from air pollution. *Science*, *384*(6691), 33–34. DOI: 10.1126/science.abo3801 PMID: 38574150

Sinan, K. I., Ak, G., Etienne, O. K., Jekő, J., Cziáky, Z., Gupcsó, K., João Rodrigues, M., Custodio, L., Mahomoodally, M. F., Sharmeen, J. B., Brunetti, L., Leone, S., Recinella, L., Chiavaroli, A., Orlando, G., Menghini, L., Tacchini, M., Ferrante, C., & Zengin, G. (2021). Deeper Insights on Alchornea cordifolia (Schumach. & Thonn.) Müll.Arg Extracts: Chemical Profiles, Biological Abilities, Network Analysis and Molecular Docking. *Biomolecules*, *11*(2), 219. DOI: 10.3390/biom11020219 PMID: 33557215

Sindhoora, D., & Bhattacharjee, A. (2020). A Brief Review on Pharmacological Profile of Zingiber officinale. *RGUHS Journal of Pharmaceutical Sciences*, *10*(2), 1230. Advance online publication. DOI: 10.26463/rjps.10_2_7

Singh, V. K., Arora, D., Ansari, M. I., & Sharma, P. K. (2019). Phytochemicals based chemopreventive and chemotherapeutic strategies and modern technologies to overcome limitations for better clinical applications. *Phytotherapy Research*, *33*(12), 3064–3089. DOI: 10.1002/ptr.6508 PMID: 31515899

Srinivas, Ch., & Singh, Dr. G. (2023). Traditional Plant uses and Indigenous Knowledge in Ethnobotany. *International Journal of Horticulture, Agriculture and Food Science*, 7(5), 01–05. DOI: 10.22161/ijhaf.7.5.1

Sun, Q., Li, Y., Shi, L., Hussain, R., Mehmood, K., Tang, Z., & Zhang, H. (2022). Heavy metals induced mitochondrial dysfunction in animals: Molecular mechanism of toxicity. *Toxicology*, *469*, 153136. DOI: 10.1016/j.tox.2022.153136 PMID: 35202761

Tagne, A. M., Marino, F., & Cosentino, M. (2018). Tithonia diversifolia (Hemsl.) A. Gray as a medicinal plant: A comprehensive review of its ethnopharmacology, phytochemistry, pharmacotoxicology and clinical relevance. *Journal of Ethnopharmacology*, *220*, 94–116. DOI: 10.1016/j.jep.2018.03.025 PMID: 29596999

Tanty, H., & Herlina, T. (2018). Antidiabetic activity test for leaves extract of Cassia siamea. lamk. MATTER. *International Journal of Science and Technology*, *3*(3), 339–348. DOI: 10.20319/mijst.2018.33.339348

Tauheed, A. M., Mamman, M., Ahmed, A., Sani, N. A., Suleiman, M. M., Sulaiman, M. H., & Balogun, E. O. (2021). Acute, sub-acute, sub-chronic and chronic toxicity studies of four important Nigerian ethnomedicinal plants in rats. *Clinical Phytoscience*, *7*(1), 1. DOI: 10.1186/s40816-020-00244-2

Thiruvengadam, M., Venkidasamy, B., Subramanian, U., Samynathan, R., Ali Shariati, M., Rebezov, M., Girish, S., Thangavel, S., Dhanapal, A. R., Fedoseeva, N., Lee, J., & Chung, I.-M. (2021). Bioactive Compounds in Oxidative Stress-Mediated Diseases: Targeting the NRF2/ARE Signaling Pathway and Epigenetic Regulation. *Antioxidants*, *10*(12), 1859. DOI: 10.3390/antiox10121859 PMID: 34942962

Togbenou, K., Idoh, K., Dosseh, K., Kpatcha, T., & Agbonon, A. (2020). Anti-Inflammatory Activity of Extract Mixture of Annona senegalensis Pers. and Piliostigma thonningii (Schum.). *Journal of Drug Delivery and Therapeutics*, *10*(6-s), 103–108. DOI: 10.22270/jddt.v10i6-s.4605

Tyuryaeva, I., & Lyublinskaya, O. (2023). Expected and Unexpected Effects of Pharmacological Antioxidants. *International Journal of Molecular Sciences*, *24*(11), 9303. DOI: 10.3390/ijms24119303 PMID: 37298254

Ukaogo, P. O., Ewuzie, U., & Onwuka, C. V. (2020). Environmental Pollution: Causes, Effects, and the Remedies. In Chowdhary, P., Raj, A., Verma, D., & Akhter, Y. (Eds.), *Microorganisms for Sustainable Environment and Health* (pp. 419–429). Elsevier., DOI: 10.1016/B978-0-12-819001-2.00021-8

Unuofin, J. O., Masuku, N. P., Paimo, O. K., & Lebelo, S. L. (2021). Ginger from Farmyard to Town: Nutritional and Pharmacological Applications. *Frontiers in Pharmacology*, *12*, 779352. Advance online publication. DOI: 10.3389/fphar.2021.779352 PMID: 34899343

Usmani, J., Wasim, M., Ansari, M. N., Hassan, M. J., Sharma, M., & Ahmad, R. (2023). Potential therapeutic effect of Carica papaya leaves extract on immune response, biochemical and hematological mechanisms on cecal ligation and puncture model of sepsis in rats: an in vivo study. *3 Biotech*, 13(5), 151, 1–17. https://doi.org/ DOI: 10.1007/S13205-023-03567-2/METRICS

Van der Merwe, J., De Beer, D., Joubert, E., & Gelderblom, W. (2015). Short-Term and Sub-Chronic Dietary Exposure to Aspalathin-Enriched Green Rooibos (Aspalathus linearis) Extract Affects Rat Liver Function and Antioxidant Status. *Molecules (Basel, Switzerland)*, *20*(12), 22674–22690. DOI: 10.3390/molecules201219868 PMID: 26694346

Vimukthi, W. P. D., Dong, S., Yang, C., Zhang, Y., Baikeri, G., Lou, T., Deng, F., Li, Z., & Cao, F. (2025). Enhancing DTT assays for reactive oxygen species detection in atmospheric particulate matter: Key factors and methodological insights. *Environmental Science: Atmospheres*, *5*(8), 865–878. DOI: 10.1039/D4EA00158C

Vongsak, B., Mangmool, S., & Gritsanapan, W. (2015). Antioxidant Activity and Induction of mRNA Expressions of Antioxidant Enzymes in HEK-293 Cells of Moringa oleifera Leaf Extract. *Planta Medica*, *81*(12/13), 1084–1089. DOI: 10.1055/s-0035-1546168 PMID: 26166137

Wagner, H., & Efferth, T. (2017). Introduction: Novel hybrid combinations containing synthetic or antibiotic drugs with plant-derived phenolic or terpenoid compounds. *Phytomedicine*, *37*, 1–3. DOI: 10.1016/j.phymed.2017.10.020 PMID: 29174652

Wang, Q., Song, H., Dong, H., Guo, S., Yao, M., Wan, Y., & Lu, K. (2025). Multiphase Radical Chemical Processes Induced by Air Pollutants and the Associated Health Effects. *Environment & Health*, *3*(1), 1–13. DOI: 10.1021/envhealth.4c00157 PMID: 39839244

Xie, J. (2022). Will the role of Indigenous Knowledge Systems help in sustaining the utilization and conservation of indigenous medicinal plants? *Planta Medica*, *88*(15), 1437. Advance online publication. DOI: 10.1055/s-0042-1759002

Yada, D., Sivakkumar, T., & Srinivas, N. (2021). Aqueous Extract of Hyptis suaveolens Whole Plant Inhibits Carrageenan-Induced Paw Edema in Rats. *Advances in Pharmacology and Pharmacy*, *9*(3), 75–80. DOI: 10.13189/app.2021.090305

Yadav, N., Chandel, S. S., Venkatachalam, T., & Fathima, S. N. (2023). *Herbal Medicine Formulation, Standardization, and Commercialization Challenges and Sustainable Strategies for Improvement*. Springer International Publishing., DOI: 10.1007/978-3-031-21973-3_40-1

Yeshi, K., Crayn, D., Ritmejerytė, E., & Wangchuk, P. (2022). Plant Secondary Metabolites Produced in Response to Abiotic Stresses Has Potential Application in Pharmaceutical Product Development. *Molecules (Basel, Switzerland)*, *27*(1), 313. DOI: 10.3390/molecules27010313 PMID: 35011546

Yuan, H., Ma, Q., Ye, L., & Piao, G. (2016). The traditional medicine and modern medicine from natural products. *Molecules (Basel, Switzerland)*, *21*(5), 559. DOI: 10.3390/molecules21050559 PMID: 27136524

Zargaran, A. (2024). Ethnopharmacology, generations experience for the future of pharmacy and medicine. *Journal of Drug Research in Ayurvedic Sciences*, *9*(2), 58–59. DOI: 10.4103/jdras.jdras_105_24

Zhang, H., Chen, L., & Wang, Y. (2021). Transition metal-mediated oxidative stress in environmental pollution. *Ecotoxicology and Environmental Safety*, *218*, 112295. DOI: 10.1016/j.ecoenv.2021.112295

Zhao, C., Wu, S., & Wang, H. (2025). Medicinal Plant Extracts Targeting UV-Induced Skin Damage: Molecular Mechanisms and Therapeutic Potential. *International Journal of Molecular Sciences*, *26*(5), 2278. DOI: 10.3390/ijms26052278 PMID: 40076896

Zhou, Q., Lin, J., & Yu, S. (2023). NADPH oxidase activation and pollutant-induced ROS: Molecular mechanisms and health effects. *Free Radical Biology & Medicine*, *197*, 49–61. DOI: 10.1016/j.freeradbiomed.2023.02.013

Zhu, H., Liu, W., Tian, B., Liu, H., & Ning, S. (2011). Inhibition of Quorum Sensing in the Opportunistic Pathogenic Bacterium Chromobacterium violaceum by an Extract from Fruiting Bodies of Lingzhi or Reishi Medicinal Mushroom, Ganoderma lucidum (W.Curt.:Fr.) P. Karst. (Higher Basidiomycetes). *International Journal of Medicinal Mushrooms*, *13*(6), 559–564. DOI: 10.1615/IntJMedMushr.v13.i6.80 PMID: 22181844

Chapter 3
Neurophytomedicine: A Critical Review of Traditional Herbal Anxiolytics

Sreya Kosanam
http://orcid.org/0000-0002-0645-5677
Dr. M.G.R. Educational and Research Institute, India

R. Praveen Javali
http://orcid.org/0009-0001-3737-5813
Sri Raghavendra College of Pharmacy, Chitradurga, India

Revathi Boyina
http://orcid.org/0000-0002-8561-724X
QIS College of Pharmacy, India

Adinarayana Andy
http://orcid.org/0000-0002-5163-1094
Weatherwax Family Pharmacies Inc., USA

A. M. T. Gurubasavaraj
http://orcid.org/0009-0008-9256-2436
YSS College of Pharmacy, India

Aman Suresh Tharayil
http://orcid.org/0009-0000-5377-7428
Dr. M.G.R. Educational and Research Institute, India

K. M. D. Muzammil
http://orcid.org/0009-0000-0362-6015
YSS College of Pharmacy, India

ABSTRACT

This chapter examines the scientific and clinical foundations of traditional herbal anxiolytics within the emerging field of neurophytomedicine. It explores the global prevalence and neurobiology of anxiety disorders, limitations of conventional pharmacological treatments, and the therapeutic potential of botanicals with historical use in anxiety relief. Emphasis is placed on phytochemical classes such as flavonoids, terpenes, alkaloids, and saponins, and their mechanisms of action on GABAergic, serotonergic, and hypothalamic pituitary adrenal systems. Comparative clinical evidence, safety considerations, herb-drug interactions, and regulatory frameworks are critically reviewed. The chapter also addresses challenges in standardization,

DOI: 10.4018/979-8-3373-5876-5.ch003

placebo effects in trials, and ethical sourcing of medicinal plants. Finally, it outlines future directions including pharmacogenomic personalization, AI-driven phytochemical discovery, and integration of validated botanicals into mainstream psychiatry.

INTRODUCTION:

Anxiety disorders rank among the most common mental health conditions globally, affecting about 4% of the population. By incorporating generalized anxiety disorders, terror disorders, social anxiety disorders and specific phobias, they often cause significant emotional crisis and functional loss. The burden is extended to the high rates of comorbidity with depression, substance use disorders, and chronic medical diseases, causing effective treatment to both a clinical and public health priority (Javaid et al., 2023).

Current medicinal options, including benzodiazepines, selective serotonin receptor inhibitors (SSRIs), and serotonin-norepinephrine reuptake inhibitors (SNRIs), remain the mainstay of treatment, but are far from ideal. Benzodiazepines, although effective, well -recognized risk dependence, withdrawal, and cognitive dull that limits long -term use. SSRIs and SNRIs avoid that damage, but require weeks to get medical benefits and often cause sexual dysfunction, gastrointestinal disturbing, and rearing problems. Even in optimal conditions, an important subgroup of patients reacts only partially, and in low-resources settings, these drugs can be inaccessible or ineffective. These intervals have demanded options that are better tolerated, culturally adaptable (Conway et al., 2024).

Traditional herbal anxiolytics have become increasingly popular in this area. Their attraction goes beyond their natural origins, drawing on centuries of ethnobotanical practice and the belief, whether true or not, in their increased safety and overall wellness benefits. Despite their widespread usage, most herbal remedies have not undergone the same rigorous pharmacological and clinical examination as conventional drugs. This underscores the need to evaluate how these treatments work, how effective they are, and whether they meet modern safety standards while giving traditional knowledge the careful, evidence-based scrutiny it deserves.

Neurophytomedicine studies plant-derived compounds that affect the nervous system, drawing on neuroscience, pharmacognosy, and ethnopharmacology. Both synthetic and plant-based anxiolytics work by targeting specific neurobiological pathways to reduce anxiety. Traditional medicine, including Ayurveda, Traditional Chinese Medicine (TCM), African traditional medicine, and other indigenous healing systems, has long relied on plants for mental health care. Understanding these perspectives allows herbal anxiolytics to be considered as potentially valuable neuroactive agents, not just as cultural artifacts (Küpeli Akkol et al., 2021).

Clinically significant anxiety goes beyond ordinary worry or fear, which can serve useful purposes. Key symptoms include restlessness, muscle tension, fatigue, difficulty concentrating, and insomnia, and they can appear in a range of disorders. Generalized anxiety disorder involves persistent, uncontrollable worry; panic disorder is marked by sudden episodes of intense fear with physical symptoms; social anxiety disorder centers on strong fear of social or performance situations; and specific phobias and agoraphobia lead to avoidance of certain triggers. Other conditions, such as obsessive-compulsive disorder (OCD) and post-traumatic stress disorder (PTSD), though classified separately, also involve high levels of anxiety (Grosso et al., 2023).

These syndromes have observable neurobiological changes: diminished gamma amino-butyric acid (GABA) activity in generalized anxiety and panic disorder; serotonergic dysregulation in social anxiety and OCD; hyperactivity of the amygdala and related limbic circuits; and overactivation of the hypothalamic-pituitary-adrenal (HPA) axis. These mechanisms suggest potential targets for pharmaceuticals and for plant-based treatments (Borrás, et al., 2021).

Despite decades of psychopharmacological developments, current medications are still leaving significant gaps. Many patients discontinue medications due to side effects, lack of response, or fear of dependency; others may have no access to anything. In many lower-resourced contexts, using traditional herbal preparations for anxiety disorders is not just complementary; it is primary care. The growing interest in herbal anxiolytics, therefore, represents both a need and an opportunity; the need for safe, effective, and accessible therapies, and an opportunity to incorporate evidenced-based traditional herbal treatments into modern practice (Motti & de Falco, 2021).

Though herbal anxiolytics have long history, scientific evidence is lacking. Clinical trails on plant-based therapy are often face hight placebo rates, particularly in anxiety disorders. Blinding is imperfect as unintentionally relevance of treatment due to taste, physiological effects, and aroma of herbal drugs. Various studies used extracts of different plant species, their preparation method and standardisation are having inconsistent phytochemical profile during trails. This variation complicates and limits the comparability between findings. Usually, traditional formulas involve multiple herbs for synergistic effect, and which makes difficult to isolate single agent. These types of issues enhance the need for careful and evidence-based evaluation of herbal anxiolytics and highlights why standardized preparations, trail design are important for strengthening the clinical credibility of neurophytomedicine.

CLASSIFICATION BY PLANT FAMILIES AND ACTIVE PHYTOCHEMICALS

Herbal anxiolytics arise from a diverse range of botanical families, many of which occupy central roles in traditional medical systems worldwide (Figure 1). These families are often rich in neuroactive phytochemicals including alkaloids, flavonoids, terpenoids, and saponins that can influence the neurochemical pathways implicated in anxiety regulation. The Lamiaceae, has well-known examples such as *Melissa officinalis* (lemon balm) (Mathews et al., 2024) and *Lavandula angustifolia* (lavender) (Naufal et al., 2023) which are widely used for their calming effects. These plants are rich in essential oils and polyphenols that modulate γ-aminobutyric acid (GABA) and serotonin signaling, pathways to anxiolytic activity.

Valerianaceae family is prominently represented by *Valeriana officinalis* (valerian), one of the most extensively studied herbal sedatives. Valerian contains valerenic acid and valepotriatvalepotriate that enhance GABAergic neurotransmission and thereby modulates hyperexcitability within the CNS. Curcuma longa (turmeric) belongs to the Zingiberaceae family, and its bioactive constituent curcumin demonstrates anti-inflammatory and neuroprotective effects. Although its anxiolytic actions are often indirect, preclinical studies suggest that modulating neuroinflammation and oxidative stress can improve mood and attenuate anxiety-like behaviors (Mungali et al., 2021).

The Solanaceae family includes *Withania somnifera* (ashwagandha) (Pandit et al., 2024), a cornerstone of Ayurvedic medicine, noted for its adaptogenic properties. Ashwagandha is rich in withanolide and appears to modulate the hypothalamic–pituitary–adrenal (HPA) axis and balance neurotransmitter systems, thereby reducing the physiological impact of chronic stress and anxiety. Passiflora *incarnata* (passionflower) (La Tempa et al., 2025) is a traditional sedative whose flavonoid content, particularly chrysina, has been linked to the modulation of GABA-A receptors and reduced neural overactivity.

Across these families, the pharmacological relevance lies not in a single "active" molecule but in the synergy among multiple phytochemical constituents. Flavonoids, such as apigenin and chrysin, terpenes like linalool, alkaloids, including harmine, and various glycosides interact with neurotransmitter systems that govern anxiety responses. These compounds can work in two main ways either directly, by binding to GABA-A or serotonin receptors, or indirectly, by helping the brain regain balance through antioxidant, anti-inflammatory, or neuroendocrine effects. This chemical variety reflects the polypharmacological nature of herbal anxiolytics, which makes them especially promising for influencing the complex, interconnected systems that drive anxiety.

Figure 1. Classification of some common herbal anxiolytic's family

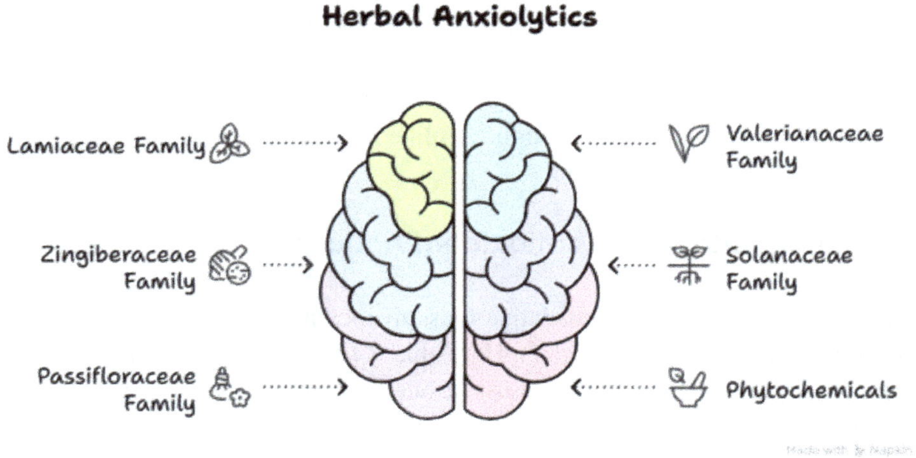

MECHANISMS OF ACTION

GABAergic Modulation

Some herbal anxiolytics act on the gammaaminobutyric acid (GABA) system, which is primary inhibitory neurotransmitter in the brain. GABAA receptor modulation is the principal mechanism behind the fast-acting effects of benzodiazepines. Herbs such as *Valeriana officinalis*, *Passiflora incarnata* (La Tempa et al., 2025), and *Matricaria chamomilla* have shown affinity for GABAA receptors or upregulation of GABA synthesis. These actions contribute to anxiolysis, sedation, and muscle relaxation without the intensity or addiction risk of synthetic GABAergic agents.

Serotonergic Activity

Several herbs influence serotonergic transmission, either by enhancing serotonin availability or modulating receptor activity. *Rhodiola rosea* and *Hypericum perforatum* (St. John's Wort) can modulate serotonin reuptake, while others, such as *Lavandula angustifolia*, may influence serotenin1A receptor expression. These effects mood stabilization and anxiety reduction, similar in principle to SSRIs, but generally with fewer side effects.

Adaptogenic Effects

Adaptogens are a class of herbs that enhance the body's resistance to physical, emotional, and environmental stress. *Withania somnifera* (Ashwagandha), *Panax ginseng*, and *Rhodiola rosea* are leading examples. These plants modulate the hypothalamicpituitaryadrenal (HPA) axis and improve stress hormone regulation, indirectly reducing anxiety and fatigue. Unlike fast acting agents, adaptogens typically build resilience over time.

Anti-inflammatory and Antioxidant Actions

Chronic inflammation and oxidative stress are increasingly recognized as contributors to anxiety and mood disorders. Herbs like *Curcuma longa*, *Camellia sinensis* (green tea), and *Ginkgo biloba* possess strong antioxidant and anti-inflammatory properties. These may exert anxiolytic effects by preserving neuronal integrity and modulating proinflammatory cytokines involved in stress responses. Some common anxiolytics and their mechanism of action are discussed below (Tabel 1):

Kava (*Piper methysticum*)

Ethnobotanical Background

Kava, derived from the root of *Piper methysticum*, is a culturally significant medicinal plant native to the South Pacific islands. It has been consumed for over 3,000 years across Polynesia, Micronesia, and Melanesia, where it plays a central role in social, spiritual, and therapeutic contexts. Traditionally, the roots are ground and mixed with water to produce a non-alcoholic, mildly psychoactive beverage used to promote calmness, communal bonding, and ceremonial solemnity.

In indigenous knowledge systems, kava is valued for its capacity to "quiet the mind," promote sociability, and ease restlessness or agitation. Medicinally, it has long been used for treating insomnia, nervous tension, headaches, and even urogenital inflammation. The local preference for peeled root and water-based preparations reflects empirical safety standards embedded in traditional practices. Over the past few decades, kava has gained international attention as a natural anxiolytic, prompting widespread commercial interest, pharmacological research, and regulatory scrutiny (Burton et al., 2023).

Pharmacological Evidence and Mechanism of Action

The pharmacological activity of kava resides primarily in a group of compounds known as kavalactones, of which six kavain, dihydrokavain, methysticin, dihydromethysticin, yangonin, and desmethoxyyangonin are considered most active. These compounds are lipophilic, enabling efficient penetration of the blood–brain barrier and interaction with central nervous system (CNS) targets. Importantly, kava does not operate through a single pathway. Its mechanism of action is multidimensional, affecting several neurotransmitter systems and neurophysiological processes that underlie anxiety, hyperarousal, and emotional dysregulation.

One of kava's primary mechanisms is its modulation of the GABAergic system. GABA (gammaaminobutyric acid) is the brain's major inhibitory neurotransmitter, and its reduced activity has been strongly linked to anxiety. Kavalactones, especially kavain and dihydrokavain, do not bind directly to the benzodiazepine site of the GABAA receptor but are believed to enhance GABA activity by increasing receptor sensitivity or promoting chloride ion flux. This results in a general dampening of neuronal excitability producing anxiolysis, muscle relaxation, and a sense of calm without the profound sedation or risk of addiction associated with benzodiazepines. Animal models have consistently shown that kava extracts reduce anxiety like behaviours in a GABA dependent manner, supporting its clinical relevance.

Beyond GABA, dopaminergic modulation plays a secondary but significant role in kava's effects. Kavalactones, such as yangonin, appear to enhance dopaminergic tone in key brain areas, such as the nucleus accumbens, which is involved in reward, motivation, and emotional regulation. This dopaminergic activity may contribute to the unique ability of kava to reduce anxiety while maintaining alertness and cognitive clarity. Enhanced dopamine transmission may also underlie the mild mood-lifting or euphoric effects sometimes described with kava use.

Kava also interacts with voltage-gated ion channels, particularly sodium and calcium channels, which regulate neuronal firing. Inhibition of these channels by kavalactones reduces neuronal excitability and neurotransmitter release, likely contributing to the anticonvulsant and muscle relaxant properties observed in preclinical studies. This ion channel modulation complements GABAergic effects, helping to stabilize neural circuits involved in fear, threat detection, and autonomic arousal.

Another pathway involves inhibition of monoamine oxidase B (MAOB), particularly through the action of yangonin. MAOB is an enzyme that breaks down dopamine and other monoamines in the brain. By mildly inhibiting this enzyme, kava may sustain dopaminergic signaling and contribute to mood stabilization. Although this effect is relatively weak compared with pharmaceutical MAO inhibitors, it adds to the plant's complex pharmacological profile and may play a subtle role in its cumulative effects on emotional tone and stress resilience.

Emerging research has also indicated possible glutamatergic modulation via NMDA receptor antagonism. Overactivation of NMDA receptors has been linked to excitotoxicity and anxiety-like behavior. Certain kavalactones may reduce this excitatory activity, leading to greater emotional regulation and stress resilience.

Although this mechanism is still under investigation, it aligns with observations of the neuroprotective and calming effects of kava.

Finally, there is growing interest in the anti-inflammatory and antioxidant properties of kava, which may indirectly support its anxiolytic action. Chronic psychological stress is associated with elevated proinflammatory cytokine and oxidative stress levels, both of which can disrupt neurotransmitter function and neuronal integrity. In vitro studies have demonstrated that kavalactones can inhibit NFκB signaling and scavenge reactive oxygen species. Although these findings are preliminary, they suggest that kava exerts broader neuroprotective effects that stabilize brain function over time.

In sum, kava acts through a polypharmacological network, engaging GABAergic, dopaminergic, and glutamatergic pathways, while also influencing ion channels, enzyme systems, and inflammatory signaling. This multitarget approach mirrors the complexity of anxiety as a disorder one that involves not a single deficit, but a dysregulated network of emotional, cognitive, and autonomic processes (Parcha et al., 2024).

Toxicology and Side Effects

The major safety concern surrounding kava is hepatotoxicity. Between 1998 and 2002, several case reports linked commercial kava products to serious liver injury, including acute hepatitis and hepatic failure. Investigations revealed that these events were often associated with nontraditional extracts those made using organic solvents or containing non-root plant parts (e.g., stems and leaves). Additionally, many affected individuals were concurrently using other hepatotoxic substances, including alcohol and acetaminophen.

Traditional water-based preparations made exclusively from peeled roots are now believed to carry far lower risk. Regulatory bodies and researchers now distinguish between traditional, pharmacologically authentic kava and improperly produced commercial products. Minor side effects can include gastrointestinal discomfort, headaches, dizziness, and, with chronic high doses, a condition known as *kava dermopathy* a reversible skin thickening and scaling (Pont-Fernandez et al., 2023).

Regulatory Status

Kava's regulatory history has been turbulent. Several European countries, including Germany and Switzerland, imposed bans on kava in the early 2000s following reports of liver toxicity. After reassessment, these bans were partially lifted under strict quality and labeling controls. In the United States, kava is available as a dietary supplement but must carry warnings about potential liver damage. Australia and New Zealand allow regulated sale of kava, though importation policies vary.

The World Health Organization (WHO) and the Food and Agriculture Organization (FAO) now recommend adherence to traditional preparation methods using peeled root only and water extraction to ensure safety. Standardization of kava cultivars and chemotypes (e.g., noble vs. nonnoble varieties) is also being pursued to reduce variability and risk in commercial products (Asare-Doku et al., 2023).

Valerian (*Valeriana officinalis*)

Ethnobotanical Background

Valeriana officinalis, commonly known as valerian, is a perennial flowering plant native to Europe and parts of Asia, now also naturalized in North America. It has been used for over 2,000 years in Western herbal traditions as a calming agent and sleep aid. The Greek physician Hippocrates is believed to have described its sedative effects, and Galen later prescribed it for insomnia. In medieval Europe, valerian was widely employed for "nervous afflictions," epilepsy, and as a general tranquilizer.

Traditional European herbal medicine recognizes valerian as a nervine tonic a substance believed to strengthen and soothe the nervous system. The root, which contains the primary active constituents, is usually dried and administered as a tea, tincture, extract, or in powdered capsule form. Valerian is also found in traditional herbal compendia such as Hildegard von Bingen's *Physica* and numerous early modern pharmacopeias, where it is consistently linked to calming the mind and easing restlessness (Malhotra et al., 2024).

Pharmacological Evidence and Mechanism of Action

The therapeutic properties of Valerian are attributed to a complex mix of phytochemicals, primarily found in the root. The key constituents include valerenic acvalerenicenal, valepotriate, isovaleric acid, borneol, and camphene. These compounds work together across several neurochemical pathways that influence both anxiety and sleep. Valerian, often thought of as just a gentle sedative, has a far more complex pharmacology than simple central nervous system depression. Its most notable effect by interacting with the GABAergic system. Valerenic acid acts as a positive allosteric modulator of the GABAA receptor, enhancing the inhibitory action of GABA in the brain. Unlike benzodiazepines, which bind at the receptor's benzodiazepine site, valerenic acid binds to a distinct site on the βsubunit of GABAA receptors. This allows it to potentiate GABAergic activity without inducing the same degree of tolerance, dependence, or sedation. Enhanced GABAergic signaling results in reduced neuronal excitability and a general calming effect, helping alleviate symptoms such as racing thoughts, physical tension, and irritability core features of anxiety.

In addition to direct GABA modulation, valerian may increase endogenous GABA levels by inhibiting its reuptake and degradation. Some studies have suggested that valerian components inhibit GABA transaminase, which is responsible for GABA catabolism. This dual mechanism boosting GABA availability while sensitizing GABAA receptors may explain the calvarian ability to reduce anxiety and promote relaxation in a balanced-suppressivessive manner.

Valerian may influence serotonin (5HT) and adenosine systems beyond that of gamma-aminobutyric acid. Preclinical data suggest that valepotriate may modulate 5HT1A receptor function, a receptor subtype linked to anxiety, mood regulation, and emotional flexibility. Though the evidence here is less robust than for GABA, the serotonergic contribution could explain valerian's mood stabilizing effects in people with stress related symptoms. Additionally, valerian's interaction with adenosine receptors, which help regulate sleep and arousal, may further support its anxiolytic and sedative profile (senn et al., 2025).

Another important aspect of valerian's mechanism is its effect on calcium and potassium ion channels. Certain valepotriates can reduce calcium influx and stabilize neuronal firing rates. By modulating excitatory transmission at the synaptic level, valerian may reduce the physiological hyperarousal that characterizes many anxiety disorders.

Notably, the valepotriates, though unstable and less well studied in humans, show potential for modulating central nervous system excitability and gene expression related to stress responses. Some animal studies have linked these compounds to hippocampal neurogenesis and HPA axis modulation, suggesting possible adaptogenic or neurotrophic effects over longer durations of use (Orhan, 2021).

In summary, valerian exhibits a poly pharmacological mechanism, acting primarily through GABAA receptor modulation, with secondary effects on serotonin signaling, adenosine pathways, and neuronal ion channels. This layered neurochemical interaction contributes to its profile as a nonaddictive, mild to moderate anxiolytic suitable for chronic use or adjunctive support.

Human Clinical Trials

Valerian has been more extensively studied for insomnia than for anxiety, but several human trials have evaluated its anxiolytic potential often in the context of stress related conditions, generalized anxiety disorder, or procedural anxiety.

In a double blind, placebo-controlled study involving 36 patients with generalized anxiety, administration of valerian extract (100 mg thrice daily) for 4 weeks resulted in significant reductions in Hamilton Anxiety Rating Scale (HAM-A) scores compared to placebo. Patients reported improved calmness without cognitive dulling or sedation. Another study assessing preoperative anxiety found that valerian (500 mg) administered 1-2 hours before surgery was as effective as low dose diazepam in reducing subjective anxiety.

Meta analyses remain cautious due to variation in study quality, extract standardization, and outcome measures. However, a pattern of modest efficacy with excellent tolerability has emerged across studies. Valerian appears most beneficial in individuals with mild to moderate anxiety, situational stress, or comorbid insomnia (Chandra Shekhar et al., 2024).

Toxicology and Side Effects

Valerian is generally regarded as safe and well tolerated when used appropriately. Side effects are typically mild and infrequent, including headache, gastrointestinal upset, drowsiness (usually mild) and vivid dreams or morning grogginess (in some individuals). There are no known cases of dependency or withdrawal associated with valerian. Unlike benzodiazepines, valerian does not appear to impair cognition, driving ability, or psychomotor coordination at recommended doses.

Animal studies and long-term human observations suggest a low toxicity profile, although high doses in rodents have shown hepatomegaly and CNS depression. These effects are not well established in human populations. Valerian may interact with CNS depressants, including alcohol, sedative medications, and anaesthetics. Caution is advised when combining with other GABAergic agents due to potential additive effects (Kenda et al., 2022).

Regulatory Status

Valerian is widely available over the counter across Europe, North America, and parts of Asia. In the European Union, it is approved as a traditional herbal medicinal product for nervous tension and sleep disorders under the Traditional Herbal Medicinal Products Directive (THMPD).

In the United States, valerian is marketed as a dietary supplement under DSHEA regulations. Although no FDA approved drug formulations exist, valerian is included in the monographs of the U.S. Pharmacopeia and the American Herbal Pharmacopoeia.

Several national and international pharmacopeias now include monographs that standardize valerian based on valerenic acid content, ensuring a consistent level of active constituents across commercial preparations (Salman et al., 2025).

Ashwagandha (*Withania somnifera*)

Ethnobotanical Background

Withania somnifera, commonly known as Ashwagandha, is a foundational herb in Ayurveda, where it has been used for over 3,000 years. The name *Ashwagandha* translates to "smell of a horse," referring both to the herb's odor and the belief that it imparts the strength and stamina of a stallion. It is classified in Ayurvedic texts as a rasayana a rejuvenate tonic used to promote longevity, vitality, and resilience against stress.

In classical formulations, Ashwagandha is used to treat conditions related to Vata imbalance, particularly those involving nervous system depletion such as anxiety, fatigue, insomnia, and cognitive decline. Its traditional applications also include use in convalescence, chronic inflammation, and fertility enhancement. The roots are the primary medicinal part, typically consumed as a powder, decoction, or extract. Ashwagandha is globally recognized herb that helps the body cope with stress by modulating the hypothalamic pituitary adrenal (HPA) axis (Mikulska et al., 2023).

Pharmacological Evidence and Mechanism of Action

Ashwagandha's pharmacological actions are attributed to a group of steroidal lactones, cawithanolidelides, sitoindosides, alkaloids, and other bioactive compounds. Whereas, synthetic anxiolytics target a single receptor, ASH works across multiple biological systems, particularly those involved in stress response, neurotransmission, and neuroinflammation.

HPA Axis Modulation and Adaptogenic Effects

Central mechanism of Ashwagandha is, modulation of the HPA axis, a primary hormonal system governing the stress response. Chronic stress leads to sustained activation of this axis, resulting in elevated cortisol levels, hippocampal atrophy, and altered mood and cognition. Ashwagandha has been shown in both animal and human studies to lower cortisol concentrations and restore HPA axis balance.

In rodent models, Ashwagandha reduces stress induced increases in plasma corticosterone and adrenal gland hypertrophy. In humans, standardized root extracts have consistently demonstrated the ability to lower serum cortisol, suggesting direct downregulation of HPA axis hyperactivity a key factor in both generalized anxiety and stress related disorders.

GABAergic Modulation

Ashwagandha also influences GABAergic signalling, a central pathway in anxiety regulation. Animal studies have shown that Ashwagandha extracts increase GABA levels in the brain and enhance GABA receptor sensitivity. Withanolides may bind indirectly to GABAA receptors, mimicking the anxiolytic effects of benzodiazepines without their sedative or addictive properties.

GABA modulation explains the calming; muscle relaxing effects observed in both preclinical and clinical settings. This action is particularly valuable because it does not suppress cognition or alertness a limitation common in pharmaceutical anxiolytics (Park et al., 2023).

Serotonergic and Dopaminergic Influence

Ashwagandha may also interact with serotonin (5HT) and dopamine systems. Some studies indicate upregulation of 5HT1A receptor expression in the cortex and hippocampus, consistent with antidepressant and anxiolytic effects. In parallel, dopamine receptor modulation has been suggested, particularly in prefrontal areas, supporting mood enhancement and mental clarity under stress.

These serotonergic and dopaminergic pathways likely contribute to Ashwagandha's dual action as a mood stabilizer and cognitive enhancer. In contrast to monoamine-based drugs, Ashwagandha's effects emerge without drastic alteration of synaptic neurotransmitter levels, offering a gentler and more balanced modulation (Della Porta et al., 2023).

Anti-inflammatory and Antioxidant Effects

Chronic anxiety is associated with increased neuroinflammation and oxidative stress, which impair neuroplasticity and neurotransmitter signaling. Ashwagandha exhibits potent anti-inflammatory effects by downregulating proinflammatory cytokines (IL6, TNFα) and inhibiting NFκB signaling.

Neurogenesis and BDNF Enhancement

Emerging evidence also points to Ashwagandha's role in enhancing brain derived neurotrophic factor (BDNF) expression. BDNF is essential for synaptic plasticity and emotional resilience. In animal models, Ashwagandha has been shown to promote neurogenesis in the dentate gyrus of the hippocampus, possibly contributing to long-term mood stability and anxiety reduction.

Human Clinical Trials

In a pivotal randomized, double blind, placebo-controlled trial (Chandrasekhar et al. 2012), 64 participants with a history of chronic stress received 300 mg of high concentration Ashwagandha root extract twice daily for 60 days. The treatment group showed a 44% reduction in stress scores (Perceived Stress Scale) and a 28% decrease in serum cortisol, compared to negligible changes in the placebo group.

Another study (Cooley et al. 2009) evaluated Ashwagandha as part of a naturopathic treatment plan for anxiety. Over 12 weeks, the group receiving Ashwagandha had significantly lower anxiety scores compared to the control group receiving psychotherapy alone.

A meta-analysis of five randomized controlled trails concluded that Ashwagandha has a statistically significant effect in reducing anxiety, particularly when standardized extracts (with ≥5% withanolides) are used at doses ranging from 250–600 mg per day. Importantly, the herb was well tolerated in all trials, with no serious adverse events reported (Akhgarjand et al., 2022).

Toxicology and Side Effects

Ashwagandha is generally considered safe and nontoxic when used at therapeutic doses. Rare reports of thyroid stimulation exist, as Ashwagandha may increase T3 and T4 levels in some individuals. Caution is advised in patients with hyperthyroidism or those taking thyroid medications.

Unlike benzodiazepines or SSRIs, Ashwagandha has not been associated with dependency, withdrawal, or cognitive dulling. Longterm safety studies are still limited but early evidence suggests good tolerability over periods of several months. Ashwagandha may interact with sedatives, thyroid medications, and immunosuppressants (Holzman et al., 2025).

Regulatory Status

Ashwagandha is legally available in most countries as an over-the-counter supplement or traditional herbal medicine. In India, it is listed in the Ayurvedic Pharmacopoeia and used widely in clinical Ayurvedic practice. In the United States, Ashwagandha is sold as a dietary supplement, often labeled as an adaptogen or stress relief aid. In the European Union, it is included in the European Medicines Agency (EMA) Herbal Monographs, although regulatory classification varies by country (Ramadoss & Koumaravelou, 2022). Germany and France allow its use under traditional herbal medicine regulations, while the UK permits it as a food supplement. Standardization by withanolide content (typically 5-10%) is becoming more common to ensure consistent clinical dosing and safety (Pandit et al., 2024).

Passionflower (*Passiflora incarnata*)

Ethnobotanical Background

Passiflora incarnata, commonly known as passionflower or maypop, is a climbing vine native to the southeastern United States and parts of Central and South America. Indigenous American tribes, including the Cherokee and Aztecs, traditionally used the plant for treating anxiety, restlessness, and insomnia. Spanish settlers adopted it into early European American herbal practice, and it later appeared in the 19thcentury U.S. Pharmacopoeia.

In traditional herbal medicine, passionflower is used as a mild sedative and nervine, employed to calm emotional agitation, relieve tension headaches, and aid sleep. The aerial parts of the plant particularly the flowers and leaves are used in teas, tinctures, or extracts. In modern herbal pharmacology, *P. incarnata* has gained attention for its potential as a gentle, nonaddictive anxiolytic, often compared to low dose benzodiazepines or herbal sedatives like valerian and lemon balm (La Tempa et al., 2025; Kera et al., 2024).

Pharmacological Evidence and Mechanism of Action

The pharmacological activity of passionflower is primarily linked to its content of flavonoids (especially chrysin, vitexin, isovitexin, and apigenin), glycosides, alkaloids, and trace harmalatype βcarbolines. These constituents exert a multitarget effect, influencing neurotransmitter systems central to anxiety regulation, particularly GABAergic, serotonergic, and dopaminergic pathways.

GABAergic Modulation

The dominant mechanism of passionflower's anxiolytic effect is through enhancement of GABAergic transmission, particularly via GABAA receptors. GABA is the main inhibitory neurotransmitter in the central nervous system, and its dysregulation is a hallmark of many anxiety disorders.

Several flavonoids in *Passiflora incarnata*, most notably chrysin, have been shown to bind to the benzodiazepine site of the GABAA receptor, enhancing GABA induced chloride influx and promoting neuronal inhibition. This mechanism mimics the effect of benzodiazepines but appears to do so with lower potency and minimal sedation, which may explain why passionflower reduces anxiety without heavily impairing cognition or motor function.

Preclinical studies support this mechanism: in mouse models, *P. incarnata* extracts produce anxiolytic behavior comparable to diazepam, and these effects are reversed by flumazenil, a benzodiazepine antagonist further confirming GABAA receptor involvement.

Monoaminergic Activity

In addition to GABAergic effects, some studies suggest modulation of monoamines, particularly serotonin (5HT) and dopamine. While the precise molecular mechanisms are still under investigation, passionflower flavonoids are believed to inhibit monoamine oxidase (MAOA and MAOB) to a mild degree, reducing the breakdown of serotonin and dopamine. These effects may contribute to mood stabilization and enhanced emotional regulation, especially in individuals with coexisting depressive symptoms.

Furthermore, the interaction with 5HT1A receptors, implicated in both anxiety and antidepressant responses, has been proposed. Although direct receptor binding studies are limited, the serotonergic tone influenced by flavonoids and alkaloids in passionflower likely plays a secondary but supportive role in its anxiolytic effect.

βCarbolines and Mild Sedative Activity

Passionflower also contains trace amounts of βcarboline alkaloids such as harman and harmaline. These compounds, structurally like those found in psychoactive plants like *Banisteriopsis caapi*, can act as reversible MAO inhibitors and may influence GABA and dopamine dynamics. At low levels, they are not hallucinogenic or psychoactive but may subtly enhance the herb's anxiolytic and sedative effects. This could explain why some users describe a dreamlike or tranquil mental state after taking passionflower, especially in combination with other calming herbs.

Additionally, the plant's mild sedative effect may stem from adenosinergic modulation, as some flavonoids interact with adenosine receptors involved in the sleep wake cycle and anxiety regulation. In sum, *Passiflora incarnata* works through a converging network of GABAergic potentiation, monoamine modulation, and ion channel regulation, producing a gentle but clinically significant reduction in anxiety without the risks associated with synthetic sedatives (Singla et al., 2025).

Human Clinical Trials

Clinical evidence supporting the anxiolytic effects of passionflower is growing, though still modest in scale. Notably, the herb has been tested both as a standalone intervention and as an adjunct to pharmaceutical treatment.

In a randomized, double blind controlled trial by (Akhondzadeh et al., 2001), *Passiflora incarnata* extract (45 drops/day) was compared to oxazepam (30 mg/day) in patients with Generalized Anxiety Disorder. After four weeks, both groups showed similar reductions in HAMA scores, but passionflower produced significantly less impairment in job performance and alertness, indicating lower sedative burden.

Another clinical study evaluated passionflower extract in the preoperative setting. In a trial involving 60 surgical patients, oral administration of passionflower (500 mg) significantly reduced anxiety before surgery compared to placebo, without impairing psychomotor performance or increasing drowsiness an outcome that benzodiazepines often fail to achieve (Movafegh et al., 2008).

A third study tested a combination formula containing passionflower, valerian, and hops in patients with adjustment disorder and mild anxiety. Participants experienced statistically significant reductions in anxiety symptoms after two weeks, with no serious side effects reported.

While more largescale trials are needed, the existing body of evidence suggests that passionflower is effective for mild to moderate anxiety, especially in contexts where sedation or impaired cognition is undesirable.

Toxicology and Side Effects

Passionflower is generally well tolerated. There are no known cases of toxicity from standard therapeutic use. Passionflower does not appear to cause tolerance, withdrawal, or dependency, making it a safe alternative for long-term or as needed anxiety support. In contrast to benzodiazepines, it maintains efficacy without cognitive dulling or rebound anxiety.

However, caution is advised in individuals taking sedatives, antidepressants, or MAO inhibitors, as there is potential for additive effects, especially if passionflower is taken in concentrated extract form. Pregnant women are typically advised to avoid high doses due to possible uterine stimulating properties observed in some in vitro models.

Regulatory Status

Passionflower is legally available in most regions as an over-the-counter dietary supplement or traditional herbal product. It is included in the European Pharmacopoeia and recognized by Germany's Commission E as a treatment for nervous restlessness and mild anxiety.

In the United States, it is sold under DSHEA guidelines, commonly found in stress relief blends, sleep aids, and single herb formulations. The American Herbal Products Association (AHPA) classifies passionflower as a botanical with a long history of safe use. Standardization of commercial extracts often focuses on total flavonoid content (usually around 1.5-4%), with chrysin or vitexin used as marker compounds.

Passiflora incarnata offers a well-rounded, evidence based herbal option for managing anxiety. Its ability to enhance GABAergic tone without heavy sedation makes it particularly suitable for daytime use and for individuals with mild to moderate anxiety, situational stress, or sleep disturbances. The synergistic effects of flavonoids, alkaloids, and trace βcarbolines contribute to a calming profile that is both gentle and effective.

With strong traditional backing, favorable safety data, and emerging clinical evidence, passionflower represents a valuable addition to the therapeutic toolkit for anxiety especially when long-term safety, cognitive clarity, and minimal drug interactions are priorities (La Tempa et al., 2025).

Chamomile (*Matricaria chamomilla*)

Ethnobotanical Background

Matricaria chamomilla commonly known as German chamomile is one of the most widely used medicinal herbs in traditional European and Middle Eastern herbalism. Its name derives from the Latin *mater* (mother), reflecting its historic association with gentle, nurturing, and healing properties. Chamomile is known primarily as a calming remedy used to treat anxiety, irritability, digestive upset, and sleep disturbances. The dried flower heads are used in teas, tinctures, infusions, and essential oils, often administered to both adults and children for their mild sedative and antispasmodic effects.

In Western herbal traditions, chamomile has been called the "herbal aspirin" and "mother of the gut," reflecting its combined actions on the nervous and gastrointestinal systems. It was described by Dioscorides, Hippocrates, and later by European monastic practitioners as a general tonic for restlessness, melancholy, and digestive disturbances caused by nervous tension. Today, chamomile remains one of the most consumed herbal teas globally and is increasingly studied in clinical contexts for anxiety, insomnia, and mood disorders (Saadatmand et al., 2024).

Pharmacological Evidence and Mechanism of Action

Chamomile owes its medicinal effects to a complex array of phytochemicals, including flavonoids (notably apigenin, luteolin, and quercetin), terpenoids (e.g., bisabolol, chamazulene), and coumarins. These constituents act synergistically across neural, endocrine, and immune pathways to produce chamomile's anxiolytic and calming effects. Unlike fastacting sedatives, chamomile's impact is gentle, cumulative, and well tolerated ideal for individuals seeking mild to moderate support without cognitive or motor impairment.

GABAergic Modulation

The principal anxiolytic mechanism of chamomile involves modulation of the GABAergic system, particularly via the flavonoid apigenin. Apigenin has been shown in vitro and in animal studies to bind to benzodiazepine receptors on GABAA receptors, enhancing the inhibitory action of GABA and promoting neuronal calm. While apigenin binds with lower affinity than diazepam, its action is sufficient to produce a measurable anxiolytic effect without the side effects typically seen with conventional benzodiazepines.

Animal studies have demonstrated that chamomile extract exerts anxiolytic and mild sedative activity like low dose benzodiazepines. These effects are blocked by flumazenil, confirming GABAA receptor involvement. However, unlike synthetic drugs, apigenin does not cause sedation or impair motor function at therapeutic doses, suggesting a safer profile for daytime use.

Anti-inflammatory and HPA Axis Regulation

Chamomile also demonstrates anti-inflammatory properties, particularly through inhibition of proinflammatory cytokines such as TNFα and IL6, and the suppression of NFκB signaling. This is relevant because chronic anxiety is often accompanied by low-grade neuroinflammation, which can alter neurotransmitter balance and promote HPA axis dysregulation.

Bisabolol and chamazulene, volatile oils in chamomile, exhibit potent anti-inflammatory activity and contribute to the herb's overall calming effect. By modulating the immune response and reducing oxidative stress, chamomile may help restore neurochemical balance and resilience under chronic psychological stress.

In addition, chamomile may indirectly regulate the hypothalamic pituitary adrenal (HPA) axis, which becomes dysregulated in anxiety states. While data here is still emerging, some animal models show a reduction in corticosterone levels after chamomile administration suggesting possible attenuation of the stress response.

Serotonergic and Noradrenergic Effects

Emerging evidence also suggests that chamomile may influence monoaminergic transmission, particularly serotonin and norepinephrine. Some flavonoids may partially inhibit monoamine reuptake, while others can influence receptor sensitivity. Although these effects are weaker when compared to synthetic antidepressants, they may help explain chamomile's dual role as an anxiolytic and a mood stabilizer. Overall, chamomile's action spans multiple pathways, including GABA-A modulation, immune regulation, mild serotonergic support, and stress hormone balance, producing a gentle yet measurable shift in both emotional state and physical tension (El Joumaa & Borjac, 2022).

Human Clinical Trials

A landmark randomized, double-blind, placebo-controlled trial conducted by (Amsterdam et al. 2009) assessed the efficacy of *Matricaria chamomilla* extract

(500–1,500 mg/day) in individuals with mild to moderate GAD. The treatment group showed significantly greater reductions in HAMA scores compared to placebo after eight weeks, with excellent tolerability and no serious adverse events. Follow-up studies confirmed these findings, with additional data showing improvements in cooccurring depressive symptoms, sleep quality, and overall wellbeing. In a 2016 long term trial, chamomile not only reduced anxiety but also demonstrated relapse prevention effects in patients who had responded to initial treatment (Mao et al., 2016).

Toxicology and Side Effects

Chamomile is considered one of the safest herbal remedies, even for long-term use. There is no evidence of dependency, withdrawal, or tolerance associated with chamomile. It does not impair cognition, driving ability, or psychomotor skills, making it suitable for use during the day or in combination with other calming strategies (Kazemi et al., 2024).

Regulatory Status

Chamomile is widely accepted in both traditional and modern medicine. It is included in the European Pharmacopoeia, as an approved treatment for gastrointestinal spasms and nervous restlessness, and recognized by the U.S. Pharmacopeia as a safe and effective botanical.

In the United States and most countries, chamomile is sold as a dietary supplement or traditional herbal product. It is available in teas, capsules, extracts, and topical formulations, and used in both conventional and complementary settings. Standardized products often measure apigenin content (typically around 1–1.2%) to ensure quality and consistency.

Matricaria chamomilla (chamomile) exemplifies the strengths of traditional herbal medicinegentle, effective, and remarkably safe. Its mechanism of action is multifaceted, centered on GABAA modulation, anti-inflammatory effects, and HPA axis support, with secondary serotonergic and antioxidant activity.

Backed by a rich ethnobotanical history and emerging clinical trials, chamomile is a viable herbal anxiolytic for individuals with mild to moderate anxiety, especially those seeking natural alternatives to pharmaceuticals. Its safety profile makes it suitable for diverse populations, including the elderly, the anxious but medication averse, and those needing daytime calming without sedation (Carvalho et al., 2025).

Bacopa (*Bacopa monnieri*)

Ethnobotanical Background

Bacopa monnieri, commonly known as Brahmi in Ayurveda, is a creeping aquatic herb found in wetlands across India, Southeast Asia, and parts of Australia. It has been used for thousands of years in Ayurvedic medicine as a medhya rasayana, a class of herbs believed to enhance intellect, memory, and emotional stability. Ancient texts of Ayurveda like *Charaka Samhita* and *Sushruta Samhita* states, Brahmi has ability in improving mental function, calming the mind, and treating conditions like anxiety, epilepsy, and insomnia.

Bacopa has long been used to restore balance in the nervous system, often alongside other nootropic and adaptogenic herbs. While best known for enhancing cognitive function, it also supports emotional regulation, making it one of the few botanicals that serves as both a nootropic and an anxiolytic. The whole plant has medicinal value, but modern extracts primarily use the leaves, which are often standardized for their bacoside content (Joshi et al., 2021).

Pharmacological Evidence and Mechanism of Action

Bacopa's therapeutic effects are primarily linked to bacosides A and B, triterpenoid saponins found only in this plant. These compounds influence the central nervous system through multiple mechanisms, including regulation of neurotransmitters, enhancement of neuroplasticity, and reduction of oxidative stress. Unlike sedatives, Bacopa's anxiolytic action works over time, helping to recalibrate the stress response and maintain neurochemical balance.

Modulation of Serotonergic and Dopaminergic Systems

Bacopa has been shown to upregulate serotonergic activity, particularly via 5-HT1A receptor expression, which plays a central role in anxiety regulation. In animal models, chronic administration of Bacopa extract increases serotonin levels in the hippocampus, cortex, and other emotion-regulating areas of the brain.

This serotonergic enhancement is not as immediate or forceful as that produced by SSRIs, but it contributes to gradual mood stabilization and emotional resilience. Additionally, Bacopa may modulate dopamine and norepinephrine levels, especially in the prefrontal cortex, contributing to improved mood, attentional control, and reward processing.

Unlike monoamine oxidase inhibitors or reuptake inhibitors, Bacopa appears to influence neurotransmitter levels through indirect modulation of enzyme activity and receptor sensitivity, resulting in a balanced, non-overstimulating effect.

Though not its primary mechanism, Bacopa may also interact with the GABAergic system. Some studies suggest increased GABA synthesis or receptor density following chronic use, supporting its anxiolytic effects. This GABAergic support is subtle but synergistic, contributing to the calming effect without producing sedation.

Bacopa's influence on the cholinergic system, particularly through acetylcholine enhancement and acetylcholinesterase inhibition, supports its cognitive-enhancing and stress-buffering properties. This overlap of cognitive and emotional support is unique among herbal anxiolytics and helps explain Bacopa's traditional classification as a "brain tonic."

Antioxidant and Neuroprotective Effects

Chronic anxiety is associated with increased oxidative stress and impaired mitochondrial function in key brain regions. Bacopa possesses strong antioxidant properties, primarily through activation of endogenous defense enzymes such as superoxide dismutase (SOD), catalase, and glutathione peroxidase. These actions help reduce neuronal damage, improve synaptic integrity, and support long-term emotional stability.

Modulation of the HPA Axis

Bacopa exhibits adaptogenic properties, modulating the hypothalamic-pituitary-adrenal (HPA) axis and reducing cortisol levels in stressed animals. In rodent models, Bacopa reverses stress-induced changes in adrenal gland size, cortisol secretion, and anxiety-like behavior. While HPA regulation in humans is still under investigation, early clinical data support its capacity to blunt physiological stress responses over time.

Neuroplasticity and BDNF Upregulation

Finally, Bacopa may promote neurogenesis and brain-derived neurotrophic factor (BDNF) expression, particularly in the hippocampus, a region critically involved in emotion regulation and cognitive processing. Enhanced BDNF supports resilience to stress and the capacity to adaptively rewire thought-emotion patterns, a core deficit in many anxiety disorders.

Taken together, Bacopa acts as a neuromodulator and neuroprotectant, gradually building a biochemical environment conducive to calmness, clarity, and emotional resilience rather than inducing sedation or rapid symptomatic relief (Fathima et al., 2022).

Human Clinical Trials

Though better known as a cognitive enhancer, Bacopa has been evaluated in several clinical trials for its anxiolytic effects often as a secondary outcome.

In a randomized, double-blind, placebo-controlled trial involving 54 healthy adults, (Stough et al. 2008) found that 300 mg/day of standardized Bacopa extract (containing 55% bacosides) significantly improved memory retention and reduced state anxiety over 12 weeks. Participants also reported improved emotional regulation and reduced nervousness.

Another study in older adults showed that Bacopa not only enhanced cognitive performance but also led to reductions in anxiety and depression scores as measured by the DASS-21 (Depression, Anxiety, and Stress Scale) (Morgan & Stevens, 2010).

More recent studies have evaluated Bacopa as part of multi-herb formulations in adolescents and adults with anxiety and attention-deficit symptoms. In most cases, Bacopa contributed to reductions in restlessness, worry, and emotional dysregulation suggesting its broader application in stress-related syndromes.

Regulatory Status

Bacopa is widely available as a dietary supplement. In India, it is officially listed in the Ayurvedic Pharmacopoeia and extensively used in traditional formulations. It is also recognized in the British Herbal Pharmacopoeia and included in monographs by the American Herbal Pharmacopoeia.

Standardized Bacopa extracts are usually titrated to 20-55% bacosides, which is considered the key bioactive marker. Quality control and standardization are important, as non-standardized products may vary significantly in potency (Hossain et al., 2022).

St. John's Wort (Hypericum perforatum)

Ethnobotanical Background

Hypericum perforatum, commonly known as St. John's Wort, is a perennial flowering herb native to Europe and Asia and now naturalized across North America and Australia. Its medicinal use dates back more than 2,000 years, appearing in texts by Hippocrates, Dioscorides, and later in medieval European herbalism where it was used for "melancholy," nervous agitation, and disturbances of the spirit. Traditionally, the aerial parts were harvested around the summer solstice (St. John's Day), believed to enhance the plant's potency. While best known for its antidepressant effects, St. John's Wort has also been used in folk medicine for anxiety, restlessness, and psychosomatic symptoms associated with stress.

Pharmacological Evidence and Mechanism of Action

It contains various bioactive compounds, such as hypericin, hyperforin, flavonoids, phenolic acids, where each contributes to neuropharmacological profile. The mechanism behind St. John's Wort's is inhibition of synaptic reuptake of serotonin, dopamine and norepinephrine. The reuptake inhibition increases monoamine presence. It also acts on GABAergic and Glutamatergic receptors, HPA Axis. It has great anti-inflammatory and neuroprotective effects.

Toxicology and Side Effects

It is strong inducer of CYP3A4, CYP2C9, CYP2C19, and P-glycoprotein and can reduce blood levels of oral contraceptives, warfarin, antiretrovirals, immunosuppressants (e.g., cyclosporine), and many cardiovascular drugs. Because many individuals self-prescribe Hypericum products, recognizing and managing these interactions is essential for safe use.

Regulatory Status

St. John's Wort is approved in several European countries (e.g., Germany) as an over-the-counter phytopharmaceutical for mild to moderate depression. It appears in the European Medicines Agency's herbal monographs and is included in WHO guidelines for herbal psychotropics.

In the United States, it is marketed as a dietary supplement under DSHEA regulations. Standardized products typically specify hypericin or hyperforin content, though significant variability across brands has been documented, underscoring the need for tighter quality control.

Magnolia Bark (*Magnolia officinalis*)

Ethnobotanical Background

Magnolia officinalis is a deciduous tree native to China, long used as classical remedy for "stagnation of Qi" and disorders involving anxiety, digestive discomfort, and insomnia. For over 2,000 years, it has been used to treat symptoms such as abdominal bloating, emotional distress, restlessness, and shortness of breath linked to stress and anxiety. It is often prescribed in formulas alongside other calming herbs like *Poria cocos*, *Ziziphus jujuba*, or *Bupleurum chinense*.

While *Magnolia officinalis* was traditionally viewed through an energetic and organ-centred framework, modern research has uncovered potent bioactive compounds in the bark that exert direct neuropharmacological effects particularly relevant for anxiety, stress, and mood disorders.

Pharmacological Evidence and Mechanism of Action

The therapeutic potential of magnolia bark lies in its key active compounds: honokiol and magnolol, two biphenolic neolignans that have shown powerful central nervous system effects in both preclinical and emerging human data. These compounds operate through multiple mechanisms, most notably GABAergic modulation, endocannabinoid system interaction, anti-inflammatory activity, and monoaminergic balance.

GABA-A Receptor Modulation

Honokiol and magnolol, the main active compounds in magnolia, help calm the nervous system by boosting the effects of GABA at its receptors by working on different sites unlike benzodiazepines. This reduces overactive nerve signaling and eases anxiety without the heavy sedation, muscle relaxation, or mental fog that often come with prescription tranquilizers. In animal studies, honokiol has eased anxiety as effectively as diazepam but without affecting movement or causing tolerance. This makes magnolia especially appealing for people who need relief during the day but want to stay clear-headed and alert.

Endocannabinoid System Interaction

Activation of the CB1 receptor modulates neurotransmitter release, reduces excitotoxicity, and regulates the HPA axis all of which are disrupted in chronic anxiety states. Honokiol interacts with cannabinoid receptors, particularly CB1 receptors, contributing to anxiolytic and neuroprotective effects. This interaction may also explain honokiol's ability to change stress responses, improve emotional regulation, and influence neuroplasticity in regions such as the amygdala and prefrontal cortex.

Monoaminergic Modulation

Although not a primary pathway, magnolia bark may also influence dopaminergic and serotonergic signaling. Some studies have observed honokiol-mediated increases in dopamine and serotonin turnover in limbic brain regions, contributing to improvements in mood and motivation. These effects are particularly relevant for anxious depression or mixed anxiety-depression states.

Interestingly, magnolia also demonstrates some acetylcholinesterase inhibition, suggesting mild cognitive-enhancing potential that may complement its anxiolytic profile.

In sum, magnolia bark exerts anxiolytic effects through a blend of GABA-A enhancement, CB1 activation, inflammation reduction, making it one of the few botanicals to target both neurotransmitter systems and neuroinflammatory pathways simultaneously (Ming-Xin Guo et al., 2023).

Human Clinical Trials

Human studies on magnolia bark remain limited but promising. Most clinical research has evaluated it as part of multi-herb or multi-nutrient formulas, often with *Phellodendron amurense* (in a common blend called Relora), used to treat stress-related eating, anxiety, and mood instability.

In a randomized, placebo-controlled trial (Talbott et al., 2013), 56 overweight individuals with chronic stress received Relora for 6 weeks. Compared to placebo, the treatment group had significant reductions in cortisol levels, perceived stress scores, and anxiety symptoms without any sedative effects.

Another double-blind study assessed Relora in premenopausal women with moderate anxiety and found significant reductions in state anxiety as early as two weeks. Sleep quality, mood, and stress reactivity were also improved (Kalman et al., 2008).

Regulatory Status

Magnolia bark is legally available in most countries as a dietary supplement or traditional herbal ingredient. In Traditional Chinese Medicine, *Magnolia officinalis* is a licensed component in hundreds of formulas, particularly those addressing mood, digestion, and lung function.

In the West, it is sold both as a single extract and in combination with other herbs under stress-support and sleep-aid labels. Standardized extracts typically contain 2–10% honokiol, though quality control can vary among commercial products.

There are no major regulatory restrictions on magnolia bark when used at appropriate doses. It is generally recognized as safe (GRAS) in the U.S., and accepted as a traditional medicine in China, Japan, and Korea (Zhang, D. 2025).

Table 1. Overview of traditional anxiolytics

Herb	Primary Mechanisms	Clinical Use Level	Sedation Risk	Dependency Risk	Regulatory Status
Kava (Piper methysticum)	GABA-A modulation, Dopamine enhancement, MAO-B inhibition	Moderate (Good evidence for GAD)	Low to Moderate (dose-dependent)	Low (with traditional prep)	Varies by country; restricted in some regions due to hepatotoxicity concerns
Valerian (Valeriana officinalis)	GABA-A modulation, Serotonin support	Moderate (Commonly used for sleep/anxiety)	Mild (less than benzodiazepines)	None	Widely approved as dietary supplement or traditional medicine
Ashwagandha (Withania somnifera)	HPA axis modulation, GABA support, BDNF upregulation	Strong (Multiple RCTs support use in anxiety and stress)	Minimal	None	Widely available; official in Ayurvedic pharmacopoeia
Passionflower (Passiflora incarnata)	GABA-A modulation, Mild MAO inhibition	Moderate (RCTs support use in mild to moderate anxiety)	Low	None	Approved as traditional medicine; dietary supplement in US/EU

continued on following page

Table 1. Continued

Herb	Primary Mechanisms	Clinical Use Level	Sedation Risk	Dependency Risk	Regulatory Status
Chamomile (Matricaria chamomilla)	GABA-A modulation, Anti-inflammatory, Serotonergic support	Mild to Moderate (Good for subclinical anxiety and sleep)	Minimal	None	Approved in EU and US; widely used OTC
Bacopa (Bacopa monnieri)	Serotonin enhancement, BDNF, HPA modulation	Mild to Moderate (Supports cognitive-emotional balance)	None	None	Approved in Ayurvedic/ Traditional systems, OTC globally
Magnolia (Magnolia officinalis)	GABA-A modulation, CB1 activation, Anti-inflammatory	Emerging (Strong preclinical, limited human data)	Low	None	Dietary supplement in US/ EU; official in TCM

SAFETY AND DRUG-HERB INTERACTIONS

Herbal anxiolytics depends on quality, dose, concurrent medications, and physiology. Though each herb has its own toxicological profile, and understanding potential interactions is important for researchers and clinicians to evaluate clinical applicability. Kava enhances GABAergic signaling and produce sedative effects when used in combination with alcohol, opioids, benzodiazepines. Excessive CNS depression is a safety concern, especially in geriatrics. Valerian is similar with risk of excessive sedatives and anesthetic agents. Clinician should be aware of Herb-drug interactions, altered drug metabolism, synergistic sedation (Le, et al., 2022). Overview of major interactions are in Table 2.

Table 2. Clinical dosing, formulations, and key drug–herb interactions of major herbal anxiolytics

Herb	Typical Standardized Dose	Common Formulations	Key Drug-Herb Interactions
Kava *(Piper methysticum)*	70–250 mg kavalactones/day	Standardized extract, traditional water infusion	Additive sedation with benzodiazepines, alcohol, opioids; avoid with hepatotoxic drugs
Valerian *(Valeriana officinalis)*	300–600 mg extract (0.8% valerenic acids)	Capsules, tinctures, teas	Additive sedation with CNS depressants and anesthetics
Ashwagandha *(Withania somnifera)*	250–600 mg extract (5–10% withanolides)	Capsules, powders, standardized extracts	Potentiation with sedatives; caution with thyroid medications and immunosuppressants
Passionflower *(Passiflora incarnata)*	200–500 mg extract or 30–60 drops tincture	Capsules, tinctures, teas	Additive effects with sedatives; theoretical MAOI interaction

continued on following page

Table 2. Continued

Herb	Typical Standardized Dose	Common Formulations	Key Drug-Herb Interactions
Chamomile *(Matricaria chamomilla)*	220–1,500 mg extract/day; tea infusions	Teas, capsules, liquid extracts	Mild interactions with anticoagulants (coumarin-sensitive individuals)
Bacopa *(Bacopa monnieri)*	300 mg/day (20–55% bacosides)	Capsules, powders, standardized extracts	Minimal; may enhance sedative effects at high doses
Magnolia *(Magnolia officinalis)*	200–400 mg extract (2–10% honokiol)	Capsules, combination formulas (e.g., Relora)	Additive sedation; caution with CNS depressants
St. John's Wort *(Hypericum perforatum)*	300 mg TID (0.3% hypericin or 2–5% hyperforin)	Capsules, tablets, teas	Strong CYP3A4 induction; dangerous interactions with SSRIs/SNRIs/MAOIs; reduces efficacy of many drugs

Evidence-Based Evaluation of Efficacy

Herbal anxiolytics have been used for centuries in traditional medicine systems, yet only in recent decades have they become the subject of formal clinical evaluation. As demand for natural alternatives to pharmaceutical anxiolytics grows, a growing number of randomized controlled trials (RCTs), observational studies, and meta-analyses have attempted to quantify the efficacy and safety of these plant-based treatments. This section reviews the clinical evidence behind major herbal anxiolytics, critically assesses their performance against standard pharmaceutical options, and explores the methodological challenges that continue to limit definitive conclusions in the field (Zhang et al., 2022).

Comparative Effectiveness vs. Standard Anxiolytics

One of the central questions in evaluating the therapeutic potential of herbal anxiolytics is how their efficacy and safety compare to standard pharmacological treatments, such as benzodiazepines, selective serotonin reuptake inhibitors (SSRIs), and buspirone. While large-scale, double-blind, head-to-head trials remain limited, several studies have explored this comparison, offering valuable insight into relative performance.

In a randomized controlled trial conducted by (Akhondzadeh et al. 2001), Passiflora incarnata (passionflower) extract was compared directly to oxazepam, a short-acting benzodiazepine. Over a 4-week treatment period for patients with generalized anxiety disorder (GAD), passionflower was found to be comparably effective in reducing anxiety symptoms. Importantly, the herbal treatment was associated with fewer reports of impairment in job performance and did not produce significant sedation an advantage over oxazepam, which commonly causes drowsiness and psychomotor slowing. Similar findings have emerged in studies of preoperative anxiety, where passionflower demonstrated comparable anxiolytic effects to midazolam (a fast-acting benzodiazepine) without inducing cognitive impairment or delayed recovery time (Movafegh et al., 2008).

Withania somnifera (ashwagandha) has not yet been evaluated in direct comparisons with benzodiazepines, but it has been studied alongside SSRIs and other standard medications. In one open-label, comparative study involving patients with mixed anxiety and depressive symptoms, ashwagandha was found to perform on par with SSRIs in reducing anxiety scores, while also displaying a more favorable tolerability profile (Cooley et al., 2009). Patients receiving ashwagandha reported fewer adverse events and better sleep quality, suggesting potential for its use in chronic or stress-related anxiety disorders where long-term safety is essential.

Matricaria chamomilla (chamomile) has consistently shown modest anxiolytic effects in individuals with GAD when compared to placebo. A notable randomized controlled trial by (Amsterdam et al. 2009) demonstrated significant symptom reduction in participants receiving chamomile extract, although the magnitude of improvement was generally smaller than what is typically observed with SSRIs in similar populations.

Overall, herbal anxiolytics tend to be less potent than prescription drugs but are generally better tolerated. They usually take longer to work, and their effects are milder, which means they may not be the best choice for acute or severe anxiety. But for ongoing, low-level anxiety, they offer advantages: less sedation, minimal risk of dependency or withdrawal, and fewer concerns about long-term harm. While the current research is encouraging, but still lack, high-quality trials in diverse populations. Future studies should focus on standardizing herbal formulations.

Limitations:

Research on herbal anxiolytics shows promise but is limited by small sample sizes, lack of product standardization, inconsistent blinding, and wide variation in dosing. Many trials on herbs like valerian, bacopa, and passionflower involve fewer than 100 participants, reducing reliability. Extracts often differ in composition due to species, sourcing, and preparation, yet studies rarely report or standardize their phytochemical profiles. Blinding is frequently inadequate, especially with herbs that have strong tastes or odors, increasing placebo risk. Doses vary widely sometimes beyond traditional use making it hard to establish effective guidelines.

To move herbal anxiolytics into mainstream care, larger, well-designed trials with standardized products and consistent dosing are essential.

Advances in Phytochemical Screening and Standardization

A major barrier to bringing herbal anxiolytics into mainstream use has been inconsistent chemical composition. Traditional remedies often use whole plants or crude extracts with little control over active ingredient levels. Modern tools like LC-MS, NMR spectroscopy, and HPTLC now allow precise mapping and measurement of phytochemicals such as withanolide from ashwagancha ensuring consistency for both efficacy and regulatory approval. Metabolomics is revealing how complex phytochemical networks work together, moving beyond the outdated "one plant–one compound" model. DNA barcoding adds another layer by confirming species identity and preventing adulteration. Together, these advances are making standardized, reliable botanical medicines a realistic goal.

Adulteration and Quality Control

The pharmacokinetic and pharmacodynamic profile of herbal anxiolytics depend on the product authenticity and chemical consistency. Hepatoxicity of kava was became an issue in early 2000s due to usage of aerial part of plants and organic solvent extracts than traditional aqueous extract of peeled roots. Even ashwagandha and bacopa are easily adulterated with saponin rich plants. DNA barcoding, a HPLC and metabolomic fingerprinting for verification and phytochemical standardization. However, some variations are common in supplement markets, making 3rd party testing and transparent labelling is needed for clinical reliability.

Integration into Mainstream Psychiatry

Psychiatry is beginning to adapt the door to evidence-based herbal treatments, though progress is gradual. Conventional options for chronic anxiety such as SS-RIs or benzodiazepines are effective for many patients, but their long-term use can bring side effects like dependence, withdrawal symptoms, and cognitive dulling. These concerns have pushed some clinicians to explore complementary strategies that offer relief without the same risks. Randomized controlled trials supports the benefits of herbs like chamomile, ashwagandha, and passionflower for reducing anxiety symptoms. Patients themselves are increasingly seeking approaches that feel safer, avoid sedation, and align with personal or cultural health traditions. At the same time, integrative and functional psychiatry is gaining ground, emphasizing lifestyle, nutrition, and phytomedicine as central to mental health care rather than peripheral additions. The aim is not to replace standard medications but to create well-designed co-therapy models in which botanicals work alongside conventional treatments. This blended approach could allow for more personalized care offering symptom relief, improving long-term tolerability, and respecting patient preferences all while staying grounded in rigorous evidence (Zhang et al., 2022).

Personalized Medicine and Pharmacogenomics

Pharmacogenomics tailoring treatment based on a person's genetic makeup is reshaping modern medicine, and its application to herbal therapy is gaining traction. Genetic variations in CYP450 enzymes, serotonin transporters, and HPA-axis genes affect how individuals metabolize and respond to plant compounds. For instance, some people may derive stronger effects from bacopa or chamomile due to variations in gut flora or receptor sensitivity. Gut bacteria can metabolize plant flavonoids into neuroactive substances, implying that the microbiome may be a key determinant of efficacy in herbal therapy. In the future, clinicians may use genomic and microbiomic profiling to predict herb responsiveness, creating a framework for truly personalized neurophytomedicine (Zhang et al., 2022).

CONCLUSION: BRIDGING TRADITION AND SCIENCE IN ANXIETY CARE

Traditional herbal anxiolytics continue to attract clinical and scientific interest because they target anxiety through multiple neurobiological pathways and offer a wider therapeutic breadth than many single-target pharmaceuticals. Across the herbs reviewed, a consistent pattern emerges: actions on GABAergic signaling, monoaminergic modulation, HPA axis regulation, neuroinflammation, and redox balance often converge to produce meaningful anxiolytic effects. This polypharmacological nature aligns well with the complex physiology of anxiety and helps explain why several botanicals show clinical promise despite their relatively gentle pharmacodynamic profile.

Among the herbs evaluated, the strongest human evidence supports Ashwagandha, Chamomile, and Kava each backed by randomized controlled trials and measurable improvements in stress or anxiety scores. Passionflower and Valerian demonstrate moderate, situational benefits, particularly where mild anxiety coexists with sleep disturbances. Bacopa and Magnolia contribute additional support for cognitive-emotional regulation, although current evidence is still emerging. St. John's Wort remains clinically relevant for mixed anxiety–depression states but requires careful monitoring due to its extensive interaction profile.

Despite these encouraging findings, important challenges remain. Variability in extract quality, incomplete phytochemical standardization, high placebo response rates, and small trial sizes continue to limit comparability and confidence. Safety considerations especially drug-herb interactions, mislabeling, and adulteration must also be taken seriously in real-world use. Standardized dosing ranges, clear contraindications, and consistent reporting of active constituents are essential steps toward improving reliability and clinical utility.

Looking forward, neurophytomedicine sits at a productive intersection of traditional practice and modern neuroscience. Advances in analytical chemistry, regulatory harmonization, pharmacogenomics, and integrative medicine offer an opportunity to develop botanical therapies that are consistent, evidence-based, and clinically actionable. The field's future lies not in replacing conventional anxiolytics but in building thoughtful, evidence-supported bridges between phytomedicine and modern psychiatric care. By integrating mechanistic insight, clinical evidence, and practical guidance, traditional herbal anxiolytics can play a meaningful role in a more holistic, patient-centered approach to anxiety management.

Opportunities and Challenges

We stand at a point of convergence. Advances in phytochemistry, AI, pharmacogenomics, and systems biology are unlocking the potential of plant-based therapies. At the same time, challenges persist particularly around standardization, regulation, safety, and ethical sourcing. Global use of herbal products demands a shared regulatory language and commitment to quality. Additionally, we must address sustainability and biopiracy, ensuring that indigenous knowledge systems and ecosystems are respected, protected, and compensated. The most promising future for neurophytomedicine lies not in rejecting modern pharmacology but in building bridges between traditional insight and scientific rigor.

REFERENCES

Akhgarjand, C., Asoudeh, F., Bagheri, A., Kalantar, Z., Vahabi, Z., Shab-bidar, S., Rezvani, H., & Djafarian, K. (2022). Does Ashwagandha supplementation have a beneficial effect on the management of anxiety and stress? A systematic review and meta-analysis of randomized controlled trials. *Phytotherapy Research, 36*(11), 4115–4124. DOI: 10.1002/ptr.7598 PMID: 36017529

Akhondzadeh, S., Naghavi, H. R., Vazirian, M., Shayeganpour, A., Rashidi, H., & Khani, M. (2001). Passionflower in the treatment of generalized anxiety: A pilot double-blind randomized controlled trial with oxazepam. *Journal of Clinical Pharmacy and Therapeutics, 26*(5), 363–367. DOI: 10.1046/j.1365-2710.2001.00367.x PMID: 11679026

Amsterdam, J. D., Li, Y., Soeller, I., Rockwell, K., Mao, J. J., & Shults, J. (2009). A randomized, double-blind, placebo-controlled trial of oral Matricaria recutita (chamomile) extract therapy for generalized anxiety disorder. *Journal of Clinical Psychopharmacology, 29*(4), 378–382. DOI: 10.1097/JCP.0b013e3181ac935c PMID: 19593179

Asare-Doku, W., Settumba Stolk, S., Peacock, A., Shakeshaft, A., Waller, E., Nathan, S., & Farrell, M. (2023). *Monitoring and evaluation of the kava pilot program*. National Drug and Alcohol Research Centre, UNSW.

Borrás, S., Martínez-Solís, I., & Ríos, J. L. (2021). Medicinal plants for insomnia related to anxiety: An updated review. *Planta Medica, 87*(10/11), 738–753. DOI: 10.1055/a-1510-9826 PMID: 34116572

Burton, N., Sneed, K., & Pathak, Y. (2023). Systemic Review of the Use of Kava Kava for the Reduction of Anxiety Disorder.

Carvalho, A. C. B., Perfeito, J. P. S., de Britto Vidal Filho, W., & Silveira, D. (2025). A decade retrospective and future prospects: How European regulatory alignment shapes Brazil's herbal medicine market. *Journal of Ethnopharmacology, 353*, 120404. DOI: 10.1016/j.jep.2025.120404 PMID: 40803612

Chandra Shekhar, H., Joshua, L., & Thomas, J. V. (2024). Standardized extract of Valeriana officinalis improves overall sleep quality in human subjects with sleep complaints: A randomized, double-blind, placebo-controlled, clinical study. *Advances in Therapy, 41*(1), 246–261. DOI: 10.1007/s12325-023-02708-6 PMID: 37899385

Chandrasekhar, K., Kapoor, J., & Anishetty, S. (2012). A prospective, randomized double-blind, placebo-controlled study of safety and efficacy of a high-concentration full-spectrum extract of ashwagandha root in reducing stress and anxiety in adults. *Indian Journal of Psychological Medicine*, *34*(3), 255–262. DOI: 10.4103/0253-7176.106022 PMID: 23439798

Conway, C. C., Grogans, S. E., Anderson, A. S., Islam, S., Craig, L. E., Wedlock, J., Hur, J., DeYoung, K. A., & Shackman, A. J. (2024). Neuroticism Is Prospectively Associated With 30-Month Changes in Broadband Internalizing Symptoms, but Not Narrowband Positive Affect or Anxious Arousal, in Emerging Adulthood. *Clinical Psychological Science*, *12*(5), 823–839. DOI: 10.1177/21677026231205270 PMID: 39359716

Cooley, K., Szczurko, O., Perri, D., Mills, E. J., Bernhardt, B., Zhou, Q., & Seely, D. (2009). Naturopathic care for anxiety: A randomized controlled trial ISRCTN78958974. *PLoS One*, *4*(8), e6628. DOI: 10.1371/journal.pone.0006628 PMID: 19718255

Della Porta, M., Maier, J. A., & Cazzola, R. (2023). Effects of Withania somnifera on cortisol levels in stressed human subjects: A systematic review. *Nutrients*, *15*(24), 5015. DOI: 10.3390/nu15245015 PMID: 38140274

El Joumaa, M. M., & Borjac, J. M. (2022). Matricaria chamomilla: A valuable insight into recent advances in medicinal uses and pharmacological activities. *Phytochemistry Reviews*, *21*(6), 1913–1940. DOI: 10.1007/s11101-022-09817-0

Grosso, C., Santos, M., & Barroso, M. F. (2023). From plants to psycho-neurology: Unravelling the therapeutic benefits of bioactive compounds in brain disorders. *Antioxidants*, *12*(8), 1603. DOI: 10.3390/antiox12081603 PMID: 37627598

Holzman, A., Brown, A. E., Kelley, J., Rappaport, D., & Martini, W. A. (2025). Unmasking Potential Withdrawal Effects of Ashwagandha: A Case Report and Review. *Cureus*, *17*(5). Advance online publication. DOI: 10.7759/cureus.83577 PMID: 40476122

Hossain, C. M., Gera, M. E. E. T. A., & Ali, K. A. (2022). Current status and challenges of herbal drug development and regulatory aspect: A global perspective. *Asian Journal of Pharmaceutical and Clinical Research*, *15*(2), 31–41. DOI: 10.22159/ajpcr.2022.v15i12.46134

Javaid, S. F., Hashim, I. J., Hashim, M. J., Stip, E., Samad, M. A., & Ahbabi, A. A. (2023). Epidemiology of anxiety disorders: Global burden and sociodemographic associations. *Middle East Current Psychiatry, Ain Shams University*, *30*(1), 44. DOI: 10.1186/s43045-023-00315-3

Joshi, T., Gupta, A., Kumar, P., Singh, A., & Kumar, A. (2021). Bacopa monnieri (brahmi). In *Naturally Occurring Chemicals Against Alzheimer's Disease* (pp. 243–256). Academic Press. DOI: 10.1016/B978-0-12-819212-2.00020-7

Kalman, D. S., Feldman, S., Feldman, R., Schwartz, H. I., Krieger, D. R., & Garrison, R. (2008). Effect of a proprietary Magnolia and Phellodendronextract on stress levels in healthy women: A pilot, double-blind, placebo-controlled clinical trial. *Nutrition Journal, 7*(1), 1–6. DOI: 10.1186/1475-2891-7-11

Kazemi, A., Shojaei-Zarghani, S., Eskandarzadeh, P., & Hashempur, M. H. (2024). Effects of chamomile (Matricaria chamomilla L.) on sleep: A systematic review and meta-analysis of clinical trials. *Complementary Therapies in Medicine, 84*, 103071. DOI: 10.1016/j.ctim.2024.103071 PMID: 39106912

Kenda, M., Kočevar Glavač, N., Nagy, M., & Sollner Dolenc, M. (2022). Medicinal plants used for anxiety, depression, or stress treatment: An update. *Molecules (Basel, Switzerland), 27*(18), 6021. DOI: 10.3390/molecules27186021 PMID: 36144755

Kera, V., Nath, S., Kotso, A., Resuh, V., & Dutta, A. (2024). Melissa Officinalis: A Review on the Antioxidant, Anxiolytic, and Anti-depressant Activity. *Biosciences Biotechnology Research Asia, 21*(2), 491–500. DOI: 10.13005/bbra/3241

Küpeli Akkol, E., Tatlı Çankaya, I., Şeker Karatoprak, G., Carpar, E., Sobarzo-Sánchez, E., & Capasso, R. (2021). Natural compounds as medical strategies in the prevention and treatment of psychiatric disorders seen in neurological diseases. *Frontiers in Pharmacology, 12*, 669638. DOI: 10.3389/fphar.2021.669638 PMID: 34054540

La Tempa, A., Ferraiuolo, G., Pranzetti, B., Pruccoli, J., & Parmeggiani, A. (2025). Passiflora Incarnata L. Herba in the Treatment of Anxiety Symptoms and Insomnia in Children and Adolescents with Feeding and Eating Disorders. *Adolescents (Basel, Switzerland), 5*(2), 24. DOI: 10.3390/adolescents5020024

Le, T. T., McGrath, S. R., & Fasinu, P. S. (2022). Herb-drug interactions in neuropsychiatric pharmacotherapy–a review of clinically relevant findings. *Current Neuropharmacology, 20*(9), 1736–1751. DOI: 10.2174/1570159X196662108091 00357 PMID: 34370637

Malhotra, P., Minocha, N., Pandey, P., Kaushik, D., & Vashist, N. (2024). A review on history, chemical constituents, phytochemistry, pharmacological activities, and recent patents of Valerian. *The Natural Products Journal, 14*(2), 98–106. DOI: 10 .2174/2210315514666230718100526

Mao, J. J., Xie, S. X., Keefe, J. R., Soeller, I., Li, Q. S., & Amsterdam, J. D. (2016). Long-term chamomile (Matricaria chamomilla L.) treatment for generalized anxiety disorder: A randomized clinical trial. *Phytomedicine*, *23*(14), 1735–1742. DOI: 10.1016/j.phymed.2016.10.012 PMID: 27912875

Mathews, I. M., Eastwood, J., Lamport, D. J., Cozannet, R. L., Fanca-Berthon, P., & Williams, C. M. (2024). Clinical efficacy and tolerability of lemon balm (Melissa officinalis L.) in psychological well-being: A review. *Nutrients*, *16*(20), 3545. DOI: 10.3390/nu16203545 PMID: 39458539

Mikulska, P., Malinowska, M., Ignacyk, M., Szustowski, P., Nowak, J., Pesta, K., Szeląg, M., Szklanny, D., Judasz, E., Kaczmarek, G., Ejiohuo, O. P., Paczkowska-Walendowska, M., Gościniak, A., & Cielecka-Piontek, J. (2023). Ashwagandha (Withania somnifera)—current research on the health-promoting activities: A narrative review. *Pharmaceutics*, *15*(4), 1057. DOI: 10.3390/pharmaceutics15041057 PMID: 37111543

Ming-Xin Guo, M. M., Wu, X., Feng, Y. F., & Hu, Z. Q. (2023). Research Progress on the structural modification of Magnolol and Honokiol and the Biological activities of their derivatives. *Chemistry & Biodiversity*, *20*(8), e202300754. DOI: 10.1002/cbdv.202300754 PMID: 37401658

Morgan, A., & Stevens, J. (2010). Does Bacopa monnieri improve memory performance in older persons? Results of a randomized, placebo-controlled, double-blind trial. *Journal of Alternative and Complementary Medicine (New York, N.Y.)*, *16*(7), 753–759. DOI: 10.1089/acm.2009.0342 PMID: 20590480

Motti, R., & de Falco, B. (2021). Traditional herbal remedies used for managing anxiety and insomnia in Italy: An ethnopharmacological overview. *Horticulturae*, *7*(12), 523. DOI: 10.3390/horticulturae7120523

Movafegh, A., Alizadeh, R., Hajimohamadi, F., Esfehani, F., & Nejatfar, M. (2008). Preoperative oral Passiflora incarnata reduces anxiety in ambulatory surgery patients: A double-blind, placebo-controlled study. *Anesthesia and Analgesia*, *106*(6), 1728–1732. DOI: 10.1213/ane.0b013e318172c3f9 PMID: 18499602

Mungali, M., Tripathi, A., & Singhal, S. (2021). Valeriana officinalis (valerian). In *Naturally Occurring Chemicals Against Alzheimer's Disease* (pp. 283–291). Academic Press. DOI: 10.1016/B978-0-12-819212-2.00023-2

Orhan, I. E. (2021). A review focused on molecular mechanisms of anxiolytic effect of Valerina officinalis L. in connection with its phytochemistry through in vitro/in vivo studies. *Current Pharmaceutical Design*, *27*(28), 3084–3090. DOI: 10.2174/1381612827666210119105254 PMID: 33463459

Pandit, S., Srivastav, A. K., Sur, T. K., Chaudhuri, S., Wang, Y., & Biswas, T. K. (2024). Effects of Withania somnifera extract in chronically stressed adults: A randomized controlled trial. *Nutrients, 16*(9), 1293. DOI: 10.3390/nu16091293 PMID: 38732539

Parcha, V., Bhandari, P., Chhetri, S., Kumar, U., & Kumar, D. (2024). on the Medicinal Use of Piper methysticum (Kava). *Medicinal Roots and Tubers for Pharmaceutical and Commercial Applications*, 140.

Park, C. W., Hong, K. B., Suh, H. J., & Ahn, Y. (2023). Sleep-promoting activity of amylase-treated Ashwagandha (Withania somnifera L. Dunal) root extract via GABA receptors. *Yao Wu Shi Pin Fen Xi, 31*(2), 278. DOI: 10.38212/2224-6614.3456 PMID: 37335157

Pont-Fernandez, S., Kheyfets, M., Rogers, J. M., Smith, K. E., & Epstein, D. H. (2023). Kava (Piper methysticum) in the United States: The quiet rise of a substance with often subtle effects. *The American Journal of Drug and Alcohol Abuse, 49*(1), 85–96. DOI: 10.1080/00952990.2022.2140292 PMID: 36410029

Ramadoss, M. S. K., & Koumaravelou, K. (2022). Regulatory Requirement Sufficiency for Registration of Traditional Herbal Medicine Based Products in Association of Southeast Asian Nations Regions: A Model Study with Ashwagandha Tablets. *Indian Journal of Pharmaceutical Sciences, 84*(2). Advance online publication. DOI: 10.36468/pharmaceutical-sciences.944

Saadatmand, S., Zohroudi, F., & Tangestani, H. (2024). The Effect of Oral Chamomile on Anxiety: A Systematic Review of Clinical Trials. *Clinical Nutrition Research, 13*(2), 139. DOI: 10.7762/cnr.2024.13.2.139 PMID: 38784853

Salman, A., Singh, A. K., & Mishra, S. B. (2025). Health Policies and Health Regulations Regarding Nutraceuticals for Sleep. In *Nutraceuticals in Insomnia and Sleep Problems* (pp. 267–299). Apple Academic Press. DOI: 10.1201/9781003560890-14

Senn, R., Schertler, L., Bussmann, H., Drewe, J., Boonen, G., & Butterweck, V. (2025). Valerenic Acid and Pinoresinol as Positive Allosteric Modulators: Unlocking the Sleep-Promoting Potential of Valerian Extract Ze 911. *Molecules (Basel, Switzerland), 30*(11), 2344. DOI: 10.3390/molecules30112344 PMID: 40509231

Singla, R., Kamboj, S., Duvey, B. K., Bhargava, A., & Chaudhary, J. (2025). Flavonoids and anxiety: Decoding their role in brain function and pathophysiology. *Medicine in Drug Discovery, 27*, 100214. DOI: 10.1016/j.medidd.2025.100214

Stough, C., Downey, L. A., Lloyd, J., Silber, B., Redman, S., Hutchison, C., Wesnes, K., & Nathan, P. J. (2008). Examining the nootropic effects of a special extract of Bacopa monniera on human cognitive functioning: 90-day double-blind placebo-controlled randomized trial. *Phytotherapy Research*, *22*(12), 1629–1634. DOI: 10.1002/ptr.2537 PMID: 18683852

Talbott, S. M., Talbott, J. A., & Pugh, M. (2013). Effect of Magnolia officinalis and Phellodendron amurense (Relora®) on cortisol and psychological mood state in moderately stressed subjects. *Journal of the International Society of Sports Nutrition*, *10*(1), 37. DOI: 10.1186/1550-2783-10-37 PMID: 23924268

Zhang, D. (2025). Exploring the versatile world of magnolias: Urban landscape enhancement and metabolite applications in drug discovery and cosmetics. *Discover Plants*, *2*(1), 139. DOI: 10.1007/s44372-025-00216-1

Zhang, W., Yan, Y., Wu, Y., Yang, H., Zhu, P., Yan, F., Zhao, R., Tian, P., Wang, T., Fan, Q., & Su, Z. (2022). Medicinal herbs for the treatment of anxiety: A systematic review and network meta-analysis. *Pharmacological Research*, *179*, 106204. DOI: 10.1016/j.phrs.2022.106204 PMID: 35378276

Chapter 4
Phytochemical and Pharmacology Effect of Piper betle L.

Bui Thi Hao
Vietnam University of Traditional Medicine, Hanoi, Vietnam

Nguyen Thi Anh Hong
VNU University of Medicine and Pharmacy, Vietnam

Nguyen Minh Khoi
National Institute of Medicinal Materials, Hanoi, Vietnam

Bui Thanh Tung
http://orcid.org/0000-0002-7308-5039
Faculty of Medicine and Pharmacy, Academy of Security Engineering and Technology, Bac Ninh, Vietnam

ABSTRACT

Piper betle L. is widely recognized for its diverse medicinal properties, including antimicrobial activity, therapeutic efficacy in dermatological disorders, analgesic effects, and its beneficial role in managing respiratory disorders. The plant contains a variety of bioactive chemical constituents, such as hydroxychavicol, chavibetol, chavibetol acetate, caryophyllene, allyl pyrocatechol diacetate, camphene, chavibetol methyl ether, eugenol, α-pinene, β-pinene, limonene, sabinene, 1,8-cineol, and allyl pyrocatechol monoacetate. These compounds exhibit notable pharmacological activities, contributing to the potential as stimulants with properties such as antiplatelet, anti-inflammatory, immunomodulatory, gastroprotective, and antidiabetic activities.

DOI: 10.4018/979-8-3373-5876-5.ch004

This review aims to provide a comprehensive overview of the phytochemical constituents and pharmacological properties of Piper betle L., with particular emphasis on its antimicrobial, antioxidant, antidiabetic, anticancer, and anti-gout potential.

INTRODUCTION

Piper betle L. (Piperaceae), commonly known as a perennial creeping plant belonging to the family Piperaceae, is native to central and eastern Peninsular Malaysia with a distribution extending to East Africa and tropical countries of Asia (Biswas, Anand, Saha, Kant, Mishra, Masih, Bar, Pandey, Jha, Majumder, Das, Gadekar, Shekhawat, Kumar, Radha, Proćków, Lastra, & Dey, 2022). *Piper betle* is notable for its yellowish-green to dark green, glossy leaves that emit a distinctive and pleasant aroma. These aromatic leaves owe their sweet to pungent flavor primarily to the presence of essential oils. Morphologically, the leaves are heart-shaped, simple, alternate, stipulate, and petiolate. Their size varies by cultivar, typically ranging from 7 to 15 cm in length and 5 to 14 cm in width. The leaf surface is smooth and leathery, with shapes ranging from ovate to oblong or elliptic, and bases that are acuminate, oblique, or rounded. Traditionally, betel leaves have been widely used as natural mouth fresheners and for treating various ailments such as colds, coughs, bronchial asthma, rheumatism, stomach pain, bad breath, abscesses, conjunctivitis, constipation, gum swelling, and minor wounds. Their essential oils exhibit significant antibacterial, antifungal, and antiprotozoal properties (Das et al., 2016). In this review, we provide a comprehensive summary of the phytochemical characteristics and pharmacological effects of the *Piper betle* L.

MATERIALS AND METHODS

This review is designed to retrieve from the databases of Google Scholar, SciFinder, PubMed, Science Direct, Web of Science, and Springer using the keywords of "Piper betle", "phytochemistry," "pharmacology," "anti-inflammatory" "gout," "acid uric" and related terms. These articles were published on scientific journals, Vietnam herbal medicine books and magazines, as well as thesis's, were obtained. This plant was utilized in the World Flora (https://www.worldfloraonline.org) database to determine the nomenclature and acquire information on *Piper* genus.

Chemical constituents of *Piper betle* L.

The pharmacological effects of medicinal plants mainly result from a diverse range of bioactive phytochemicals that have important biomedical and pharmaceutical applications. (Biswas, Anand, Saha, Kant, Mishra, Masih, Bar, Pandey, Jha, Majumder, Das, Gadekar, Shekhawat, Kumar, Radha, Proćków, Lastra, & Dey, 2022). *Piper betle* contains a wide range of phytochemicals, whose composition varies according to the plant's botanical origin and the type of solvent used for extraction (Nayaka et al., 2021). Nutritionally, the leaves contain essential macronutrients such as proteins (3.0–3.5%), carbohydrates (0.5–6.1%), minerals (2.3–3.3%), and tannins (0.1–1.3%). They are also rich in micronutrients, including calcium, phosphorus, iron, iodine, potassium, and vitamins A, B, and C. Phytochemical analyses have revealed a complex mixture of volatile and non-volatile constituents. Among these, major aromatic and phenolic compounds include eugenol, hydroxychavicol, chavibetol, chavibetol acetate, and safrole. In essential oil derived from common betel leaves, safrole (up to 48.7%) and chavibetol acetate (approximately 12.5%) have been identified as dominant components (Rekha et al., 2014), (Azahar et al., 2020). Additional compounds reported include 4-terpineol, β-caryophyllene, camphene, chavibetol methyl ester, α-pinene, β-pinene, limonene, 1,8-cineole, and allylpyrocatechol derivatives. A study using hydro-distillation identified 65 constituents in the essential oil, with 5-(2-propenyl)-1,3-benzodioxole (25.67%), eugenol (18.27%), and 2-methoxy-4-(2-propenyl) acetate-phenol (8.0%) as the predominant compounds. Ether-soluble fractions further confirmed chavibetol (53.1%) and chavibetol acetate (15.5%) as major constituents. Additionally, GC-MS analysis of solvent fractions revealed other bioactives such as 4-chromanol, which was found in high concentrations in aqueous extracts (27.81%) and ethanol extracts, along with squalene and tocopherol, which were exclusive to the aqueous fraction. The non-volatile fractions include various flavonoids (e.g., quercetin), tannins, and long-chain aliphatic compounds like pentadecyl 6-hydroxytridecanoate and methyl hexacos-7-enoate, isolated via silica gel and column chromatography. These phytoconstituents collectively contribute to the plant's broad-spectrum pharmacological properties. Among these, eugenol and hydroxychavicol—both classified as propenylphenols—have been particularly noted for their antioxidant, anti-inflammatory, and antifungal activities. Meanwhile, chavibetol not only adds to the bioactivity profile but also imparts the characteristic spicy aroma of *Piper betle* essential oil (Umar et al., 2018).

Table 1. Phytochemical constituents of P. betle

Plant part/Extract/ Essential oil	Techniques	Chemical compounds
Aqueous extract of leaves	GC/MS	2,3-bis(hydroxy)propyl ester, 2-monopalmitin, α-hydroxy, alpha-hydroxyphenyl, benzeneacetic acid, benzeneacetic acid, hexadecanamide, hexadecanoic acid, hexadecanoic acid, hydroxychavicol, myristic acid, octadecanoic acid, octadecanoic acid (Biswas, Anand, Saha, Kant, Mishra, Masih, Bar, Pandey, Jha, Majumder, Das, Gadekar, Shekhawat, Kumar, Radha, Proćków, Lastra, & Dey, 2022)
Essential oil from leaves	GC/MS	4-allyl-1,2-diacetoxybenzene, acetyleugenol, bicyclo(4.1.0) hept-3-en- camphene, chavicol, cis-ocimene, cyclohexene,4-methyl-decanal, eugenol, germacrene B, germacrene D, globulol, ledene, linalyl acetate, l-limonene, methyl-eugenol, phenyl acetylaldehyde, t-caryophyllene, t-ocimene, undecanal, α –humulene, α-pinene, β-elemene, β-myrcene, γ-cadinene, γ-ionene, γ-muurolene (Biswas, Anand, Saha, Kant, Mishra, Masih, Bar, Pandey, Jha, Majumder, Das, Gadekar, Shekhawat, Kumar, Radha, Proćków, Lastra, & Dey 2022)
Leaf extract	DART-MS	chavicol, allylpyrocatechol, chavibetol, phenyl alanine, chavicol acetate, allylpyrocatechol acetate, chavibetol acetate, allylpyrocatechol, diacetate(Biswas, Anand, Saha, Kant, Mishra, Masih, Bar, Pandey, Jha, Majumder, Das, Gadekar, Shekhawat, Kumar, Radha, Proćków, Lastra, & Dey, 2022)
Acetone extract and different fractions of leaf	UV/VIS/NIR, NMR, HR-ESI-MS, GC/MS	Sphingolipids - pipercerebroside A pipercerebroside B(Biswas, Anand, Saha, Kant, Mishra, Masih, Bar, Pandey, Jha, Majumder, Das, Gadekar, Shekhawat, Kumar, Radha, Proćków, Lastra, & Dey, 2022)
Volatile oil from leaves	GC/MS	β- caryophyllene, α-farnesene, α-humulene, germacrene b, germacrene d(Biswas, Anand, Saha, Kant, Mishra, Masih, Bar, Pandey, Jha, Majumder, Das, Gadekar, Shekhawat, Kumar, Radha, Proćków, Lastra, & Dey, 2022)
Hexane extract of leaves	GC/MS	2,3-dihydro-3,5-dihydroxy-6-methyl-4h-pyran-4-one, phellandrene, α-terpinene, p-cymene, sabinene, γ-terpinene, o-guaiacol, linalool, tujene, terpine-1-ol, terpine-4-ol, α-terpineol, safrole, eugenol, isoeugenol, α-copaene, β –bourbonene, methyleugenol, β –caryophyllene, β –cubebene, γ-cadinene, α-humulene, β-selinene, α-selinene, caryophyllene oxide, camphene, germacrene b, longifolene, phytol(Biswas, Anand, Saha, Kant, Mishra, Masih, Bar, Pandey, Jha, Majumder, Das, Gadekar, Shekhawat, Kumar, Radha, Proćków, Lastra, & Dey, 2022)
Ethanol extract of leaves	GC/MS	heptafluorobutyrate, ethyl diazoacetate, 4-(2-propenyl)phenol, 3-fluoro-2-propynenitrite, eugenol, tris(trifluoromethyl) phosphine(Biswas, Anand, Saha, Kant, Mishra, Masih, Bar, Pandey, Jha, Majumder, Das, Gadekar, Shekhawat, Kumar, Radha, Proćków, Lastra, & Dey, 2022)

continued on following page

Table 1. Continued

Plant part/Extract/ Essential oil	Techniques	Chemical compounds
Aqueous and ethanol extracts of leaves	GC/MS	amino acid: alanine, valine, isoleucine, proline fatty acids: palmitic acid, linoleic acid, linolenic acid, oleic acid, stearic acid, palmitic acid derivatives sterols: cholesterol, cholesterol derivatives, stigmasterol, β -sitosterol(Biswas, Anand, Saha, Kant, Mishra, Masih, Bar, Pandey, Jha, Majumder, Das, Gadekar, Shekhawat, Kumar, Radha, Proćków, Lastra, & Dey, 2022)
Ethanol extract of leaves	GC/MS	1-phenylpropene-3,3-diol diacetate, eugenol, 4-chromanol, 4-allyl-1,2-diacetoxybenzene, hydroxychavicol (1-allyl-3, 4-dihydroxybenzene) (Biswas, Anand, Saha, Kant, Mishra, Masih, Bar, Pandey, Jha, Majumder, Das, Gadekar, Shekhawat, Kumar, Radha, Proćków, Lastra, & Dey, 2022)
Chloroform extract of leaves	1D NMR, 2D NMR, ESI-MS, FT-IR and HR-ESI-MS	s 1-n-dodecanyloxy resorcinol (H1) and desmethylenesqualenyl deoxy-cepharadione-A(Biswas, Anand, Saha, Kant, Mishra, Masih, Bar, Pandey, Jha, Majumder, Das, Gadekar, Shekhawat, Kumar, Radha, Proćków, Lastra, & Dey, 2022)
Ultrasound-assisted extract of leaves	GC/MS	hydroxychavicol, eugenol, isoeugenol, and 4-allyl-1,2-diacetoxybenzene(Biswas, Anand, Saha, Kant, Mishra, Masih, Bar, Pandey, Jha, Majumder, Das, Gadekar, Shekhawat, Kumar, Radha, Proćków, Lastra, & Dey, 2022)

Pharmacological activities of *Piper betle L*

This plant has been extensively researched for its diverse pharmacological properties, including its potent antimicrobial activity, which encompasses both antibacterial and antifungal effects (Biswas, Anand, Saha, Kant, Mishra, Masih, Bar, Pandey, Jha, Majumder, Das, Gadekar, Shekhawat, Kumar, Radha, Proćków, Lastra, & Dey, 2022). Additionally, it exhibits significant antioxidant potential, contributing to cellular protection against oxidative stress. Its anti-diabetic properties help regulate blood glucose levels and improve metabolic health, while its anticancer activity has shown promise in inhibiting tumor growth and promoting apoptosis in cancer cells (Azahar et al., 2020). Moreover, betel leaf exhibits anti-inflammatory properties, supporting gout treatment. These findings highlight the therapeutic potential of this plant in addressing various health conditions.

Antibacterial activity

Piper betle L. leaf extract shows strong potential as a natural therapeutic agent for bacterial infections, particularly conjunctivitis, by inhibiting Gram-positive bacteria such as *Brevibacillus brevis*, *Micrococcus luteus*, and *Staphylococcus cohnii*, as well as Gram-negative bacteria including *Escherichia coli*, *Pseudomonas aeruginosa*, and *Salmonella enterica* (Lubis & Wahyuni, 2020),(Chan & Wong, 2014).

The antimicrobial effects of *P. betle* are attributed to a diverse array of phytochemicals, including alkaloids, phenols, flavonoids, tannins, saponins, glycosides, terpenoids, and steroids. Among these, phenolic compounds play a central role due to their dual bacteriostatic and bactericidal actions. These compounds, through their carboxyl groups, form complexes with bacterial proteins, disrupting membrane function and ultimately compromising cell wall integrity—especially in Gram-positive bacteria (Lubis & Wahyuni, 2020).

In addition, a key phenolic constituent, hydroxychavicol (also known as allylpyrocatechol), has been shown to inhibit the growth of *Streptococcus sanguinis* by targeting Muramylpentapeptide-UDP-N-acetylglucosamine dehydrogenase (MurA is an essential enzyme in the bacterial cell wall synthesis process, particularly in the production of peptidoglycan), a key enzyme involved in peptidoglycan biosynthesis. This mechanism leads to bacterial cell wall disruption. Hydroxychavicol also exhibits dose-dependent antibacterial activity against *Streptococcus intermedius* and *S. mutans*, both of which are implicated in oral infections such as caries, gingivitis, and periodontitis (Nayaka et al., 2021).

Moreover, tannin and flavonoid compounds also contribute to the antibacterial activity of *Piper betle* L. leaf extract. Flavonoids exert their antibacterial effects by disrupting the potassium balance in Gram-positive bacteria, leading to cytoplasmic membrane dysfunction. The antibacterial activity of tannins, attributed primarily to tannic acid, is proposed to involve alterations in potassium concentration, inhibition of enzyme production, and suppression of enzymatic reactions. (Lubis & Wahyuni, 2020). In conclusion, the antibacterial properties of *Piper betle* L. make it a promising candidate for the treatment of various bacterial infections. Natural products are highly sought after due to their broad biological activities and their role as valuable sources for the discovery of effective bioactive compounds. *Piper betle* L., in particular, has been recognized for its diverse pharmacological activities, including significant antibacterial effects (Subashkumar et al., 2013).

Antifungal activity

Betel leaves demonstrate potential antifungal activity through various solvent extracts (Biswas, Anand, Saha, Kant, Mishra, Masih, Bar, Pandey, Jha, Majumder, Das, Gadekar, Shekhawat, Kumar, Radha, Proćków, Lastra, & Dey, 2022). The antifungal and aflatoxin-suppressing activities of Betel Leaf Essential Oil (BLEO) are primarily attributed to its major constituent, eugenol. Eugenol possesses a hydroxyl group capable of forming hydrogen bonds with the active sites of fungal enzymes involved in aflatoxin production, leading to enzyme denaturation. Additionally, eugenol has been reported to cause morphological abnormalities in fungi by disrupting the fungal cell wall structure, increasing cell membrane fluidity and permeability, and interfering with the functions of key regulatory proteins (Nayaka et al., 2021). Furthermore, docking simulations of eugenol acetate and chavicol acetate, components of BLEO, revealed strong interactions with amino acids involved in fungal protein structures. These interactions are predicted to impair fungal metabolism and promote biomass degradation, thereby reducing fungal virulence (Nayaka et al., 2021).

Moreover, hydroxychavicol, isolated from the chloroform fraction of the aqueous leaf extract of *Piper betle* L. (Piperaceae), was evaluated for its antifungal activity against 124 strains of selected fungi (Ali et al., 2010). Hydroxychavicol was capable of completely killing *Candida albicans* at a minimum concentration of 400 μg/mL, with its fungicidal activity against *C. albicans* and *Candida glabrata* shown to be dose-dependent. Hydroxychavicol also exhibited fungicidal effects against various clinical fungal isolates, with minimum inhibitory concentrations (MICs) ranging from 7.81 to 62.5 μg/mL for dermatophytes, 15.62 to 500 μg/mL for yeasts, and 125 to 500 μg/mL for *Aspergillus* species. The minimum fungicidal concentrations (MFCs) were observed to be equal to or up to two-fold higher than the corresponding MICs. Additionally, hydroxychavicol was able to inhibit biofilm formation and facilitate biofilm eradication. Biofilm development, characterized by a dense network of microbial cells adhering to mucosal surfaces, is associated with severe infections (Nayaka et al., 2021). In conclusion, *Piper betel* has shown the highest antifungal activity among all the plant fractions (Nazmul, 2011).

Antioxidant activity

Antioxidants are substances that either directly scavenge reactive oxygen species (ROS) or indirectly enhance antioxidant defenses or inhibit ROS production. They play a crucial role in protecting humans from serious diseases such as cardiovascular disorders, cancer, and neurodegenerative diseases including Parkinson's and Alzheimer's. Antioxidant supplements or antioxidant-rich foods can help reduce oxidative damage caused by free radicals and reactive oxygen species. Synthetic antioxidants, such as butylated hydroxytoluene (BHT), butylated hydroxyanisole (BHA), and Trolox, are widely used in the pharmaceutical and food industries; however, they have been associated with toxic and mutagenic effects. Consequently, there is increasing interest in the development and isolation of natural antioxidants from plant sources. Among these, phenolic compounds are major contributors to antioxidant activity due to their abundance, synergistic effects, and their ability to donate hydrogen atoms, act as reducing agents, and scavenge free radicals (Jaiswal et al., 2014).

Piper betel L. has some antioxidant activity. The phenolic constituent allyl pyrocatechol from the leaves showed activity against obligate oral anaerobes responsible for halitosis. The leaf extract of *Piper betle* has demonstrated a significant stimulatory effect on pancreatic lipase activity in experimental rats. It also inhibited radiation-induced lipid peroxidation and enhanced superoxide dismutase (SOD) activity in a dose-dependent manner, indicating an improvement in the antioxidant status of Swiss albino mice. Additionally, *P. betle* leaves exhibited notable hepatoprotective effects, improving tissue antioxidant capacity by increasing the levels of nonenzymatic antioxidants (reduced glutathione, vitamin C, and vitamin E) and enhancing the activities of free radical-detoxifying enzymes in the liver and kidneys of ethanol-treated rats. Furthermore, *P. betle* leaf extract inhibited platelet aggregation through both antioxidative mechanisms and modulation of thromboxane B_2 (TXB_2) and prostaglandin D_2 (PGD_2) production. Compounds isolated from *P. betle* — including piperbetol, methylpiperbetol, piperol A, and piperol B — were found to be effective platelet-activating factor (PAF) receptor antagonists in vitro. (Dasgupta & De, 2004).

Moreover, the 1,1-diphenyl-2-picrylhydrazyl (DPPH) assay of the ethanol extracts of *Piper betel* possesses the best antioxidant activity (Rathee et al., 2006). DPPH is a stable free radical that accepts an electron or a hydrogen atom to form a stable diamagnetic molecule, and it is commonly used as a substrate for evaluating the antioxidant activity of compounds (Alam et al., 2013). In summary, *Piper betle L.* exhibits significant antioxidant properties due to its rich content of phenolic compounds, flavonoids, and polyphenols, making it a valuable natural source for combating oxidative stress and supporting overall health.

Antidiabetic activity

Diabetes mellitus is a chronic metabolic disorder and a major public health concern, characterized by elevated blood glucose levels resulting from impaired insulin secretion or insulin resistance (Saravanabhavan, 2018). Diabetes mellitus is classified into two main types: Type I and Type II. Type I diabetes, often referred to as juvenile diabetes, is insulin-dependent and accounts for approximately 5% of the diabetic population. Type II diabetes, which is non-insulin dependent, typically develops in adults over the age of 40. Chronic hyperglycemia associated with diabetes has been well established to cause long-term damage, dysfunction, and eventual failure of various organs, particularly the eyes, kidneys, nerves, heart, and blood vessels. Conventional pharmacological treatments aim to manage diabetes by improving insulin sensitivity, enhancing insulin secretion, and reducing blood glucose levels. However, these therapies are often associated with adverse effects and may not consistently maintain normal blood glucose levels. As a result, there has been considerable interest in medicinal plants as potential sources of antidiabetic compounds. Numerous traditional medical systems worldwide have utilized plant-based treatments for diabetes, many of which have shown promising efficacy. The hypoglycemic effects of active plant components are believed to involve inhibition of α-amylase activity and modulation of various blood parameters implicated in the development of diabetes. Although a wide range of antidiabetic drugs is currently available, no definitive cure for the disease exists. Moreover, concerns regarding the side effects and efficacy of existing drugs have spurred the demand for safer and more effective therapeutic alternatives. In recent years, the interest in herbal medicines for diabetes management has grown significantly, both in developing and developed countries, due to their natural origin and lower incidence of adverse effects (Mamun-or-Rashid et al., 2014).

The ethanolic *P. betle L.* extract showed good antidiabetic activity (Saravanabhavan, 2018). The betel leaf extracts have remarkable hypoglycemic activity. The suspension of leaf can significantly lower the blood glucose level and glycosylated hemoglobin and decrease the activity of liver fructose-1,6-bisphosphatase and glucose-6- phosphatase, but in Streptozocin (STZ) diabetic rats, liver hexokinase increased in comparison with the untreated diabetic rats. In addition, alkaloids exhibit a variety of medicinal properties including anti-hyperglycemic hyperglycemic activities and extracted anti from the Piperaceae family. It aimed to investigate the inhibitory potentials of different varieties of *P. betle* leaf extracts on α-glucosidase, one of the key enzymes involved in carbohydrate hydrolysis. Besides the n-hexane extract of different *P. betle* leaf extracts exhibited the highest role in α-glucosidase inhibition which can be considered as a potential pharmaceutical therapeutic to treat diabetes (Sarker et al., 2024). Besides, betel leaf extract inhibited α-amylase and α-glucosidase activities through competitive inhibition (Alam et al., 2023). *Piper betle* extract also helped maintain stable body weight without significant weight loss, likely by enhancing glucose uptake in peripheral tissues or by inhibiting the catabolism of fat and protein through improved glycemic control (Azahar et al., 2020).

In conclusion, diabetes mellitus remains a major public health challenge, with current pharmacological treatments often accompanied by side effects and limited efficacy in fully controlling blood glucose levels. In this context, natural compounds from medicinal plants have gained increasing attention as alternative or complementary therapies. Betel leaf (*Piper betle* L.) has demonstrated significant antidiabetic potential, including hypoglycemic effects, inhibition of key carbohydrate-hydrolyzing enzymes, and improved glycemic control. Its ability to regulate blood glucose levels and support metabolic balance highlights its promise as a potential therapeutic agent for diabetes management. Further research is needed to fully elucidate its mechanisms of action and optimize its clinical application

Anticancer activity

Piper betle leaves and their active phenolic compound, eugenol, exhibited strong anticancer activity against KB oral carcinoma cells. The anticancer effects of the extract were primarily attributed to its phenolic constituents, particularly eugenol, which demonstrated significant cytotoxicity toward cancer cells (Preethi & Padma, 2016). KB cell lines are widely used in research on oral squamous cell carcinoma, as they are presumed to have originated from an epidermoid carcinoma of the oral cavity (Veettil et al., 2019). Moreover, hydroxychavicol (HC), an active compound from *Piper betle* leaves, inhibited the attachment of KB cells to type I collagen and fibronectin, leading to cell cycle arrest at the S and G_2/M phases (Veettil et al., 2019).

Moreover, hydroxychavicol, a component of *Piper betle* leaves, has demonstrated anti-proliferative effects against oral carcinoma cell lines. Antioxidants may inhibit carcinogenesis not only through their radical-scavenging activities but also via non-antioxidant mechanisms, such as modulating signaling pathways involved in cell proliferation, growth, and differentiation, as well as influencing the activities of cancer-related enzymes like cyclooxygenase-2 and phase I or II metabolizing enzymes, or by inducing cell cycle arrest. The antitumor properties of *Piper betle* are likely attributable to its rich phytochemical content, including polyphenols and alkaloids, many of which are potent free radical scavengers. Phenolic compounds such as epigallocatechin gallate, catechin, genistein, and quercetin have been shown to suppress the growth of breast cancer cells, highlighting the role of antioxidants in mediating anti-proliferative effects. Anti-cancer agents with antioxidant properties may exert therapeutic effects by balancing reactive oxygen species (ROS) levels—preventing excessive proliferation of cancer cells while still permitting apoptosis (Roy & Vijayalaxmi, 2013).Becauses tumor cells exhibit elevated production of reactive oxygen species (ROS), resulting in oxidative stress and disruption of the redox balance, which leads to DNA damage, mutations, and altered gene expression—factors that contribute to carcinogenesis. Simultaneously, cancer cells often possess a compromised antioxidant defense system, reducing their capacity to eliminate excess ROS. However, ROS also play a crucial role in inducing apoptosis, suggesting a dual role in both promoting and inhibiting cancer progression. Therefore, achieving an optimal balance between ROS levels and antioxidant defenses is essential to inhibit tumor growth while preserving the ability to trigger apoptosis. One potential mechanism underlying the antiproliferative effects of *Piper betle* extract may involve the upregulation of antioxidant enzyme activities, thereby helping to maintain redox homeostasis. Furthermore, previous studies have proposed several mechanisms contributing to the antiproliferative properties observed (Veettil et al., 2019).

In conclusion, the anticancer potential of *Piper betle* leaves is attributed to its bioactive compounds, particularly eugenol and hydroxychavicol, which exhibit strong cytotoxic and antiproliferative effects against oral carcinoma cells. By modulating oxidative stress, inducing cell cycle arrest, and inhibiting cancer-related pathways, *Piper betle* emerges as a promising natural therapeutic agent for cancer treatment, warranting further investigation into its clinical applications.

Anti-inflammation activity

Inflammation is a complex biological response of vascular tissues to harmful stimuli such as pathogens, damaged cells, or irritants. It serves as a key mechanism of innate immunity and is characterized by the classical signs of pain, heat, redness, swelling, and loss of function (Rintu et al., 2015). Various endogenous mediators, such as histamine, serotonin, bradykinin, and prostaglandins, are abundantly present in inflammatory cells. Among these, prostaglandins are ubiquitous molecules that initiate and modulate cellular and tissue responses during inflammation. Even at low concentrations, these mediators can trigger pain responses. Pain leads to reduced muscular activity and is associated with the generation of free radicals and reactive oxygen species (ROS), which activate second messenger pathways and contribute to the sensitization of dorsal horn neurons—an essential mechanism underlying neuropathic pain (Alam et al., 2013).

Betel leaf has been traditionally used as a natural remedy for oral inflammation, and modern research supports its potent anti-inflammatory properties. Studies have shown that ethanolic extracts of betel leaf exhibit significant anti-inflammatory activity at non-toxic concentrations. Among its bioactive constituents, eugenol has been extensively studied for its anti-inflammatory effects in various animal models exposed to different inflammatory agents (Dasgupta & De, 2004). Additionally, hydroxychavicol (HC), a key phytochemical in betel leaf, has demonstrated multiple pharmacological benefits. HC has been found to inhibit platelet aggregation, function as a potent COX-1/COX-2 inhibitor, and act as a reactive oxygen species (ROS) scavenger. Furthermore, HC plays a crucial role in modulating platelet calcium signaling, making it a promising therapeutic candidate for cardiovascular diseases. Notably, its anti-inflammatory properties contribute to cardiovascular health without adversely affecting normal hemostatic functions. Another, P. betle extracts inhibit platelet aggregation through antioxidant effects and by modulating the production of pro-inflammatory mediators, notably Thromboxane B_2 (TXB_2) and Prostaglandin D_2 (PGD_2) (Rintu et al., 2015). These findings highlight the therapeutic potential of betel leaf and its bioactive compounds in inflammation-related disorders, warranting further investigation into their clinical applications.

Moreover, betel leaf has been found to gradually reduce uric acid levels in the blood, making it a safe and effective option for long-term use. Its essential oils, including eugenol, chavibetol, chavicol, and estragole, contribute to its anti-inflammatory and analgesic properties. These bioactive compounds help combat arthritis, promote the recovery of damaged joints, and support metabolic processes by enhancing detoxification mechanisms in the body. Due to its ability to alleviate joint inflammation and reduce nerve pain associated with gout, betel leaf has been traditionally used in Vietnam as a natural remedy for managing the disease. Its effectiveness in restoring joint function and mitigating gout-related discomfort makes it a valuable therapeutic option. Notably, with an essential oil content of approximately 2.4%, betel leaf is a potent natural anti-inflammatory agent, further supporting its role in gout treatment and joint health (Hoi, 2020).

In conclusion, inflammation plays a critical role in the body's immune response but can contribute to chronic diseases when uncontrolled. Betel leaf, with its rich composition of bioactive compounds, has demonstrated significant anti-inflammatory, analgesic, and antioxidant properties. Its ability to modulate inflammatory pathways, reduce uric acid levels, and support joint health highlights its therapeutic potential in managing inflammatory disorders like arthritis and gout. Further research is warranted to fully explore its clinical applications and optimize its use in modern medicine.

Anti- gout

Hyperuricemia and gout effect of *Piper betle* L. extract were demonstrated in some previous research. Studies showed that betel leaf extract significantly reduced uric acid levels in broiler chickens and mice (Vikrama Chakravarthi et al., 2022) (Faizal et al., 2019). The mechanism of hyperuricemia in this plant was involved in suppressing xanthine oxidase activity, thereby reducing the biosynthesis of uric acid and supporting its traditional use in Gout management (Vikrama Chakravarthi et al., 2022). Comparative studies in reducing uric acid levels indicated that betel leaf is more effective than breadfruit leaf (Faizal et al., 2019). While P. betle is generally considered safe in traditional medicine, comprehensive preclinical toxicology data, including in vivo acute and chronic toxicity tests, are often insufficiently documented in modern literature. Research suggests that the extract may be a safe option for long-term use in chronic conditions like Gout, but systematic studies are necessary. These limited findings suggest that *Piper betle* L. extract could be a potential herbal drug that has both anti-gout benefits and fewer side effects.

FUTURE DIRECTIONS AND RESEARCH PRIORITIES

Despite the immense pharmacological potential of Piper betle, its transition to modern clinical application faces several significant challenges. The greatest hurdle lies in the substantial chemical variability observed among different chemotypes, geographical origins, and extraction methodologies, which severely impedes product standardization. Future research must, therefore, prioritize the development of robust quantitative and qualitative standardization methods for extracts, using key bioactive markers like Hydroxychavicol and Eugenol. A critical knowledge gap in the translational pipeline is the lack of comprehensive Pharmacokinetics (PK) studies, particularly concerning the absorption, distribution, metabolism, and excretion (ADME) profiles of the main lipophilic active compounds. To enhance efficacy and bioavailability, a major research focus should be placed on developing Advanced Drug Delivery Systems, such as nanoemulsions, nanostructured lipid carriers (NLCs), or liposomes, aimed at improving the solubility and stability of the hydrophobic constituents of P. betle. Ultimately, the pivotal step for converting ethnobotanical promise into a validated therapeutic reality is the execution of rigorous, randomized, and controlled human clinical trials. These trials are essential to confirm safety, establish optimal dosages, and definitively validate therapeutic efficacy against target pathologies, including diabetes, cancer, and gout, thereby laying a solid foundation for the integration of P. betle into evidence-based modern medicine

CONCLUSION

In conclusion, the important chemical constituents of *Piper betle* include chavibetol, chavibetol acetate, caryophyllene, allyl pyrocatechol diacetate, camphene, chavibetol methyl ether, eugenol, α-pinene, β-pinene, limonene, sabinene, 1,8-cineol, and allyl pyrocatechol monoacetate. *Piper betle* exhibits significant biological activities such as antifungal, antibacterial, antioxidant, antidiabetic, and anticancer properties, making it a valuable natural resource for therapeutic applications. These multifaceted benefits highlight its potential for further research and development in the pharmaceutical and healthcare industries.

ACKNOWLEDGMENTS

This research has been done under the research project QG 23.70, "Study on formulation and evaluation of the therapeutic support effect for acute gout treatment in experimental model of hard capsules containing quantified extract of *Piper betle* L., Piperaceae" of Vietnam National University, Hanoi. This study was funded by Vietnam National University Hanoi, Vietnam, with grant number QG 23.70

REFERENCES

Alam, B., Akter, F., & Parvin, N.. (2013). Antioxidant, analgesic and anti-inflammatory activities of the methanolic extract of Piper betle leaves. *Avicenna Journal of Phytomedicine*, *3*(2), 112–125. PMID: 25050265

Alam, M. J., Mahmud, T., Hasan, R., & Islam, K. (2023). Inhibition of Key Digestive Enzymes Linked to Type 2 Diabetes Mellitus by Piper betle L. Leaf Extracts to Manage Diabetes in an Alternative Way. *Current Nutrition and Food Science*, *18*(6), 651–658. DOI: 10.2174/1573401318666220928091823

Ali, I., Khan, F. G., Suri, K. A., Gupta, B. D., Satti, N. K., Dutt, P., Afrin, F., Qazi, G. N., & Khan, I. A. (2010). In vitro antifungal activity of hydroxychavicol isolated from Piper betle L. *Annals of Clinical Microbiology and Antimicrobials*, *9*(1), 7. DOI: 10.1186/1476-0711-9-7 PMID: 20128889

. Azahar N.I., Mokhtar N.M., and Arifin M.A. (2020). Piper betle: a review on its bioactive compounds, pharmacological properties, and extraction process. 991, 012044.

Biswas, P., Anand, U., Saha, S. C., Kant, N., Mishra, T., Masih, H., Bar, A., Pandey, D. K., Jha, N. K., Majumder, M., Das, N., Gadekar, V. S., Shekhawat, M. S., Kumar, M., Radha, , Proćków, J., Lastra, J. M. P., & Dey, A. (2022). Betelvine (Piper betle L.): A comprehensive insight into its ethnopharmacology, phytochemistry, and pharmacological, biomedical and therapeutic attributes. *Journal of Cellular and Molecular Medicine*, *26*(11), 3083–3119. DOI: 10.1111/jcmm.17323 PMID: 35502487

Biswas, P., Anand, U., Saha, S. C., Kant, N., Mishra, T., Masih, H., Bar, A., Pandey, D. K., Jha, N. K., Majumder, M., Das, N., Gadekar, V. S., Shekhawat, M. S., Kumar, M., Radha, , Proćków, J., Lastra, J. M. P., & Dey, A. (2022). Betelvine (Piper betle L.): A comprehensive insight into its ethnopharmacology, phytochemistry, and pharmacological, biomedical and therapeutic attributes. *Journal of Cellular and Molecular Medicine*, *26*(11), 3083–3119. DOI: 10.1111/jcmm.17323 PMID: 35502487

Chan, E. W. C., & Wong, S. K. (2014). Phytochemistry and pharmacology of three Piper species: An update. *International Journal of Pharmacognosy : a Journal of Crude Drug Research*, (9), 534–544.

Das, S., Parida, R., Sandeep, I. S., Nayak, S., & Mohanty, S. (2016). Biotechnological intervention in betelvine (Piper betle L.): A review on recent advances and future prospects. *Asian Pacific Journal of Tropical Medicine*, *9*(10), 938–946. DOI: 10.1016/j.apjtm.2016.07.029 PMID: 27794386

Dasgupta, N., & De, B. (2004). Antioxidant activity of Piper betel L. Leaf extract in vitro | Request PDF. *Food Chemistry*, *88*(2), 219–224. DOI: 10.1016/j.foodchem.2004.01.036

. Faizal F., Nauphar D., Pratamawati T.M., et al. (2019). Effectiveness of betel leaves (piper betle l.) and breadfruit leaves (Artocarpus atilis) in reducing uric acid levels in hyperuricemic male white rats (Rattus norvegicus). 1146, 012007.

Hoi, H. (2020). Vietnamese Medicinal Plants Useful in Treatments of Gout. *Pharmacognosy Journal*, *12*(6s), 1693–1697. DOI: 10.5530/pj.2020.12.228

Jaiswal, S., Patel, M., & Saxena, D.. (2014). Antioxidant Properties of Piper Betel (L) Leaf Extracts from Six Different Geographical Domain of India. *J Bioresour Eng Technol*, *2*(2), 12–20.

Lubis, R. R., & Wahyuni, D. D. (2020). Antibacterial activity of betle leaf (Piper betle l.) extract on inhibiting Staphylococcus aureus in conjunctivitis patient. *American Journal of Clinical and Experimental Immunology*, *9*(1), 1.

Mamun-or-Rashid, A. N. M., Hossain, M. S., Hassan, N., Dash, B. K., Sapon, M. A., & Sen, M. K. (2014). A review on medicinal plants with antidiabetic activity. *Journal of Pharmacognosy and Phytochemistry*, *3*(4), 149–159.

Nayaka, N. M. D. M. W., Sasadara, M. M. V., Sanjaya, D. A., Yuda, P. E. S. K., Dewi, N. L. K. A. A., Cahyaningsih, E., & Hartati, R. (2021). Piper betle (L): Recent Review of Antibacterial and Antifungal Properties, Safety Profiles, and Commercial Applications. *Molecules (Basel, Switzerland)*, *26*(8), 2321. DOI: 10.3390/molecules26082321 PMID: 33923576

Nazmul, M. H. M. (2011). In-vitro screening of antifungal activity of plants in Malaysia. *Biomedical Research*, *22*(1), 28–30.

Preethi, R., & Padma, P. R. (2016). Anticancer activity of silver nanobioconjugates synthesized from Piper betle leaves extract and its active compound eugenol. *International Journal of Pharmacy and Pharmaceutical Sciences*, *8*(9), 201. DOI: 10.22159/ijpps.2016.v8i9.12993

Rathee, J. S., Patro, B. S., Mula, S., Gamre, S., & Chattopadhyay, S. (2006). Antioxidant activity of piper betel leaf extract and its constituents. *Journal of Agricultural and Food Chemistry*, *54*(24), 9046–9054. DOI: 10.1021/jf061679e PMID: 17117789

Rekha, V., Kollipara, M., & Gupta, B.. (2014). A Review on Piper betle L.: Nature's Promising Medicinal Reservoir. *Am J Ethnomedicine*, *1*(5), 276–289.

Rintu, D., Shinjini, M., Kaustab, M., Pramathadhip, P., Umesh, P. S., & Banerjee, E. R. (2015). Anti-oxidant and anti-inflammatory activities of different varieties of Piper leaf extracts (Piper betle L.). *Journal of Nutrition & Food Sciences*, *5*(415), 2.

Roy, U. B., & Vijayalaxmi, K. K. (2013). Evaluation of cytotoxic activity of Piper betle Linn. using murine and human cell lines in vitro. *International Journal of Scientific and Engineering Research*, *4*(9), 221–233.

Saravanabhavan, K. (2018). Antidiabetic and Antioxidant Activities of Ethanolic Extract of Piper Betle L. Leaves in Catfish, Clarias Gariepinus. *Asian Journal of Pharmaceutical and Clinical Research*, *11*(3), 194–198. DOI: 10.22159/ajpcr.2018.v11i3.22393

Sarker, M., Sharmin, T., & Akter, R.. (2024). A Comparative Analysis of Phytoconstituents, Cytotoxicity and Antidiabetic Activity of Three Regional Piper betle Varieties: First Report from Bangladesh. *South Asian Res J Nat Prod*, *7*(1), 20–29.

Subashkumar, R., Sureshkumar, M., Babu, S., & Thayumanavan, T. (2013). Antibacterial effect of crude aqueous extract of Piper betle L. against pathogenic bacteria. *International Journal of Research in Pharmaceutical and Biomedical Sciences*, *4*, 42–46.

Umar, R. A., Zahary, M. N., Rohin, M. A. K., & Ismail, S. (2018). Chemical composition and the potential biological activities of Piper betel–a Review. *Malaysian Journal of Applied Sciences*, *3*(1), 1–8.

. Veettil S.R., Sunil E.A., Mukunda A., et al. (2019). Anticancer effect of Piper betle leaf extract on KB cell lines – an in vitro study. 13(1).

Vikrama Chakravarthi, P., Murugesan, S., Arivuchelvan, A., Sukumar, K., Arulmozhi, A., & Jagadeeswaran, A. (2022). Therapeutic antigout and antioxidant activity of Piper betle L. in gout-induced broilers. *British Poultry Science*, *63*(3), 324–331. DOI: 10.1080/00071668.2021.1998365 PMID: 34859728

Chapter 5
Integrating Spectroscopy and Bioassays for Scientific Evaluation of Herbal Formulations

Taye Temitope Alawode
http://orcid.org/0000-0002-8671-8632
Federal University Otuoke, Nigeria

ABSTRACT

This chapter discusses the critical need for scientific validation of complex traditional herbal formulations, particularly those widely used in Africa, which frequently lack established efficacy, safety, and consistency. It offers a comprehensive framework that integrates advanced chemical profiling and biological assays. Various spectroscopic and hyphenated techniques used for characterization of herbal medicines are discussed, as well as common assays used for validating herbal formulations' medicinal properties. The use of spectroscopy for standardization, quality control, and safety assessment of herbal formulations is also covered. The chapter demonstrates how bridging indigenous knowledge with modern evidence-based healthcare can help researchers, regulators, and healthcare providers realize the full potential of the world's botanical heritage in disease treatment.

BACKGROUND

Herbal formulations are inherently complex, containing thousands of compounds whose concentrations vary widely across geographical regions (Ogwu et al., 2025), making their standardization difficult. About 60-80% of the world population, es-

DOI: 10.4018/979-8-3373-5876-5.ch005

pecially among the rural populace of Africa and other developing countries, rely on traditional medicine to meet their healthcare needs (Ekor, 2014). Traditional remedies, which include decoctions, tinctures, powders, ointments, and pastes, often lack scientific validation regarding their efficacy, safety, and consistency, thereby impeding their incorporation into modern evidence-based healthcare.

This chapter outlines a scientific framework for evaluating herbal mixtures, aiming to bridge indigenous herbal knowledge with modern pharmacological understanding. It details the processes of plant material authentication, extraction, isolation, and characterization using various spectroscopic techniques. Chemical profiling methodologies, such as HPLC, LC-MS/MS, GC-MS, and metabolomics, are discussed for identifying and quantifying the constituents within complex herbal mixtures. When this detailed chemical understanding is combined with the assessment of biological effects through standard assays, a clear correlation can be established between chemical profiles and observed therapeutic outcomes. This integrated approach provides a robust blueprint for the standardization of herbal products, implementation of quality control measures, and comprehensive assessment of efficacy and safety, ultimately facilitating the integration of herbal products into contemporary healthcare systems.

The Place of Herbal Formulations in Traditional Medicine

Traditional medicine is inextricably linked to the religious beliefs, cultural identity, and ancestral wisdom of different ethnic groups. Its continued relevance in many parts of the world, particularly in Africa and other developing regions, is due to a number of factors, including limited access to allopathic medicine, the perceived efficacy of treatments supported by generations of empirical observations, and deep cultural trust (Mensah et al., 2019).

These formulations arose from empirical knowledge accumulated over thousands of years by ancient civilizations. Through meticulous observation, these civilizations discovered the potential effects of plants, both singly and, more importantly, in combination, resulting in the creation of complex recipes. These recipes, which specify precise plant ratios, preparation methods, and administration techniques for maximum pharmacological effect, have been passed down through oral tradition or ancient texts (Izah et al., 2024). They are used to treat a wide range of conditions, from infectious diseases like malaria and respiratory infections to chronic conditions like diabetes and hypertension, and they frequently approach treatments holistically by addressing the root cause of illness. Traditional healers also anticipate potential synergy between herbal constituents, with the goal of enhancing therapeutic action, or antagonism, in which one herb may counteract the negative effects of another (Karole et al., 2019).

Issues in Herbal Formulations: Complexity, Safety, Efficacy and Standardization

Numerous scientific studies have found that herbal mixtures are effective in treating diseases. These formulations have several advantages over single-herb preparations, including increased efficacy through synergistic interactions, lower toxicity via antagonistic modulations, broad-spectrum activity, pharmacokinetic modulation, and improved chemical stability. Despite widespread acceptance, herbal formulations face significant scientific and regulatory challenges. The main roadblocks are phytochemical complexity, safety concerns, questionable efficacy, lack of reproducibility, and standardization challenges (Fong et al., 2006).

Phytochemical Complexity and Variability

Herbal formulations are inherently complex, containing hundreds to thousands of phytochemicals, such as alkaloids, flavonoids, and terpenoids. Isolating specific therapeutic compounds from these mixtures is challenging due to their diverse nature and potential for synergistic and antagonistic interactions. Furthermore, the compositional profiles of individual herbs can vary significantly based on environmental conditions (e.g., soil quality, rainfall, sunlight), genetic variability, plant age, and post-harvest handling (such as drying methods and storage duration) (Ogwu et al., 2025). For instance, the antimalarial alkaloids in the Nigerian medicinal plant *Cryptolepis sanguinolenta* have been observed to vary from 0.8 to 2.4 mg/g across different regions, directly impacting the dosage and efficacy of herbal products derived from it (Biernacki et al., 2020). The inherent variability in plant composition, influenced by environmental and genetic factors, means that the chemical fingerprint of a single herb, let alone a herbal formulation, is not static. This presents a dynamic challenge for standardization.

Safety Concerns

Several serious adverse side effects have been documented in patients taking herbal products, including hallucinations, convulsions, cerebral hemorrhage, perforation of the gastrointestinal tract, congestive heart failure, renal failure, liver damage, respiratory arrest, and even cancer (Başaran et al., 2022). Fatal cases have been reported due to the cardiotoxicity of certain herbal products, with heart-related problems such as hypertension, hypotension, ventricular fibrillation, myocardial infarction, and cardiac arrest associated with traditional medicinal herbs like *Don* quai (*Angelica sinensis*) and Yohimbe (*Pausinystalia johimbe*) (Brown, 2017).

Also, the presence of intrinsic toxic compounds, contaminants, and the possibility of herb-drug interactions all raise serious concerns about the safety of herbal formulations. Some plants contain toxic constituents such as pyrrolizidine alkaloids, which have been linked to hepatotoxicity and veno-occlusive disease (Yee & Roth, 2018), as well as aristolochic acids, which have been linked to nephrotoxicity and urothelial carcinomas. Beyond intrinsic toxicity, contamination and adulteration are widespread problems, with synthetic pharmaceuticals, heavy metals, pesticide residues, and aflatoxin B1 all posing serious health risks.

Efficacy

Despite numerous anecdotal claims and ethnobotanical records, scientific validation of herbal formulation efficacy remains insufficient. Furthermore, while the multi-herb synergy central to traditional formulations is conceptually appealing, current scientific methods such as checkerboard assays and isobolograms fail to accurately simulate the complex interactions that occur in human physiology (Kemegne et al., 2021). As a result, even when therapeutic potential exists, the inability to adequately evaluate and quantify these effects calls into question the scientific credibility of such formulations.

EXTRACTION, ISOLATION AND PURIFICATION STRATEGIES

To ensure that herbal formulations meet the stringent regulatory requirements for inclusion in modern evidence-based healthcare systems, they must be collected, authenticated, and extracted using acceptable protocols. Following these protocols is critical for understanding the chemistry of herbal mixtures and developing a strong framework for standardization and quality control.

Herbal Formulations: Plant Preparation and Authentication

The proper identification of plant materials is critical to ensuring the safety and efficacy of herbal formulations. Incorrect identification can result in ineffective treatment and negative side effects, as well as compromising quality control and facilitating adulteration. Plant materials are authenticated using a variety of methods, including macroscopic and microscopic evaluation, chromatographic fingerprinting (TLC and HPLC), chemical profiling (HPLC, GC-MS, NMR), and DNA barcoding. Chromatographic fingerprinting, using techniques like TLC and HPLC, can confirm the presence of specific marker compounds or active ingredients, ensuring consistency and quality, and assisting in the detection of adulterants or contaminants (Malherbe et al., 2012). DNA barcoding involves sequencing a specific region of the herb's DNA unique to each species, allowing for genetic identity determination and exposure of potential adulteration (Senapati et al., 2022). Similarly, chemical profiling of herbs using techniques like HPLC, GC-MS, or NMR, and comparing the profiles with established reference profiles, helps verify authenticity, consistency, and quality (Gainza et al., 2020).

Combining these techniques creates a comprehensive quality control approach for herbal products (Yin et al., 2022; Hu et al., 2021). After authentication, samples are cleaned and dried (air or oven) to remove moisture and prevent microbial growth, noting that the drying method can influence the chemical profile of the final extract. The dried parts are then pulverized to increase their surface area, facilitating more efficient extraction of compounds.

Extraction Techniques

Extraction techniques are critical for extracting the desired active compounds from herbs during the manufacturing of herbal products (Abeillé et al., 2020). Optimizing these techniques is crucial in ensuring the efficient recovery of compounds responsible for herbal products' potency and efficacy. Key factors to consider in extraction include the pre-extraction steps (drying and grinding methods), solvent choice, extraction temperature and pressure, and method of extraction.

After selecting an extraction protocol, it must be validated by comparing it to reference samples, performing analytical testing, and conducting statistical analysis. This ensures that the process meets predetermined quality standards for yield and the presence of desired bioactive compounds, as well as being consistent and reproducible. Common extraction methods include decoction, infusion, percolation, Soxhlet extraction, supercritical fluid extraction (SFE), microwave-assisted extraction (MAE), and ultrasound-assisted extraction. A summary of the distinct advantages and limitations of each method concerning cost, scalability, selectivity, and environmental impact are presented in Table 1.

Table 1. Common extraction techniques in herbal product development

Technique	Principle	Key Advantages	Key Limitations
Decoction/Infusion	Traditional, using boiling water or steeping.	Simple, inexpensive, traditional applicability.	Low selectivity, extracts primarily polar compounds, may degrade thermolabile compounds.
Soxhlet	Continuous solvent cycling/reflux	Highly exhaustive, high yield.	High solvent consumption, long extraction time, unsuitable for thermolabile compounds.
Supercritical Fluid Extraction (SFE)	Uses supercritical CO_2 as solvent	Highly selective, non-toxic solvent (CO_2), no residual solvent in the final product	High equipment cost, limited to non-polar/moderately polar compounds unless modifiers are used.
Microwave-Assisted Extraction (MAE)	Microwave energy heats solvent and plant cells	Rapid, reduced solvent consumption, high yield	Not all solvents are suitable, requires optimization
Ultrasound-Assisted Extraction (UAE)	Ultrasonic cavitation disrupts cell walls	Fast, efficient, operates at low temperatures	Scaling up can be challenging

CHROMATOGRAPHY

The inherent complexity of herbal extracts, often containing hundreds of unique metabolites, presents a significant analytical challenge. Chromatography is the cornerstone technique for deconvoluting this complexity, serving two primary strategic purposes in herbal medicine: 1) fingerprinting for quality control and 2) isolating bioactive compounds for identification and validation.

No single chromatographic method can resolve all constituents in a typical herbal extract. Therefore, a sequential, strategic approach is employed, moving from broad fractionation to high-resolution purification. The choice of technique is a trade-off between resolution, speed, scalability, and cost, as detailed in Table 2.

Chromatographic profiles serve as indicators of the phytoconstituents present in a herbal mixture. Chromatography serves two primary strategic purposes in herbal medicine: fingerprinting for quality control (e.g. in plant samples identification and targeted detection of adulterants (Simmler et al., 2018)) and isolating bioactive compounds from samples. Successful separation of herbal mixtures into individual components is the initial step towards identifying and evaluating the bioactivity of these constituents. Isolating compounds responsible for specific biological effects establishes a direct link between phytoconstituents and observed biological activity, providing scientific validation for the use of herbs in treating diseases and aiding their subsequent incorporation into modern evidence-based healthcare systems. Bioassay-guided fractionation, a key strategy for this purpose, is discussed in detail later.

Given the wide range of compounds found in herbal mixtures, no single chromatographic technique can successfully profile all constituents; thus, a combination of techniques is often necessary. A sequential, strategic approach is employed, moving from broad fractionation to high-resolution purification. The technique adopted is a trade-off between resolution, speed, scalability, and cost (Table 2).

The first steps usually involve the use of column chromatography (CC), vacuum liquid chromatography (VLC), or flash chromatography. These techniques are useful for processing large quantities of crude extract, separating it into broader fractions based on polarity. The value of these techniques lies in their scalability and ability to handle complex matrices, making them ideal for the first stage of bioassay-guided fractionation. Monitoring these separations and performing initial quality control requires the use of Thin-Layer Chromatography (TLC) and its advanced counterpart, High-Performance TLC (HPTLC).

TLC is a fast, simple, and inexpensive method for isolating bioactive compounds from plants and other natural sources. It requires minimal instrumentation, making it ideal for low-resource laboratories (Bele & Khale, 2011). TLC has many applications in natural products chemistry, such as monitoring column chromatography fractions, identifying compounds by comparing Rf values to reference standards, fingerprinting for authentication, standardization, and quality control in herbal drug development, and determining the purity of isolated compounds. While popular, TLC is a manual method with low reproducibility due to humidity, chamber saturation, and temperature (Upton et al., 2020).

HPTLC, is widely used for regulatory quality control due to its high reproducibility, ability to analyze multiple samples simultaneously, and its power in creating definitive chromatographic fingerprints for authentication and batch-to-batch consistency. Once a fraction shows promising biological activity, high-resolution purification is required to obtain pure compounds. This is typically achieved using Preparative High-Performance Liquid Chromatography (Prep-HPLC). Prep-HPLC offers unparalleled separation power for isolating individual compounds from complex fractions on a scale suitable for subsequent structural elucidation and biological testing (Jadhav et al., 2014). For simpler mixtures or low-resource settings, Preparative TLC provides a low-cost, effective alternative for small-scale purification. PrepTLC is inexpensive and simple; the separation can be visually monitored, and no specialized equipment is required. Common chromatographic techniques used for isolation are compared in Table 2.

Table 2. Chromatographic techniques for isolation of bioactive compounds

Technique	Principle	Key Applications & Advantages
Column Chromatography (CC)	Gravity-driven separation on a packed stationary phase	Versatile, scalable for initial broad fractionation of crude extracts; low equipment cost
Vacuum Liquid Chromatography (VLC)	CC accelerated by vacuum for faster solvent flow	Rapid initial fractionation; faster and more efficient than gravity CC (Maurya et al., 2018)
Flash Chromatography	Medium-pressure liquid chromatography	Faster and higher resolution than VLC; suitable for finer separations; can be automated (Sravani, 2018)
Preparative Thin-Layer Chromatography (Prep TLC)	Separation on a thick-layer plate; bands are scraped and eluted	Low-cost, small-scale purification; ideal for isolating mg quantities of compounds
Preparative HPLC (Prep-HPLC)	High-pressure liquid chromatography on a large scale	High-resolution purification of complex mixtures; highly reproducible and automatable

SPECTROSCOPIC TECHNIQUES

The next important task after isolation is characterization of the bioactive compounds responsible for the observed biological activities. This is achieved through spectroscopic techniques, which are also indispensable in direct profiling of entire extracts (where they provide comprehensive information on the structure of compounds within the mixture). This information is crucial for implementing quality control and standardization, and for understanding the mechanisms of action of herbal formulations. The technique selected for characterization depends on a number of factors including the information required, the available infrastructure, and the nature of the sample (Table 3).

Nuclear Magnetic Resonance (NMR) spectroscopy is the most critical tool for unambiguous structural elucidation of novel compounds (or confirming the structure of known ones). It leverages the interaction of atomic nuclei with an external magnetic field to generate detailed spectral data that reveal a molecule's connectivity and functional groups. Additionally, NMR is also invaluable for fingerprinting complex botanical formulations, allowing differentiation between closely related species, distinguishing herbal mixtures from adulterants, and assisting in maintaining batch-to-batch consistency and implementing quality control for herbal formulations. However, the high capital and maintenance costs of high-field NMR instruments (requiring specialized, controlled environments, expensive consumables, and frequent, and highly technical maintenance), coupled with the need for specialized expertise, can be a significant barrier. This limitation highlights the importance of collaborative networks between research institutions and industries in developing countries and well-equipped central facilities.

Mass Spectrometry, especially when coupled with chromatographic techniques (e.g., LC-MS, GC-MS), provides invaluable data for chemical profiling, quantification, and structural elucidation of constituents in herbal formulations, thereby aiding in quality control and safety assessment. It is exceptionally sensitive and excels at determining molecular weight and providing clues about structure through fragmentation patterns. With the advent of High-Resolution Mass Spectrometry (HRMS), it is possible to obtain the exact molecular mass of unknown compounds and hence their precise elemental composition which is a critical step identification in structural elucidation. This makes HRMS invaluable for *dereplication*—the rapid identification of known compounds to avoid redundant research. It is a cornerstone of metabolomics studies, where accurate mass is vital for identifying thousands of metabolites in complex biological samples (Wallace and McCord, 2020). However, like NMR, HRMS represents a major investment and requires significant operational costs. In resource-limited settings, a strategic approach is crucial. Lower-resolution LC-MS or GC-MS systems, which are more widely available, can still provide invaluable data for fingerprinting, quantifying marker compounds, and dereplication when supported by well-established reference libraries and methods.

Fourier-Transform Infrared (FT-IR) Spectroscopy offers a rapid and cost-effective means to identify functional groups in a compound. It measures the absorption of infrared radiation by molecules, with the absorbed energy corresponding to the vibrational modes of specific chemical bonds within the molecule (Pasieczna-Patkowska et al., 2005). While it rarely provides a full structure alone, its value in herbal medicine lies in its speed and use as a fingerprinting technique. Its affordability, minimal sample preparation, and ease of use make it an exceptionally accessible tool for routine quality control on the ground. FT-IR finds applications in the quality control of herbal formulations; by comparing the IR spectra of different batches of the same formulation, variations in composition can be identified, ensuring product consistency. Furthermore, FT-IR can monitor chemical changes in herbal products over time, assessing their stability and shelf-life by observing changes in functional group absorption bands (Bunaciu et al., 2011). The technique can also be used to monitor various stages of processing, such as extraction or drying, to ensure optimal conditions for retaining desired constituents. Since FT-IR spectra of complex extracts form a fingerprint of functional groups, differences in peak patterns can indicate plant identity or adulteration.

Table 3. Spectroscopic techniques for herbal formulation analysis

Technique	Principle	Key Applications in Herbal Medicine	Key Considerations
Nuclear Magnetic Resonance (NMR)	Absorption of radiofrequency energy by atomic nuclei in a magnetic field	Unambiguous structural elucidation of pure compounds; fingerprinting for batch-to-batch consistency and detecting adulteration.	Low sensitivity; requires pure compounds for full structure elucidation; high equipment cost and expertise
Mass Spectrometry (MS)	Measures mass-to-charge (m/z) ratio of ionized molecules.	Molecular weight determination; fragmentation pattern analysis; quantification	Often coupled with separation techniques (LC-MS, GC-MS)
High-Resolution MS (HRMS)	High-precision mass measurement (to 4-5 decimal places)	Exact molecular formula determination; dereplication (rapid ID of knowns); cornerstone of metabolomics	Higher cost than low-resolution MS; crucial for metabolomics.
Fourier Transform Infrared (FT-IR)	Absorption of infrared radiation corresponding to vibrational modes of chemical bonds.	Rapid functional group fingerprinting; quality control (batch consistency); detection of gross adulteration	Low-to-Moderate capital cost; widely accessible.

CHEMICAL PROFILING OF HERBAL FORMULATIONS

Chemical profiling is a systematic approach for characterizing the chemical composition of herbal formulations. Given the inherent complexity of these mixtures, strong analytical strategies are required. Chemical profiling aims to identify and quantify the constituents, understand their relative proportions, and establish a chemical fingerprint that can be correlated with biological activity, geographical origin, processing methods, and overall quality. This is crucial for standardization, quality control, and ensuring the safety and efficacy of herbal products.

Hyphenated Techniques

Hyphenated techniques involve the coupling of two or more analytical techniques, typically a separation technique with a spectroscopic technique, to achieve enhanced separation efficiency, specificity, and sensitivity. This combination allows for the resolution of complex mixtures into individual components and their subsequent identification and quantification, addressing the challenges posed by the intricate nature of herbal formulations.

Gas Chromatography-Mass Spectrometry (GC-MS)

Gas Chromatography-Mass Spectrometry (GC-MS) couples the high separation efficiency of gas chromatography (GC) with mass spectrometry (MS). GC-MS is a critical tool for establishing characteristic fingerprints of essential oils and other volatile fractions of herbal formulations (Chevalier and Sommerer, 2011). This profile can be used as a reference standard to ensure consistency across different batches of raw material or finished products, with deviations indicating potential quality issues or adulteration. Furthermore, GC-MS enables the identification and quantification of specific volatile bioactive compounds, assisting in defining quantitative standards for formulations. It can also identify and quantify volatile organic contaminants (e.g., pesticide residues, residual solvents) and synthetic adulterants. A main limitation of GC-MS is that many plant metabolites are non-volatile or thermally unstable (e.g., sugars, organic acids, amino acids, some phenolic compounds), requiring chemical derivatization to convert them into more volatile and thermally stable forms amenable to GC analysis (Valle-Algarra et al., 2014).

Liquid Chromatography-Mass Spectrometry (LC-MS)

Liquid Chromatography-Mass Spectrometry (LC-MS) is a powerful hybrid technique that combines the separation capability of liquid chromatography (LC) with the identification and quantification power of mass spectrometry (MS). It is ideal for the analysis of non-volatile, thermally labile, and polar compounds, making it essential for profiling plant metabolites (Zeki et al., 2020).

LC-MS can detect a wide range of plant metabolites, even at trace levels, resulting in a comprehensive chemical fingerprint of the herbal formulation. By combining chromatographic retention time, accurate mass data (from high-resolution MS), and fragmentation patterns (from tandem MS, MS/MS), known and novel plant compounds can be confidently identified and structurally elucidated. LC-MS is the primary platform for both untargeted and targeted metabolomics, allowing for the investigation of global metabolic changes in plants or biological systems treated with herbal extracts. LC-MS profiles can also be used to compare different batches of raw material or finished products, ensuring consistency and identifying deviations in chemical composition or detecting adulteration.

Metabolomic Techniques

Metabolomics is the systematic study of the complete set of metabolites within a biological system (e.g., a plant, tissue, or organism) at a specific time. In the context of herbal formulations, metabolomics provides a comprehensive snapshot of the chemical constituents, allowing for a deeper understanding of their composition, biological effects, and potential variations.

Untargeted Metabolomics

Untargeted metabolomics aims to capture a comprehensive metabolic profile of a sample without prior knowledge of its composition, detecting as many metabolites as possible (Wishart et al., 2022). Techniques like LC-MS offer high sensitivity and broad coverage for a wide range of polar and semi-polar metabolites, with data typically involving retention time and m/z features used for statistical analysis and metabolite identification (Zeki et al., 2020). GC-MS is excellent for volatile and semi-volatile metabolites, providing highly reproducible fragmentation patterns for compound identification against spectral libraries, often complementing LC-MS data. NMR Spectroscopy provides quantitative and highly reproducible data with minimal sample preparation; it is non-destructive, and can analyze a wide range of metabolites simultaneously. NMR is particularly strong for identifying major and moderately abundant compounds and their structural elucidation. The rich datasets generated using these techniques, can be used for comparative analysis, biomarker discovery, and holistic assessment of herbal mixtures. This approach is especially useful for distinguishing samples based on geographical origin, harvest season, or preparation method, and is a powerful tool for identifying novel compounds or unexpected contaminants (Wishart et al., 2022).

Targeted Metabolomics

Targeted metabolomics focuses on the accurate and precise quantification of a predefined set of metabolites. Unlike untargeted approaches, it aims to measure specific compounds of interest, often known bioactive markers or compounds relevant to a specific metabolic pathway (McMillen et al., 2023). This approach helps standardize herbal products by quantifying marker compounds (e.g., specific flavonoids, alkaloids) to ensure consistent quality and potency. It assists in routine monitoring of key constituents to confirm product specifications and identify batch variations, and aids in establishing dose-response relationships.

Chemometric Tools for Herbal Medicine

Chemometrics is an interdisciplinary field that applies mathematical and statistical methods to chemical data to extract meaningful information. In the context of herbal medicine, where chemical profiles are often complex and information-rich, chemometrics is an invaluable tool for data interpretation and quality control. The tools of chemometrics extend beyond simple data visualization and are used to perform more advanced tasks like clustering, classification, and prediction. Some of the most common techniques include: Hierarchical Cluster Analysis (HCA), Principal Component Regression (PCR), and Artificial Neural Networks (ANNs).

By applying these chemometric tools, researchers can transform complex chemical data into actionable understandings, enabling better quality control, improved batch consistency, and a more robust scientific basis for the development and use of herbal products. The integration of metabolomics and chemometrics represents a data science revolution in natural products research. It moves beyond simply identifying individual compounds to understanding the entire network of chemical interactions and their collective biological effects. This shift is critical for developing "systems pharmacology" approaches to herbal medicine, where the focus is on the holistic impact of a complex mixture rather than isolated components.

BIOLOGICAL ASSAYS

Biological assays are experimental procedures used to determine the biological activity or potency of a substance, such as an herbal extract or an isolated compound. In the context of herbal formulations, bioassays are crucial for scientifically validating traditional claims, identifying specific therapeutic effects, and guiding the isolation of bioactive compounds. These assays typically involve exposing biological systems (e.g., microorganisms, enzymes, cell lines) to the herbal formulation and observing the resulting biological response.

Common *In Vitro* Assays Used for Bioactivity Evaluation

In vitro assays are conducted in a controlled environment outside of a living organism, typically using cells, tissues, or biochemical components. They are cost-effective, high-throughput, and provide valuable preliminary data on the potential biological activities of herbal formulations.

Antimicrobial Assay

Antimicrobial assays assess the ability of a substance to inhibit the growth or kill microorganisms (bacteria, fungi, viruses). Common assays used in antimicrobial assays include the Agar Disc Diffusion Assay, Broth Microdilution Assay (MIC, MBC/MFC), and the Time-Kill Kinetics (Hossain, 2024).

Anti-inflammatory Assays

Herbal medicines are widely used to treat inflammation-related conditions, and anti-inflammatory assays help elucidate their mechanisms of action. Common anti-inflammatory assays include: enzyme inhibition assays, cellular assays, and protein denaturation inhibition assay (Peiris et al., 2025). These methods help link traditional anti-inflammatory claims with specific molecular targets and pathways, reinforcing the scientific foundation of herbal medicine.

Antioxidant Assays

Antioxidant assays assess the ability of a substance to neutralize free radicals or prevent oxidative damage, as oxidative stress is implicated in numerous diseases. Common *in vitro* antioxidant assays include the DPPH (2,2-Diphenyl-1-Picryl-Hydrazyl Hydrate) Assay, Ferric Reducing Antioxidant Potential (FRAP) Assay and Hydrogen Peroxide Free Radical Scavenger Assay (Munteanu and Apetrei, 2021).

Anticancer Assays

Anticancer assays evaluate the cytotoxic or antiproliferative effects of substances on cancer cell lines. Examples of these assays include the MTT (3-(4,5-dimethylthiazol-2-yl)-2,5-diphenyltetrazolium bromide) assay, the XTT (2,3-Bis-(2-methoxy-4-nitro-5-sulfophenyl)-2H-tetrazolium-5-carboxanilide) assay, the Trypan Blue Dye Exclusion assay, and Sulforhodamine B (SRB) Assay (Sanjai et al., 2024).

Table 4 contains categories of bioassays and their common uses in herbal medicine.

Table 4. Categories of bioassays and their common use cases in herbal medicine

Bioassay Category	Principle of Action	Common Use Cases in Herbal Medicine	Examples of Assays
Antioxidant Activity	Measures the capacity of compounds to neutralize free radicals or reduce oxidative species.	Standardization based on total antioxidant potential; assessing radical scavenging for anti-aging or protective formulations	DPPH assay, FRAP assay, Oxygen Radical Absorbance Capacity (ORAC) assay.
Anti-inflammatory Activity	Measures the inhibition of pro-inflammatory mediators (e.g., cytokines, enzymes) or the reduction of cellular inflammation markers.	Validation of traditional uses for arthritis, pain management, and chronic inflammatory diseases.	COX-1/COX-2 inhibition assays, measurement of nitric oxide (NO) production in macrophages (e.g., RAW 264.7 cells)
Antimicrobial/ Antifungal	Measures the ability of the extract or compound to inhibit the growth or kill microorganisms (bacteria, fungi).	Screening for natural preservatives; discovering novel antibiotics/ antiseptics; validation of traditional use for infections	Minimum Inhibitory Concentration (MIC), Minimum Bactericidal Concentration (MBC), Disk diffusion methods.
Cytotoxicity & Anticancer	Measures the toxicity of the extract towards cancer cells (cytotoxicity) versus normal cells	Discovery of novel chemotherapy agents; assessment of safety margins for high-dose traditional remedies	MTT assay, Sulforhodamine B (SRB) assay, Flow cytometry for apoptosis induction
Enzyme Inhibition	Measures the inhibition of specific target enzymes related to disease pathways.	Screening for diabetes (α-amylase, α-glucosidase), hypertension (ACE), or neurological disorders (AChE, BChE).	Spectrophotometric assays targeting specific enzyme substrates (e.g., pNPG for α-glucosidase)
Receptor Binding & Modulation	Measures the binding affinity of a compound to a specific cellular receptor or its ability to activate/inhibit a pathway.	Identifying compounds that target hormone receptors, neurotransmitter receptors, or immune signaling pathways.	Luciferase reporter assays, Radioligand binding assays, Calcium flux assays.
Toxicology & Safety	Measures acute or chronic toxicity in various *in vitro* (cell) or *in vivo* (animal) models.	Essential for regulatory submission; establishing a safe dosage range; identifying genotoxic or hepatotoxic risks	Ames test (mutagenicity), Hepatotoxicity assays (e.g., HepG2 cells), Acute oral toxicity studies.

Bioassay-Guided Fractionation

Bioassay-guided fractionation is a strategic approach that couples bioactivity testing with chromatographic separation to isolate active constituents from complex herbal mixtures. The process begins with a crude extract, which is partitioned or fractionated using solvents or chromatographic techniques (e.g., column chromatography). Each fraction is then subjected to biological assays to identify those with the desired activity. Active fractions are further purified and re-tested, eventually leading to the isolation of pure bioactive compounds. The chemical structure of the isolated active compound(s) is then determined using advanced spectroscopic techniques (NMR, MS, IR, UV-Vis).

This iterative process enables the identification of pharmacologically relevant constituents and the elucidation of structure-activity relationships. It also provides a rational basis for standardization and quality control, ensuring that therapeutic claims are linked to specific, measurable bioactive compounds. Bioassay-guided fractionation has been instrumental in the discovery of plant-derived drugs like artemisinin and paclitaxel and remains a cornerstone of natural product research. However, challenges associated with this technique include potential loss of activity if the pharmacological properties exhibited by the medicinal plant are due to synergistic interactions between multiple compounds. The active compounds may also be unstable during purification, and the process is often labor-intensive, especially when dealing with complex extracts (Malviya and Malviya, 2017).

MULTI-COMPONENT EFFECTS IN HERBAL FORMULATIONS

Herbal formulations are characterized by their polyherbal nature—combinations of multiple plant species or phytochemical constituents that collectively contribute to therapeutic outcomes. This multi-component composition is deeply rooted in traditional medical systems, where the blending of herbs is intended to maximize efficacy, broaden the therapeutic spectrum, reduce toxicity, and correct imbalances. However, understanding and scientifically validating how these components interact (whether synergistically, additively, or antagonistically) is critical for both product development and regulatory acceptance.

Synergy, Additivity, and Antagonism

When two or more compounds are combined, their joint effect can differ from the sum of their individual effects. These interactions are fundamental to understanding the pharmacological basis of herbal formulations.

Synergy

Synergy (or synergism) occurs when the combined effect of two or more compounds is greater than the sum of their individual effects. This implies that the compounds enhance each other's activity, leading to a more potent therapeutic outcome at lower concentrations than would be achieved by individual components. Synergy can arise through various mechanisms, including multi-target effects (different compounds acting on distinct but related molecular targets), improved bioavailability (one compound enhancing the absorption or stability of another), reduction of resistance, mitigation of side effects (one compound reducing the toxicity of another), and complementary mechanisms (compounds affecting different stages of a pathological process). Synergy is often cited as a key advantage of traditional herbal medicine, where the complex mixture is believed to offer superior therapeutic benefits, often with reduced side effects due to balanced interactions (Roell et al., 2017).

For example, *Artemisia annua* (Asteraceae), is usually considered as a substitute treatment for malaria in regions where people lack access to or cannot afford effective anti-malarials, including artemisinin combination therapy (Hirt & M'Pia, 2008). According to studies, the anti-plasmodial IC_{50} values of *A. annua* herb extracts obtained by manually wringing out the juice or by pounding the fresh herb to a pulp and then squeezing out the juice (Wright et al., 2010) were 6 to 18 times lower than expected in terms of their artemisinin content, indicating that the extracts' activity could not be fully explained by their artemisinin content. For instance, in *Plasmodium berghei*-infected mice, the pounded juice (two doses of 500 μL, spaced 12 hours apart) equivalent to 18 mg/kg artemisinin lowered parasitaemia by 95%, while a single treatment of 30 mg/kg artemisinin suppressed parasitaemia by 88% (Wright et al., 2010). Additionally, in mice infected with *P. berghei* given a crude ethanolic extract of *A. annua* formulated with oil in a soft gel capsule, the ED_{50} value with respect to the artemisinin content was 35.1 mg/kg whereas the ED_{50} of pure artemisinin was 122 mg/kg (Wan et al., 1992). These results suggest that compounds present in *A. annua*, especially flavonoids, may act synergistically to enhance the action of artemisinin (Liu et al., 1992; Elford et al., 1987; Liu et al., 1989). The flavone casticin enhances the *in vitro* activity of artemisinin by 3-5 fold (Elford et al., 1987). Some other hydroxy-polymethoxy flavone constituents (artemetin, chrysosplenetin, chrysosplenol-D, cirsilineol, eupatorin) also produce enhancement of 1.1-2.2 fold (Liu et al., 1992).

In another eample, Curcumin, the primary active compound in turmeric, has poor oral bioavailability. On the other hand, Piperine, a major component of black pepper, is a known bioavailability enhancer. When co-administered, piperine inhibits the metabolic glucuronidation of curcumin in the liver and intestine, significantly increasing its serum concentration. This is an example of pharmacokinetic synergy where one compound (without intrinsic activity) dramatically improves the systemic exposure of the other (Shoba *et al.*, 1998).

Additivity

Additivity occurs when the combined effect of two or more compounds is equal to the sum of their individual effects. The compounds act independently or on the same target with similar mechanisms, and their combined effect is predictable from their individual potencies. While less dramatic than synergy, additive effects are common in herbal mixtures (Roell et al., 2017). For example, Eugenol in combination with ampicillin, penicillin or erythromycin had an additive effect against *E. coli* (Palaniappan and Holley, 2010).

Antagonism

Antagonism occurs when the combined effect of two or more compounds is less than the sum of their individual effects, or even less than the effect of the most active single component. This means that one compound reduces or nullifies the activity of another. Antagonism can occur through various mechanisms, including competitive binding (one compound competing for the same receptor without eliciting a strong response), metabolic inactivation (one compound promoting the degradation of another), and opposing physiological effects (compounds having contrary actions on different biological pathways) (Roell et al., 2017).

St. John's Wort (*Hypericum perforatum*), used for depression, is a well-documented example of pharmacokinetic antagonism or interference. Its long-term use induces the cytochrome P450 enzyme system (particularly CYP3A4) and the drug efflux pump P-glycoprotein. This can accelerate the metabolism and reduce the plasma concentrations of a wide range of conventional drugs, including anticoagulants (e.g., warfarin), immunosuppressants (e.g., cyclosporine), and oral contraceptives, effectively antagonizing their intended therapeutic effects (Henderson et al., 2002).

APPLICATIONS OF SPECTROSCOPIC CHARACTERIZATION IN HERBAL FORMULATIONS

Spectroscopic techniques (NMR, MS, FT-IR, UV-Vis) are not merely tools for structural elucidation of isolated compounds; they are central to the scientific evaluation of whole herbal formulations. Their comprehensive capabilities for chemical profiling underpin efforts in standardization, quality control, safety assessment, validation of ethnomedicinal claims, and the development of improved herbal products.

Standardization and Quality Control

Standardization aims to ensure consistency in the chemical composition and, consequently, the biological activity of herbal formulations. Quality control involves monitoring this consistency throughout the production process, from raw material to finished product. Spectroscopic characterization provides the foundation for both.

Establishment of Reference Standards and Chemical Fingerprints

For each bioactive compound isolated from herbal formulations, spectroscopic techniques (especially FTIR, NMR, and HRMS) are indispensable for their unambiguous structural elucidation and purity assessment. These authenticated pure compounds then serve as reference standards for quantitative analysis in quality control programs. Furthermore, herbal formulations are complex, and their therapeutic effects often arise from the combined action of multiple constituents. Rather than quantifying every single compound, chemical fingerprinting aims to establish a characteristic chromatographic or spectroscopic profile that represents the entire chemical complexity of a genuine, high-quality herbal product (Custers et al., 2017). This "fingerprint" serves as a benchmark for comparison. Any deviation from this established fingerprint in subsequent batches indicates a potential quality issue (e.g., different species, poor growth conditions, improper processing, degradation). For instance, the World Health Organization recognizes chromatographic fingerprinting for identity and quality control of many herbal drugs (Alaerts et al., 2014)

Detection of Adulterants and Contaminants

Adulteration, whether intentional (e.g., substitution with cheaper or ineffective plant material, addition of synthetic drugs) or unintentional (e.g., misidentification of plants), poses significant risks to consumer health and undermines the credibility of herbal medicine. Spectroscopic fingerprints (e.g., from FT-IR, NMR, LC-MS) can rapidly differentiate authentic herbal materials from adulterants (Kucharska-Ambrożej and Karpinska, 2020). Distinct chemical profiles or the presence of unexpected compounds immediately flag an adulterated sample.

Furthermore, herbal products can be contaminated with pesticides, heavy metals, mycotoxins, or microbial impurities (Shaban et al., 2015). While heavy metals and microbial contaminants often require specific analytical methods, GC-MS is widely used for the detection and quantification of pesticide residues and volatile organic contaminants (VOCs), and high-resolution MS can also be employed to detect a broad range of environmental contaminants (Kardani et al., 2023; Putri et al., 2022; Muter and Bartkevics, 2020).

Safety Assessment

Beyond efficacy, the safety of herbal formulations is paramount. Spectroscopic characterization plays a growing role in predicting potential toxicities and undesirable interactions.

Prediction of Toxicity by Chemical Profiling

Comprehensive chemical profiling (metabolome) of an herbal formulation using LC-MS, GC-MS, or NMR, aids the detection of compounds known to be toxic and the proactive dentification of new risks. Examples of established and well-documented chemical classes with severe clinical toxicity (often subject to stringent regulatory warnings or outright bans) include Aristolochic Acids and Pyrrolizidine Alkaloids. Aristolochic Acids are potent nephrotoxins and human carcinogens, associated with Aristolochic Acid Nephropathy (AAN) (Wang et al., 2021), while Pyrrolizidine Alkaloids are hepatotoxic compounds.. Spectroscopic techniques can detect these toxins at trace levels in herbal samples, allowing for the immediate rejection of contaminated batches (Tabuas et al., 2024).

Beyond chemical classes where toxicities are well-established, other emerging safety concerns involve less predictable risks. These include unintentional contaminants such as mycotoxins (e.g., aflatoxins from improper storage), and the intentional addition of non-natural components, such as synthetic pharmaceutical agents (e.g., sildenafil analogs) in herbal formulations. Complex LC-MS fingerprinting is crucial for the detection of these unexpected toxic or adulterating components. Furthermore, chemometric analysis of metabolic profiles can correlate specific chemical signatures in the herbal product with observed toxicological endpoints in preclinical studies, leading to the identification of chemical markers associated with toxicity (Das and Ojha, 2025).

Herbal-Drug Interaction (HDI) Prediction

Spectroscopy-guided identification of constituents with known cytochrome P450 enzyme inhibition or induction profiles can forecast possible herb-drug interactions (HDIs). For example, LC-MS can quantify hyperforin in St. John's Wort, a compound known to induce CYP3A4 and reduce the efficacy of many drugs (Riedel et al., 2004). Understanding the concentration and behavior of such compounds enables mitigation strategies in formulation design and patient guidance.

Validation of Ethnomedicinal Claims on Efficacy of Herbal Formulations

Traditional ethnomedicinal claims, passed down through generations, often describe specific therapeutic uses for herbal remedies. Spectroscopic characterization plays a vital role in providing scientific evidence for these claims. Bioactivity-Guided Fractionation directly links the chemical constituents to the observed biological activity. When an extract shows activity aligned with an ethnomedicinal claim (e.g., anti-inflammatory activity for a plant traditionally used for pain), spectroscopic techniques are used to identify the specific compounds responsible for this effect. This provides molecular validation for the traditional use. Additionally, comparing the chemical fingerprints of batches of herbal formulations proven efficacious (either clinically or in robust preclinical models) against those that are less effective can identify specific chemical markers associated with efficacy. These markers can then serve as quality control parameters.

The comprehensive applications of spectroscopy collectively form a regulatory bridge that can transform anecdotal traditional knowledge into evidence-based medicine acceptable to modern healthcare systems. By providing quantitative, reproducible, and verifiable data on identity, purity, safety, and efficacy, spectroscopy addresses the core concerns of regulatory bodies and healthcare professionals. This implies that investment in spectroscopic infrastructure and expertise is not merely a scientific luxury but a strategic necessity for countries aiming to integrate traditional medicine into their national health systems and participate in the global natural products market. It also suggests that future regulatory frameworks will increasingly rely on these advanced analytical fingerprints rather than just botanical names.

An integrated workflow for the standardization and quality control of herbal formulations is shown in Figure 1.

Figure 1. Integrated workflow for the standardization and quality control of herbal formulations

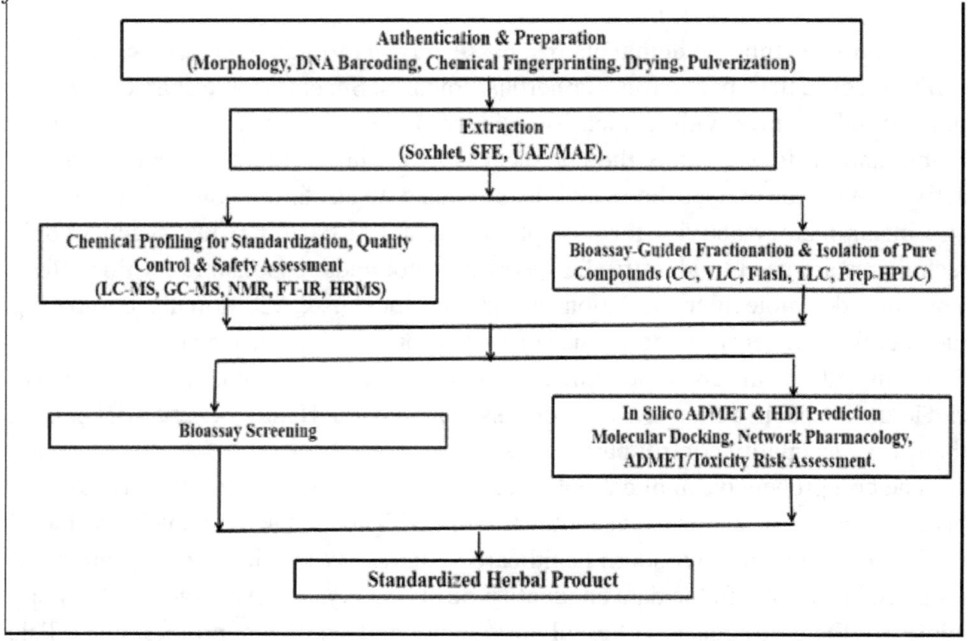

CASE STUDIES FROM TRADITIONAL MEDICINE

To concretize the scientific principles and methodologies discussed, this section presents illustrative case studies of herbal formulations rooted in traditional medicine. These cases demonstrate how modern spectroscopic, metabolomic, and bioassay-guided approaches can be successfully applied to evaluate, standardize, and validate complex herbal mixtures used in managing prevalent diseases such as inflammation, cancer, and pain. The studies reinforce the feasibility of integrating traditional knowledge with evidence-based approaches for improved healthcare delivery.

Case Study on Characterization and Bioactivity of Traditional Herbal Formulations for Diarrheal Diseases

In a previous study, Gholkar et al. (2021) developed a prototype for standardization of plant extracts with respect to efficacy, using the anti-diarrheal activity of *Psidium guajava* (guava) leaf extract as an example (Gholkar et al., 2021).

Ninety samples of mature guava leaves were collected from distinct regions across different seasons to account for environmental variations. ^{1}H NMR spectroscopy was used for holistic "fingerprinting" of metabolites. LC-MS/MS analysis confirmed the presence of quercetin, ferulic acid, and gallic acid in the samples. Eight *in vitro* bioassays reflecting different stages of diarrheal pathogenesis (e.g., antibacterial activity, effect on bacterial colonization/invasion, effect on bacterial enterotoxins) were undertaken for each extract, with empirical cut-off limits to classify activity as 'good' or 'poor'. The ^{1}H NMR spectral data were correlated with the bioactivity results using unsupervised Principal Component Analysis (PCA) and supervised Orthogonal Partial Least Square-Discriminant Analysis (OPLS-DA) and OPLS-Regression Analysis (OPLS-RA).

PCA and OPLS-DA showed clear seasonal and regional segregation of extracts based on their metabolic profiles, indicating significant environmental influence on chemical composition. Significant OPLS models identified specific ^{1}H NMR signals that correlated with either good or poor anti-diarrheal activity. While quercetin, ferulic acid, and gallic acid were confirmed, they did not consistently correlate with the specific peaks that segregated extracts with good and poor activity, suggesting that overall efficacy is likely due to the interplay of several compounds rather than a single biomarker. This case study successfully demonstrated that ^{1}H NMR-based spectral fingerprinting, combined with multivariate analysis, can serve as a robust prototype for standardizing herbal extracts based on their efficacy, even when specific active principles are unidentified or act synergistically. It emphasizes the importance of a holistic fingerprinting approach over reliance on single marker compounds for standardization.

Case Study on the Adulteration of Herbal Products

Adulteration poses serious risks to consumers because the efficacy, safety, and toxicological data of these modified compounds are often unknown. A study by Oh et al. (2006) investigated herbal products marketed for erectile dysfunction to screen for the presence of sildenafil and its analogues.

Bulk powders of marketed products were extracted with methanol and characterized using High-Performance Liquid Chromatography-Diode Array Detection

(HPLC-DAD), Liquid Chromatography-Tandem Mass Spectrometry (LC-MS/MS), Infrared (IR) Spectroscopy, and Nuclear Magnetic Resonance (NMR) Spectroscopy.

The study successfully detected several sildenafil analogues, including Homosildenafil, Hydroxyhomosildenafil, and Acetildenafil, in the herbal products. This demonstrated that manufacturers of illicit herbal products are modifying the chemical structures of prescription drugs to create new compounds that are difficult to detect using standard screening methods. The increasing occurrence of these modified structures poses a significant and potentially life-threatening risk to consumers. The study highlights the urgent need for greater collaboration among health authorities, professionals, and researchers, as well as public education, to address this growing trend of adulteration, as the efficacy and safety of these analogues are largely unknown.

Integrated Approach for Scientific Validation of a Traditional Herbal Formulation for Diabetes Management

This case study (Singh et al., 2022) presents an integrated approach for the scientific validation of a herbal formulation traditionally used for diabetes management.

Extracts of the herbal mixture were characterized using FT-IR and High-Resolution Liquid Chromatography-Mass Spectrometry (HR-LC/MS). The identified phytochemical compounds were further analyzed for their physiochemical, drug-likeness, and pharmacokinetic properties using an online server.

FT-IR analysis aided the identification of the various functional groups in the extracts. HR-LC/MS analysis identified 51 compounds, providing a detailed profile of the chemical constituents of the sample. In silico analysis of the identified compounds revealed that 25 of them satisfied Lipinski's rule of five and exhibited drug-like characteristics, with 16 demonstrating good oral bioavailability. The study provides a comprehensive framework for the scientific validation of traditional herbal formulations by combining phytochemical screening, spectroscopic analysis, and in silico studies to confirm the presence of numerous bioactive compounds with pharmaceutical potential. This integrated approach not only scientifically validates a traditional remedy but also identifies specific compounds with favorable drug-like properties, which can serve as a foundation for future drug discovery and the development of standardized herbal products.

CHALLENGES, FUTURE PERSPECTIVES, AND CONCLUSIONS

Current Challenges

Despite remarkable progress in applying modern analytical and biological tools to evaluate herbal formulations, several critical challenges persist. A major limitation is the scarcity of expertise in interdisciplinary techniques that combine natural products chemistry, pharmacology, metabolomics, and bioinformatics. The complexity of herbal formulations demands highly trained personnel who can interpret advanced spectral data, develop validated bioassays, and perform sophisticated data analysis. However, many research institutions, especially in developing countries where traditional medicine is most practiced, lack such cross-disciplinary capacity. Another persistent hurdle is the high cost and limited accessibility of advanced instrumentation such as LC-MS/MS, HRMS, NMR, and FT-IR. Many laboratories, particularly in Africa, lack the infrastructure to support these techniques, impeding efforts to standardize and validate traditional formulations.

Future Perspectives

Application of In Silico Techniques to Aid ADMET and HDI Risk Predictions, Molecular Docking, and Network Pharmacology

In silico tools offer a cost-effective and time-saving approach to complement experimental methods. Computational models for ADMET (Absorption, Distribution, Metabolism, Excretion, and Toxicity) prediction and herb-drug interaction (HDI) risk assessments can prioritize compounds for further study. Molecular docking can simulate the interaction of phytochemicals with biological targets, providing insights into mechanisms of action. Network pharmacology, which explores the interactions between multiple constituents and multiple targets, aligns well with the polyherbal nature of traditional formulations. Together, these tools can inform the rational development of safer and more effective herbal products.

Sustainable Sourcing and Biotechnological Production

The increasing interest in traditional herbal medicine necessitates sustainable sourcing of medicinal plants to prevent overharvesting and loss of biodiversity. Cultivation of medicinal plants under controlled conditions, coupled with the use of biotechnological approaches such as plant tissue culture and metabolic engineering, can ensure a stable supply of bioactive compounds. Biotechnological production also opens the door for the heterologous expression of plant biosynthetic pathways, allowing for the scalable production of rare or endangered phytochemicals.

CONCLUSION

The scientific evaluation of traditional herbal formulations represents a transformative shift in natural products research, driven by the adoption of a unified analytical paradigm where high-throughput spectroscopic profiling and functional bioassays are combined with predictive *in silico* modeling. These integrative strategies are essential to align traditional medicine with contemporary healthcare standards and must be formally adopted into regulatory pathways. This means moving beyond single-marker standardization to complex chemical fingerprinting and requiring ADMET/HDI prediction for product licensing. Futhermore, regulatory bodies should incorporate data derived from network pharmacology and metabolomics,into herbal monographs, so that they can reflect the true multi-component nature of such remedies. This chapter has illustrated how modern analytical frameworks can unravel the complex phytochemical matrix of herbal mixtures, identify bioactive compounds, assess synergy and toxicity, and ensure reproducibility. This resonates with the mission of the African Centre for Herbal Research, Ilorin (ACHRI), which advocates for the responsible and evidence-based utilization of Africa's rich botanical heritage. However, the envisaged transformation depends on robust capacity building, especially in resource-limited environments. Strategic investments must be made in affordable, rugged analytical platforms (like FT-IR and benchtop LC-MS systems) and cross-disciplinary training programs must be implemented. Prioritizing accessible analytical tools and shared knowledge networks, would empower local research institutions to validate and standardize herbal formulation, enabling a safe utilization of Africa's rich botanical heritage, and aligning traditional medicine with contemporary global healthcare standards.

REFERENCES

Abeille, A., Hemforth, B., Winckel, E., & Gibson, E. (2020). Extraction from subjects: Differences in acceptability depend on the discourse function of the construction. *Cognition*, *204*, 104293. DOI: 10.1016/j.cognition.2020.104293 PMID: 32731004

Alaerts, G., Pieters, S., Logie, H., Van Erps, J., Merino-Arévalo, M., Dejaegher, B., Smeyers-Verbeke, J., & Heyden, Y. V. (2014). Exploration and classification of chromatographic fingerprints as additional tool for identification and quality control of several Artemisia species. *Journal of Pharmaceutical and Biomedical Analysis*, *95*, 34–46. DOI: 10.1016/j.jpba.2014.02.006 PMID: 24637050

Başaran, N., Pasli, D., & Başaran, A. (2022). Unpredictable adverse effects of herbal products. *Food and Chemical Toxicology*, *159*, 112762. DOI: 10.1016/j.fct.2021.112762 PMID: 34896186

Bele, A. A., & Khale, A. (2011). An overview on thin layer chromatography. *International Journal of Pharmaceutical Sciences and Research*, *2*(2), 256.

Biernacki, M., Kuczyńska, B., & Wawrzeńczyk, A. (2020). The Antimalaria Alkaloids in the Nigerian Medicinal Plant, Cryptolepis sanguinolenta. *Journal of Ethnopharmacology*, *250*, 112445.

Brown, A. C. (2017). Heart toxicity related to herbs and dietary supplements: Online table of case reports. *Journal of Dietary Supplements*. PMID: 28981338

Bunaciu, A. A., Aboul-Enein, H. Y., & Fleschin, S. (2011). Recent Applications of Fourier Transform Infrared Spectrophotometry in Herbal Medicine Analysis. *Applied Spectroscopy Reviews*, *46*(4), 251–260. DOI: 10.1080/05704928.2011.565532

Chevalier, F., & Sommerer, N. (2011). Analytical Methods: Mass Spectrometric Methods. In Fuquay, J. W. (Ed.), *Encyclopedia of Dairy Sciences* (2nd ed., pp. 198–205). Academic Press. DOI: 10.1016/B978-0-12-374407-4.00019-4

Custers, D., Van Praag, N., Courselle, P., Apers, S., & Deconinck, E. (2017). Chromatographic fingerprinting as a strategy to identify regulated plants in illegal herbal supplements. *Talanta*, *164*, 490–502. DOI: 10.1016/j.talanta.2016.12.008 PMID: 28107963

Das, S., & Ojha, P. K. (2025). Bridging chemistry and toxicology: Chemometric-driven prediction and prioritization of various drugs addressing hazardous effects for human safety. *Journal of Hazardous Materials*, *495*, 139134. DOI: 10.1016/j.jhazmat.2025.139134 PMID: 40633349

Ekor, M. (2014). The growing use of herbal medicines: Issues relating to adverse reactions and challenges in monitoring safety. *Frontiers in Pharmacology*, *4*, 177. DOI: 10.3389/fphar.2013.00177 PMID: 24454289

Elford, B. C., Roberts, M. F., Phillipson, J. D., & Wilson, R. J. (1987). Potentiation of the antimalarial activity of qinghaosu by methoxylated flavones. *Transactions of the Royal Society of Tropical Medicine and Hygiene*, *81*(3), 434–436. DOI: 10.1016/0035-9203(87)90161-1 PMID: 3318019

Fong, H. H. S., Pauli, G. F., Bolton, J. L., Van Breemen, R. B., Banuvar, S., Shulman, L., & Farnsworth, N. R. (2006). Evidence-based herbal medicine: Challenges in efficacy and safety assessments. In *Current review of Chinese medicine: Quality control of herbs and herbal material* (pp. 11-26).

Gainza, P., Sverrisson, F., Monti, F., Rodol, E., Boscaini, D., Bronstein, M. M., & Limonciel, L. (2020). Deciphering interaction fingerprints from protein molecular surfaces using geometric deep learning. *Nature Methods*, *17*(2), 184–192. DOI: 10.1038/s41592-019-0666-6 PMID: 31819266

Gholkar, M. S., Jain, P., Sharma, S., & Bhamare, V. (2021). 1H nuclear magnetic resonance-based metabolite profiling of guava leaf extract: An attempt to develop a prototype for standardization of plant extracts. *Journal of Applied Pharmaceutical Science*, *11*(01), 11–19. PMID: 33736648

Henderson, L., Yue, Q. Y., Bergquist, C., Gerden, B., & Arlett, P. (2002). St John's wort (*Hypericum perforatum*): Drug interactions and clinical outcomes. *British Journal of Clinical Pharmacology*, *54*(4), 341–448. DOI: 10.1046/j.1365-2125.2002.01683.x PMID: 12392581

Hirt, H. M., & M'Pia, B. (2008). *Natural medicine in the tropics 1: foundation text: tropical plants as a source of health care: production of medicines and cosmetics*. Anamed.

Hossain, T. J. (2024). Methods for screening and evaluation of antimicrobial activity: A review of protocols, advantages, and limitations. *European Journal of Microbiology & Immunology*, *14*(2), 97–115. DOI: 10.1556/1886.2024.00035 PMID: 38648108

Hu, G., Li, X., Zhang, J., Zhang, L., Qi, J., & Yu, B. (2021). An integrated strategy for the identification and screening of anti-allergy components from natural products based on calcium fluctuations and cell extraction coupled with HPLC-Q-TOF-MS. *Analytical and Bioanalytical Chemistry*, *413*(25), 6253–6266. DOI: 10.1007/s00216-021-03580-5 PMID: 34415362

Izah, S. C., Ogidi, O. I., Ogwu, M. C., Salimon, S. S., Yusuf, Z. M., Akram, M., & Iyingiala, A. A. (2024). Historical perspectives and overview of the value of herbal medicine. In *Herbal medicine phytochemistry: Applications and trends* (pp. 3–35). Springer International Publishing. DOI: 10.1007/978-3-031-43199-9_1

Jadhav, B. G., Jadhav, A. M., Shirode, A. R., & Kadam, V. J. (2014). A Comprehensive Review for the Learners and Users: Preparative High Performance Liquid Chromatography. *IJCPA*, *1*(3), 121–129.

Kardani, F., Jelyani, A. Z., Hashemi, M., Rashedinia, M., Shariati, S., Mirzaei, R., & Noori, S. M. A. (2023). Determination of 323 pesticide residues in Iran's cereal by GC-MS and HPLC-UV combined with QuEChERS extraction and mixed-mode SPE clean-up method. *Journal of Food Composition and Analysis*, *124*, 105670. DOI: 10.1016/j.jfca.2023.105670

Karole, S., Shrivastava, S., Thomas, S., Soni, B., Khan, S., Dubey, J., & Jain, D. K. (2019). Polyherbal Formulation Concept for Synergic Action: A Review. *Journal of Drug Delivery and Therapeutics*, *9*(1-s, 3-s), 499–503. DOI: 10.22270/jddt.v9i1-s.2339

Kemegne, G. A., Kamdem, S. L. S., Nyegue, M. A., Menut, C., & Etoa, F. X. (2021). Comparing checkerboard, isobologram and CCD methods for drug combination: A case study of ciprofloxacin and plant extracts on Escherichia coli and Shigella. *Journal of Medicinal Plants Research*, *5*(10), 479–489.

Kucharska-Ambrożej, K., & Karpinska, J. (2020). The application of spectroscopic techniques in combination with chemometrics for detection adulteration of some herbs and spices. *Microchemical Journal*, *153*, 104278. DOI: 10.1016/j.microc.2019.104278

Liu, K. C. S., Yang, S. L., Roberts, M. F., Elford, B. C., & Phillipson, J. D. (1989). The contribution of flavonoids to the antimalarial activity of *Artemisia annua*. *Planta Medica*, *55*(7), 654–655. DOI: 10.1055/s-2006-962242

Liu, K. S., Yang, S. L., Roberts, M., Elford, B., & Phillipson, J. (1992). Antimalarial activity of *Artemisia annua* flavonoids from whole plants and cell cultures. *Plant Cell Reports*, *11*(12), 637–640. DOI: 10.1007/BF00236389 PMID: 24213368

Malherbe, C. J., De Beer, D., & Joubert, E. (2012). Development of on-line high performance liquid chromatography (HPLC)-biochemical detection methods as tools in the identification of bioactives. *International Journal of Molecular Sciences*, *13*(3), 3101–3133. DOI: 10.3390/ijms13033101 PMID: 22489144

Malviya, N., & Malviya, S. (2017). Bioassay guided fractionation-an emerging technique influence the isolation, identification and characterization of lead phytomolecules. *International Journal of Hospital Pharmacy, 2*(5). Advance online publication. DOI: 10.28933/ijhp-2017-07-0901

Maurya, A., Kalani, K., Verma, S. C., Singh, R., & Srivastava, A. (2018). Vacuum Liquid Chromatography: Simple, Efficient and Versatile Separation Technique for Natural Products. *Organic and Medicinal Chemistry International Journal, 7*(5).

McMillen, T. S., Leslie, A., Chisholm, K., Penny, S., Gallant, J., Cohen, A., Drucker, A., Fawcett, J. P., & Pinto, D. M. (2023). A large-scale, targeted metabolomics method for the analysis and quantification of metabolites in human plasma via liquid chromatography-mass spectrometry. *Analytica Chimica Acta, 1279*, 341791. DOI: 10.1016/j.aca.2023.341791 PMID: 37827685

Mensah, M. L., Komlaga, G., Forkuc, A. D., Firempong, C., Anning, A. K., & Dickson, R. A. (2019). Toxicity and Safety Implications of Herbal Medicines. *Herbal Medicine, 63*.

Munteanu, I. G., & Apetrei, C. (2021). Analytical Methods Used in Determining Antioxidant Activity: A Review. *International Journal of Molecular Sciences, 22*(7), 3380. DOI: 10.3390/ijms22073380 PMID: 33806141

Muter, O., & Bartkevics, V. (2020). Advanced analytical techniques based on high-resolution mass spectrometry for the detection of micropollutants and their toxicity in aquatic environments. *Current Opinion in Environmental Science & Health, 18*, 1–6. DOI: 10.1016/j.coesh.2020.05.002

Ogwu, M. C., Izah, S. C., & Joshua, M. T. (2025). Ecological and environmental determinants of phytochemical variability in forest trees. *Phytochemistry Reviews, 24*(6), 1–29. DOI: 10.1007/s11101-025-10066-0

Oh, S. S.-Y., Zou, P., Low, M.-Y., & Koh, H.-L. (2006). Detection of sildenafil analogues in herbal products for erectile dysfunction. *Journal of Toxicology and Environmental Health. Part A., 69*(22), 1951–1958. PMID: 16982533

Palaniappan K. & Holley R. A. (2010). Use of natural antimicrobials to increase antibiotic susceptibility of drug resistant bacteria. Int J Food Microbiol. 15;140(2-3):164-8. .DOI: 10.1016/j.ijfoodmicro.2010.04.001

Pasieczna-Patkowska, S., Cichy, M., & Flieger, J. (2005). Application of Fourier Transform Infrared (FTIR) Spectroscopy in Characterization of Green Synthesized Nanoparticles. *Molecules (Basel, Switzerland), 30*(3), 684. DOI: 10.3390/molecules30030684 PMID: 39942788

Peiris, D. S. H. S., Fernando, D. T. K., Senadeera, S. P. N. N., & Ranaweera, C. B. (2025). Assessment of In Vitro Anti-Inflammatory Activity: A Comprehensive Review of Methods, Advantages, and Limitations. *Asian Journal of Research in Biochemistry*, *15*(2), 37–52. DOI: 10.9734/ajrb/2025/v15i2365

Putri, S. P., Ikram, M. M. M., Sato, A., Dahlan, H. A., Rahmawati, D., Ohto, Y., & Fukusaki, E. (2022). Application of gas chromatography-mass spectrometry-based metabolomics in food science and technology. *Journal of Bioscience and Bioengineering*, *133*(5), 425–435. DOI: 10.1016/j.jbiosc.2022.01.011 PMID: 35184928

Riedel, K.-D., Rieger, K., Martin-Facklam, M., Mikus, G., Haefeli, W. E., & Burhenne, J. (2004). Simultaneous determination of hypericin and hyperforin in human plasma with liquid chromatography-tandem mass spectrometry. *Journal of Chromatography. B, Analytical Technologies in the Biomedical and Life Sciences*, *813*(1-2), 27–33. DOI: 10.1016/j.jchromb.2004.09.061 PMID: 15556512

Roell, K. R., Reif, D. M., & Motsinger-Reif, A. A. (2017). An Introduction to Terminology and Methodology of Chemical Synergy-Perspectives from Across Disciplines. *Frontiers in Pharmacology*, *8*, 158. DOI: 10.3389/fphar.2017.00158 PMID: 28473769

Sanjai, C., Hakkimane, S. S., Guru, B. R., & Gaonkar, S. L. (2024). A comprehensive review on anticancer evaluation techniques. *Bioorganic Chemistry*, *142*, 106973. DOI: 10.1016/j.bioorg.2023.106973 PMID: 37984104

Senapati, A., Basak, S., & Rangan, L. (2022). A review on application of DNA barcoding technology for rapid molecular diagnostics of adulterants in herbal medicine. *Drug Safety*, *45*(2), 193–213. DOI: 10.1007/s40264-021-01133-4 PMID: 34846701

Shaban, N. S., Abdou, K. A., & Hassan, N. E. Y. (2015). Impact of toxic heavy metals and pesticide residues in herbal products. *Beni-Suef University Journal of Basic and Applied Sciences*, *5*(2), 102–106.

Shoba, G., Joy, D., Joseph, T., Majeed, M., Rajendran, R., & Srinivas, P. S. (1998). Influence of piperine on the pharmacokinetics of curcumin in animals and human volunteers. *Planta Medica*, *64*(4), 353–356. DOI: 10.1055/s-2006-957450 PMID: 9619120

Simmler, C., Graham, J. G., Chen, S. N., & Pauli, G. F. (2018). Integrated analytical assets aid botanical authenticity and adulteration management. *Fitoterapia*, *129*, 401–414. DOI: 10.1016/j.fitote.2017.11.017 PMID: 29175549

Singh, T. P., Singh, H. L., & Singh, R. M. (2022). Phytochemical Screening, Quantification, FT-IR Analysis, and In Silico Characterization of Potential Bio-active Compounds Identified in HR-LC/MS Analysis of the Polyherbal Formulation from Northeast India. *Pharmacognosy Journal*, *14*(3), 570–579. PMID: 36157760

Sravani, A. (2018). A Review Article on Flash Chromatography. *Asian Journal of Research in Chemistry*, *11*(5), 815–818. DOI: 10.5958/0974-4150.2018.00144.X

Tabuas, B., Cruz Barros, S., Diogo, C., Cavaleiro, C., & Sanches Silva, A. (2024). Pyrrolizidine Alkaloids in Foods, Herbal Drugs, and Food Supplements: Chemistry, Metabolism, Toxicological Significance, Analytical Methods, Occurrence, and Challenges for Future. *Toxins*, *16*(2), 79. DOI: 10.3390/toxins16020079 PMID: 38393157

Upton, R., David, B., Gafner, S., & Glasl, S. (2020). Botanical ingredient identification and quality assessment: Strengths and limitations of analytical techniques. *Phytochemistry Reviews*, *19*(5), 1157–1177. DOI: 10.1007/s11101-019-09625-z

Valle-Algarra, F. M., Mateo-Castro, R., Mateo, E. M., Gimeno-Adelantado, J. V., & Jiménez, M. (2014). MYCOTOXINS | Detection and Analysis by Classical Techniques. In Batt, C. A., & Tortorello, M. L. (Eds.), *Encyclopedia of Food Microbiology* (2nd ed., pp. 862–868). Academic Press. DOI: 10.1016/B978-0-12-384730-0.00232-9

Wallace, M. A. G., & McCord, J. P. (2020). Chapter 16 - High-resolution mass spectrometry. In J. Beauchamp, C. Davis, & J. Pleil (Eds.), *Breathborne Biomarkers and the Human Volatilome* (2nd ed., pp. 253-270). Elsevier.

Wan Y. D., Zang Y. D. & Wang J. S. (1992). Studies on the antimalarial action of gelatin capsule of *Artemisia annua*. Zongguo ji sheng chong xue yu ji sheng chong bing za shi (*Chinese Journal of Parasitology and Parasitic Diseases*). 10:290–294.

Wang, Y.-K., Li, W. Q., Xia, S., Guo, L., Miao, Y., & Zhang, B.-K. (2021). Metabolic activation of the toxic natural products from herbal and dietary supplements leading to toxicities. *Frontiers in Pharmacology*, *12*, 758468. DOI: 10.3389/fphar.2021.758468 PMID: 34744736

Wishart, D. S., Cheng, L. L., Copi, V., Edison, A. S., Eghbalnia, H. R., Hoch, J. C., Gouveia, G. J., Pathmasiri, W., Powers, R., Schock, T. B., Sumner, L. W., & Uchimiya, M. (2022). NMR and Metabolomics-A Roadmap for the Future. *Metabolites*, *12*(8), 678. DOI: 10.3390/metabo12080678 PMID: 35893244

Wright, C. W., Linley, P. A., Brun, R., Wittlin, S., & Hsu, E. (2010). Ancient Chinese methods are remarkably effective for the preparation of artemisinin-rich extracts of Qing Hao with potent antimalarial activity. *Molecules (Basel, Switzerland)*, *15*(2), 804–812. DOI: 10.3390/molecules15020804 PMID: 20335947

Yee, S. B., & Roth, R. A. (2018). Pyrrolizidine alkaloid-induced hepatotoxicity. In McQueen, C. A. (Ed.), *Comprehensive Toxicology* (3rd ed., pp. 522–537). Elsevier. DOI: 10.1016/B978-0-12-801238-3.02114-0

Yin, F., Song, Z., He, Z., Qin, B., John, G. F., Zhang, L., & Guo, D. A. (2022). Chemical fingerprinting and characterization of spilled oils and burnt soot particles - a case study on the Sanchi oil tanker collision in the East China Sea. *The Science of the Total Environment, 824*, 153896. DOI: 10.1016/j.scitotenv.2022.153896 PMID: 35182621

Zeki, Ö. C., Eylem, C. C., Reçber, T., Kır, S., & Nemutlu, E. (2020). Integration of GC–MS and LC–MS for untargeted metabolomics profiling. *Journal of Pharmaceutical and Biomedical Analysis, 190*, 113509. DOI: 10.1016/j.jpba.2020.113509 PMID: 32814263

KEY TERMS AND DEFINITIONS

Additivity: This is a condition in which the combined effect of two or more compounds precisely equals the sum of their individual effects.

Antagonism: The opposite of synergism; a situation where the combined effect of two or more compounds is less than the sum of their individual effects.

Bioassay-guided fractionation: This is a strategic method that combines bioactivity testing with chromatographic separation to isolate active constituents from complex herbal mixtures.

Chemical profiling: This is a systematic method used for characterizing and quantifying the chemical composition of samples.

Herb-drug interactions: This refers to the possibility that an herbal constituent may alter the pharmacologic effects of a conventional drug given concurrently or vice versa.

Metabolomics: The comprehensive and systematic study of all metabolites present within a biological system at a specific point in time.

Standardization: The process of ensuring consistent chemical composition and, consequently, predictable biological activity across different batches of herbal formulations.

Synergism: A phenomenon where the combined effect of two or more compounds exceeds the sum of their individual effects.

Chapter 6
Herbal Remedies in Nigeria:
Friend or Foe

Damilare Rotimi
http://orcid.org/0000-0003-3721-8065
Landmark University, Nigeria

Victor Oluwadamilare Adeogun
Landmark University, Nigeria

Oluyomi Stephen Adeyemi
http://orcid.org/0000-0001-9342-8505
Bowen University, Nigeria

ABSTRACT

Herbal medicine involves the use of medicinal plants for treatment of diseases in developing and developed countries. Plants have been used for medical purposes in human history and it's still widely practiced today. Herbal remedies have active constituent/ingredient which is known to have curative effects on the body. They are used as treatment and relief for various diseases such as diabetes, low sperm count, anemia as well as cancer. Herbal remedies in Nigeria have become popular and are majorly classified into monoherbal and polyherbal remedies. The use of herbal remedies tends to affect humanity both positively and negatively. Some positive importance reported includes high level of effectiveness of the herb, cheap and readily availabile with numerous health benefits and vitality. The disadvantages however are the observed side effects, high percentage of alcohol content, and lack of dosage regulation of the herbs.

DOI: 10.4018/979-8-3373-5876-5.ch006

INTRODUCTION

Herbal remedies represent the oldest form of medical care and have been used for centuries, particularly in developing countries. Historically, humans relied on nature not only for food and clothing but also for remedies to treat various ailments (Nontokozo & Mthokozia, 2018). Across time, medicinal plants and herbs have been widely employed worldwide for disease prevention and treatment. Extracted herbs and their isolated active compounds have played a significant role in the development of modern pharmacotherapy, with many of these natural compounds serving as templates for the synthesis of contemporary drugs (Djordjevic, 2017).

With the advancement of science, the popularity of herbal remedies has grown significantly, with over 80% of the world's population incorporating them into their healthcare (Alostad et al., 2018). In response to increasing demand and concerns over quality and potential toxicity, several countries, including Germany, France, and Austria, have implemented strict regulations and established comprehensive herbal remedy registration systems to ensure safety. However, in many countries, including Nigeria, herbal products are often used indiscriminately, which can lead to harmful effects and, in extreme cases, death (Yusuf et al., 2019). While herbal remedies offer numerous therapeutic benefits, improper use poses risks. Once considered "ancient" medicine by Western standards, modern research has validated many of their medicinal properties, and numerous pharmaceuticals have been developed based on phytochemicals derived from these plants (Ezekwesili & Okaka, 2019).

Herbal Remedies

The World Health Organization (WHO) defines herbal remedies as practices involving the use of plants, herbal materials, preparations, and finished herbal products that contain active ingredients derived from plant parts or other plant components for the prevention or treatment of diseases (Nontokozo & Mthokozia, 2018).

Herbal remedies typically contain active constituents from plant materials in either raw or processed forms, often combined with excipients such as solvents, diluents, or preservatives. These bioactive compounds help protect plants against pests and diseases and contribute to characteristic properties such as aroma, flavour, and colour. Scientifically, these active constituents—known as phytochemicals—are classified into major groups including flavonoids, glycosides, tannins, alkaloids, terpenoids, and others.

History Of Herbal Remedies

Herbal remedies—also known as medicinal herbs or medicinal plants—have been used in traditional medicine since prehistoric times. Early records from the Sumerian civilization list numerous therapeutic plants on clay tablets (Ahn, 2017). Many plants now used as culinary herbs and spices originally served medicinal purposes (Tapsell et al., 2006). Even animals such as primates, monarch butterflies, goats, and sheep have been observed consuming medicinal plants when ill (Sumner, 2000). Archaeological evidence dates herbal use to the Paleolithic era, about 60,000 years ago, with written documentation appearing around 5,000 years ago among the Sumerians. Major civilizations advanced this knowledge: Ayurveda in India employed herbs like turmeric as early as 4000 BC; Egypt's Ebers Papyrus listed over 850 plant medicines; and in China, Emperor Shennong reportedly catalogued 365 medicinal herbs during the Shang dynasty.

Classifications Of Active Constituents In Herbal Remedies

These active constituents are known to exert therapeutic effects in the body. They are broadly classified into several phytochemical groups, including anthocyanins, anthraquinones, alkaloids, cardiac glycosides, coumarins, flavonoids, cyanogenic glycosides, phenolic compounds, tannins, silymarin, glucosinolates, and others.

Common Herbal Remedies And Uses

Echinacea

Echinacea, commonly known as coneflower, is a flowering plant and widely used herbal remedy. Native to North America, it has been employed in traditional Native American medicine to treat wounds, burns, toothaches, sore throat, and digestive issues (Ansley, 2020). The plant contains a diverse range of bioactive compounds, including caffeic acid, alkamides, phenolic acids, rosmarinic acid, and polyacetylenes (Jahanian et al., 2017).

Echinacea is reported to have multiple therapeutic effects, such as lowering blood sugar, reducing anxiety, providing anti-inflammatory benefits, treating certain skin conditions, and offering potential protective effects against cancer. Common side effects, particularly in individuals with flower allergies, include rashes, swelling of body parts, and nausea.

Figure 1. Echinacea plant

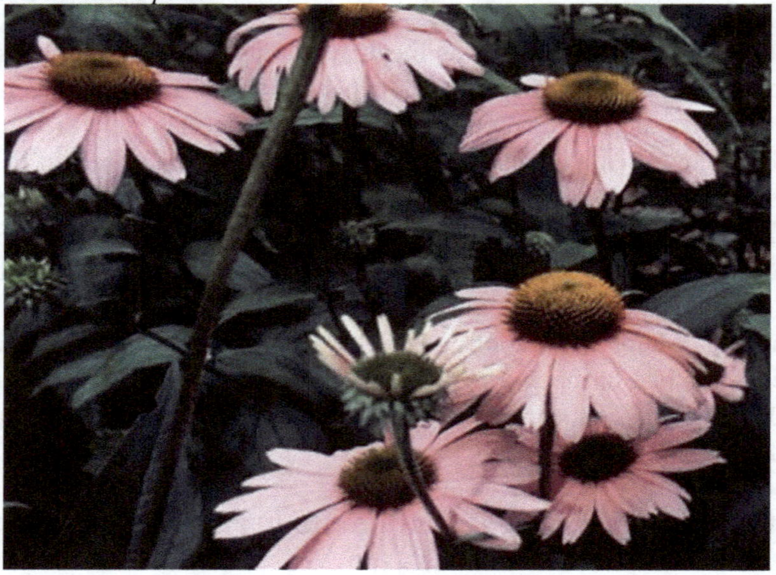

Ginkgo Biloba

Ginkgo biloba, commonly known as ginkgo, is an herbal remedy derived from the maidenhair tree. Used for thousands of years, it remains one of the most popular herbal supplements today. Ginkgo contains a variety of potent antioxidants, which are believed to contribute to its therapeutic effects. It is commonly used to support heart health, improve cognitive function in dementia, address mental difficulties, and manage certain sexual dysfunctions. Possible side effects include headaches, heart palpitations, and skin reactions.

Figure 2. Ginkgo biloba plant

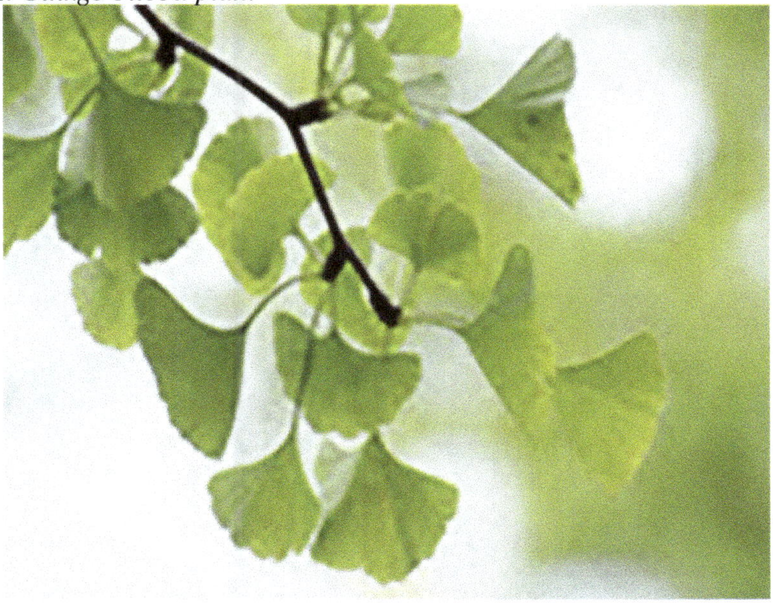

Chamomile

Chamomile is a flowering plant and one of the most widely used herbal remedies globally. The flowers are primarily used to prepare tea, while the leaves can be dried for medicinal extracts or topical compresses. For centuries, chamomile has been employed to treat nausea, diarrhea, constipation, stomach pain, urinary tract infections, wounds, and upper respiratory infections. It contains over 100 bioactive compounds (Ompal, 2011).

Laboratory and animal studies have shown that chamomile possesses anti-inflammatory, antimicrobial, and antioxidant properties; however, there is currently limited clinical evidence from human studies to fully support these effects (Sepide, 2016).

Figure 3. Chamomile plant (Ompal. 2011)

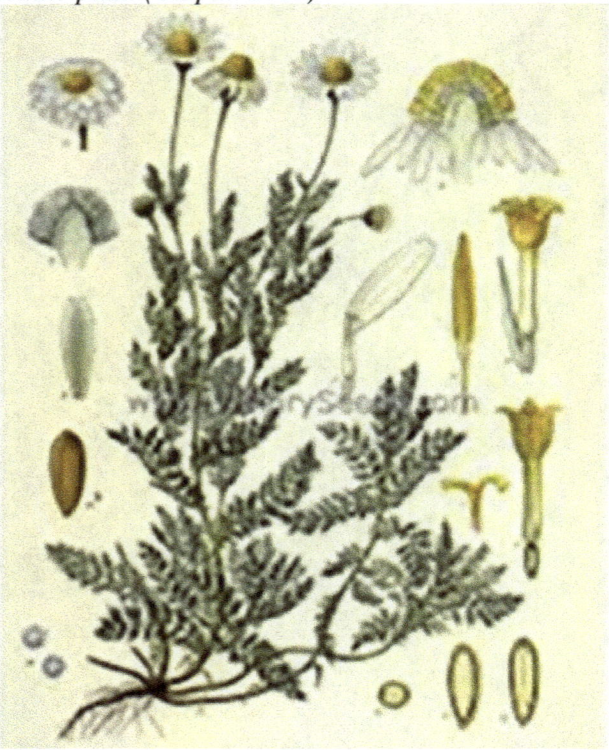

Milk Thistle

Milk thistle (*Silybum marianum*) is an herbal remedy derived from the milk thistle plant, recognizable by its purple flowers and distinctive white veins. Its primary active component is silymarin, which is believed to have hepatoprotective properties. Milk thistle is commonly used to support liver health, particularly in cases of alcohol-induced liver damage, non-alcoholic fatty liver disease, hepatitis, and liver cancer (Alessandro, 2017).

Beyond liver support, milk thistle is also used for other potential health benefits, including prevention of age-related cognitive decline, bone protection, enhancement of breast milk production, acne treatment, and lowering blood sugar in individuals with diabetes.

Figure 4. Milk thistle

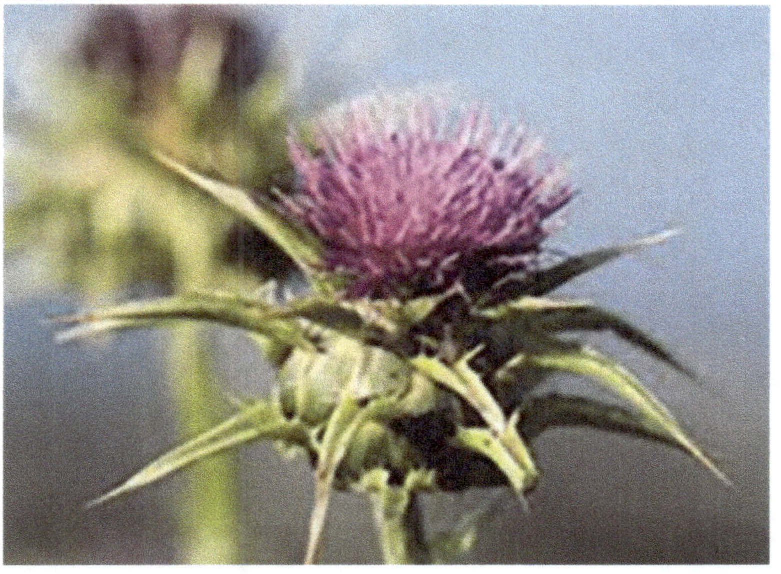

Turmeric

Turmeric is a bright yellow remedy and spice used for its medicinal, antioxidant, and anti-inflammatory components for thousands of years. Turmeric contains curcumin, a substance with powerful antioxidants and anti-inflammatory. Turmeric is used to ease arthritis symptoms, prevent Alzheimer's diseases, and prevent cancer, boost the immune system, and lowers cholesterol.

Figure 5. Turmeric

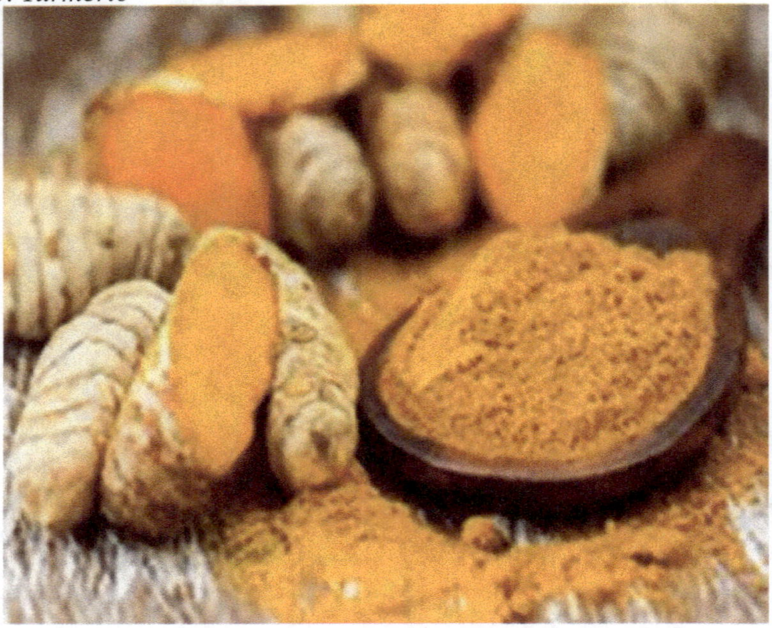

Green Tea

Green tea is another herbal remedy that is filled with polyphenol antioxidants, it is said to be one of the healthiest beverages on earth. The benefit of green tea are numerous, some include improvement of brain functionality, increase fat burning, lower the risk of cancers (breast, prostate, and colorectal cancer), reduce bad breath, prevent type 2 diabetes, and prevents cardiovascular disease.

Figure 6. Green tea

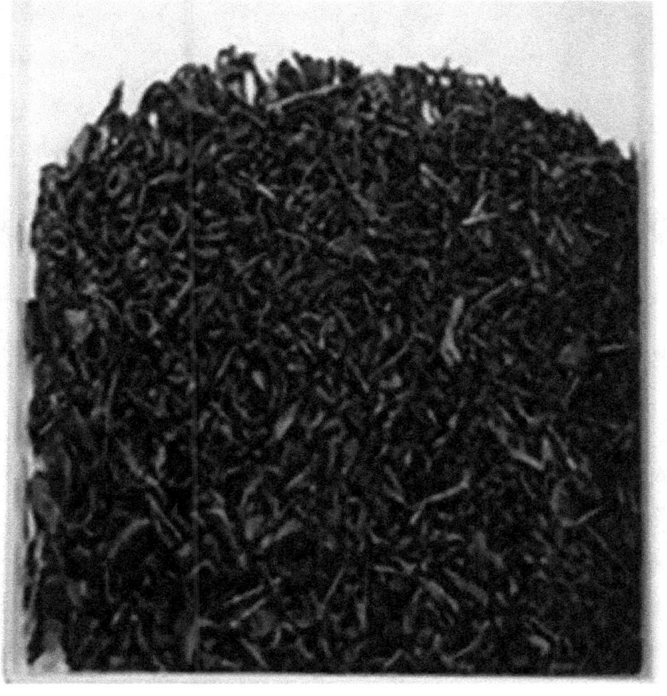

Garlic

Garlic is an aromatic herbaceous that is used worldwide as a food and herbal remedy for various ailments, it has been recorded to possess numerous biological properties, the medical uses of garlic are anti-carcinogenic, antioxidant, antidiabetic, antibacterial, antihypertensive, and anti-atherosclerotic (Gaber et al, 2020). Garlic is known for treating cold and infection, used as a natural blood thinner, used to control blood pressure, treat diabetes mellitus, and many more ailments (Shakya et al, 2017).

Figure 7. Garlic (Gaber et al, 2020)

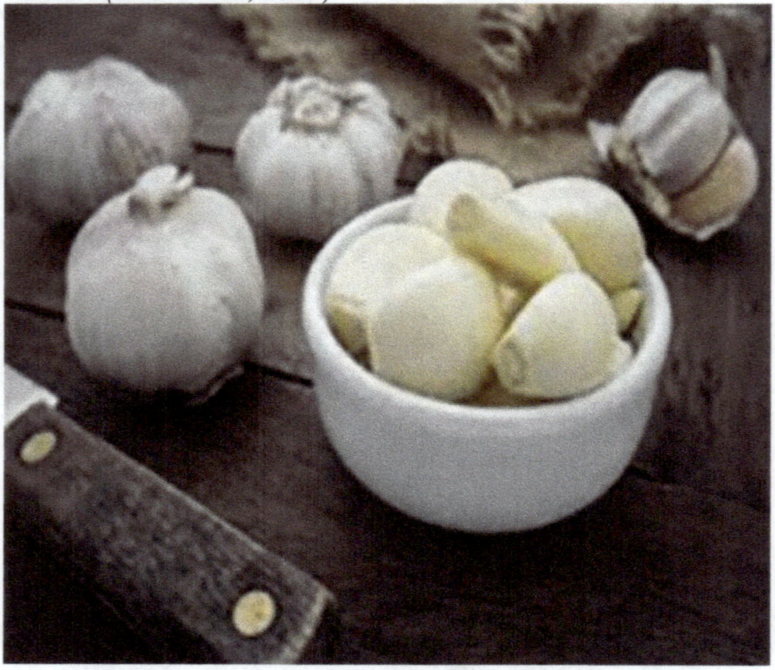

Dong Quai

Dong Quai is a plant which roots are used to make remedies, they are also called female ginseng and Dang Gui. It is rich in compounds with anti-inflammatory and immune-stimulating effects, it helps in treating ailments from allergies, constipation to high blood pressure, and even more (Chao & Lin, 2011). Dong Quai is used to build blood health, boost or activate blood circulation, treat blood deficiency, regulate the immune system, relieve pain and relax bowels.

Figure 8. Dong Quai leaves stem, and root

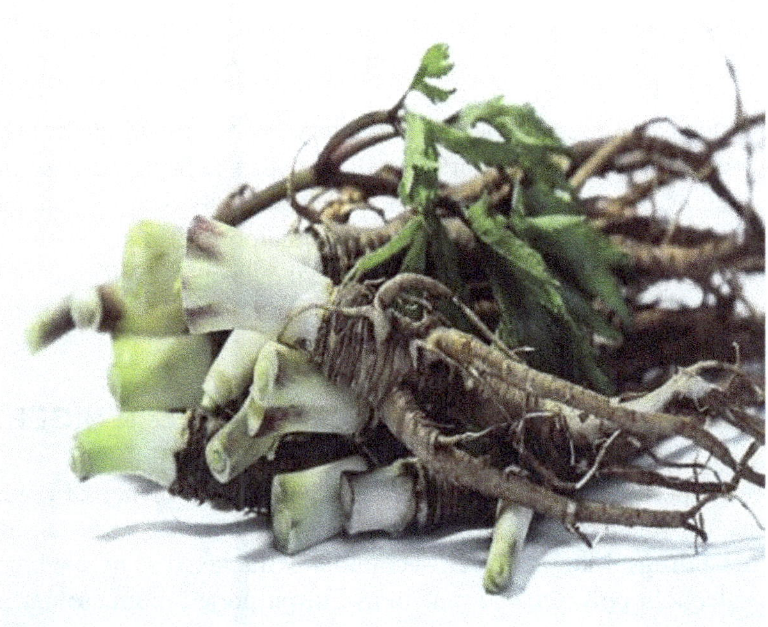

HERBAL REMEDIES IN NIGERIA

The use of herbal remedies constitutes an important supplementary component of healthcare delivery in Nigeria. In many developing countries, including Nigeria, traditional herbal practice contributes to expanding health coverage for the population (Chukwuma et al., 2015). Across West Africa—and particularly in Nigeria—studies consistently report a high prevalence of herbal medicine use (Odedina et al., 2020).

Herbal medicines are commonly employed in Nigeria for the management of conditions such as cancer, hypertension, diabetes, toothache, mental disorders, epilepsy, asthma, and sickle cell disease (Oshikoya et al., 2008). Growing public reliance has also stimulated biomedical evaluation of their efficacy, with some Nigerian herbal formulations demonstrating antimalarial activity (Lawal et al., 2015). Their widespread use is largely attributed to accessibility, perceived effectiveness, and affordability (Krah et al., 2018).

Nigeria has long relied on the practical skills of herbal practitioners, including herb sellers, traditional birth attendants, and traditional surgeons, whose botanical knowledge of plant ecology, species, and availability is invaluable (Cunningham,

1993). This expertise has been preserved and transmitted across generations through oral traditions such as storytelling and, more recently, through formal education at universities including Obafemi Awolowo University (Osun State), University of Nigeria (Nsukka, Enugu State), and University of Ibadan, which offer programs in herbal medicine (Lawal et al., 2015).

Despite this extensive knowledge, regulatory oversight and quality control of herbal remedies in Nigeria remain limited. Research indicates that some herbal products contain dangerously high levels of heavy metals such as lead, cadmium, and mercury, while others are contaminated with microorganisms at levels exceeding World Health Organization standards (Ezekwesili & Okaka, 2019). These findings highlight the urgent need for stricter regulation and quality assurance.

MONOHERBAL AND POLYHERBAL REMEDIES IN NIGERIA

A large proportion of Nigerians use monoherbal and polyherbal remedies for disease management, largely due to the perception that they produce fewer side effects than synthetic drugs. Many products—commonly marketed as herbal bitters—are aqueous or alcoholic polyherbal formulations with purported antimicrobial, immune-boosting, detoxifying, and hepatoprotective properties (Imaga & Valentine, 2013; Anionye & Onyeneke, 2016). Several local manufacturers produce remedies for conditions such as malaria, hypertension, diabetes, piles, and infertility. Widely used preparations include commercial bitters and plant-based remedies such as Cymbopogon citratus, Garcinia kola, Moringa oleifera, Zingiber officinale, and Vernonia amygdalina (Kale et al., 2018). The following section reviews key herbal remedies used in Nigeria, covering both monoherbal and polyherbal formulations.

Lemongrass (*Cymbopogon citratus*)

Lemongrass is a popular monoherbal remedy used in Nigeria and various parts of the world, it is an ample source of lignocellulose substance containing 22.6% hemicellulose, 39.5% cellulose and 28.5% lignin (Bekele et al., 2017). Lemongrass is said to have antioxidant, antimicrobial, anti-inflammatory properties, researcher have found out it is a good herb for reduction of cancer, promotion of healthy digestion, reduction of high systolic blood pressure, regulation of cholesterol, a remedy for menstrual cramps and a good cure for malaria and fever (Olsen, 2019).

Figure 9. Cymbopogon citratus (Olsen, 2019)

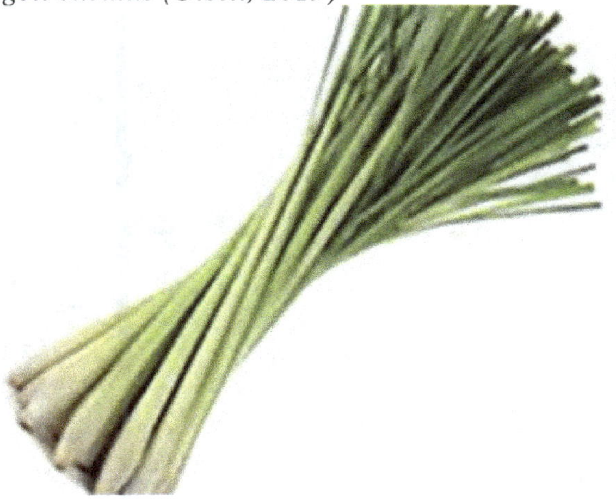

Garcinia Kola (*Bitter Kola*)

Popularly known as bitter kola, *Garcina kola* is popular in the southern part of Nigeria. It is usually found in the tropical rainforest of West Africa (Okwu, 2007). Exact confirmation and developing exploration recommend that it is safe helpful, particularly when used as herbal remedies, numerous pharmacological impacts have been shown for *Garcinia kola*, among them anti-inflammatory, antihepatotoxic, a bronchodilator, and antiviral properties. *G. kola* is claimed to be effective in the treatment of food poisoning, diarrhea, stomachache, and aphrodisiac (Vincent, 2018).

Figure 10. Garcinia kola (Okwu, 2007)

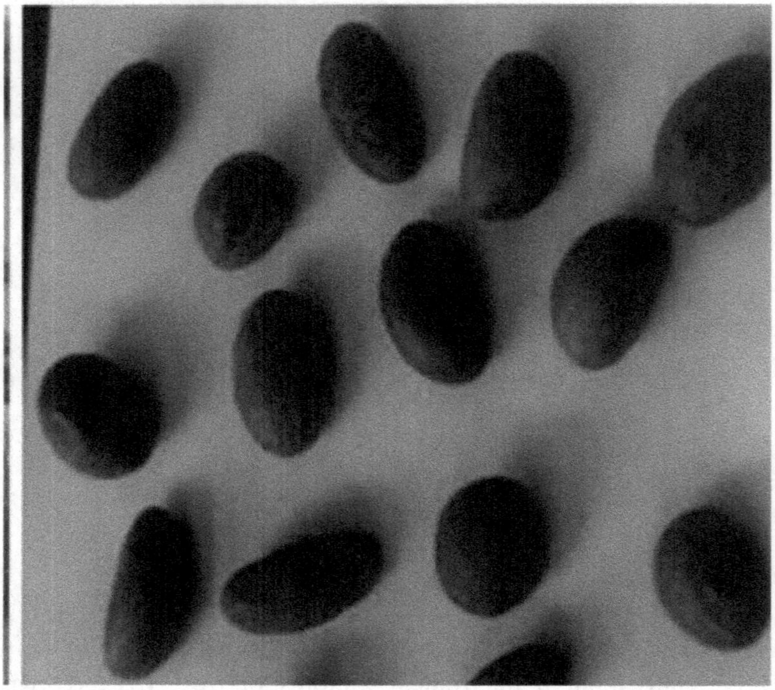

Moringa oleifera

Moringa is a plant that is common to areas of Nigeria, India, Pakistan, Afghanistan, and Bangladesh. The flowers, bark, leaves, fruits, roots, and seeds are all medicinal. *Moringa oleifera* contains protein, vitamins, and minerals, as an antioxidant, it helps to protect cells from damages and it is used to treat various ailments such as constipation, high blood pressure, kidney stones, obesity, epilepsy, and many others (Ibitoye et al., 2019).

Figure 11. Moringa oleifera (Ibitoye et al., 2019)

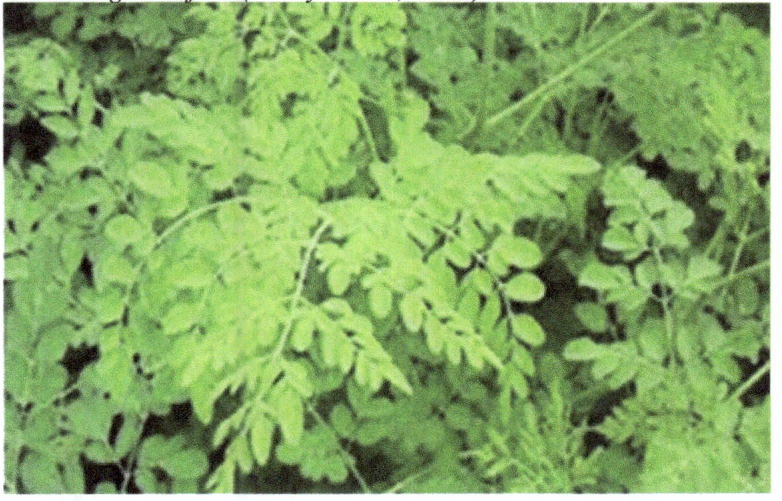

Yoyo Bitters

Yoyo bitters is an oral polyherbal liquid-based remedy in the class of herbal bitters popularly used in the southwest of Nigeria, it was released into the Nigerian market in 2003 by Abllat Company Nigeria limited (Igbokwe et al., 2017). Yoyo bitters contains different remedial herbs such as *Citrus aurantifola, Cinnamum aromaticum, Aloe vera, Citrus aurantifola, Chenopodium murale*, and *Acinos arvensis*, which are used to cure different ailments such as infertility, cough, lack of proper digestion, and plenty more (Kumdi et al, 2011; Igbokwe et al., 2017).

Figure 12. Yoyo bitters (Igbokwe et al., 2017)

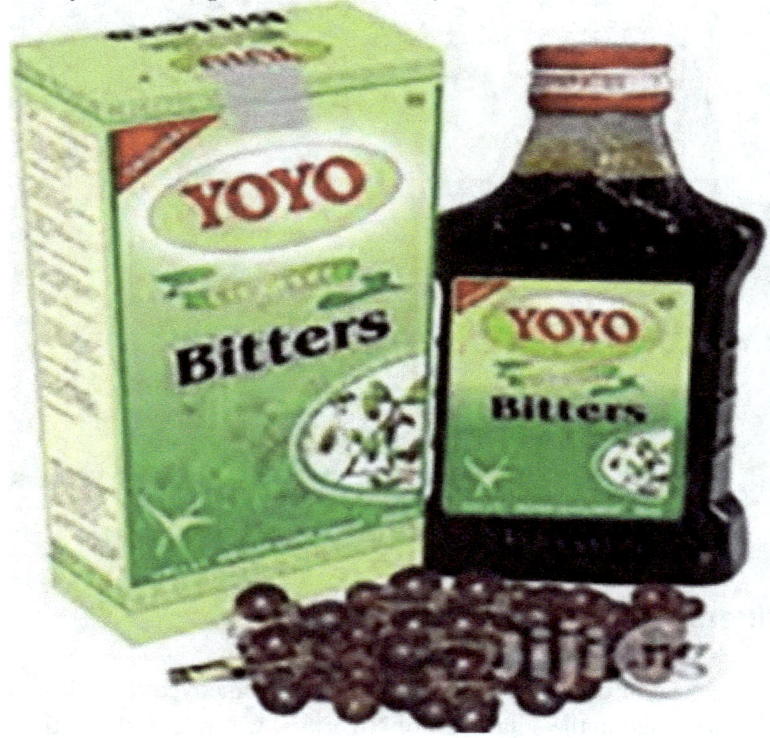

The formulation is also indicated for the treatment of kidney and bladder infection, normalization of intestine movement, helping regulate blood pressure, facilitate digestion, and to control weight.

Yoyo bitters is believed to have antioxidant, hepatoprotective, immunity enhancing and a detoxifying property like other bitters.

OROKI HERBAL MIXTURE

Oroki herbal mixture is a polyherbal preparation produced in Nigeria by Nured industrial and commercial company Ltd. It contains numerous herbs such as *Sorghum bicolar* stem, *Khaya grandifoliola, Cassia siberiana, Staudtia stipitata* root, *Alsotonia congenesis* bark, *Ocimun basidicum* leaves, *Magifera indica* leaves, *Cyathula prostrate* leaves, *Securidaca longepeduncalata* root, and *Sacchurum officinarum* stem (Bamidele et al., 2018). Oroki herbal mixture is famous for the treatment of pile, waist pain, stomach pain, dysentery, blood stooling, menstrual problems, deworming, and turgidity (Emikpe et al., 2018).

Figure 13. Oroki herbal mixture (Bamidele et al., 2018)

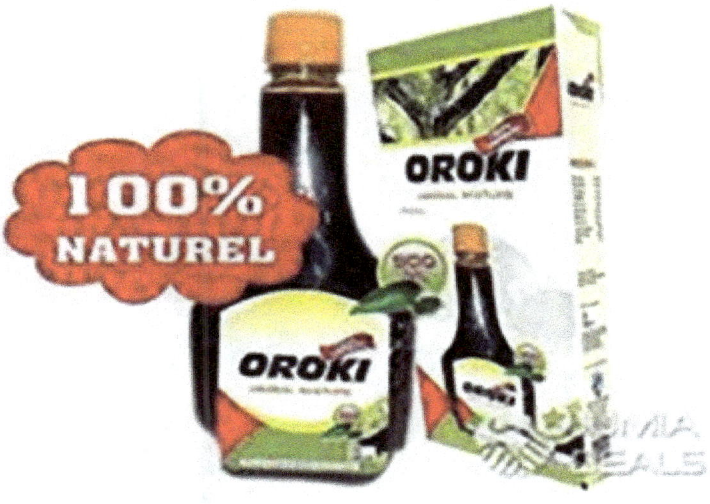

Ruzu Bitters

Ruzu bitters is another polyherbal remedy fast-growing and widely used in Nigeria, known for its greenish-brown appearance with a bitter taste and ginger-like smell, as claimed by the manufacturers, it is a naturally pure marvel with the ability to aid in the treatment of various ailments (Francis et al., 2017). Ruzu bitters contains 40% *Curculigo pilosa* roots, 40% colocynthis bark, and 20% *Uvaria chamae* stem. Ruzu herbal bitters is widely uses as an anti-obesity, hypertension, diabetes, arthritis, and infertility among others (Ogunlana et al., 2020).

Figure 14. Ruzu bitters (Ogunlana et al., 2020)

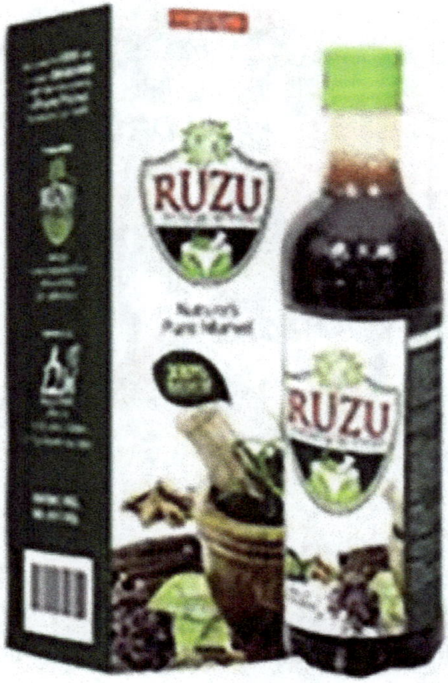

Alomo Bitters

Aloma bitters, which is primarily produced in Ghana is an herbal combination containing alcohol of 42% v/v and is widely uses as a social drink or herbal remedy in Nigeria (Adegbolagun & Nwabuife, 2018). It is reported to contain carefully picked tropical herbs extract consisting *Treculia africana*, *Khaya ivorensis, Lecaniodiscus cupanoides, Diallum guineense*, and *Capparis arythrocarpus* (Subair et al 2018). Alomo bitters is proudly known to clean the bowel, relieve body pain, improve vitality and general wellbeing reduce menstrual cramps/pains in women with anti-malaria and aphrodisiac properties.

Figure 15. Alomo bitters (Adegbolagun & Nwabuife, 2018)

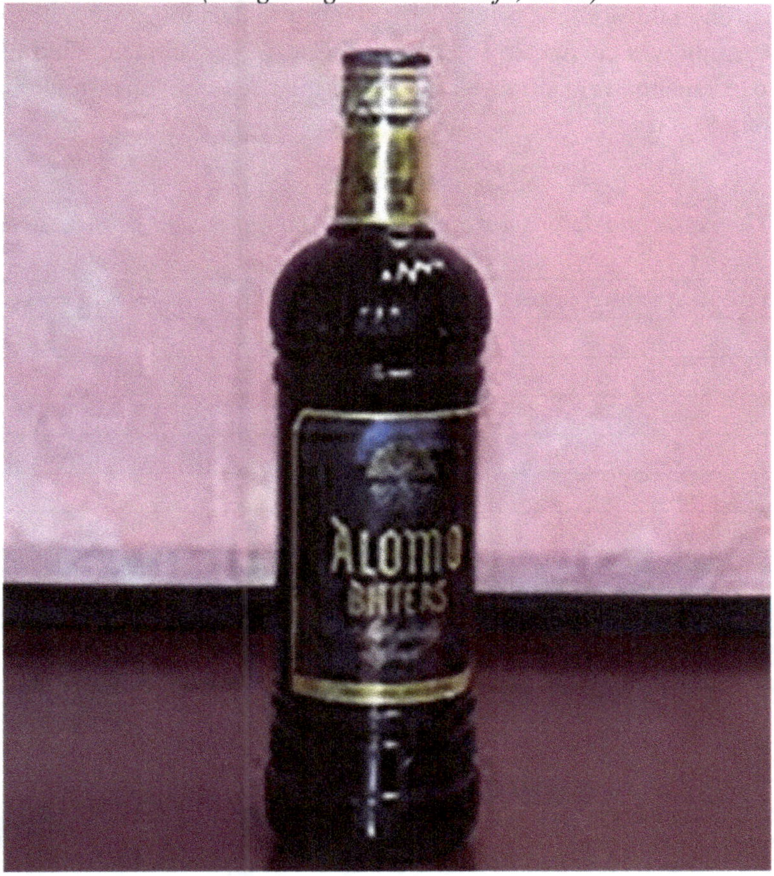

COMMON USES OF HERBAL REMEDIES IN NIGERIA

Herbal remedies in Nigeria have become the first line of treatment in many households. Given this widespread reliance, it is important to examine the common patterns and reasons for their use.

The use of herbal remedies has been extensively documented in Nigeria. Many users reportedly rely on them for conditions such as epilepsy (Danesi & Adetunji, 1994), hypertension (Amira & Okunbadejo, 2007), diabetes mellitus (Ogbera et al., 2010), cancer (Ezeome & Anarado, 2007), sickle cell anaemia, and asthma (Oshikoya et al., 2008). They are also commonly used for malaria, fever, diarrhoea, piles, menstrual pain, and dysentery. Notably, some individuals report using herbal remedies even in the absence of a specific medical indication.

A case study was conducted in Surulere LGA, Lagos, in which 388 randomly selected participants were surveyed regarding their reasons for using herbal remedies (Table 1).

Table 1. The common reasons for the use of herbal remedies by the respondents in Surulere Lagos

Reason for the use of herbal remedies	Number of herbal remedy users	Percentage (%)
No reason	62	25.9
Malaria	54	20.8
Reduction of the blood level	42	16.2
Fever	26	10.0
Prophylaxis	16	6.2
Body pain relieve	12	4.6
Diarrhea	9	3.5
Fatigue	9	3.5
Self-protection	4	1.5
Skincare	3	1.2
General illness	3	1.2
Dysentery	3	1.2
Energy-boosting	2	0.8
Blood cleansing	2	0.8
Cholera	2	0.8
Blood enrichment	1	0.4
	388 participants	100%

(Kazeem et al., 2011)

FACTORS INFLUENCING THE USE HERBAL REMEDIES

Several studies have been conducted to elucidate why individuals turn to alternative forms of medicine, particularly herbal remedies. Evidence suggests that many people prefer to maintain personal control over their health. In addition, dissatisfaction with conventional treatments, their perceived lack of a holistic approach, and concerns about potential side effects of orthodox medications have been identified as key drivers of herbal remedy use (Adeosun, 2017).

Studies show that many users choose herbal remedies because they believe these therapies align better with their personal beliefs, values, and views of health. Use is also influenced by social pressure, dissatisfaction with hospital staff attitudes, reluctance to prescribe drugs, and lack of privacy in hospitals. Additionally, withdrawal of some prescription medicines and the marketing of herbal products as "all-natural" (often perceived as safe) encourage their use. High healthcare costs and the perception that providers prioritize profit further drive consumers toward herbal remedies as a cheaper alternative.

Herbal Remedies: Friend

- Different herbal remedies contain numerous healing properties such as *Cymbopogon citratus* having anti-inflammatory properties, *Garcinia kola* having anti-hepatotoxic, anti-viral properties, and *Moringa oleifera* having anti-oxidant properties. Other herbs contain properties such as anti-hyperglycemic, anti-tumor activities, anti-pyretic, anti-apoptotic, anti-platelet, anti-tumorigenic, antioxidant, anti-tumor activities, analgesic properties, and anti-clotting (Mohamad et al 2019).

Figure 16. Anti-diabetic plants and their mechanism

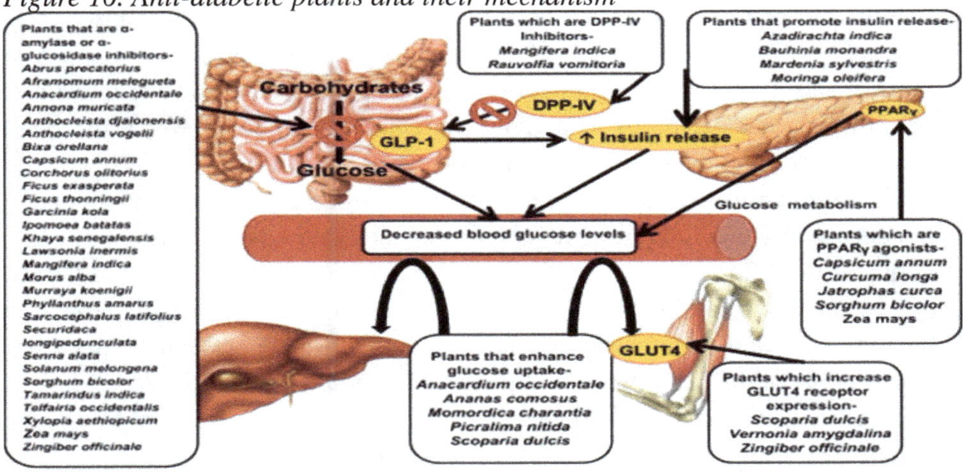

- Cost of effectiveness and affordability: Modern medicals and orthodox drugs are becoming highly cost the common masses can hardly pay for them, a common man will rather take herbal remedies such as *Cymbopogon citratus* (lemongrass) for malaria which is affordable than going to the pharmacy to buy pharmaceutical malaria drugs. The growing testimonies of increasing the efficacy of herbal medicine, together with lower incidents of reactions, have made herbal remedies a ready alternative to pharmaceuticals medicine.
- Readily available: Herbal remedies are known to be widely available since they can be cultivated by various individuals in the society, this enables the individual to have easy access to these remedies when need, for example, people in rural areas where there is no hospitals, pharmacist or chemist can have easy access to these herbs to meet their health care for the moment (Ekeopara & Ugoha, 2017).

Herbal Remedies: Foe

- Irrespective of the increase in the usage of these remedies for its use in different medicinal products still there are several problems associated with their safety. Very little information is available regarding the toxicity of these products. Some plants produce toxic constituents for defense purposes. These harmful herbs are not distinguished from therapeutically active constituents.
- **Side effects**: The majority of herbal remedy user's experiences side effects such as anemia, blurred vision, weight loss, vomiting. It is noted that some remedies may contribute possible effects such as vomiting and nausea (bitters), heartburn, skin reactions (Ginger) paralysis (extracts of moringa roots) there was a statistically significant relationship between a side effect and use of these remedies, this explained that these herbs contain different active constituent causing the side effects (Illumuanya et al., 2017).
- **The high volume of alcohol content**: It has become worrisome and a major concern that many brands of herbal remedies, most herbal bitters are frequently soaked in alcohol or distilled. This implies that most users of herbal remedies consume a sizeable proportion of alcohol. Most herbal remedies contain as high as 35% concentration of alcohol. Related research has shown that some herbal remedies have up to 40% alcohol volume. Therefore, intake of herbal remedies with a higher percentage of alcohol may lead to further ailments instead of preventing or curing these ailments.

CONCLUSION

The rising demand for herbal remedies in Nigeria and beyond reflects strong public confidence in their perceived benefits for disease prevention and treatment. However, this growing use has also raised concerns about the quality, standardization, and safety of products available in the market. Without adequate regulation, the potential benefits of herbal remedies cannot be reliably safeguarded, given their capacity to produce both positive and adverse health effects. Since the safety of these products depends largely on effective policy oversight, governments, international organizations, and relevant stakeholders must strengthen regulatory frameworks and enforcement. In the absence of proper regulation, herbal remedies in Nigeria risk becoming a public health concern rather than a reliable therapeutic option.

REFERENCES

Adegbolagun, O. M., & Nwabuife, J. C. (2018). Comparative pharmaceutical and physicochemical equivalence of some brands of chlorphenamine maleate tablets. *Nigerian Journal of Pharmaceutical Research, 14*(2), 197–202.

Adeosun, F. (2017). *Use of herbal remedies for infants by nursing mothers in Ibadan South East Local Government Area*. Population and Reproductive Health Education.

Ahn, K. (2017). The worldwide trend of using botanical drugs and strategies for developing globally. *BMB Reports, 50*(3), 111–116. DOI: 10.5483/BMBRep.2017.50.3.221 PMID: 27998396

Alessandro, F. (2017). Silymarin/silybin and chronic liver diseases: A marriage of many years, pp. 5–7.

Alostad, A., Steink, D., & Schafhuette, E. (2018). International comparison of the herbal medicine registration system to inform regulation development. *Pharmaceutical Medicine*, •••, 39–49. DOI: 10.1007/s40290-018-0223-0 PMID: 29456449

Amira, C. O., & Okubadejo, N. U. (2007). Frequency of complementary and alternative medicine utilization in hypertensive patients attending an urban tertiary care centre in Nigeria. *BMC Complementary and Alternative Medicine, 7*(1), 1. DOI: 10.1186/1472-6882-7-30 PMID: 17903257

Anionye, J. C., & Onyeneke, E. C. (2016). Composition and in vitro antioxidant capacity of super bitters. *European Journal of Applied Sciences, 8*(5), 289–296.

Bamidele, O. D., Adegbolagun, O. M., Subair, H. G., & Emikpe, B. O. (2018). Pharmaco-epidemiologic survey and experimental study of co-administration of three herbal products with paracetamol. *African Journal of Biomedical Research*, •••, 153–159.

Bekele, F., Tefera, T., Biresaw, G., & Yohannes, T. (2017). Parasitic contamination of raw vegetables and fruits collected from selected local markets in Arba Minch town, Southern Ethiopia. *Infectious Diseases of Poverty, 6*(1), 19. DOI: 10.1186/s40249-016-0226-6 PMID: 28264707

Chao, W., & Lin, B. (2011). *Bioactivities of major constituents isolated from Angelica sinensis*. China Medical. DOI: 10.1186/1749-8546-6-29

Chukwuma, E. C., Soladoye, M. O., & Feyisola, R. T. (2015). Traditional medicine and the future of medicinal Plants in Nigeria. *Journal of Medicinal Plants Studies, 3*(4), 23–29.

Cunningham, A. B. (1993). *African medicinal plants*. United Nations Educational, Scientific and Cultural Organization.

Danesi, M. A., & Adetunji, J. B. (1994). Use of alternative medicine by patients with epilepsy: A survey of 265 epileptic patients in a developing country. *Epilepsia*, *35*(2), 344–351. DOI: 10.1111/j.1528-1157.1994.tb02442.x PMID: 8156955

Djordjevic, S. M. (2017). From medicinal plant raw materials to herbal remedies. In *Aromatic and Medicinal Plants* (pp. 269–288). Back to Nature. DOI: 10.5772/66618

Ekeopara, C. A., & Ugoha, A. (2017). The contribution of African traditional medicine to Nigeria's healthcare delivery system. *Journal of the Humanities and Social Sciences*, *22*, 32.

Ezekwesili, J., & Okaka, A. (2019). Herbal medicines in African traditional medicine. *Herbal Medicine*, *10*, 191–214.

Ezeome, E. R., & Anarado, A. N. (2007). Use of complementary and alternative medicine by cancer patients at the University of Nigeria Teaching Hospital, Enugu, Nigeria. *BMC Complementary and Alternative Medicine*, *7*(1), 28. DOI: 10.1186/1472-6882-7-28 PMID: 17850665

Francis, E., Amaeza, U., & Aniyaka, E. (2017). Ruzu bitters and glibenclamide tablets: Dissolution and in-vitro release kinetic studies. *The Nigerian Journal of Pharmacy : the Official Organ of the Pharmaceutical Society of Nigeria*, •••, 73–82.

Ibitoye, O., Shafiq, O., & Matrawy, A. (2019, December). Analyzing adversarial attacks against deep learning for intrusion detection in IoT networks. In *2019 IEEE global communications conference (GLOBECOM)* (pp. 1-6). IEEE. DOI: 10.1109/GLOBECOM38437.2019.9014337

Imaga, N. A., & Valentine, O. J. (2013). Analyses of the effects of Swedish bitters on selected metabolic profiles.

Jahanian, H. R., Shafabakhsh, G. H., & Divandari, H. (2017). Performance evaluation of Hot Mix Asphalt (HMA) containing bitumen modified with Gilsonite. *Construction & Building Materials*, *131*, 156–164. DOI: 10.1016/j.conbuildmat.2016.11.069

Krah, E., de Kruijf, J., & Ragno, L. (2018). Integrating traditional healers into the health care system: Challenges and opportunities in rural northern Ghana. *Journal of Community Health*, *43*(1), 157–163. DOI: 10.1007/s10900-017-0398-4 PMID: 28681282

Lawal, B., Shittu, O. K., Kabiru, A. Y., Jigam, A. A., Umar, M. B., Berinyuy, E. B., & Alozieuwa, B. U. (2015). Potential antimalarials from African natural products: A reviw. *Journal of Intercultural Ethnopharmacology*, *4*(4), 318. DOI: 10.5455/jice.20150928102856 PMID: 26649238

Nontokozo, Z. M., & Mthokozisi, S. (2018). *Herbal medicine*. Herbal Medicine.

Ogbera, A. O., Dada, O., & Adeyeye, F. (2010). Complementary and alternative medicine use in diabetes mellitus. *West African Journal of Medicine*, *29*, 158–162. PMID: 20665458

Ogunlana, O. O., Ogunlana, O. E., Tobi, S., Adekunbi, B. O., Adetuyi, B. O., & Adegboye, B. E. (2020). Anti-inflammatory mechanism of Ruzu bitters on diet-induced non-alcoholic fatty liver disease in male Wistar rats. *Evidence-Based Complementary and Alternative Medicine*. *Article ID*, *5246725*, 8.

Okwu, D. E. (2007). Nigerian medicinal plants I. *Medicinal and Aromatic Plant Science and Biotechnology*, *1*(1), 90–96.

Ompal, S. (2011). Chamomile: An overview. *Matricaria chamomilla*, pp. 70–71.

Oshikoya, K. A., Senbanjo, I. O., Njokanma, O. F., & Soipe, A. (2008). Use of complementary and alternative medicines for children with chronic health conditions in Lagos, Nigeria. *BMC Complementary and Alternative Medicine*, *8*(1), 66. DOI: 10.1186/1472-6882-8-66 PMID: 19113999

Sepide, M. (2016). A systematic review of therapeutic effects of *Matricaria recutita* (chamomile). *Electronic Physician*, *8*(9), 3024. DOI: 10.19082/3024 PMID: 27790360

Shakya, P., Shrestha, D., Maharjan, E., Sharma, V. K., & Paudyal, R. (2017). ESBL production among E. coli and Klebsiella spp. causing urinary tract infection: A hospital based study. *The Open Microbiology Journal*, *11*(1), 23–30. DOI: 10.2174/1874285801711010023 PMID: 28553414

Sunmer, J. (2000). *The natural history of medicinal plants*. Timber Press.

Vincent, P. (2018). A descriptive cross-sectional study on various uses and outcomes of *Garcinia kola* among people in Oshimili North, Delta State, Nigeria. *International Quarterly Journal of Research in Ayurveda*, p. 25.

Yusuf, K., Aykut, P., Zemzem, O., & Neslihan, P. (2019). Herbal drug usage habits of patients attending Balcali Hospital of Cukurova University. *Turkish Journal of Family Medicine and Primary Care*, *13*(4), 457–461. DOI: 10.21763/tjfmpc.651395

Chapter 7
Ethnopharmacology and Toxicological Profiles of Anti-Inflammatory and Analgesic Herbs

Chhan Kumar Kalita
http://orcid.org/0009-0006-8447-4538
Mizoram University, India

Awadhesh Kumar
Mizoram University, India

ABSTRACT

Inflammation in the body might be viewed as a cascade (driven by the immune, vascular, and signaling systems) whenever the body is affected by some foreign agents. This cascade boils and terminates at activated repair mechanisms when the host detects the offending stimulus. The persistence of states of drug resistance and toxicological effects in the human body stimulates the search for new therapeutic agents that can combat inflammation and analgesia. Ethnopharmacological research of plants with traditional uses as anti-inflammatory and analgesic agents demonstrates an extensive variety of bioactive constituents that have been utilized traditionally by various tribal communities to alleviate pain and restrain the inflammatory processes. Phytochemical analysis of these ethnomedicinal herbs has revealed that be contain secondary metabolites such as curcumin, ursolic acid, escin, withaferin A, etc., often showing the ability to inhibit important inflammatory mediators, viz., cyclooxygenase-2 (COX-2), nuclear factor-κB (NF-κB), and pro-inflammatory cytokines, e.g., TNF-α and IL-1β.

DOI: 10.4018/979-8-3373-5876-5.ch007

INTRODUCTION

Inflammation can be defined as an instinctive response to injury, infection, irritants, or harmful stimuli. Foreign antigen exposure triggers an integrated cascade involving the immune, vascular, and signaling systems that culminates in host-initiated repair mechanisms upon stimulus recognition. Symptoms such as pain, increased body temperature, localized swelling, and organ dysfunction can result from the dilation of venules and the subsequent leakage of plasma into the affected tissue, which is facilitated by specific biological mediators, including histamine, prostaglandins, and cytokines. At the same time, the immune cells (i.e., WBCs) are deputed to the injured location to restore the tissues (*Figure 1*). A prolonged reaction (chronic) could continue for up to a year or more. The neutrophils and macrophages release mediators, i.e., histamine, bradykinin, PGE_2, LTB_4, TNF-α, IL-1β, and IL-6 to perform phagocytosis. Ultimately, the resolution takes place via *a*) debris clearance, *b*) collagen deposition, or can progress to chronic inflammation. Although acute inflammation transpires decisively and endures for a brief duration due to a wound or infection, chronic inflammation is typically triggered by the immune system striking the infected tissues, which may ultimately lead to abnormalities such as tumors, cardiovascular disease, type 2 diabetes, asthma, and arthritis, such as rheumatoid arthritis etc.

Figure 1. Diagrammatic representation of the inflammation mechanism. Initiation leads to leukocyte adhesion and migration. The neutrophils and macrophages release mediators, i.e., histamine, bradykinin, PGE_2, LTB_4, TNF-α, IL-1β, and IL-6 to perform phagocytosis. Resolution takes place via a) debris clearance, b) collagen deposition, or can progress to chronic inflammation

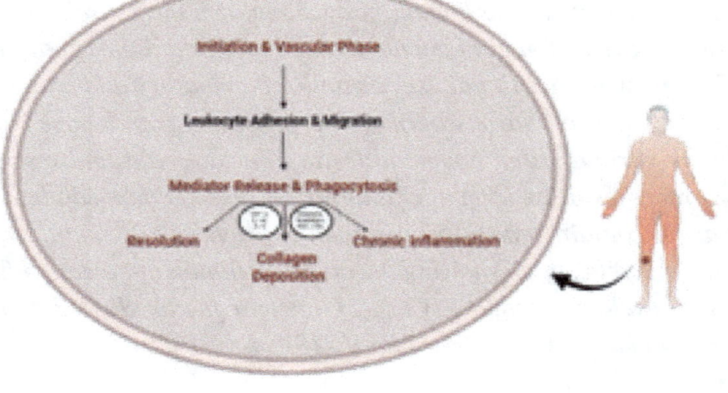

Non-steroidal anti-inflammatory drugs (NSAIDs) and steroidal anti-inflammatory drugs (SAIDs) are complementary in use to dampen the chronic inflammatory conditions. However, aside from their positive response to the infected parts, long-term application of the same has been linked to serious adverse reactions, *e.g.*, uncontrolled gastrointestinal bleeding (Li et al., 2003). According to research, the more up-to-date selective drugs targeted at cyclooxygenase-2 (COX-2) are likewise not encouraged for prolonged administration since they interfere with the production of the most effective antithrombotic and vasodilator prostacyclin (PGI_2). These types of cases may ultimately increase the cardiovascular and renal risks. Given such limitations of conventional anti-inflammatory drugs, researchers are increasingly turning to ethnopharmacology to explore plant-based alternatives. Since the earliest time, medicinal plants have been employed in conventional treatment methods for a range of human ailments, and the global demand for their application has remained constant (Kalita et al., 2024).

The multifaceted rigor of the ethnopharmacology methodically examines the traditional plant-based healing strategies of indigenous communities. Evaluation of these ethnobotanical leads is ultimately practiced in modern drug discovery. Emerging drug-resistance behavior of the living body over time has triggered the need to search for alternative medicines to cure various ailments, where potential ethnobotanical information is highly emphasized (Kalita et al., 2025). Recent reports by the World Health Organization (WHO) suggest that the primary reliance on ethnobotanical knowledge to cure health problems in developing nations has increased by 80%. Traditional healers around the globe have been using various herbs like *Curcuma longa* (turmeric), *Zingiber officinale* (ginger), and *Urtica dioica* (stinging nettle) etc., for ages to tackle inflammation and ease pain. Standardized extracts from these plants often show the ability to inhibit important inflammatory mediators, viz., cyclooxygenase-2 (COX-2), nuclear factor-κB (NF-κB), and pro-inflammatory cytokines, *e.g.*, TNF-α and IL-1β (Elisha et al., 2016; Vogl et al., 2013). Curcumin is the main bioactive in *Curcuma longa* that acts as a reducer of inflammation by suppressing NF-κB and blocking COX and lipoxygenase pathways (de Cássia da Silveira e Sá et al., 2013). Gingerol and shogaol are the compounds present in *Zingiber officinale* that possess analgesic activity by reducing prostaglandin production and inhibiting the transient receptor potential vanilloid-1 (TRPV1) channel (Mashhadi et al., 2013). Despite the promising pharmacodynamic profiles, ethnopharmacological research strongly calls for careful toxicological evaluations. There is a school of thought that herbal medicines don't reflect side effects, but case reports and systematic studies have shown a variety of adverse effects, viz., hepatotoxicity, nephrotoxicity, cardiotoxicity, and even carcinogenicity, etc. For instance, *Aristolochia* species, which were once used to treat arthritis and gout, contain aristolochic acids that have been linked to serious kidney damage and bladder cancer (Debelle et al., 2008). Standardized extracts along with close monitoring of pyrrolizidine alkaloid toxicity are of paramount importance, as extracts from the shrub *Piper methysticum* have been similarly attributed to severe liver toxicity (Teschke et al., 2011). Acute toxicity studies are commonly centered on establishing an herb's median lethal dose (LD_{50}). In the case of many anti-inflammatory plant extracts, the LD_{50} values are shown to exceed 2,000 mg/kg in rodent models, suggesting low acute toxicity when prepared appropriately. The case with sub-acute and chronic toxicity indicates potential cumulative impacts; for instance, long-term intake of poorly processed *Albizia procera* extracts caused a slight elevation of liver enzymes in rats, which advocates the necessity of dose control and duration limits. Furthermore, genotoxicity and reproductive toxicity studies are crucial, especially for herbs that may be consumed by at-risk demographics, including expectant mothers and minors (Yesilada & Gürbüz, 2016). The cutting-edge ethnopharmacological research incorporates an array of in vitro experiments, viz., cytotoxicity and enzyme inhibition, in vivo animal models, viz., carrageenan-induced paw oedema and the formalin pain test, and 'multi-omics' to characterize phytochemical accounts and forecast adverse responses to guarantee both efficacy and safety (Siriwatanametanon et al., 2010; Burford et al., 2022). This comprehensive approach fills the gap between conventional knowledge and evidence-based treatments by making it easier to identify responsible bioactive compounds, elucidating molecular pathways of action, and establishing toxicological thresholds. This chapter mainly discusses the in-hand primary reports of the utilization of several herbs as anti-inflammatory and analgesic agents, highlighting their mechanism of action, toxicity, safety considerations, and advocating their utmost scientific validation.

INDIGENOUS USES OF HERBS AS ANTI-INFLAMMATORY AND ANALGESIC AGENTS

Studies of the usage of medicinal herbs by tribal communities or ethnopharmacology is a cross-disciplinary concept that challenges the ethnobotany of plants as it is influenced by the cultural population, and as such, a source of bioactive compounds to modern medicine. Such an effort combines ethnobotany with phytochemical and pharmacological studies. This is usually followed by ethnobotanical surveys comprising guides, field walks, semi-structured interviews, and focus-group discussions in recording the species used, parts of the plants used, the methods used to prepare, and the therapeutic indications of indigenous or local communities (Tadesse et al., 2025). The quantitative indicators like Informant Consensus Factor (IcF), Use Value (UV), and Fidelity Level (FL), etc., are used to prioritize the species with high consensus values and high utilization, helping in further profound inquiry

(Tsioutsiou et al., 2023). Phytochemical analyses are conducted using sequential separation, extraction, and analytical processes, such as gas chromatography-mass spectrometry (GC-MS), liquid chromatography mass spectrometry (LC-MS), two-dimensional liquid chromatography (2D-LC), thin layer chromatography (TLC), high performance liquid chromatography (HPLC), and spectral methods to separate and recognize secondary metabolites in plants with respect to their bioactivity. After that, they are processed in subsequent bioassays (both in vitro and in vivo) to authorize the primary traditional usage that may be of an analgesic characteristic, anti-inflammatory, antimicrobial, anti-oxidative, as well as cytotoxicity (Abat et al., 2017). Different medicinal plants are represented as manifold. For instance, *Curcuma longa* and *Nigella sativa* are two of the well-known plants with scientific credit. Their major components, viz., curcuminoids and polyphenol antioxidants, have been found to have amazing biological properties such as anti-inflammatory, analgesic, antioxidant, antitumoral, and immunomodulatory actions (Abat et al., 2017; Dogara et al., 2025).

Traditional healers and tribal communities employ several plants to cure inflammatory conditions (*Table 1*), and analgesic (*Table 2*) conditions can be considered as preliminary data for full-fledged drug discovery. The Khampti tribe of Lohit District of Arunachal Pradesh, India, utilizes a number of potential plants with healing potential for the primary treatment of wounds and inflammation-related conditions. According to available literature, 34 species of 32 genera and 22 families were documented for the same, where the members from the Asteraceae, Euphorbiaceae, Zingiberaceae, Lamiaceae, and Mileaceae families were represented to be highly used, respectively (Namsa et al., 2009). About 43 medicinal plants, diversified into 28 families, were reported to be used to treat inflammation-related conditions by the Aboriginals of the western province of Sri Lanka. With a Relative frequency of citation (RFC) of 0.23, Coriandrum sativum is reported as the most commonly used plant to heal such conditions, followed by *Coscinium fenestratum* and *Adhatoda vasica* with RFC values of 0.13 and 0.12, respectively (Napagoda et al., 2018). The plant species from these taxonomic families were also found to be used as a source of anti-inflammatory and wound healing agents in other tribal communities of the world (Namsa et al., 2009). The Karbi tribe of West Karbi-anglong of Assam uses the paste of the leaves of *Adiantum capillus-veneris* L., and the paste of the leaves or whole plant of *Mentha piperita* L. to combat the inflammatory conditions. The powder of dried leaves of *Ocimum tenuiflorum* L. and *Oxalis corniculata* L. is dissolved in warm water and consumed in some tribal villages of the area (Kalita et al., 2025). A variety of plants are utilized as anti-inflammatory agents in North East India, such as *Alpinia galanga* L., *Curcuma caesia*, *Globba clarkei* Baker, and *Zingiber montanum* (Koen.) Link ex A. Dietr. etc., mixing with some other plants. For a long *Amomum dealbatum* has been used as an analgesic agent, but for the treatment of rheumatic joint inflammation, it has been reported as new (Basak et al., 2010). A cross-cultural study of the anti-inflammatory activity, e.g., asthma, arthritis, rheumatism, fever, edema, infections, snakebite, etc., of some Australian and Chinese medicinal plants, such as *Abrus precatorious*, *Clematis pickeringii*, *Euphorbia australis*, *Euphorbia drummondii*, *Tinospora sinensis*, *T. smilacina*, *Verbena officinalis,* etc., was validated for their traditional healing claims (Li et al., 2003). Ethnobotanical surveys in the North-central Morocco regions revealed the use of 104 medicinal plants belonging to 49 families for the traditional healing against inflammation and inflammatory pain. Medicinal plants belonging to the Lamiaceae family are utilized mostly, followed by Apiaceae and Asteraceae. In many remotest areas of the region, external poultice of *Carpobrotus edulis* L. (skin & gastric inflammation), *Aloe vera* (L.) Burm.f., (cutaneous inflammation & gastric pain), decoction of *Glycyrrhiza glabra* L. (mouth & gastric inflammation), decoction of *Centaurium erythraea* Rafn with olive oil (inflammatory bronchitis), *Trigonella foenum-graecum* L., *Ceratonia siliqua* L. (analgesic & stomach inflammation), *Pistacia lentiscus* L., *Calamintha officinalis* Moench., *Lavandula angustifolia* P. Mill. (analgesic) etc., are reported to be used as the traditional healing strategy (Lefrioui et al., 2024).

Table 1. Primary reports of the use of herbs as anti-inflammatory herbs around the globe

Sl No.	Plant Name	Mode of administration	Used Region/ Country	Method of data acquisition	Reference
1	*Abutilon indicum* (L.) Sweet	Taken orally as a soup	China	SSI	Hong et al., 2015
2	*Abrus precatorius* L.	NM	China	NM	Li et al., 2003
3	*Achillea nigrescens* (E. Mey.) Rydb.	Decoction of the Applied	Turkey	SI	Polat et al., 2015
4	*Achyranthes aspera* L.	Chew and spit the juice	Ethiopia	SSI	Teklay et al., 2013
5	*Acmella paniculata* (Wall.ex DC.) R.K.Jansen	Crushed and rubbed	Tripura	SSQ	Choudhury et al., 2015
6	*Adiantum capillus-veneris* L.	Paste of the leaves	West Karbi-Anglong	SSQ	Kalita et al., 2025
7	*Aerva javanica* (Burm. F.) Juss. ex Schult	Crushed and rubbed	Tripura	SSQ	Choudhury et al., 2015
8	*Ageratum conyzoides* Linn.	Boil with water and take orally	Arunachal Pradesh	SI	Namsa et al., 2009

continued on following page

Table 1. Continued

Sl No.	Plant Name	Mode of administration	Used Region/ Country	Method of data acquisition	Reference
9	*Allium fistulosum* L.	Decoction	China	SSI	Hong et al., 2015
10	*Allium sativum* L.	Infusion of blub is applied	Western Province of Sri Lanka	SSQ	Napagoda et al., 2018
11	*Alocasia macrorrhizos* (L.) G.Don	Crushed and rubbed	Tripura	SSQ	Choudhury et al., 2015
12	*Aloe vera* (L.) Burm.f.	Paste of leaves	Western Province of Sri Lanka	SSQ	Napagoda et al., 2018
13	*Alpinia galanga* L.	Powder of Rhizome	Arunachal Pradesh, Assam, Manipur, Mizoram, Nagaland	SI	Basak et al., 2010
14	*Amaranthus retroflexus* L.	Infusion	Turkey	SI	Polat et al., 2015
15	*Ammi visnaga* (L.) Lam.	Dried fruits mixed with dried fruits of *Bunium persicum*	Pakistan	SSQ	Ahmed et al., 2014
16	*Amomum subulatum* Roxb	By boiling 2-3 pods in water for 30 minutes. Strain and drink the extract	Arunachal Pradesh, Assam	SI	Basak et al., 2010
17	*Androsace umbellata* (Lour.)Merr.	Taken orally	China	SSI	Hong et al., 2015
18	*Arisaema heterophyllum* Blume	Taken orally	China	SSI	Hong et al., 2015
19	*Artemisia japonica* Thunb.	Decoction	China	SSI	Hong et al., 2015
20	*Artemisia nilagirica* (Clarke) Pamp. L	Hot water extracted the juice of the leaves	Arunachal Pradesh	SI	Namsa et al., 2009
21	*Atropa acuminate* Royle ex Lindl.	Powdered roots, leaves, and floral parts are taken with milk	Pakistan	SSQ	Ahmed et al., 2014
22	*Azadirachta indica* A. Juss (Linn.)	Stem juice and leaves are applied on a strained muscle	Arunachal Pradesh	SI	Namsa et al., 2009
23	*Bidens pilosa* Linn	Fresh paste of the leaves is applied to the infected area	Arunachal Pradesh	SI	Namsa et al., 2009
24	*Blumea balsamifera* (L.) DC.	Taken orally	China	SSI	Hong et al., 2015
25	*Blumea fistulosa* (Roxb.) Kurz	Juice of the leaves is applied	Arunachal Pradesh	SI	Namsa et al., 2009

continued on following page

Table 1. Continued

Sl No.	Plant Name	Mode of administration	Used Region/ Country	Method of data acquisition	Reference
26	*Bombax ceiba* Linn.	Bark paste combined with cow excrement and applied	Arunachal Pradesh	SI	Namsa et al., 2009
27	*Canarium strictum* Roxb.	Melted fresh resins are applied to the caterpillar larvae's skin where the toxic hairs are present	Arunachal Pradesh	SI	Namsa et al., 2009
28	*Cassia tora* Linn.	Decoction	China	SSI	Hong et al., 2015
29	*Centella asiatica* Linn.	Stem juice is applied to the strained muscle 3-4 times a day	Arunachal Pradesh	SI	Namsa et al., 2009
30	*Chirita eburnea* Hance	Decoction and taken orally	China	SSI	Hong et al., 2015
31	*Clematis chinensis* Osbeck	NM	China	NM	Li et al., 2003
32	*Clematis pickeringii* A.Gray	NM	Australia	NM	Li et al., 2003
33	*Coccinia grandis* (L.)	Decoction of leaves is used to drink	Tripura	SSQ	Choudhury et al., 2015
34	*Commelina communis* L	Decoction and taken orally	China	SSI	Hong et al., 2015
35	*Coriandrum sativum* L.	Infusion of seed is applied	Western Province of Sri Lanka	SSQ	Napagoda et al., 2018
36	*Curculigo orchioides* Gaertn.	Decoction and taken orally	China	SSQ	Hong et al., 2015
37	*Curcuma caesia* Roxb.	*Andrographis paniculata* powdered seeds is blended with desiccated rhizome powder and coated	Arunachal Pradesh; Assam, Mizoram	SI	Namsa et al., 2009; Basak et al., 2010
38	*Curcuma domestica* (Medik)	The dried powder of the rhizome	Arunachal Pradesh, Assam, Manipur, Nagaland	SI	Basak et al., 2010
39	*Curcuma longa* L	Before eating, mashed rhizomes are consumed orally	Arunachal Pradesh, Assam, Manipur, Meghalaya, Mizoram, Nagaland, Tripura	SI	Basak et al., 2010
40	*Curcuma zedoaria* (Christm.) Roscoe	Poultice of rhizome	Western Province of Sri Lanka; China	SSQ	Napagoda et al., 2018; Hong et al., 2015

continued on following page

Table 1. Continued

Sl No.	Plant Name	Mode of administration	Used Region/ Country	Method of data acquisition	Reference
41	*Cynanchum atratum* Bunge	Juice of the root	China	SSI	Hong et al., 2015
42	*Cyperus rotundus* L.	Infusion of leaves or stems	Western Province of Sri Lanka	SSQ	Napagoda et al., 2018
43	*Datura stramonium* L.	Leaves crushed and rubbed	Tripura	SSQ	Choudhury et al., 2015
44	*Datura stramonium* L.	Young leaves are crushed and applied to the affected part	Ethiopia	SSI	Teklay et al., 2013
45	*Desmodium triflorum* (L.) DC	Paste of leaves	Western Province of Sri Lanka	SSQ	Napagoda et al., 2018
46	*Drynaria propinqua* (Wall.exMett.) J.Sm.	Juice of the rhizome taken orally	China	SSI	Hong et al., 2015
47	*Dysosma versipellis* (Hance) M.ChengexT.S.Ying	Taken orally	China	SSI	Hong et al., 2015
48	*Elettaria cardamomum* Maton	Infusion, powder, or milk decoction	Arunachal Pradesh, Assam	SI	Basak et al., 2010
49	*Eleusine indica* (L.) Gaertn.	Poultice of whole plant; decoction	Western Province of Sri Lanka; China	SSQ	Napagoda et al., 2018; Hong et al., 2015
50	*Emilia sonchifolia* (L.) DC.	Taken orally	China	SSI	Hong et al., 2015
51	*Epimedium brevicornum* Maximowicz Trudy	Juice is taken	China	SSI	Hong et al., 2015
52	*Equisetum telmateia* Ehrh.	Infusion	Turkey	SI	Polat et al., 2015
53	*Eupatorium adenophorum* Spreng	Decoction of leaves in hot water	Arunachal Pradesh	SI	Namsa et al., 2009
54	*Eupatorium odoratum* Linn.	Decoction of leaves in hot water	Arunachal Pradesh	SI	Namsa et al., 2009
55	*Euphorbia drummondii* Boiss.	NM	Australia	NM	Li et al., 2003
56	*Euphorbia helioscopia* L.	NM	China	NM	Li et al., 2003
57	*Gerbera piloselloides* (L.) Cass	Decoction	China	SSI	Hong et al., 2015
58	*Gomphocarpus purpurascens* A. Rich.	Fluid from the rhizome is taken orally	Ethiopia	SSI	Teklay et al., 2013

continued on following page

Table 1. Continued

Sl No.	Plant Name	Mode of administration	Used Region/ Country	Method of data acquisition	Reference
59	*Gynostemma pentaphyllum* (Thunb.) Makino	Decoction	China	SSI	Hong et al., 2015
60	*Hedera nepalensis* K. Koch	Leaves that have been crushed and seasoned in water are consumed orally	Pakistan	SSQ	Ahmed et al., 2014
61	*Hedychium coccineum* Buch.-Ham. ex Sm	Rhizome paste applied over the swollen part	Arunachal Pradesh, Mizoram	SI	Basak et al., 2010
62	*Hedychium spicatum* SM.	Powder of Rhizome	Arunachal Pradesh, Manipur, Meghalaya, Mizoram	SI	Basak et al., 2010
63	*Hedyotis diffusa* Willd	Taken orally	China	SSI	Hong et al., 2015
64	*Homalomena occulta* (Lour.) Schott	Decoction or taken orally	China	SSI	Hong et al., 2015
65	*Hypericum perforatum* L.	Decoction	Turkey	SI	Polat et al., 2015
66	*Hypoestes forskaolii* (Vahl) Roem.& Schult.	Chew and swallow the fluid	Ethiopia	SSI	Teklay et al., 2013
67	*Ipomoea pescaprae* (L.) R.Br.	Taken orally	China	SSI	Hong et al., 2015
68	*Kaempferia pulchra* Ridl.	Steamed rhizomes, stems, and leaves	Assam, Mizoram	SI	Basak et al., 2010
69	*Kalanchoe laciniata* (L.) DC.	Infusion of leaves	Western Province of Sri Lanka	SSQ	Napagoda et al., 2018
70	*Kalanchoe pinnata* (Lam.) Pers.	Crushed leaves applied directly	Arunachal Pradesh	SI	Namsa et al., 2009
71	*Kalimeris indica* (L.) Sch.Bip.	Taken orally	China	SSI	Hong et al., 2015
72	*Laggera alata* (D.Don) Sch.Bip. ex Oliv.	Decoction	China	SSI	Hong et al., 2015
73	*Laportea cuspidata* (Wedd.) Friis	Juice of leaves taken orally	China	SSI	Hong et al., 2015
74	*Lobelia sequinii* Levl. et Vant.	Boiled with water and taken orally	China	SSI	Hong et al., 2015
75	*Malva neglecta* Wallr.	Boil or infusion	Turkey	SI	Polat et al., 2015

continued on following page

Table 1. Continued

Sl No.	Plant Name	Mode of administration	Used Region/ Country	Method of data acquisition	Reference
76	*Maytenus royleana* (Wall. ex M.A. Lawson) Cufod	Fresh leaves are crushed and the extract is used as eye drops	Pakistan	SSQ	Ahmed et al., 2014
77	*Mentha piperita* L.	Leaf paste or the entire plant is eaten	West Karbi Anglong	SSQ	Kalita et al., 2025
78	*Mollugo cerviana* (L.) Ser.	Infusion of stem or leaves	Western Province of Sri Lanka	SSQ	Napagoda et al., 2018
79	*Ocimum sanctum* Linn.	Paste of the leaves applied to the infected part	Arunachal Pradesh	SI	Namsa et al., 2009
80	*Ocimum tenuiflorum* L.	The powder of dried leaves is boiled in water and consumed	West Karbi Anglong	SSQ	Kalita et al., 2025
81	*Origanum vulgare* L.	Decoction	Turkey	SI	Polat et al., 2015
82	*Oxalis corniculata* L.	The entire plant's extract is consumed	West Karbi Anglong	SSQ	Kalita et al., 2025
83	*Paeonia emodi* Royle	Dried ground roots are fried and taken orally	Pakistan	SSQ	Ahmed et al., 2014
84	*Piper longum* L.	Infusion or decoction of fruits	Western Province of Sri Lanka	SSQ	Napagoda et al., 2018
85	*Plantago lanceolata* L.	Boil or infusion	Turkey	SI	Polat et al., 2015
86	*Plantago major* Linn.	Decoction of the whole plant is used for stomach inflammation,	Arunachal Pradesh	SI	Namsa et al., 2009
87	*Platycodon grandiflorus* (Jacq.) A.DC.	Decoction	China	SSI	Hong et al., 2015
88	*Ricinus cummunis* Linn	To reduce swelling and inflammation, fresh leaves that have been burned on a hob are placed all over the body	Arunachal Pradesh	SI	Namsa et al., 2009
89	*Sambucus chinensis* Lindl.	Taken orally	China	SSI	Hong et al., 2015
90	*Sida acuta* Burm.f.	Decoction of roots	Western Province of Sri Lanka	SSQ	Napagoda et al., 2018
91	*Solanum lyratum* Thunb.	NM	China	NM	Li et al., 2003

continued on following page

Table 1. Continued

Sl No.	Plant Name	Mode of administration	Used Region/ Country	Method of data acquisition	Reference
92	*Solanum surattense* Burm. f.	Porridge or the smoke of leaves	Western Province of Sri Lanka	SSQ	Napagoda et al., 2018
93	*Solanum xanthocarpum* Schrad.&H.Wendl	Infusion of leaves	Western Province of Sri Lanka	SSQ	Napagoda et al., 2018
94	*Swertia chirayita* Roxb. H. Karst.	An infusion of the herb is generally employed	Pakistan	SSQ	Ahmed et al., 2014
95	*Trigonella foenum-graecum* L.	Poultice of seeds	Western Province of Sri Lanka	SSQ	Napagoda et al., 2018
96	*Urtica dioica* L.	Decoction	Turkey	SI	Polat et al., 2015
97	*Verbena officinalis* L.	NM	Australia	NM	Li et al., 2003
98	*Vitis vinifera* L.	Infusion	Turkey	SI	Polat et al., 2015
99	*Woodwardia japonica* (L.f.) Sm.	Taken orally	China	SSI	Hong et al., 2015
100	*Zingiber cassumunar* Roxb.	Rhizome paste with salt is taken orally	Assam, Manipur, Mizoram, Meghalaya, Arunachal Pradesh	SI	Basak et al., 2010
101	*Zingiber montanum* (Koen.) Link ex A. Dietr.	Rhizome of *Z. officinale* and *Kaempferia galanga* used together as a paste	Arunachal Pradesh, Assam	SI	Basak et al., 2010
102	*Zingiber officinale* Roscoe	Infusion of rhizome	Western Province of Sri Lanka; Arunachal Pradesh, Assam, Manipur, Meghalaya	SSQ	Napagoda et al., 2018; Basaak et al., 2010
103	*Zingiber zerumbet* Rosc. EX SM.	Ground rhizome material is mixedwith water and taken orally	Manipur	SI	Basak et al., 2010

Aberrations: *Used Part:* L-Leaf; S-Stem; Se-Seed; R-Root; Rh-Rhizome; Wp-Whole plant; Ap-Aerial parts; Fr-Fruit; Fl-Flower; T-Tuber; Ys-Young shoot; La-Latex; B-Bark. *Method of Data Acquisition*: Semi-structured questionnaire-SSQ; Semi-structured interviews-SSI; Spot interview-SI; Semi-structured survey-SSS; Not mentioned-NM

Table 2. Primary reports of the use of herbs as analgesic herbs around the globe

Sl No.	Plant Name	Used part	Mode of administration	Used Region/ Country	Method of data acquisition	Reference
1	*Aconitum chasmanthum* Stapf ex Holmes	Rh	Powder of the rhizome	Pakistan	SSQ	Ahmed et al., 2014
2	*Ajuga integrifolia* Buch-Ham.	L	Crushed leaves taken with water	Ethiopia	SSI	Teklay et al., 2013
3	*Alpinia officinarum* Hance	R	Decoction	Morocco	SSS	Lefrioui et al., 2024
4	*Amaranthus retroflexus* L.	Ap	Infusion	Turkey	SI	Polat et al., 2015
5	*Ammi visnaga* L.	Fr	Decoction	Morocco	SSS	Lefrioui et al., 2024
6	*Ammodaucus leucotrichus* Coss.	Se	Decoction or infusion and taken orally	Morocco	SSS	Lefrioui et al., 2024
7	*Amomum subulatum* Roxb.	Se	Boil of seeds	Arunachal Pradesh	SI	Basak et al., 2010
8	*Anacyclus pyrethrum* L.	R	Crushed and taken with water	Morocco	SSS	Lefrioui et al., 2024
9	*Anemone vesicatoria* (L.f.) Prantl.	L	Infusion	South Africa	SR	Aremu & Pendota, 2021
10	*Asclepias crispa* P.J.Bergius.	R	Decoction	South Africa	SR	Aremu & Pendota, 2021
11	*Baccharoides adoensis* (Sch.Bip. Ex Walp.) H.Rob.L,S,R		Decoction	South Africa	SR	Aremu & Pendota, 2021
12	*Ballota africana* (L.) Benth.	L	Infusion	South Africa	SR	Aremu & Pendota, 2021
13	*Bidens pilosa* L.	L,Se	Decoction of leaves or seeds, crushed and applied	South Africa	SR	Aremu & Pendota, 2021
14	*Bistorta amplexicaulis* (D.Don) Greene	R	Powder of root	Pakistan	SSQ	Ahmed et al., 2014
15	*Boesenbergia rotunda* (L.) Mansf.	R	Infusion	Thailand	SSI	Pikulthong et al., 2022
16	*Boophone disticha* (L. f.) Herb.	B	Decoction	South Africa	SR	Aremu & Pendota, 2021
17	*Cannabis sativa* L.	Wp	Decoction of leaves	South Africa	SR	Aremu & Pendota, 2021
18	*Carum carvi* L.	Se	Decoction	Morocco	SSS	Lefrioui et al., 2024

continued on following page

Table 2. Continued

Sl No.	Plant Name	Used part	Mode of administration	Used Region/ Country	Method of data acquisition	Reference
19	*Catharanthus roseus* (L.) G.Don.	L,R	Decoction of leaves, root crushed, and applied	South Africa	SR	Aremu & Pendota, 2021
20	*Centella asiatica* (L.) Urb.	Wp,L	Decoction of leaves	South Africa	SR	Aremu & Pendota, 2021
21	*Clitoria ternatea* L.	Se	Infusion	Thailand	SSI	Pikulthong et al., 2022
22	*Cotyledon orbiculata* L.	L	Decoction or juice of leaves	South Africa	SR	Aremu & Pendota, 2021
23	*Crinum macowanii* Baker.	B	Decoction	South Africa	SR	Aremu & Pendota, 2021
24	*Cucumis ficifolius* A. Rich.	R	Juice of the root after crushing	Ethiopia	SSI	Teklay et al., 2013
25	*Curcuma longa* L.	R	Infusion	Thailand	SSI	Pikulthong et al., 2022
26	*Cynanchum officinale* (Hemsl.) Tsiang&H.D.Zhang	R	Taken orally	China	SSI	Hong et al., 2015
27	*Dicoma capensis* Less.	L	Infusion	South Africa	SR	Aremu & Pendota, 2021
28	*Dracaena elliptica* Thunb. & Dalm	S	Stem crushed and applied directly	Tripura	SSQ	Choudhury et al., 2015
29	*Drimia elata* Jacq.	B	Poultice of the bulb	South Africa	SR	Aremu & Pendota, 2021
30	*Elettaria cardamomum* L.	Se	Decoction	Morocco	SSS	Lefrioui et al., 2024
31	*Foeniculum vulgare* Mill.	L	Decoction	South Africa	SR	Aremu & Pendota, 2021
32	*Fumaria indica* (Hausskn.) Pugsley	Wp	Decoction	Pakistan	SSQ	Ahmed et al., 2014
33	*Galium boreo-aethiopicum* Puff	R	Roots, after being crushed, the fluid is taken	Ethiopia	SSI	Teklay et al., 2013
34	*Galium tomentosum* Thunb.	L	Powdered leaves are taken with water	South Africa	SR	Aremu & Pendota, 2021
35	*Globba multiflora* Baker.	Rh	Crushed rhizome applied locally to the infected area	Arunachal Pradesh	SI	Basak et al., 2010

continued on following page

Table 2. Continued

Sl No.	Plant Name	Used part	Mode of administration	Used Region/ Country	Method of data acquisition	Reference
36	*Gnidia kraussiana* Meisn.	R	Decoction or infusion	South Africa	SR	Aremu & Pendota, 2021
37	*Helichrysum cymosum* (L.) D.Don.	L	Vapor of the boiled leaves	South Africa	SR	Aremu & Pendota, 2021
38	*Helichrysum odoratissimum* (L.) Sweet.	Wp	Infusion	South Africa	SR	Aremu & Pendota, 2021
39	*Kaempferia parviflora* Wallich. ex Baker.	R	Brew in liquor and drink	Thailand	SSI	Pikulthong et al., 2022
40	*Lepidium sativum* L.	Se	Crushed seeds are drunk with water	Ethiopia	SSI	Teklay et al., 2013
41	*Leucas aspera* (Willd.) Link	L	Leaves crushed and rubbed	Tripura	SSQ	Choudhury et al., 2015
42	*Ligusticum sinense* Oliv.	Wp	Juice of the leaves	China	SSI	Hong et al., 2015
43	*Linum usitatissimum* L.	Se	Decoction of seeds	Morocco	SSS	Lefrioui et al., 2024
44	*Mentha longifolia* (L.) Huds.	L	Paste of leaves	South Africa	SR	Aremu & Pendota, 2021
45	*Mentha longifolia* (L.) L	L,S, Fl	Dried leaves are taken with water	Pakistan	SSQ	Ahmed et al., 2014
46	*Mentha villosa* Huds.	L	Infusion	Thailand	SSI	Pikulthong et al., 2022
47	*Ocimum africanum* Lour	L	Taken directly	Thailand	SSI	Pikulthong et al., 2022
48	*Ocimum basilicum* L.	L	Infusion	Thailand	SSI	Pikulthong et al., 2022
49	*Ocimum tenuiflorum* L.	L	Leaves crushed and rubbed	Tripura	SSQ	Choudhury et al., 2015
50	*Origanum vulgare* L.	Wp	Juice of the crushed plant	Pakistan	SSQ	Ahmed et al., 2014
51	*Orthosiphon aristatus* (Blume) Miq.	S	Infusion	Thailand	SSI	Pikulthong et al., 2022
52	*Paeonia emodi* Royle	R	Dried root powder	Pakistan	SSQ	Ahmed et al., 2014
53	*Pajanelia longifolia* (Willd.) K.Schum.	B	Juice of the crushed bark	Tripura	SSQ	Choudhury et al., 2015

continued on following page

Table 2. Continued

Sl No.	Plant Name	Used part	Mode of administration	Used Region/ Country	Method of data acquisition	Reference
54	*Pennisetum typhoides* (Burm.) Stapf. & Hubb.	Se	Powder of the seeds taken with milk	Morocco	SSS	Lefrioui et al., 2024
55	*Pentanisia prunelloides* subsp. *Latifolia* (Hochst.) Verdc.	L,R	Decoction of leaves	South Africa	SR	Aremu & Pendota, 2021
56	*Petasites hybridus* (L.) Gaertn., Mey. & Scherb.	Ap	Infusion	Turkey	SI	Polat et al., 2015
57	*Plantago major* L.	L	Powder of the leaves taken with water	Morocco	SSS	Lefrioui et al., 2024
58	*Platycarpha glomerata* (Thunb.) Less.	R	Juice of the root after crushing	South Africa	SR	Aremu & Pendota, 2021
59	*Podophyllum emodi* Wall. ex Royle	R	Decoction	Pakistan	SSQ	Ahmed et al., 2014
60	*Rheum australe* D. Don	Wp	Powder of the whole plant	Pakistan	SSQ	Ahmed et al., 2014
61	*Satureja spicigera* (C.Koch) Boiss.	L	Infusion	Turkey	SI	Polat et al., 2015
62	*Solanum panduriforme* E. Mey.	Fr,R	Powder of the fruits or roots taken with water	South Africa	SR	Aremu & Pendota, 2021
63	*Sutherlandia frutescens* (L.) R.Br.	L	Leaves are clean and chewed directly	South Africa	SR	Aremu & Pendota, 2021
64	*Thymus schimperi* Ronniger	Wp	Boil and take orally	Ethiopia	SSI	Teklay et al., 2013
65	*Trichodesma trichodesmoides* (Bunge) Gurke	L	Crushed seeds are drunk with water	Ethiopia	SSI	Teklay et al., 2013
66	*Trigonella foenum-graecum* (Bunge) Gurke.	Se	Crushed seeds drunk with water	Ethiopia	SSI	Teklay et al., 2013
67	*Tulbaghia violacea* Harv.	L	Leaves are crushed and rubbed on the forehead	South Africa	SR	Aremu & Pendota, 2021
68	*Turbina oblongata* A. Meeuse.	L	Poultices of leaves	South Africa	SR	Aremu & Pendota, 2021
69	*Urtica dioica* L.	L,Se,Fl	Decoction	Turkey	SI	Polat et al., 2015

continued on following page

Table 2. Continued

Sl No.	Plant Name	Used part	Mode of administration	Used Region/ Country	Method of data acquisition	Reference
70	*Valeriana jatamansi* Jones	Rh	Dried rhizome taken with milk	Pakistan	SSQ	Ahmed et al., 2014
71	*Verbascum thapsus* L.	L,S	Decoction of seeds is taken orally	Pakistan	SSQ	Ahmed et al., 2014
72	*Verbena officinalis* L	Wp	Crushed and fluid taken directly	Ethiopia	SSI	Teklay et al., 2013
73	*Viola inconspicua* Blume	Wp	Taken orally	China	SSI	Hong et al., 2015
74	*Viola pilosa* Blume	L,Fl	Decoction	Pakistan	SSQ	Ahmed et al., 2014
75	*Zantedeschia aethiopica* (L.) Spreng	L	Decoction	South Africa	SR	Aremu & Pendota, 2021
76	*Zingiber montanum* (Koenig) Link ex Dietr.	R	Infusion	Thailand	SSI	Pikulthong et al., 2022
77	Zingiber officinale Roscoe	R	Taken directly	Thailand	SSI	Pikulthong et al., 2022

Aberrations: *Used Part*: L-Leaf; S-Stem; Se-Seed; R-Root; Rh-Rhizome; Wp-Whole plant; Ap-Aerial parts; Fr-Fruit; B-Bark. *Method of Data Acquisition*: Semi-structured questionnaire-SSQ; Semi-structured interviews-SSI; Spot interview-SI; Semi-structured survey-SSS; Systematic review-SR.

MAJOR CLASSES OF PHYTOCHEMICALS IN ANTI-INFLAMMATORY AND ANALGESIC HERBS

The primary anti-inflammatory and analgesic effects of all medicinal herbs are based on their content of a set of secondary metabolites that are split into some major classes. Members of the flavonoid family, namely flavones (*Fig: 2A-C*) (e.g., apigenin, luteolin, baicalin), flavonols (*Fig: 3A-B*) (quercetin, kaempferol), flavanones (*Fig: 4A-B*) (naringenin, hesperidin), isoflavones (*Fig: 5A-B*) (genistein, puerarin), and catechins (*Fig: 6*) (epigallocatechin gallate) as well as anthocyanidins (cyanidin-3-O-glycoside) exert their effects via regulating major signalling pathways, namely NF-kB, MAP. In the same vein, phenolic acids (rosmarinic, ellagic, gallic, protocatechuic, vanillic acids, 6-gingerol, and caffeic acid phenethyl ester) play the role of inhibiting the activity of NF-kB in addition to increasing the Nrf2/ HO-1 pathway, thus reducing oxidative stress and the production of inflammatory compounds (Nisar et al., 2023). Terpenoids, including monoterpenes (*Fig. 7A-B*) (cineole, paeoniflorin), sesquiterpenes (parthenolide, zerumbone), diterpenoids (ginkgolides), and triterpenoids (ursolic acid, escin, withaferin A, sitosterol), regulate PPAR-gamma, NF-kappa, MAPKs, and Nrf2 pathway to inhibit cytokine secretion and recruitment of leukocytes (Linghu et al., 2019; Nisar et al., 2023). The saponins and more specifically steroidal saponins (*Fig. 8A-C*) (e.g., diosgenin, guggulsterones, and solasodine) are structurally related to glucocorticoids and inhibit PLA 2 and proinflammatory cytokines, having potent effects with limited side effects (Patel & Savjani, 2015). Alkaloids such as tetrandrine, berbamine, and a range of isoquinolines can interfere with the COX and LOX pathways and act to reduce TNF-alpha, PGE2, and leukocyte activity (Gomes et al., 2008; Ahmadiani et al., 2001; Beg et al., 2011). Tannin and coumarin are found alongside the flavonoids that bind to and block inflammatory enzymes, especially COX-2 and LP, and inhibit vascular leakiness (Ahmadiani et al., 2001; Musa et al., 2008). Glycosides (e.g., harpagoside, arbortristoside-A) prevent arachidonic acid metabolism and synthesis of prostanoids, showing some central and peripheral analgesia, as well as showing muscle relaxant effects (Arul et al., 2005; Nisar et al., 2023). Anthraquinones, iridoids, and phenylpropanoids (e.g., aloe-emodin, iridoid glycosides, salicin) complement them in suppressing neuroinflammation, facilitated by glia and the central pain pathways (Jha et al., 2025). Monoterpene and sesquiterpene-rich essential oils quickly achieve analgesia and anti-inflammatory effects through TRP channel modulation and proinflammatory mediator suppression (Pinho-Ribeiro et al., 2016). All of these phytochemical classes have a synergistic and multi-targeted nature, which includes the ion channel modulation, suppression of cytokines, and redox homeostasis, justifying the therapeutic value of these as complementary or alternative agents in analgesia and inflammation (Arul et al., 2005; Beg et al., 2011).

Figure 2. A-8C. Major phytochemicals present in the anti-inflammatory and analgesic herbs

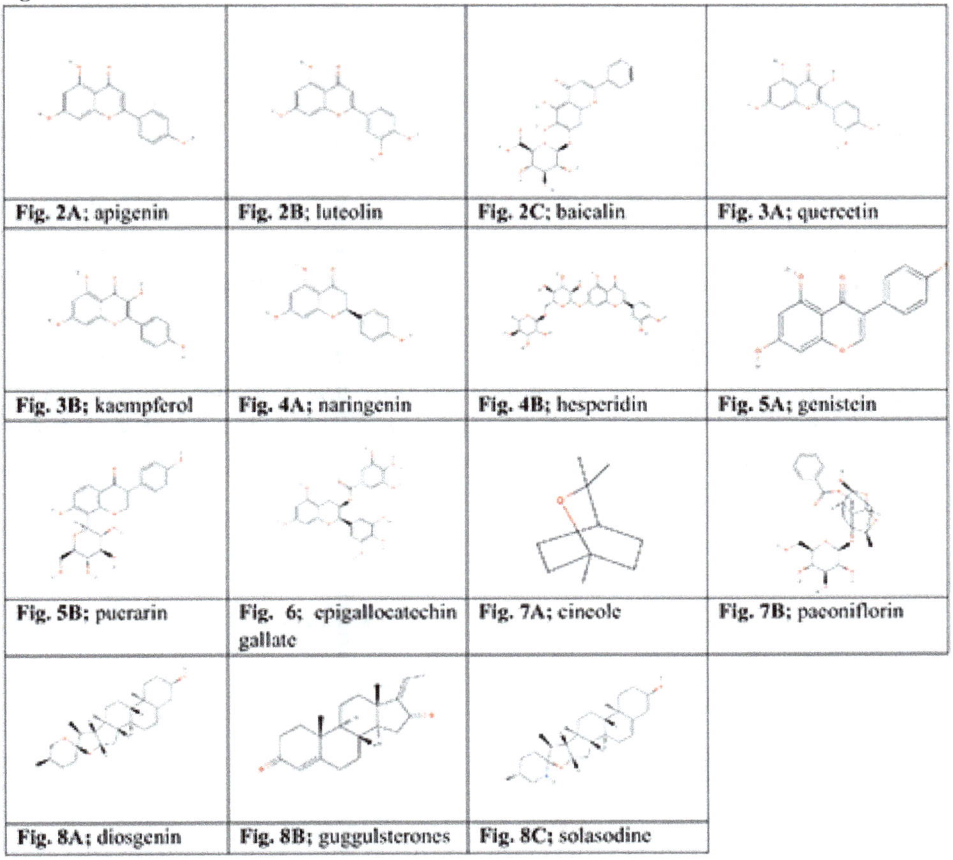

KEY SIGNALING PATHWAYS INVOLVED IN ANTI-INFLAMMATORY AND ANALGESIC ACTIVITY

Medicinal herbs contain anti-inflammatory properties that involve modifying conserved intracellular pathways for the transmission of signals, which control the activity and verbalism of pro-inflammatory enzymes, cytokines, and transcription factors (*Fig. 9*). Multimodal analgesia can be obtained through the use of analgesic herbs which act on central target enzymes (COX/LOX), ion channels (TRP, calcium), neurotransmitter receptors (opioid, cannabinoid, monoamine, GABA, adrenergic), intracellular signal cascades (NF- kB, MAPK, JAK-STAT), and oxidative/nitrosative pathways. Their pharmacology profile justifies their involvement as an adjuvant or unorthodox approach in the treatment of acute, chronic, and neuropathic pain.

Figure 3. Diagrammatic representation of the interaction with membrane receptors, upstream kinases, transcription factors, and their downstream mRNA targets in overall signaling pathways. Curcumin blocks the canonical Toll-like receptor 4 (TLR4) pathway by disrupting the TLR4-MyD88-IkappaB-alpha (IKK) complex, thus preventing IkappaB-alpha (IkB-alpha) phosphorylation and translocation to the nucleus of NF-kappaB. Resveratrol mediates a controlled stimulation of reactive oxygen species (ROS) that can directly oxidize Keap1 cysteine residues, thereby releasing Nrf2 as it activates antioxidant response element (ARE)-dependent expression of heme oxygenase-1 (HO-1) and NAD(P)H quinone dehydrogenase 1 (NQO1). Andrographolide-keto-beta-alanine (AKBA) can thus bind fatty-acid-activated protein (FLAP), inhibit 5-lipoxygenase (5-LOX) dependent leukotriene production, and inhibit NF-kappaB-, mitogen-activated protein kinase (MAPK) dependent cyclooxygenase 2 (COX-2) expression

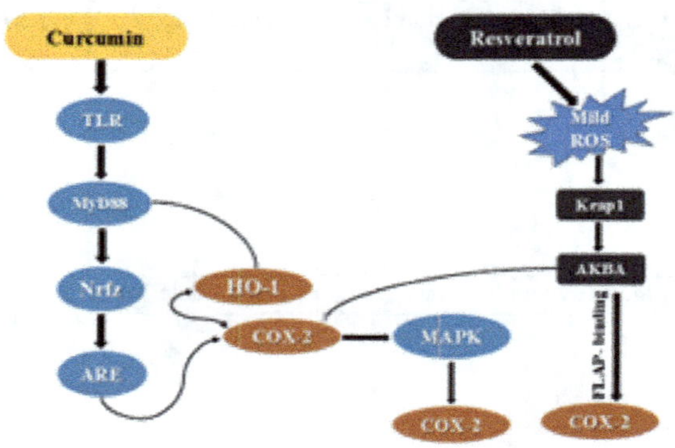

1) **Nuclear factor-kappa B (NF-kappa B) pathway:** The NF-kappa B dimers (p65/p50) are bound in the cytoplasm by the inhibitor of kappa B alpha (I kappa B alpha). After it is stimulated with pro-inflammatory cytokines (e.g., IL-11 beta, TNF-alpha), the I kappa B kinase (IKK) phosphorylates I x B alpha on Ser 32/36, which is targeted with ubiquitination and degradation in the proteasome. After the liberation, NF-kB translocates into nuclear cells, anchors to 3B regions,

and stimulates the expression of COX-2, iNOS, M MPs, TNF-1, and ILs-1 and 6 (Buhrmann et al., 2011). For example, Curcumin is a diarylheptanoid found in the root of *Curcuma longa,* and it inhibits IL-1activation of the NF-κB in human tenocytes by:

i. A direct inhibition of IKK activity results in the prevention of IKK-mediated phosphorylation/degradation of IkBa.
ii. It prevents the phosphorylation (Ser536) activation and nuclear translocation of p65.
iii. It prevents p65 acetylation, which is essential to affect its full transcriptional activity.

2) **Nrf2/HO-1 antioxidant pathway**: Nrf2 in quiescent cells is kept in the cytoplasm in an inactive form in the form of Nrf2 interaction with the cytoplasmic inhibitor Keap1 that helps in ubiquitinating Nrf2 via Cullin3-E3 ligase complex. Oxidative or electrophilic injury provokes a reaction that alters the cysteine residues of Keap1 and thus interrupts this interaction, which translates to redistribution of Nrf2 Nuclear translocation. Nrf2 can form heterodimers with small Maf proteins and binds antioxidant response elements (ARE), thereby stimulating a number of protective genes and enzymes such as heme oxygenase-1 (HO-1), NAD (P)H quinone oxidoreductase-1 (NQO1), glutathione S-transferases, and 2-glutamylcysteine ligase. *Vitis vinifera-derived* stilbene resveratrol acts by activating Nrf2 by causing low ROS accumulation, whereupon transient thiol oxidation of Keap1 favors Nrf2 dissociation and binding to ARE. The inhibition of nuclear factor-kappa B (NF-kB) and pro-inflammatory agents results in the promotion of the enzymatic activity of superoxide dismutase (SOD) and catalase (Alavi et al. 2021).

3) **Arachidonic acid metabolism (5-lipoxygenase/5-LOX) and cyclooxygenase/ COX pathways**: Phospholipase A_2 encourages the liberation of arachidonic acid (AA) from membrane phospholipids. Further processing of AA by 5-lipoxygenase (5-LOX) splits up into pro-inflammatory leukotrienes, e.g., $LTB_{4,}$ and through cyclooxygenase-2 (COX-2), the formation of prostaglandins such as PGE_2 occurs. FLAP is the activating protein of 5-LOX, is essential to the action of the former. The boswellic acids, especially the acetyl-11-keto-β-boswellic acid (AKBA) present in *Boswellia serrata* are noncompetitive inhibitors of 5-LOX and FLAP, and they inhibit the formation of LTB_4. Besides, AKBA suppresses the expression and synthesis of COX-2 and PGE_2. In an osteoarthritic rat model, AKBA-rich extract formulations suppressed the levels of TNF-alpha, IL-1-beta, IL-6, the metalloproteinases-2 (MMP-2) and metalloproteinases-13 (MMP-13), and this reduction was found to reduce synovial inflammation and cartilage-degradation (Shin et al., 2022).

TOXICOLOGICAL PROFILES OF ANTI-INFLAMMATORY AND ANALGESIC HERBS

Examination of the toxicity is a critical aspect of ethnopharmacology and ensures safe integration of conventional medicinal plants into the modern health care systems. However, a great proportion of herbal preparations have bioactive ingredients that can result in toxicity, adverse reactions, and disease damage when used in the wrong way or in large quantities (Prajapati, 2024; Rehman et al., 2022; Zhang et al., 2015). Toxicity assessments form a vital part of the differentiation between the therapeutic and harmful drug concentration, the determination of safe dosing arrangements, and the reduction of unwanted health effects. Systematic toxicity profiling provides a scientific foundation in proving the safety and efficacy of traditional remedies to pave the way towards precise risk-benefit analysis and develop evidence-based facts that can be referred to by healthcare professionals and regulatory specialists (Prajapati, 2024; Rehman et al., 2022). These assessments are usually an extensive analysis of animal models and in vitro experiments involving acute, subacute, and chronic exposures as required by the internationally agreed-upon guidelines, such as OECD guidelines (Rehman et al., 2022). All of these studies work towards the prevention of incidents of toxicity associated with these products and help in the safe use and development of herbal medicines, creating trust in its therapeutic properties in both traditional and modern health settings (Prajapati, 2024; Rehman et al., 2022; Zhang et al., 2015).

Acute and chronic toxicity

Toxicological characterization of botanicals that address anti-inflammatory functions and analgesic features is imperative towards establishing the safe level of dosage and the general adverse impact of this exposure, which is both acute and repeated. The water-soluble extract of *Curcuma longa* leaf demonstrated low acute oral toxicity (LD_{50} of 2,154 mg/kg) in Swiss albino mice, with some mild clinical signs, viz., salivation and reduced locomotor activity; nonetheless, mortality was observed till 1,600 mg/kg (Chourasiya et al., 2024). Essential oil of *C. longa* demonstrated minimal acute oral toxicity in Wistar rats, with LD_{50} exceeding 5,000 mg/kg and no alterations in body weight, food consumption, hepatic markers (AST, ALT, ALP), renal function (urea, creatinine), or serum electrolytes at the highest dose tested (0.5 g/kg) (Liju et al., 2013). Similarly, a water-soluble *Boswellia serrata* gum resin extract (LI51202F1) exhibited low acute toxicity in Sprague Dawley rats and white rabbits, with LD_{50} exceeding 2,000 mg/kg, and no mortality, systemic toxicity, dermal irritation, or ocular toxicity was observed (Dodda et al., 2022).

Long-term toxicity studies are fundamental in establishing safety in sustainable therapy. Another 28-day repeated-dose study of *B. serrata* resin extract (LI13019F1) in Wistar rats revealed dose-independent results on body weight, organ weight, hematology, clinical chemistry, and determination of a no-observed-adverse-effect level (NOAEL) of 1,000 mg/kg/day (Alluri et al., 2019). In another 90-day gavage study of *B. serrata* in Wistar rats at doses 100, 500, and 1,000 mg/kg/day, a slight and temporary body-weight reduction occurred in the 1,000 mg/kg/day group, but no clinical, histological, or biochemical abnormalities were seen in the 500 mg/kg/day group; accordingly, the latter dose was the NOAEL (Singh et al., 2012). Similarly, 90 days study with a standardized NR-INF-02 at a dosage of 250, 500 and 1,000 mg/kg/day did not result in mortality, clinical toxicity effects and also no significant changes in body weights, food consumption, hematology, serum biochemistry, urinary parameters and organ histopathology, which confidently supports a NOAEL of 1,000 mg/kg/day (Murugan et al., 2021). A 28-day study of 250-1,000 mg/kg/day ethanol extract of *Curcuma* sp. rhizome exhibits no adverse effects on liver and kidney functions in parallel studies in rats and showed heightened antioxidant-enzyme activities, as well as high-density lipoprotein cholesterol boosted, signifying both safety and potential pharmacological effects (John et al., 2024).

Comparison of in vivo acute toxicities revealed that the therapeutically used anti-inflammatory turmeric, boswellia, and willow bark remarkably possess very high LD_{50} values (>2,000 mg /kg). This level of safety is recommended in the studies of chronic and sub-chronic administration. NOAELs are in the range of 500-1000 mg/kg/day, revealed no mutagenicity or clastogenicity, no toxicity and organ-specificity, as well as no significant alterations of biochemical parameters (Singh et al., 2012; Dodda et al., 2022; Alluri et al., 2019; Murugan et al., 2021).

Organ-specific toxicity

C. longa and *B. serrata* are two of the most widely used botanical anti-inflammatories and analgesics, with remarkably unique top organ-specific toxicities that should be thoroughly investigated. The most widely studied turmeric polyphenol, viz., curcumin, tends to have a good tolerability profile. However, very bioavailable formulations and involving piperine as a co-administrator or nanoparticle delivery have also shown at least transient hepatocellular lesions. Information obtained by the U.S. Drug-Induced Liver Injury Network also shows that the time between the onset of the drug and expression of symptoms (fatigue, anorexia, dark urine, jaundice) is 1-4 months, and very often the serum alanine aminotransferase (ALT) levels are more than 1,000 U/L, and bilirubin is 2-10 mg/dL. Complications of liver failure follow in about 10% of cases of jaundice, and fatality is possibly 5%. Toxicity is idiosyncratic and closely related to HLA-B 35:01 (>70% of individuals with the condition versus 10-15% of the population), resolving self-limiting within a period of 1-3 months after termination of treatment in the majority of subjects. It is typically displayed histologically as hepatocellular necrosis, eosinophilic infiltration, classical autoimmune hepatitis, but a small amount of fibrosis. In comparison, the gum resin of *B. serrata,* rich in pentacyclic triterpenic boswellic acids. This has not been reported to have any clinically evident hepatotoxicity in humans, despite extensive use, and serum enzyme increases are uncommon even in prolonged usage (Eltahir et al., 2024). Preclinical studies indicate that high-dose oral administration (up to 1,000 mg/kg/day) during 90 90-day study in rodents shows no perceptible effects on the enzymes in the liver, serum bilirubin, or pathological lesions and hence propagates a no observed adverse effect level (NOAEL) of 1,000 mg/kg/day at 90 days after taking orally.

Renal safety has also been established in a carbon tetrachloride (CCl4)-induced nephrotoxicity model wherein *B. serrata* extract was administered at 150 mg/kg/day for 2 weeks beginning post-injury achieved serum creatinine (0.67 +/- 0.06 mg/dl) and urea (53.50 +/- 3.14 mg/dl) measurements that were equal to those obtained in control animals (0.66 +/- 0.05 mg The activity of antioxidant enzymes (catalase, total antioxidant rate) was normalized and histopathological changes of fibrosis were improved (Eltahir et al., 2024). Such results highlight liver and kidney safety in non-rodents.

CONCLUSION & RECOMMENDATIONS

The convergence of ethnopharmacological investigation with rigorous toxicological assessment represents a paradigmatic approach to establishing the therapeutic credibility and safety profiles of traditional anti-inflammatory and analgesic herbs. This ethnobotanical knowledge is refined through generations of practical application and continues to provide invaluable leads for identifying therapeutically active plant species worthy of scientific validation. Contemporary research has demonstrated that numerous medicinally used herbs exhibit substantial anti-inflammatory and analgesic properties mediated through bioactive phytochemicals that modulate inflammatory pathways at both molecular and cellular levels. Nonetheless, the transition from folk medicine to evidence-based therapeutics necessitates a comprehensive toxicological evaluation to ensure patient safety and regulatory compliance. Acute toxicity assessments following standardized protocols have revealed that most commonly used anti-inflammatory and analgesic herbs display favorable safety profiles with LD_{50} values exceeding therapeutic dose ranges. However, emerging evidence identifies specific toxicological concerns that demand careful attention. Nephrotoxicity represents a significant adverse effect, particularly with botanicals containing aristolochic acids, anthraquinones, and certain saponins that precipitate dose-dependent renal damage through mechanisms of tubular injury and interstitial inflammation. Hepatotoxicity manifests through hepatobiliary dysfunction and elevated transaminases with prolonged exposure to specific plant constituents. Subacute and chronic toxicity evaluations further reveal organ-specific accumulation effects and potential alterations in hematological parameters that warrant extended safety assessment protocols.

A critical challenge impeding clinical integration of ethnopharmacologically validated herbs involves inadequate standardization and quality control at the mode of preparation. In addition to that, environmental variability was observed to influence the phytochemical composition and quality. The implementation of comprehensive quality assurance strategies, such as high-performance liquid chromatography (HPLC), gas chromatography-mass spectrometry (GC-MS), and DNA barcoding techniques, is crucial for ensuring product authenticity and chemical consistency. Establishment of standardized extraction protocols, quantification of marker compounds, and rigorous contamination testing for heavy metals, aflatoxins, and mycotoxins represents prerequisites for pharmaceutical-grade herbal formulations. These quality control measures should align with international guidelines viz., Good Manufacturing Practices (GMP), Good Agricultural Practices (GAP), and World Health Organization recommendations to facilitate global recognition and regulatory approval. Implementation of rigorous pharmacovigilance systems and post-market surveillance strategies may constitute an essential framework for monitoring adverse events and establishing long-term safety profiles in clinical contexts. Documentation of adverse effects, pharmacokinetic interactions, and organ toxicity across diverse populations and dosage parameters will strengthen the understanding of risk-benefit ratios. The specific molecular processes underlying the anti-inflammatory and analgesic properties of herbs can be elucidated through the application of network pharmacology techniques in conjunction with systems biology tools. By effectively combining traditional methods with thorough scientific research and structured toxicological evaluations, anti-inflammatory and analgesic herbs can evolve from being complementary therapies to evidence-based pharmaceutical solutions that meet the unfulfilled requirements in pain management and the treatment of inflammatory diseases.

REFERENCES

Abat, J. K., Kumar, S., & Mohanty, A. (2017). Ethnomedicinal, phytochemical and ethnopharmacological aspects of four medicinal plants of Malvaceae used in Indian traditional medicines. *Revista de Medicina (São Paulo)*, *4*(4), 75. PMID: 29057840

Ahmadiani, A., Javan, M., Semnanian, S., Barat, E., & Kamalinejad, M. (2001). Anti-inflammatory and antipyretic effects of *Trigonella foenum-graecum* leaves extract in the rat. *Journal of Ethnopharmacology*, *75*(2-3), 283–286. DOI: 10.1016/S0378-8741(01)00187-8 PMID: 11297864

Alavi, M., Farkhondeh, T., Aschner, M., & Samarghandian, S. (2021). Resveratrol mediates its anti-cancer effects by Nrf2 signalling pathway activation. *Cancer Cell International*, *21*(1), 579. DOI: 10.1186/s12935-021-02280-5 PMID: 34717625

Alluri, V. K., Dodda, S., Kilari, E. K., Golakoti, T., & Sengupta, K. (2019). Toxicological assessment of a standardized Boswellia serrata gum resin extract. *International Journal of Toxicology*, *38*(5), 423–435. DOI: 10.1177/1091581819858069 PMID: 31234670

Aremu, A. O., & Pendota, S. C. (2021). Medicinal plants for mitigating pain and inflammatory-related conditions: An appraisal of ethnobotanical uses and patterns in South Africa. *Frontiers in Pharmacology*, *12*, 758583. DOI: 10.3389/fphar.2021.758583 PMID: 34744737

Arul, V., Miyazaki, S., & Dhananjayan, R. (2005). Studies on the anti-inflammatory, antipyretic and analgesic properties of the leaves of *Aegle marmelos* Corr. *Journal of Ethnopharmacology*, *96*(1-2), 159–163. DOI: 10.1016/j.jep.2004.09.013 PMID: 15588665

Basak, S., Sarma, G. C., & Rangan, L. (2010). Ethnomedical uses of *Zingiberaceous* plants of Northeast India. *Journal of Ethnopharmacology*, *132*(1), 286–296. DOI: 10.1016/j.jep.2010.08.032 PMID: 20727402

Beg, S., Swain, S., Hasan, H., Barkat, M. A., & Hussain, M. S. (2011). Systematic review of herbals as potential anti-inflammatory agents: Recent advances, current clinical status and future perspectives. *Pharmacognosy Reviews*, *5*(10), 120. DOI: 10.4103/0973-7847.91102 PMID: 22279370

Buhrmann, C., Mobasheri, A., Busch, F., Aldinger, C., Stahlmann, R., Montaseri, A., & Shakibaei, M. (2011). Curcumin modulates nuclear factor κB (nf-κB)-mediated inflammation in human tenocytes in vitro: Role of the phosphatidylinositol 3-kinase/Akt pathway. *The Journal of Biological Chemistry*, *286*(32), 28556–28566. DOI: 10.1074/jbc.M111.256180 PMID: 21669872

Burford, N., Shipilov, A. V., & Furr, N. R. (2022). How ecosystem structure affects firm performance in response to a negative shock to interdependencies. *Strategic Management Journal*, *43*(1), 30–57. DOI: 10.1002/smj.3318

Choudhury, P. R., Choudhury, M. D., Ningthoujam, S. S., Das, D., Nath, D., & Talukdar, A. D. (2015). Ethnomedicinal plants used by traditional healers of North Tripura district, Tripura, North East India. *Journal of Ethnopharmacology*, *166*, 135–148. DOI: 10.1016/j.jep.2015.03.026 PMID: 25794807

Chourasiya, P., Gour, R., & Patel, A. K. (2024). Qualitative Phytochemical Investigation and Acute Oral Toxicity Study on Ethanolic Extract of Curcuma longa Leaves. *Journal of Drug Delivery and Therapeutics*, *14*(2), 73–78. DOI: 10.22270/jddt.v14i1.6244

De Cássia da Silveira e Sá, R., Andrade, L., & De Sousa, D.de Cássia da Silveira e Sá. (2013). A review on anti-inflammatory activity of monoterpenes. *Molecules (Basel, Switzerland)*, *18*(1), 1227–1254. DOI: 10.3390/molecules18011227 PMID: 23334570

Debelle, F. D., Vanherweghem, J. L., & Nortier, J. L. (2008). Aristolochic acid nephropathy: A worldwide problem. *Kidney International*, *74*(2), 158–169. DOI: 10.1038/ki.2008.129 PMID: 18418355

Dodda, S., Madireddy, R. K., Alluri, V. K., Golakoti, T., & Sengupta, K. (2022). Safety assessment of a novel water-soluble extract of *Boswellia serrata* gum resin: Acute toxicity, 90-day sub-chronic toxicity, Ames' bacterial reverse mutation, and in vivo micronucleus assays. *Toxicology Mechanisms and Methods*, *32*(5), 362–372. DOI: 10.1080/15376516.2021.2012545 PMID: 34886755

Dogara, A. M., Bradosty, S. W., Al-Zahrani, A. A., Hamad, S. W., & Almalki, H. D. (2025). Ethnobotany, bioactive compounds and pharmacology of *Syzygium guineense* (Willd.) DC: A review. *Journal of Ethnopharmacology*, *339*, 119149. DOI: 10.1016/j.jep.2024.119149 PMID: 39603399

Elisha, I. L., Dzoyem, J. P., McGaw, L. J., Botha, F. S., & Eloff, J. N. (2016). The anti-arthritic, anti-inflammatory, antioxidant activity and relationships with total phenolics and total flavonoids of nine South African plants used traditionally to treat arthritis. *BMC Complementary and Alternative Medicine*, *16*(1), 307. DOI: 10.1186/s12906-016-1301-z PMID: 27554099

Eltahir, H. M., Shalkami, A. G. S., Shehata, A. M., Almikhlafi, M., Aldhafiri, A. J., Alalawi, A., & Abouzied, M. M. (2024). *Boswellia serrata* Gum Resin Mitigates Renal Toxicity: Role of TNF-α, Interleukins, TGF-β, and Lipid Peroxidation. *Life (Chicago, Ill.)*, *14*(12), 1669. PMID: 39768376

Gomes, A., Fernandes, E., Lima, J. L., Mira, L., & Corvo, M. L. (2008). Molecular mechanisms of anti-inflammatory activity mediated by flavonoids. *Current Medicinal Chemistry*, *15*(16), 1586–1605. DOI: 10.2174/092986708784911579 PMID: 18673226

Hong, L., Guo, Z., Huang, K., Wei, S., Liu, B., Meng, S., & Long, C. (2015). Ethnobotanical study on medicinal plants used by Maonan people in China. *Journal of Ethnobiology and Ethnomedicine*, *11*(1), 1–35. DOI: 10.1186/s13002-015-0019-1 PMID: 25925830

Jha, P. K., Pandey, B., Yadav, R. K., Sindhu, K. C., Poudel, S., & Panta, S. (2025). Anti-inflammatory, analgesic, antioxidant, and alpha-amylase inhibitory effects of the hydroethanolic leaf extract of *Aleuritopteris bicolor* (Roxb.) Fraser-Jenk. *PLoS One*, *20*(6), e0326808. DOI: 10.1371/journal.pone.0326808 PMID: 40549787

John, O. C., Kalu, A. N., Christopher, O. O., & Amarachi, O. C. (2024). Phytochemical composition and toxicological profiling of *Curcuma longa* (turmeric) root extract in rats. *International Journal of Biochemistry Research & Review*, *33*(1), 1–12. DOI: 10.9734/ijbcrr/2024/v33i1847

Kalita, C. K., Das, P., Mech, B., Das, S., & Mili, C. (2025). A study on ethnomedicinal plants used by Karbi tribes in West Karbi Anglong district of Assam, India. *Vegetos*, •••, 1–15. DOI: 10.1007/s42535-025-01311-0

Kalita, C. K., Mili, C., Deka, M. J., Das, P., & Das, S. N. (2024). Study on ethnoveterinary medicinal plants used by local people inhabiting char area, Kamrup District, Assam, North-East India. *Ecological Questions*, *35*(4), 1–18. DOI: 10.12775/EQ.2024.048

Lefrioui, Y., Chebaibi, M., Bichara, M. D., Mssillou, I., Bekkari, H., Giesy, J. P., & Bousta, D. (2024). Ethnobotanical survey of medicinal plants used in north-central Morocco as natural analgesic and anti-inflammatory agents. *Scientific African*, *25*, e02275. DOI: 10.1016/j.sciaf.2024.e02275

Li, R. W., Myers, S. P., Leach, D. N., Lin, G. D., & Leach, G. (2003). A cross-cultural study: Anti-inflammatory activity of Australian and Chinese plants. *Journal of Ethnopharmacology*, *85*(1), 25–32. DOI: 10.1016/S0378-8741(02)00336-7 PMID: 12576199

Liju, V. B., Jeena, K., & Kuttan, R. (2013). Acute and subchronic toxicity as well as mutagenic evaluation of essential oil from turmeric (*Curcuma longa* L). *Food and Chemical Toxicology*, *53*, 52–61. DOI: 10.1016/j.fct.2012.11.027 PMID: 23201370

Linghu, K. G., Wu, G. P., Fu, L. Y., Yang, H., Li, H. Z., Chen, Y., Yu, H., Tao, L., & Shen, X. C. (2019). 1, 8-Cineole ameliorates LPS-induced vascular endothelium dysfunction in mice via PPAR-γ dependent regulation of NF-κB. *Frontiers in Pharmacology*, *10*, 178. DOI: 10.3389/fphar.2019.00178 PMID: 30930772

Mashhadi, N. S., Ghiasvand, R., Askari, G., Hariri, M., Darvishi, L., & Mofid, M. R. (2013). Anti-oxidative and anti-inflammatory effects of ginger in health and physical activity: Review of current evidence. *International Journal of Preventive Medicine*, *4*(Suppl 1), S36. PMID: 23717767

Murugan, S., Solanki, H., Purusothaman, D., Bethapudi, B., Ravalji, M., & Mundkinajeddu, D. (2021). Safety evaluation of standardized extract of *Curcuma longa* (NR-INF-02): A 90-day subchronic oral toxicity study in rats. *BioMed Research International*, *2021*(1), 6671853. DOI: 10.1155/2021/6671853 PMID: 34337042

Musa, Y. M., Haruna, A. K., Ilyas, M., Yaro, A. H., Ahmadu, A. A., & Usman, H. (2008). Phytochemical, analgesic, and anti-inflammatory effects of the ethylacetate extract of the leaves of *Pseudocedrella kotschyii*. *African Journal of Traditional, Complementary, and Alternative Medicines : AJTCAM*, *5*(1), 92–96. DOI: 10.4314/ajtcam.v5i1.31261 PMID: 20162060

Namsa, N. D., Tag, H., Mandal, M., Kalita, P., & Das, A. K. (2009). An ethnobotanical study of traditional anti-inflammatory plants used by the Lohit community of Arunachal Pradesh, India. *Journal of Ethnopharmacology*, *125*(2), 234–245. DOI: 10.1016/j.jep.2009.07.004 PMID: 19607898

Napagoda, M. T., Sundarapperuma, T., Fonseka, D., Amarasiri, S., & Gunaratna, P. (2018). An ethnobotanical study of the medicinal plants used as anti-inflammatory remedies in Gampaha District, Western Province, Sri Lanka. *Scientifica*, *2018*(1), 9395052. DOI: 10.1155/2018/9395052 PMID: 29974006

Nisar, A., Jagtap, S., Vyavahare, S., Deshpande, M., Harsulkar, A., Ranjekar, P., & Prakash, O. (2023). Phytochemicals in the treatment of inflammation-associated diseases: The journey from preclinical trials to clinical practice. *Frontiers in Pharmacology*, *14*, 1177050. DOI: 10.3389/fphar.2023.1177050 PMID: 37229273

) Patel, S. S., & Savjani, J. K. (2015). Systematic review of plant steroids as potential anti-inflammatory agents: Current status and future perspectives.

Pikulthong, V., Bhirompan, S., Dechkla, M., Mokkapan, K., Boonman, N., Wanna, C., MacHana, K., & Phakpaknam, S. (2022). Local herbs for pain relief in the area of Tumbon Khao Hin Son, Chachoengsao, Thailand. *Biodiversitas (Surakarta)*, *23*(10). Advance online publication. DOI: 10.13057/biodiv/d231007

Pinho-Ribeiro, F. A., Zarpelon, A. C., Fattori, V., Manchope, M. F., Mizokami, S. S., Casagrande, R., & Verri, W. A.Jr. (2016). Naringenin reduces inflammatory pain in mice. *Neuropharmacology, 105*, 508–519. DOI: 10.1016/j.neuropharm.2016.02.019 PMID: 26907804

Polat, R., Cakilcioglu, U., Kaltalioğlu, K., Ulusan, M. D., & Türkmen, Z. (2015). An ethnobotanical study on medicinal plants in Espiye and its surrounding (Giresun-Turkey). *Journal of Ethnopharmacology, 163*, 1–11. DOI: 10.1016/j.jep.2015.01.008 PMID: 25614105

Prajapati, A. K. (2024). Profiling the toxicological landscape of herbal drugs. *Journal of Preventive Medicine and Holistic Health, 10*(1), 6–9. DOI: 10.18231/j.jpmhh.2024.003

Rehman, M. H. U., Saleem, U., Ahmad, B., & Rashid, M. (2022). Phytochemical and toxicological evaluation of *Zephyranthes citrina. Frontiers in Pharmacology, 13*, 1007310. DOI: 10.3389/fphar.2022.1007310 PMID: 36210854

Shin, M. R., Kim, H. Y., Choi, H. Y., Park, K. S., Choi, H. J., & Roh, S. S. (2022). *Boswellia serrata* Extract, 5-Loxin®, Prevents Joint Pain and Cartilage Degeneration in a Rat Model of Osteoarthritis Through Inhibition of Inflammatory Responses and Restoration of Matrix Homeostasis. *Evidence-Based Complementary and Alternative Medicine : eCAM, 2022*(1), 3067526. DOI: 10.1155/2022/3067526 PMID: 36310623

Singh, P., Chacko, K. M., Aggarwal, M. L., Bhat, B., Khandal, R. K., Sultana, S., & Kuruvilla, B. T. (2012). A-90 days gavage safety assessment of *Boswellia serrata* in rats. *Toxicology International, 19*(3), 273. DOI: 10.4103/0971-6580.103668 PMID: 23293466

Siriwatanametanon, N., Fiebich, B. L , Efferth, T., Prieto, J. M., & Heinrich, M. (2010). Traditionally used Thai medicinal plants: In vitro anti-inflammatory, anticancer and antioxidant activities. *Journal of Ethnopharmacology, 130*(2), 196–207. DOI: 10.1016/j.jep.2010.04.036 PMID: 20435130

Tadesse, D., Lulekal, E., & Masresha, G. (2025). Ethnopharmacological study of traditional medicinal plants used by the people in Metema district, northwestern Ethiopia. *Frontiers in Pharmacology, 16*, 1535822. DOI: 10.3389/fphar.2025.1535822 PMID: 40129938

Teklay, A., Abera, B., & Giday, M. (2013). An ethnobotanical study of medicinal plants used in Kilte Awulaelo District, Tigray Region of Ethiopia. *Journal of Ethnobiology and Ethnomedicine, 9*(1), 1–23. DOI: 10.1186/1746-4269-9-65 PMID: 24011232

Teschke, I., Cartmill, E. A., Stankewitz, S., & Tebbich, S. (2011). Sometimes tool use is not the key: No evidence for cognitive adaptive specializations in tool-using woodpecker finches. *Animal Behaviour*, *82*(5), 945–956. DOI: 10.1016/j.anbehav.2011.07.032

Tsioutsiou, E. E., Cheilari, A., & Aligiannis, N. (2023). Ethnopharmacological study of medicinal plants used against skin ailments on Mount Pelion, central Greece. *Frontiers in Pharmacology*, *14*, 1225580. DOI: 10.3389/fphar.2023.1225580 PMID: 37583900

Zhang, J., Onakpoya, I. J., Posadzki, P., & Eddouks, M. (2015). The safety of herbal medicine: From prejudice to evidence. *Evidence-Based Complementary and Alternative Medicine : eCAM*, *2015*, 316706. DOI: 10.1155/2015/316706 PMID: 25838831

Chapter 8
Polyphenol-Rich Formulations and Their Multi-Target Interactions With Molecular Pathways in Cancer Cells

Emmanuel Henry Ezenabor
http://orcid.org/0009-0009-0231-7734
Bowen University, Nigeria

Aminat Abisola Afolabi
http://orcid.org/0009-0003-1011-2110
Bowen University, Nigeria

Oluwafemi Adeleke Ojo
http://orcid.org/0000-0001-9331-396X
University of Turku, Finland

Oluyomi Stephen Adeyemi
http://orcid.org/0000-0001-9342-8505
Bowen University, Nigeria

ABSTRACT

Cancer remains the second leading cause of death globally, with classical therapies limited by selectivity, toxicity, and resistance. This review examines polyphenol-rich preparations and their multi-target interactions in cancer cells. Polyphenols (flavonoids, phenolic acids, stilbenes, lignans) simultaneously modulate multiple targets, addressing key cancer hallmarks: sustained proliferative signaling, apoptosis

DOI: 10.4018/979-8-3373-5876-5.ch008

evasion, replicative immortality, and angiogenesis. Key pathways include PI3K/Akt/mTOR, MAPK, RAS, and p53. Notable compounds like curcumin, resveratrol, quercetin, and EGCG induce apoptosis, inhibit angiogenesis, arrest cell cycle, and modulate epigenetics. Despite encouraging preclinical evidence, clinical translation faces challenges from low bioavailability, rapid metabolism, and conflicting data. Strategies include stable derivatives, nano-encapsulation, personalized medicine, and combination with established drugs. Polyphenolic compounds emerge as promising multi-target anticancer agents with low toxicity. Further research on bioavailability and trials is needed.

1. INTRODUCTION

Cancer continues to pose a significant global health burden, ranking as the second leading cause of death worldwide and accounting for nearly one in six deaths annually (World Health Organization, 2025). It encompasses a wide range of diseases characterized by abnormal and uncontrolled cell division, the ability to invade surrounding tissues, and, in many cases, metastasize to distant organs. The pathophysiology of cancer is complex and involves genetic mutations, epigenetic alterations, and dysregulation of multiple cellular signaling pathways (Chillón-Pino et al., 2024). Over time, cancer cells acquire several biological capabilities collectively referred to as the hallmarks of cancer which include sustained proliferative signaling, evasion of growth suppressors, resistance to cell death, replicative immortality, induction of angiogenesis, and activation of invasion and metastasis (Hanahan & Weinberg, 2011).

Traditional cancer treatments such as surgery, chemotherapy, and radiotherapy, while effective in many cases, suffer from significant drawbacks. Chemotherapeutic agents, for instance, are often non-selective, attacking both cancerous and healthy cells, leading to toxic side effects and reduced quality of life. Moreover, tumors can develop resistance to these therapies through various mechanisms such as efflux pumps, DNA repair activation, or pathway redundancy (Farhan, 2023; Emran et al., 2022). The limited specificity and adaptability of these therapies have underscored the need for novel, multi-targeted, and less toxic therapeutic alternatives. In this context, natural products, especially polyphenols, have gained substantial attention for their potential role in cancer prevention and treatment. Polyphenols are a diverse class of bioactive compounds naturally found in plants, and are abundant in fruits (such as berries, grapes, and apples), vegetables, teas, coffee, red wine, cocoa, herbs, and spices (Cháirez-Ramírez et al., 2021). Structurally, they are characterized by the presence of multiple phenol units and can be broadly categorized into flavonoids, phenolic acids, stilbenes, and lignans. These compounds are part of the plant's defense mechanisms against pathogens and environmental stressors, but in humans, they exhibit a range of pharmacological properties. Among the most intriguing features of polyphenolic compounds is their ability to modulate multiple molecular targets simultaneously. Unlike conventional drugs that are designed to act on a single receptor or enzyme, polyphenols exert pleiotropic effects, influencing a wide array of cellular processes including oxidative stress response, inflammation, apoptosis, angiogenesis, immune modulation, and signal transduction pathways (Issinger & Guerra, 2021; Singaravelan & Tollefsbol, 2025; Jantan et al., 2021). This multi-targeted mechanism is especially advantageous in cancer therapy, where tumor progression is driven by multiple deregulated pathways that often compensate for one another when one is inhibited.

Moreover, polyphenols could act on not only tumoral cells but the tumor microenvironment, including stromal cells, immune cells, and the extracellular matrix, which make them have wider therapeutic potentials. They have much less toxicity compared with chemotherapeutics and are suitable for long-term treatment and in combination with other antitumor drugs, which may enhance efficacy and minimize side effects (Zhang et al., 2022). However, these exciting features notwithstanding, it is not without some challenges in clinical development. But their clinical application is hindered by their low bioavailability, rapid degradation and poor stability. Several formulation strategies, including nano-encapsulation, liposomal delivery systems and adjuvants, are being studied to improve their pharmacokinetic profiles and biological potential in order to overcome these challenges (Liu et al., 2024; Lu et al., 2025). The objective of the present review is to sum up how polyphenolic-rich preparations regulate different molecular pathways in cancer cells. This review will also emphasize their anticancer mechanisms, multi-target property and recent progress in formulations technologies for overcoming pharmacokinetic challenges. By fusing *in vitro*, *in vivo* and clinical data, this review will present polyphenols as a driver to the new wave of integrative oncology approaches.

2. OVERVIEW OF POLYPHENOLIC COMPOUNDS

Polyphenols are also a large group of plant secondary metabolites characterized by having one or more hydroxyl groups directly attached to aromatic hydrocarbon rings and are ubiquitous in the plant kingdom (Swallah et al., 2020). These molecules are widespread in fruits, vegetables, herbs, spices, seeds, and beverages (Tea, wine), and they have a major function in defending plants against ultraviolet radiation, pathogens and herbivores (Kim et al., 2023). Among the polyphenolics, polyphenols have been receiving much attention from scientists in recent years owing to their strong anti-oxidant activity, anti-inflammatory properties, and most importantly, their potential anticancer effects. It has been suggested that the polyphenols are capable to modulate various molecular targets relevant to hallmarks of cancer, and they might become potential cancer preventive and complementary agents (Pandey et al., 2025, Ko et al., 2017). Nevertheless, there is still quite a lot needs to be done in order to fully understand and utilize the therapeutic application of those microenvironments; including their classification, natural origin, and the particular obstacles related to their delivery and absorption in human body (Hao et al., 2024).

2.1. Classification of Polyphenols

Chemically, polyphenolic compounds can be divided into subgroups according to the number of phenolic rings and to the structural elements that connect these rings. The most popular classification that is becoming generally accepted contains four main categories: flavonoids, phenolic acids, stilbenes, and lignans. Each class is comprised of a number of compounds with unique molecular structures, dietary sources, and biological activities (Swallah et al., 2020; Pandey & Rizvi, 2009).

Figure 1. Classification of Polyphenol (Ciupei et al., 2024)

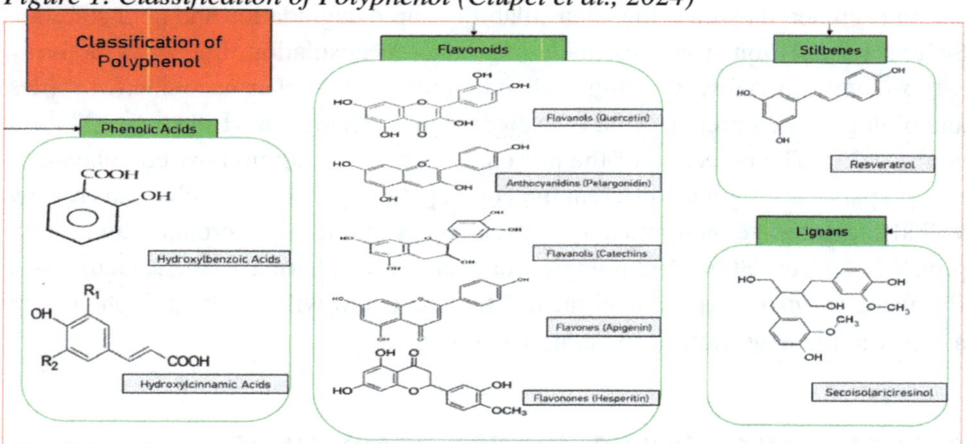

2.1.1. Flavonoids

Flavonoids are the largest and most thoroughly studied group of polyphenols, which represent about 60 per cent of all polyphenols in the diet. Structurally, flavonoids are built on a 15-carbon skeleton and based on a C6-C3-C6 carbon framework containing two benzene rings and a heterocyclic ring (three carbon atoms) as a bridge. Flavonoids are divided into six primary classes, including flavonols, flavones, flavanones, flavanols (also called catechins), anthocyanins, and isoflavones. They are found most frequently in foods like onions, kale, apples, broccoli and tea. Studies have shown that these compounds may have antiproliferative activity on cancer cells by controlling pathways (MAPK, PI3K/Akt), by preventing the cell cycle progression and by promoting apoptosis. Parsley, celery and chamomile contain high levels of flavones such as apigenin and luteolin. These molecules are known to possess anti-inflammatory and antiangiogenic activities, at least in part, because of the inhibition of NF-κB and through the downregulation of proinflammatory enzymes, including cyclo-oxygenase-2 (COX-2). Flavanones, among them naringenin and hesperidin, are mainly found in citrus fruits (e.g., oranges, lemons, and grapefruits). They have been known to boost detoxification pathways, scavenge free radicals and modulate immune reaction. These flavanols, also known as catechins, including epicatechin, epigallocatechin and epigallocatechin gallate (EGCG), are highly abundant in green tea and cocoa. Of particular interest, EGCG has strong biological activities such as anti-angiogenesis, anti-tumor invasion, anti-DNA methylation. Anthocyanins responsible for the red, purple and blue colors of berries, grapes, and red cabbage are potent antioxidants that prevent DNA oxidative damage, cancer cell replication and inflammation (Shankar et al., 2008; Proença et al., 2023).Isoflavones including genistein and daidzein are mainly present in soy products. These compounds have the structure similar to human estrogens so that they can bind to estrogen receptors; these compounds also are crucial factors to prevent hormone-dependent cancers such as breast and prostate cancer (Lin et al., 2017).

2.1.2. Phenolic Acids

They are made up of a simpler structure known as a single aromatic ring and can typically be categorized into two groups: hydroxybenzoic acids and hydroxy-cinnamic acids. Less complex compared to flavonoids, phenolic acids are important due to their antioxidant, antimicrobial, and anticancer activities. Hydroxybenzoic acids such as gallic acid and pouchetin mediate in tea, berries and red wine. These molecules have the potential to decrease oxidative stress, attenuate inflammation pathways and block cancer cell growth by apoptosis. Hydroxycinnamic acids such as caffeic, ferulic and p-coumaric acids are widely present in coffee, whole grains and a variety of fruits and vegetables. For example, Ferulic acid has been reported to prevent free radical damage, lipid peroxidation and angiogenesis in tumor models (Bastidas et al., 2022).

2.1.3. Stilbenes

Stilbenes present a smaller subset but are very bioactive polyphenols that contain two aromatic rings joined by an ethylene bridge. The most researched stilbene is resveratrol, which comes from grapes, red wine, peanuts and a few berries. These pathways include signaling via AMPK, Wnt/β-catenin and NF-κB, and resveratrol affects several of these pathways (Singh et al., 2011) (a phenomenon that is commonly referred to as pleiotropic activity).

2.1.4. Lignans

Lignans comprise diphenolic structures that are derived from dimerization of two phenylpropanoid moieties. They are especially rich in flaxseeds, sesame seeds, whole grains, legumes and certain vegetables. Typical lignans include secoisolariciresinol, matairesinol and pinoresinol. They are converted by intestinal bacteria to enterolactone and enterodiol, which have weak estrogenic activity and may lower the risk of hormone-related cancers. Lignans also have antioxidant properties and have been found to have potential anti-angiogenic and apoptosis inducing effects against cancer cells (Azrad et al., 2013).

3. HALLMARKS OF CANCER – MOLECULAR PATHWAYS

It is important to understand the basic molecular characteristics of cancer development and progression to appreciate how polyphenolic-rich preparations interact with cancer cells. Cancer is not single disease, but a complex disorder catapulting through a series of genetic, epigenetic, biochemical alterations allowing cells to surpass normal growth controls. Such modifications provide tumour cells with diverse biological features contributing to evolution to a malignant status. Hanahan and Weinberg proposed in 2000 a conceptual model called the “Hallmarks of Cancer” that describes the fundamental characteristics that cancer cells must acquire to adapt, survive, proliferate, and spread (Hanahan & Weinberg, 2000). These hallmarks were later updated in 2011 and remain the guiding framework of experimental cancer research and the discovery, and development of new cancer therapies (Hanahan & Weinberg, 2011). Each signature is based on specific molecular signaling circuits that govern cell behavior. Deregulation of these pathways permits cancer cells to escape normal cellular control (Hanahan, 2022). Interesting, polyphenolic compounds, a group of naturally phytochemicals available in fruits, vegetables, teas, and traditional medicinal plants have shown the potential to modulate many of these key pathways and sometimes multiple pathways at a same time (Ahmed et al., 2025; Talib et al., 2024). This multicomponent mechanism is at the very core of their potential as anticancer drugs. Below we present a specific review for each hallmark and the corresponding manner by which polyphenols may modulate the participative pathways.

3.1. Sustained Proliferative Signaling

One of the most elementary characteristics of a tumor is the capacity of tumor cells to maintain continuous proliferation. Growth is normally kept under severe control by extracellular signals, i.e. growth-factors. However, cancer cells acquire the ability to produce their own signals to grow, or become over-sensitive to natural ones. This is typically induced by the over-activation of growth promoting pathways, such as the epidermal growth factor receptor (EGFR) and the mitogen-activated protein kinase (MAPK) pathway. Polyphenols such as curcumin (from turmeric) and resveratrol (from grapes/red wine) have demonstrated the ability to prevent EGFR signaling and dampen the MAPK pathway, hence several fold minimizing the proliferative ability tumour cells (Rajeeve et al., 2025).

3.2. Evading Growth Suppressors

Under normal circumstances, tumor suppressor proteins, like p53 and Rb, act to inhibit cellular proliferation when cells are exposed to stress or DNA damage by causing cell cycle arrest or initiating apoptosis. In most forms of cancer, these tumor suppressors have been lost either by mutation or via interaction with viral oncoproteins. Certain tumor suppressors can be inactivated or mimicked with some polyphenols. For instance, it has been found that Quercetin can increase the induction of the tumour suppressor p53, which can result in cell cycle blockade in cancer cells. This re-establishes a fraction of the intrinsic fail-safe machinery restraining unrestricted cell replication (Nguyen et al., 2017; Rauf et al., 2018).

3.3. Resisting Cell Death (Apoptosis)

Apoptosis, or programmed cell death, is part of the body's way of getting rid of damaged or unnecessary cells. However, cancer cells become resistant to apoptosis via overexpression of anti-apoptotic proteins (for example, Bcl-2) and/or suppression of pro-apoptotic ones (for example, Bax). This leads to some condition under which they would normally die. Polyphenols like green tea-epigallocatechin gallate (EGCG) and parsley-apigenin are known to regulate these apoptotic modulators. These agents can downregulate Bcl-2, upregulate Bax, and stimulate the activation of caspases, enzymes that play a central role in the implementation of apoptosis.

And these two modulations render the apoptotic apparatus of cancerous cells active again (Mohammad et al., 2015).

3.4. Enabling Replicative Immortality

Somatic cells generally have a limited lifespan owing to the gradual shortening of telomeres (protective chromosome ends) during replication of cells. Cancer cells, on the other hand, frequently turn on telomerase, an enzyme that prevents telomeres from shortening, allowing an unlimited number of replications. This allows for limitless growth of the tumor. Certain polyphenolic compounds such as genistein, a soy isoflavone, have been demonstrated to suppress telomerase activity in cancer cells. Because they repress telomerase expression, polyphenols may also help to curb uncontrolled replication that is one of the hallmarks of cancer cells (Khaw et al., 2012).

3.5. Inducing Angiogenesis

For tumors to grow beyond a certain size and metastasize, they have to make a new blood supply, what is called angiogenesis. This is generally mediated by an upregulation of pro-angiogenic factors including VEGF. Dysregulated angiogenesis facilitates oxygen and nutrient delivery to the tumor and an avenue for the metastatic dissemination. Polyphenols (e.g., luteolin, kaempferol, and curcumin) have been found to exert anti-angiogenesis effects by lowering VEGF level and interfering with new capillary structure formation. By inhibiting angiogenesis, those polyphenols in fact deprived tumors of their "lifeblood" (Almatroudi et al., 2023; Cai et al., 2022).

4.0 KEY SIGNALING PATHWAYS MODULATED BY POLYPHENOLS

Polyphenols, a heterogeneous group of naturally found compounds present in fruits, vegetables, tea, and other plant-based foods, have received increasing attention due to their anticancer effect (Zughaibi et al., 2021). A key feature underlying their efficacy is their capacity to engage and modulate several molecular signaling pathways controlling cancer cell behaviour (Rahman et al., 2021). It is this multi-target action potential that may permit polyphenols to interfere in cancer evolution at different levels, namely proliferation, survial, metastasis and therapy resistance. Some of the major signaling pathways that are affected by polyphenols include the PI3K/Akt/mTOR pathway, MAPK signaling cascades, RAS pathway, and the tumor suppressor p53 network. All these paths are involved in the physiology of cancer cells and can be interesting targets for the therapy (Issinger et al., 2021; Chimento et al., 2023).

4.1. PI3K/Akt/mTOR Pathway

The phosphatidylinositol 3-kinase (PI3K)/Akt/mammalian target of rapamycin (mTOR) pathway is a key intracellular signaling pathway involved in cell growth, metabolism, proliferation, survival, and angiogenesis (Silva-Pinto et al., 2025). Aberrant activation of this pathway has been implicated in a wide variety of malignancies including breast, lung, colorectal and glioblastoma among others. This pathway is usually activated when growth factors bind receptor tyrosine kinases (RTKs), leading to PI3K activation. PI3K phosphorylates phosphatidylinositol 4,5-bisphosphate (PIP_2) to generate phosphatidylinositol 3,4,5-trisphosphate (PIP_3), which binds to Akt on the plasma membrane. Akt is phosphorylated and activated at the membrane by phosphoinositide-dependent-kinase-1 (PDK1) and mTOR complex 2 (mTORC2). Phosphorylated Akt targets several downstream proteins such as mTORC1 (mTOR complex 1), which is involved in promoting protein synthesis and cell growth by phosphorylating various regulatory proteins including the p70 ribosomal S6 kinase and the 4E-binding protein 1 (4EBP1) (Kopustinskiene et al., 2020).

Polyphenols have shown a strong ability to repress several key points in the pathway. Resveratrol, a stilbenoid molecule originated from grapes and berries, down-regulates PI3K/Akt signaling pathway in glioblastoma cells by inhibiting the phosphorylation of both PI3K and Akt, resulting in down-modulation of survivals signals as well as invasion and proliferation through the pathway. Quercetin, a flavonoid, that is rich in onions and apples blocks phosphorylation of Akt in mice with lymphoma which is associated with inhibition of tumor growth and angiogenesis ((Zhang et al., 2023; Hedayati et al., 2025).

Curcumin, the main curcuminoid in turmeric, is widely studied for its ability to modulate the PI3K/Akt/mTOR signaling pathway. In models of non-small cell lung cancer, curcumin promotes the expression of miR-206, which downregulates the activity of the PI3K pathway by directly targeting the pathway proteins, resulting in the inhibition of both Akt and mTOR and leads to cell cycle arrest and apoptosis. This highlights the multi-targeted anti-proliferative properties of polyphenols (Wang et al., 2019; Papavassiliou et al., 2025). In addition, polyphenols inhibit mTOR, thereby reducing hypoxia-inducible factor-1 alpha (HIF-1α) activation that induces angiogenesis and metabolic reprogramming in cancer cells. Polyphenols repress both VEGF expression (needed for angiogenesis) and new vessel formation through HIF-1α suppression (Qian et al., 2021). At the molecular level, polyphenols may interact directly with PI3K or Akt, impair its membrane localization, or influence the function of upstream modulators, including PTEN, a tumor suppressor and negative regulator of PI3K signaling. This several pronged inhibition of the signaling pathway results in inhibition of tumor cell proliferation and survival, and could be of high potential value for combination therapies. Considering specific tumorigenic nature of PI3K/Akt/mTOR pathway, therapeutic targeting inhibitors for this axis in clinical practice have great toxicity and resistance limitation (Dong et al., 2021). Polyphenols are emerging as a potential adjunct or alternative therapeutic option due to their natural origin, multi-target mode of action, and the possibility of less side effects. Their multi-target action on different key nodes of the pathway as well as on parallel pathways makes their therapeutic potential significantly more enhanced (Izzo & Stefanska, 2025).

Figure 2. PI3K/Akt/mTOR pathway (Cháirez-Ramírez et al., 2021)

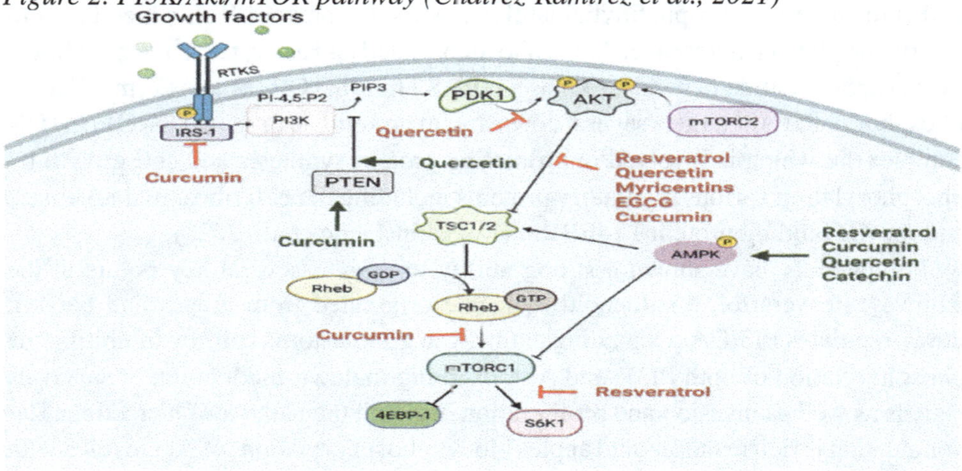

4.2. MAPK Signaling Cascades Interaction

The mitogen-activated protein kinase (MAPK) cascades are required signalling transduction pathways that transmit extracellular stimuli to target cell responses (Kubatka et al., 2025). The regulation of proliferation, differentiation, stress response and apoptosis are a few of the various responses to which these three major MAPK (ERK, JNK, and p38 MAPK) cascades are associated. Abnormal MAPK signaling is commonly present in cancer and promotes tumorigenesis (Wang et al., 2019). Polyphenols can regulate MAPK pathways according to the context, however they frequently shift the balance towards apoptosis for cancer cells. For instance, epigallocatechin-3-gallate (EGCG), the most abundant catechin in green tea, has been found to suppress ERK and JNK activation in breast cancer cells inducing cell cycle arrest and apoptosis. EGCG's modulation of these kinases disrupts proliferative signals and enhances sensitivity to chemotherapeutic agents (Oh et al., 2023).

On the other hand, polyphenols, such as curcumin, may also activate stress-sensitive MAPKs, such as p38 and JNK, which induce apoptotic pathways. Curcumin induces programmed cell death in a range of cancer cells, including pancreatic and colorectal cancers, by activating pro-apoptotic proteins, and by suppressing anti-apoptotic molecules via p38 MAPK activation. Given MAPK cascade pathways can exhibit both pro-survival and pro-apoptotic effects, polyphenols effect can vary depending on the cell line and tumor type (Keskin, 2023). Such selective modulation is partially associated with polyphenol-induced reactive oxygen species (ROS) generation that serves as a second messenger in the process of stress kinase (e.g., c-Jun N-terminal protein kinase (JNK) and p38) activation and hence apoptosis. Moreover, polyphenols may also affect events located upstream the MAPK cascades like Ras and Raf kinases with the result that MAPK signaling is further embedded in other cell signaling pathways, such as thePI3K/Akt. This cross-talk enhances the anti-cancer activity of polyphenols working together in multiple signaling systems (Wu et al., 2022; López-Gómez et al., 2024).

Figure 3. MAPK signaling cascades (Cháirez-Ramírez et al., 2021)

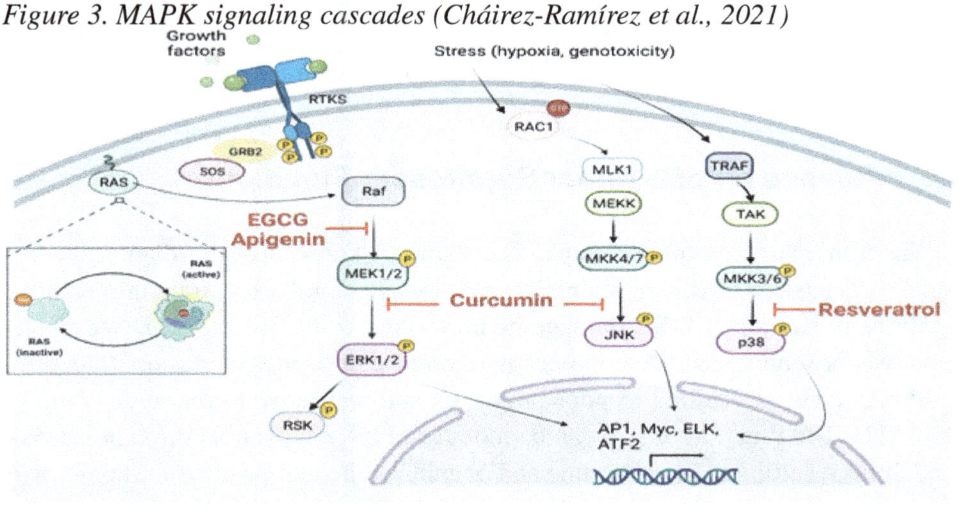

4.3. RAS Pathway Modulation

The small GTPases of the RAS family-H-Ras, K-Ras and N-Ras-are central components of oncogenic signalling. RAS point mutations are the most frequent mutations detected in human cancer, particularly in pancreatic, colorectal, and lung cancers. These mutations render RAS constitutively active, trapped in the GTP-bound state, activating downstream signaling effectors (e.g.RAF/MEK/ERK and PI3K/Akt pathways) that support uncontrolled proliferation, survival and metastatic potential. It has been previously difficult to drug mutant RAS directly because it has a high GTP/GDP binding affinity and no druggable pockets for small molecules. Yet, polyphenols provide an indirect yet novel way for the modulation of RAS signal transduction. It has been demonstrated that curcumin can inhibit the RAS/RAF/MEK/ERK pathway in colorectal cancer cells, and thus inhibit cell proliferation and promote apoptosis. It does so by preventing the phosphorylation of RAF and MEK kinases leading to the downstream ERK activation (Alam et al., 2018; De et al., 2023).

Moreover, the effects of polyphenols could be due to blocking RAS from post-translational modifications (i.e., farnesylation) required for its membrane-associated activity. Polyphenols interfere with these modifications and prevent RAS from localizing to the plasma membrane where it is needed to activate downstream signaling (Ahearn et al., 2012). Furthermore, polyphenols may influence upstream regulators and positive loops that maintain RAS stimulation. For example, they block receptor tyrosine kinases or lower levels of guanine nucleotide exchange factors (GEFs) that mediate RAS activation. This "multi-target" inhibition of RAS signaling by polyphenols is of particular interest, since targeting with conventional drugs of mutant RAS is challenging. Their potential to indirectly silence RAS-activated oncogenic signaling pathways raises their therapeutic promise to RAS-mutated cancers (Chu, 2022).

4.4. Influence on p53 Tumor Suppressor Function

The tumor suppressor protein p53 is commonly known as "guardian of the genome", because of its role in maintaining genomic stability. It coordinates cellular reactions to stress and DNA damage by promoting cell cycle arrest, DNA repair, apoptosis or senescence. Deletion or mutation of p53 is present in more than 50% of human cancers, leading to poor prognosis and resistance to therapy (Wang et al., 2023). The function of p53 can be modulated by polyphenols through various modalities resulting in repositioning and or enhancement of its tumour-suppressive attributable activities. They control p53 at the transcriptional level, enhance protein stability and facilitate post-translational processes, including phosphorylation and acetylation, both of which are necessary for its activation (Cháirez-Ramírez et al., 2021). In fact, a wide range of polyphenolic compounds (e.g.resveratrol) have been shown to increase p53 phosphorylation on serine 15, acetylation and accumulation of this protein in the nucleus, events which protectp53from proteasomal degradation (Ferraz da Costa et al., 2018). This activated form of p53 then transcribes pro-apoptotic genes including Bax, PUMA, and Noxa, and results in the development of tumor cell mitochondrial-driven apoptosis (Brady & Attardi, 2010). Several studies also indicated that quercetin could suppress the binding of p53 with MDM2 (an E3 ubiquitin ligase of p53 that leads it to proteasomal degradation). Quercetin causes stabilization of the level of p53 protein by inhibiting its degradation by MDM2, which enhances the lifetime of p53 protein in the cell (Ramli et al., 2024).

Polyphenols can determine the localization of p53, by directing it to the nucleus as a transcription factor. This is important since cytoplasmic localization of p53 is a frequent means by which cancer cells escape apoptosis. In addition, polyphenols can sensitize cancer cells to DNA-damaging agents by increasing p53-mediated checkpoint activation, which in turn can promote chemotherapy and radiotherapy effectiveness (Fetoni et al., 2022; Liu et al., 2024). In cancers with mutant p53, some polyphenols may have p53-independent anticancer properties or could also rescue mutant threats by causing a re-folding action in the mutant p53, topic that has still to be clearly investigated (de la Garza-Kalife et al., 2025; Lewis, 2015).

5. CHALLENGES AND LIMITATIONS

Although the mechanisms of anticancer actions of polyphenols have been widely explored in numerous *in vitro* and *in vivo* studies promising direct translation from bench to bed site has been accompanied with substantial difficulties. These limitation are multifaceted, extending across pharmacokinetics, molecular selectivity, interindividual variability and heterogeneity in the outcomes of the clinical trials. Overcoming these limitations is essential for the development of polyphenol-based treatments in clinical oncology practice. This part includes in-depth analysis of the key shortcomings that deprive polyphenols from clinical progress as targeted anticancer agents (Asensi et al., 2011; Rogovskii, 2022; Sharma et al., 2022).

5.1 Poor Bioavailability and Pharmacokinetics

The low oral bioavailability is arguably the most characterized and relevant obstacle for the clinical administration of polyphenols. The majority of polyphenols, like curcumin, quercetin, and resveratrol, have poor aqueous solubility, rapid first pass metabolism and fast clearance from systemic circulation resulting in low plasma and tissue levels after oral administration (Luca et al., 2020). For instance, curcumin, although exhibiting powerful anticancer activity in preclinical models, is extremely low in its absorption through the liver and intestines and fast in its metabolization. Upon oral administration, curcumin is conjugated to form glucuronide and sulfate derivatives, which are largely inactive, and potentially minimizes its therapeutic application (Cheng et al., 2025).

Resveratrol also faces similar limitations. It has rapid gastro-intestinal absorption but very low systemic bioavailability after metabolism into glucuronide and sulfate conjugates. This PK profile requires excessive dose demand to reach therapeutic levels, possibly toxic, or the need of new delivery systems and formulation strategies meant to painstakingly increase already high costs and regulatory challenges (Warias et al., 2024). Furthermore, most polyphenols have a short half-life, which means that they need to be administered over short intervals in order to reach therapeutic levels. This is not only detrimental to patient adherence, but also complicates clinical logistics. In addition, polyphenols they are sensitive to light, heat, and pH variations occurring during storage and through the passage through the gastrointestinal tract, also contributing to their stability and shelf life (Zhou et al., 2021).

5.2 Lack of Molecular Specificity

Polyphenols have a spectrum of activity against cancer by targeting various signaling pathways i.e., PI3K/AKT, NF-κB, STAT3 and MAPK. This lack of specificity at the molecular level can work both ways. This has advantages in terms of pleiotropic action which can potentially translate into efficacy across many tumor types. On the contrary, however, it can lead to an off-target effects and can interfere unintentionally with normal, non-cancerous biological processes (Colomer et al., 2017). The pro-apoptotic and anti-apoptotic pathways can be regulated by polyphenols depending on the cellular background, concentration and time of exposure. For example, low levels of quercetin have been found to function as antioxidants and cytoprotective agents in normal cells, but paradoxically may stimulate survival signals in some cancer cells in certain context. In one demonstration from resveratrol, it has shown to both promote and suppress tumors in different model systems, creating some ambiguity relative to its potential therapeutic use as an anticancer agent (Kiemlian, 2016). This non-specificity also makes it difficult to discover accurate and specific biomarkers indicative of treatment response. In contrast to targeted therapy drugs that target specific molecular alterations (e.g., EGFR inhibitors in EGFR-mutant lung cancer), polyphenols do no have a single target, therefore, it is problematic to identify which patients may benefit from therapy. This precluded the possibility of designing biomarker-driven clinical trials, which are necessary to obtain regulatory approval and clinical acceptance (Rogovskii et al., 2022).

5.3 Inconsistencies in Clinical Evidence

There are, however, many contradictions in clinical studies, showing that the effects are still uncertain and in many cases unexplainable. Several clinical trial studies on polyphenols (such as curcumin, green tea catechins, resveratrol) provide equivocal data concerning efficacy, safety, pharmacokinetic parameters and a net translation into clinical application (López-Gómez & Uranga, 2024). For instance, although new drugs such as curcumin appear to be promising in early-phase colon, pancreas and breast cancer trials, the results of prospective, randomized controlled large trials (RCTs) have frequently not resulted in an statistically significant benefit to progression-free survival (PFS) or overall survival (OS). In a phase II trial of curcumin in patients with pancreatic cancer, curcumin was found to be safe, but there was little evidence for objective tumor response in the majority of patients. Resveratrol supplementation studies also have shown mixed results where some studies found a decrease in biomarkers of inflammation, whereas other did not observe significant decrease in tumor burden or patient outcome (Gupta et al., 2013). These discrepancies are likely due to various reasons, such as heterogeneous patient populations, variations in dosage and formulation, no uniform endpoints and lack of sufficient treatment duration. Furthermore, the use of dietary supplements instead of pharmaceutical-grade compounds in most studies results in variability in purity, stability, and bioactivity, which lowers the reliability and reproducibility of clinical results (Kwok et al., 2024).

5.4 Potential Toxicity and Drug Interactions

Although polyphenols are found to be safe and well-tolerated under dietary conditions, high doses or chronic intake might cause toxic effects or negative interactions, for example in the cancer patient group which generally are immunocompromised or receive numerous drugs (Duda-Chodak & Tarko, 2023). Some polyphenols may inhibit cytochrome P450 enzymes (particularly CYP3A4) and could influence drug metabolism of chemotherapeutics, anticoagulants and immunosuppressants. For instance, quercetin has been found to block CYP2C8 and CYP3A4 affecting drugs such as paclitaxel or tamoxifen pharmacokinetics. Excessive consumption of green tea catechins may also decrease folate absorption and interfere in proteasome inhibitors like bortezomib leading to their reduced efficiency. These interactions could be an indicator that appropriate pharmacodynamic drug-drug interaction studies need to be performed prior to the safe use of polyphenol-based therapies in the context of cancer (Bhamre et al., 2022). Additionally, some polyphenols may also have pro-oxidant activities, when they reach higher levels in the system under some circumstances. This paradoxical side effect can be responsible for the oxidative stress and the DNA damage in the normal cells, which can subsequently cause cytotoxicity. The double nature of polyphenols as they are both antioxidative and pro-oxidative has context specific nature and mechanism that needs to be further elucidated when considering the best dosages and therapeutic period (Mao et al., 2017).

5.5 Regulatory and Manufacturing Hurdles

Last but not least, issues related to regulation and manufacturing can also hamper the clinical use of polyphenols. As polyphenols are not typical drugs originated from a well-established pharmaceutical route, they frequently stand in a gray zone between drugs and dietary supplements. This ambiguity confuses the regulatory approval also, for these derivatives may be below the level of pharmacokinetics, toxicity profiling, and clinical efficacy demanded from a drug (Ashrafpour & Ashrafpour, 2025; Silpi, 2025). In addition, an extensive batch-to-batch variation, no GMP compliance in the production, the lack of patentable protection contribute to diminish the commercial interest of the pharmaceutical industry in the mass development of polyphenol-based drugs. In the absence of specific regulatory guidance and compelling financial interest, the majority of potential polyphenols are lurking in the preclinical and early clinical stage, unable to crossover as standard of care (Adhikari & Venkatesh, 2025).

6. EMERGING RESEARCH DIRECTIONS ON POLYPHENOLS IN CANCER THERAPY

The field of polyphenol in oncology is very dynamic and new tendency are on the horizon that will increase the therapeutic value of these bioactive compounds. These lines guide future research to create novel derivatives, innovative vehicles and personalized solution to improve the anticancer potential of polyphenolic compounds (Oriol-Caballo et al., 2025; Lu et al., 2015). Below is an elaboration on these key areas.

6.1. Novel Derivatives of Polyphenols

The development and characterization of new derivatives as structures for anticancer action is one of the leading ways in the field of polyphenols studies. Most of the natural polyphenols are disadvantaged of their poor *in vivo* bioavailability, rapid metabolism and insufficient biological activity. To circumvent these difficulties, there is a substantial body of scientific evidence on the chemical modification of naturally occurring polyphenolic compounds to produce analogs more active, more stable (Davatgaran-Taghipour, 2017). For instance, new studies have described the synthesis of analogues from natural lignans, such as machilin C and D that have been shown to have antiproliferative activity much greater than that of the parent compound. The optimized lignans were demonstrated to have better cytotoxicity against cancer cells, indicating the structural diverse derivation will result in more potential-specific and potent analogues (Hui et al., 2012). Novel designed polyphenols have also exhibited potential for inhibiting the colon cancer cell growth by acting on the cancer cell metabolism targeting the important pathways of glycolysis part that is crucial for the surviving the tumor. These new derivatives not only enhance the anticancer properties, but also assist in understanding the structure activity relationship, serving as guidance for the development of new drugs (Gupta et al., 2023). Based on a tailored number of molecular features as the position of hydroxyl groups and conjugation patterns, new ligands exhibiting increased interaction with key cancer-related targets which may result in overall improved efficacy and reduced off-targeting (Colomer et al., 2017).

6.2. Advanced Delivery Systems for Polyphenols

Poor water solubility, low stability, and rapid body clearance have become severe obstacles to the clinical application of polyphenols because of restricted therapeutic levels achieved in the tumor sites. In order to tackle these problems, smart delivery systems, especially nanocarriers, have been created to enhance delivery efficiency, stability and site-specific targeting. Nanoformulations consists of nanosuspensions, solid lipid nanoparticles, liposomes, polymeric nanoparticles, and gold nanoparticles. These carriers are useful in preventing polyphenols from premature degradation and improving the solubility, as well as facilitating the controlled release of polyphenols at the tumor site (Jia et al., 2023). For example, the nano-encapsulation of resveratrol, curcumin, and epigallocatechin-3-gallate (EGCG) has been shown to lead to higher intracellular concentrations and superior pro-apoptotic activity in cancerous cells than those of the free compounds (Vieira et al., 2023). Further, Nano-delivery systems may be designed for active targeting through the functionalization of nanoparticles with ligands which are specific to tumor markers, increasing the selective uptake by cancer cells and reducing extended systemic toxicities (Anand et al., 2022). In addition, recent progress also involves exosome carrier-based delivery systems that utilize these natural vesicles for an active delivery of polyphenols to tumor site, providing new directions for the precision nanomedicine. The significance of such naotherapeutic apc has been improved not only by pharmacokinetics and bio distribution of polyphenols, but also in combination of polyphenols with chemotherapeutic agents in order to possibly reverse drug resistance and enhance synergistic effects (Bhat et al., 2024).

6.3. Personalized Approaches Based on Cancer Subtypes

Cancer is a complex disease of heterogeneity, which has the different response to treatment according to molecular subtypes. Recent studies have highlighted the relevance of personalized medicine approaches in the use of polyphenols, and want treatment to be "optimized" based on the established genetics and epigenetics of each specific tumor. In studying this, there is an increasing attention to interactions between polyphenols and genes to find markers with potential predictive value. For instance, p53 tumor suppressor modulation by polyphenols, including resveratrol and quercetin, is mediated through intricate post-translational modifications that differ among cancer types and suggest diverse effects on treatment response. These molecular interactions allow the development of subtype-specific polyphenol-based therapeutics with high efficacy and low toxicity profiles (Merlin et al., 2021; Lyubitelev & Studitsky, 2023). In addition, epigenetic profiling studies show that the benefits of polyphenols to be reversing abnormal DNA methylation and histone modification patterns in cancer cells to a more physiological gene expression profile. Such an epigenetic reprogramming is particularly important in cancers characterized by known epigenetic dysregulation, and it is possible to envision the inclusion of polyphenols in personalized protocols for drugs directed to such targets. The computation biology and high-throughput screening based method speed up the identification of patient-specific polyphenols targets and the optimal combination with conventional drugs. These personalized strategies are expected to increase the therapeutic index of polyphenols and broaden their clinical translation (do Valle et al., 2021).

6.4. Preservation of Polyphenol Bioactivity during Processing and Formulation

One main obstacle to the use of polyphenols as therapeutic agents is maintaining their bioactivity during extraction, sterilization and formulation (Sejbuk et al., 2024). The anticancer activity of polyphenols commonly deteriorates in conventional sterilization technologies. Novel methods such as pharmaceutical processing have been introduced more recently that preserve as much as 90% of the anti-inflammatory, antioxidant, and immune-modulatory qualities of polyphenols and flavonoids found naturally (Ammendola et al., 2020, Ozon et al., 2023). For instance, research has also addressed the retention of polyphenols in caplet handling. *In vitro* data have shown preserved gayuba and caá-avare formulations are able to inhibit aggressive cancers, such as glioblastoma, with less toxicity in normal cells, evidencing their potential as safe natural adjuvant for cancer treatment (Vieira et al., 2023).

6.5. Combination Therapies and Synergistic Effects

Novel studies also are investigating adjunct treatment using polyphenols with traditional chemotherapeutic agents and/or other phytochemicals to increase anticancer effectiveness and decrease adverse effects (Cacciola et al., 2023). Polyphenols may sensitize cancer cells to chemotherapy by influencing mechanisms of drug resistance (e.g., efflux pump inhibition, and cell survival pathways). Indeed, both *in vitro* and *in vivo* data have indicated that the combination of resveratrol with the anticancer drug, cisplatin, exerts a cytotoxic synergy in ovarian cancer, which increases tumor cell apoptosis and decreases necessary drug doses. These combinations exploit the multi-target ability of polyphenols to modulate cancer hallmarks more efficiently than single drugs alone (Thaklaewphan et al., 2024; Jakobušić Brala et al., 2023). In addition, the immunomodulatory and anti-inflammatory effects of polyphenols also support cytotoxic treatments, by modulating the tumor microenvironment and strengthening the immune surveillance. This approach by integration is being considered as a promising strategy to address the shortcomings of standard of care and to enhance the clinical effectiveness in cancer patients (Vladu et al., 2022).

8. CONCLUSION AND RECOMMENDATIONS

Polyphenols are still emerging as the most well investigated class of bioactive natural compounds with great potential in cancer prevention and treatment. The ability of polyphenols to modulate several hallmarks of cancer including apoptosis, angiogenesis, oxidative stress, immune surveillance and epi-genetic alterations, brings them in a unique position in integrative and conventional oncology in the role of adjuvants. The multi-targeted nature of polyphenols presents distinct theoretical advantages, particularly for addressing tumor heterogeneity and circumventing compensatory pathways frequently responsible for the failure of single-target therapies.

Nevertheless, there are severe limitations that hinder the overall clinical translation of polyphenols. Bad bioavailability, fast metabolism, erratic intestinal absorption, inter-individual differences and regulatory skepticism are still barriers to the implementation of polyphenolic compounds into conventional cancer therapeutics. Addressing these issues will necessitate continued, multidisciplinary, collaborative research including natural product chemists, molecular biologists, pharmacologists, clinical oncologists, and regulatory scientists.

To advance the field and facilitate the effective integration of polyphenols into cancer therapy, the following recommendations are proposed:

1. Design and synthesis of improved polyphenol derivatives with enhanced stability, potency, and target specificity.
2. Development of advanced delivery systems, including nano-formulations, liposomes, and exosome-based carriers, to enhance tumor-specific accumulation and bioavailability.
3. Comprehensive pharmacokinetic and pharmacodynamics studies to determine optimal dosing strategies, treatment schedules, and synergistic combinations with existing chemotherapeutic agents.
4. Identification and validation of predictive biomarkers that can guide personalized polyphenol-based interventions and improve patient selection.
5. Implementation of robust clinical trials, incorporating standardized polyphenol preparations, clearly defined endpoints, and adequate follow-up to evaluate long-term efficacy and safety.
6. Establishment of clear regulatory frameworks that differentiate polyphenol-based pharmaceuticals from dietary supplements, ensuring quality control, safety, and therapeutic consistency.

Furthermore, integrating systems biology, network pharmacology, and multi-omics approaches will be critical for unraveling the complex mechanisms underlying polyphenol activity and designing more informed clinical studies. Progress in this area will depend on strong interdisciplinary collaboration among researchers, clinicians, regulatory agencies, and industry partners.

REFERENCES

Adhikari, B., & Venkatesh, D. N. (2025). The nutraceutical market: Intellectual property, clinical research, and future insights. *International Journal of Applied Pharmaceutics*, *17*(2), 39–52. DOI: 10.22159/ijap.2025v17i2.53278

Ahearn, I., Haigis, K., Bar-Sagi, D., & Philips, M. R. (2012). Regulating the regulator: Post-translational modification of RAS. *Nature Reviews. Molecular Cell Biology*, *13*(1), 39–51. DOI: 10.1038/nrm3255

Ahmed, Z. S. O., Khan, E., Elias, N., Elshebiny, A., & Dou, Q. (2025). Updated review on natural polyphenols: Molecular mechanisms, biological effects, and clinical applications for cancer management. *Biomolecules*, *15*(5), 629. DOI: 10.3390/biom15050629

Alam, M. N., Almoyad, M., & Huq, F. (2018). Polyphenols in colorectal cancer: Current state of knowledge including clinical trials and molecular mechanism of action. *BioMed Research International*, *2018*, 4154185. DOI: 10.1155/2018/4154185

Almatroudi, A., Allemailem, K. S., Alwanian, W. M., Alharbi, B. F., Alrumaihi, F., Khan, A. A., Almatroodi, S. A., & Rahmani, A. H. (2023). Effects and mechanisms of kaempferol in the management of cancers through modulation of inflammation and signal transduction pathways. *International Journal of Molecular Sciences*, *24*(10), 8630. DOI: 10.3390/ijms24108630

Ammendola, M., Haponska, M., Balik, K., Janda, K., & Rosiak, D. (2020). Stability and anti-proliferative properties of biologically active compounds extracted from *Cistus L.* after sterilization treatments. *Scientific Reports*, *10*(1), 6521. DOI: 10.1038/s41598-020-63444-3

Anand, S., Sowbhagya, R., Ansari, M. A., Alzohairy, M. A., Alomary, M. N., Almalik, A. I., Ahmad, W., Tripathi, T., & Elderdery, A. Y. (2022). Polyphenols and their nanoformulations: Protective effects against human diseases. *Life (Basel, Switzerland)*, *12*(10), 1639. DOI: 10.3390/life12101639

Asensi, M., Ortega, A., Mena, S., Feddi, F., & Estrela, J. M. (2011). Natural polyphenols in cancer therapy. *Critical Reviews in Clinical Laboratory Sciences*, *48*(5–6), 197–216. DOI: 10.3109/10408363.2011.631268

Ashrafpour, S., & Ashrafpour, M. (2025). The double-edged sword of nutraceuticals: Comprehensive review of protective agents and their hidden risks. *Frontiers in Nutrition*, *12*, 1524627. DOI: 10.3389/fnut.2025.1524627

Azrad, M., Vollmer, R. T., Madden, J., Dewhirst, M., Polascik, T. J., Snyder, D. C., Ruffin, M. T., Moul, J. W., Brenner, D. E., & Demark-Wahnefried, W. (2013). Flaxseed-derived enterolactone is inversely associated with tumor cell proliferation in men with localized prostate cancer. *Journal of Medicinal Food*, *16*(4), 357–360. DOI: 10.1089/jmf.2012.0159

Bastidas, H., Araya-Valdés, G., Cortés, G., Jara, J. A., & Catalán, M. (2022). Pharmacological effects of caffeic acid and its derivatives in cancer: New targeted compounds for the mitochondria. *Advances in Experimental Medicine and Biology*, *1401*, 213–225. DOI: 10.1007/5584_2022_718

Bhamre, V. G., Deore, P. D., Amrutkar, R. D., & Patil, V. R. (2022). Polyphenols: The interactions with CYP isoenzymes and effect on pharmacokinetics of drugs. *Current Trends in Pharmacy and Pharmaceutical Chemistry*, 4(1).

Bhat, A. A., Gupta, G., Afzal, M., Thapa, R., Ali, H., Alqahtani, S. M., almalki, W. H., Kazmi, I., Alzarea, S. I., Saleem, S., & Subramaniyan, V. (2024). Polyphenol-loaded nano-carriers for breast cancer therapy: A comprehensive review. *BioNano-Science*, *14*(4), 4219–4237. DOI: 10.1007/s12668-023-01288-7

Brady, C. A., & Attardi, L. D. (2010). p53 at a glance. *Journal of Cell Science*, *123*(15), 2527–2532. DOI: 10.1242/jcs.064501

Cacciola, N. A., Cuciniello, R., Petillo, G. D., Piccioni, M., Filosa, S., & Crispi, S. (2023). An overview of the enhanced effects of curcumin and chemotherapeutic agents in combined cancer treatments. *International Journal of Molecular Sciences*, *24*(16), 12587. DOI: 10.3390/ijms241612587

Cai, Z., Mao, C., Wang, Y., Zhu, Z., Xu, S., Chen, D., Chen, Y., Ruan, W., & Fang, B. (2022). Phytochemistry and pharmacology of traditional Chinese medicine: Review research progress with luteolin as an anti-tumor agent. *Natural Product Communications*, *17*(11), 1–7. DOI: 10.1177/1934578X221133579

Cháirez-Ramírez, M. H., de la Cruz-López, K. G., & García-Carrancá, A. (2021). Polyphenols as antitumor agents targeting key players in cancer-driving signaling pathways. *Frontiers in Pharmacology*, *12*, 710304. DOI: 10.3389/fphar.2021.710304

Chillón-Pino, D., Badonyi, M., Semple, C. A., & Marsh, J. A. (2024). Protein structural context of cancer mutations reveals molecular mechanisms and candidate driver genes. *Cell Reports*, *43*(11), 114905. DOI: 10.1016/j.celrep.2024.114905

Chimento, A., De Luca, A., D'Amico, M., De Amicis, F., & Pezzi, V. (2023). The involvement of natural polyphenols in molecular mechanisms inducing apoptosis in tumor cells: A promising adjuvant in cancer therapy. *International Journal of Molecular Sciences*, *24*(2), 168. DOI: 10.3390/ijms24021680

Chu, A. J. (2022). Quarter-century explorations of bioactive polyphenols: Diverse health benefits. [Landmark Edition]. *Frontiers in Bioscience (Landmark Edition)*, *27*(4), 134. DOI: 10.31083/j.fbl2704134

Ciupei, D., Colişar, A., Leopold, L., Stănilă, A., & Diaconeasa, Z. M. (2024). Polyphenols: From classification to therapeutic potential and bioavailability. *Foods*, *13*(24), 4131. DOI: 10.3390/foods13244131

Colomer, R., Sarrats, A., Lupu, R., & Puig, T. (2017). Natural polyphenols and their synthetic analogs as emerging anticancer agents. *Current Drug Targets*, *18*(2), 147–159. DOI: 10.2174/1389450117666160112113930

Davatgaran-Taghipour, Y., Masoomzadeh, S., Farzaei, M. H., Bahramsoltani, R., Karimi-Soureh, Z., Rahimi, R., & Abdollahi, M. (2017). Polyphenol nanoformulations for cancer therapy: Experimental evidence and clinical perspective. *International Journal of Nanomedicine*, *12*, 2689–2702. DOI: 10.2147/IJN.S131973

De, S., Paul, S., Manna, A., Majumder, C., Pal, K., Casarcia, N., Mondal, A., Banerjee, S., Nelson, V. K., Ghosh, S., Hazra, J., Bhattacharjee, A., Mandal, S. C., Pal, M., & Bishayee, A. (2023). Phenolic phytochemicals for prevention and treatment of colorectal cancer: A critical evaluation of *in vivo* studies. *Cancers (Basel)*, *15*(3), 993. DOI: 10.3390/cancers15030993

de la Garza-Kalife, D. A., Loaiza-Gutiérrez, V. L., Hernández-Tobías, E. A., González-Villarreal, C. A., Islas, J. F., Santoyo-Suárez, M. G., Garza-Treviño, E. N., & Delgado-Gonzalez, P. (2025). Polyphenols in pancreatic cancer management: Exploring the roles and mechanisms of resveratrol and epigallocatechin. *Oncology Research*, *33*(9), 2243–2262. DOI: 10.32604/or.2025.065222

do Valle, F., Roweth, G., Malloy, W., Chavarria, C., Moco, S., Barron, D., Andres-Lacueva, C., Kacprowski, T., Krumsiek, J., Barabási, L., & Menichetti, G. (2021). Network medicine framework shows that proximity of polyphenol targets and disease proteins predicts therapeutic effects of polyphenols. *Nature Food*, *2*(3), 143–155. DOI: 10.1038/s43016-021-00243-7

Dong, C., Wu, J., Chen, Y., Nie, J., & Chen, C. (2021). Activation of PI3K/AKT/mTOR pathway causes drug resistance in breast cancer. *Frontiers in Pharmacology*, *12*, 628690. DOI: 10.3389/fphar.2021.628690

Duda-Chodak, A., & Tarko, T. (2023). Possible side effects of polyphenols and their interactions with medicines. *Molecules (Basel, Switzerland)*, *28*(6), 2536. DOI: 10.3390/molecules28062536

Emran, T. B., Shahriar, A., Mahmud, A. R., Rahman, T., Abir, M. H., Siddiquee, M. F.-R., Ahmed, H., Rahman, N., Nainu, F., Wahyudin, E., Mitra, S., Dhama, K., Habiballah, M. M., Haque, S., Islam, A., & Hassan, M. M. (2022). Multidrug resistance in cancer: Understanding molecular mechanisms, immunoprevention and therapeutic approaches. *Frontiers in Oncology*, *12*, 891652. DOI: 10.3389/fonc.2022.891652

Farhan, M. (2023). Insights on the role of polyphenols in combating cancer drug resistance. *Biomedicines*, *11*(6), 1709. DOI: 10.3390/biomedicines11061709

Ferraz da Costa, D. C., Campos, N. P. C., Santos, R. A., Guedes-da-Silva, F. H., Martins-Dinis, M. M. D. C., Zanphorlin, L., Ramos, C., Rangel, L. P., & Silva, J. L. (2018). Resveratrol prevents p53 aggregation in vitro and in breast cancer cells. *Oncotarget*, *9*(49), 29112–29122. DOI: 10.18632/oncotarget.25631

Fetoni, A. R., Paciello, F., & Troiani, D. (2022). Cisplatin chemotherapy and cochlear damage: Otoprotective and chemosensitization properties of polyphenols. *Antioxidants & Redox Signaling*, *36*(16–18), 1229–1245. DOI: 10.1089/ars.2021.0183

Gupta, N., Singh, S., Chauhan, D., Srivastava, R., & Singh, V. K. (2023). Exploring the anticancer potentials of polyphenols: A comprehensive review of patents in the last five years. *Recent Patents on Anti-Cancer Drug Discovery*, *18*(1), 3–10. DOI: 10.2174/1574892817666220512220036

Gupta, S. C., Patchva, S., & Aggarwal, B. B. (2013). Therapeutic roles of curcumin: Lessons learned from clinical trials. *The AAPS Journal*, *15*(1), 195–218. DOI: 10.1208/s12248-012-9432-8

Hanahan, D. (2022). Hallmarks of cancer: New dimensions. *Cancer Discovery*, *12*(1), 31–46. DOI: 10.1158/2159-8290.CD-21-1059

Hanahan, D., & Weinberg, R. A. (2000). The hallmarks of cancer. *Cell*, *100*(1), 57–70. DOI: 10.1016/S0092-8674(00)81683-9

Hanahan, D., & Weinberg, R. A. (2011). Hallmarks of cancer: The next generation. *Cell*, *144*(5), 646–674. DOI: 10.1016/j.cell.2011.02.013

Hao, B., Yang, Z., Liu, H., Liu, Y., & Wang, S. (2024). Advances in flavonoid research: Sources, biological activities, and developmental prospectives. *Current Issues in Molecular Biology*, *46*(4), 2884–2925. DOI: 10.3390/cimb46040181

Hedayati, N., Safari, M. H., Milasi, Y. E., Kahkesh, S., Farahani, N., Khoshnazar, S. M., Dorostgou, Z., Alaei, E., Alimohammadi, M., Rahimzadeh, P., Taheriazam, A., & Hashemi, M. (2025). Modulation of the PI3K/Akt signaling pathway by resveratrol in cancer: Molecular mechanisms and therapeutic opportunity. *Discover. Oncology*, *16*(1), 669. DOI: 10.1007/s12672-025-02471-w

Hui, J., Zhao, Y., & Zhu, L. (2012). Synthesis and in vitro anticancer activities of novel aryl-naphthalene lignans. *Medicinal Chemistry Research*, *21*(12), 3994–4001. DOI: 10.1007/s00044-011-9937-1

Issinger, O. G., & Guerra, B. (2021). Phytochemicals in cancer and their effect on the PI3K/AKT-mediated cellular signalling. *Biomedicine and Pharmacotherapy*, *139*, 111650. DOI: 10.1016/j.biopha.2021.111650

Izzo, A., & Stefanska, B. (2025). Natural products and cancer: From drug discovery to prevention and therapy. *British Journal of Pharmacology*, *182*(10), 2069–2074. DOI: 10.1111/bph.70014

Jakobušić Brala, C., Karković Marković, A., Kugić, A., Torić, J., & Barbarić, M. (2023). Combination chemotherapy with selected polyphenols in preclinical and clinical studies - An updated overview. *Molecules (Basel, Switzerland)*, *28*(9), 3746. DOI: 10.3390/molecules28093746

Jantan, I., Haque, A., Arshad, L., Harikrishnan, H., Septama, W., & Mohamed-Hussein, A. (2021). Dietary polyphenols suppress chronic inflammation by modulation of multiple inflammation-associated cell signaling pathways. *The Journal of Nutritional Biochemistry*, *93*, 108634. DOI: 10.1016/j.jnutbio.2021.108634

Jia, W., Zhou, L., Li, L., Zhou, P., & Shen, Z. (2023). Nano-based drug delivery of polyphenolic compounds for cancer treatment: Progress, opportunities, and challenges. *Pharmaceuticals (Basel, Switzerland)*, *16*(1), 101. DOI: 10.3390/ph16010101

Keskin, A. (2023). Impact of polyphenolic compounds on the MAPK signaling pathway against carcinogenesis. *Journal of Clinical Practice and Research*, *45*(3), 217–221.

Khaw, K., Yong, W., Kalthur, G., & Hande, P. (2012). Genistein induces growth arrest and suppresses telomerase activity in brain tumor cells. *Genes, Chromosomes & Cancer*, *51*(10), 961–974. DOI: 10.1002/gcc.21979

Kiemlian Kwee, J. (2016). Yin and yang of polyphenols in cancer prevention: A short review. *Anti-cancer Agents in Medicinal Chemistry*, *16*(7), 832–840. DOI: 10.2174/1871520616666151116124549

Kim, H., Ki, R., Min, H., & Pack, P. (2023). Advanced delivery system of polyphenols for effective cancer prevention and therapy. *Antioxidants*, *12*(5), 1048. DOI: 10.3390/antiox12051048

Ko, H., Sethi, G., Um, Y., Shanmugam, K., Arfuso, F., Kumar, P., Bishayee, A., & Ahn, K. S. (2017). The role of resveratrol in cancer therapy. *International Journal of Molecular Sciences*, *18*(12), 2589. DOI: 10.3390/ijms18122589

Kopustinskiene, M., Jakstas, V., Savickas, A., & Bernatoniene, J. (2020). Flavonoids as anticancer agents. *Nutrients*, *12*(2), 457. DOI: 10.3390/nu12020457

Kubatka, P., Bojkova, B., Nosalova, N., Huniadi, M., Samuel, M., Sreenesh, B., Hrklova, G., Kajo, K., Hornak, S., Cizkova, D., Bubnov, R., Smokovski, I., Büsselberg, D., & Golubnitschaja, O. (2025). Targeting the MAPK signaling pathway: Implications and prospects of flavonoids in 3P medicine as modulators of cancer cell plasticity and therapeutic resistance in breast cancer patients. *The EPMA Journal*, *16*(2), 437–463. DOI: 10.1007/s13167-025-00407-6

Kwok, R., Einbond, S., Tantawi, H., Strange, T., Smith, C., Dhar, M., Bershadskiy, A., & Castellanos, R. (2024). Effects of common nutraceutical supplements marketed for cancer prevention on tumor cell growth. *Journal of Clinical Oncology*, *42*(16), e22504. DOI: 10.1200/JCO.2024.42.16_suppl.e22504

Lewis, E. J. (2015). PRIMA-1 as a cancer therapy restoring mutant p53: A review. *Bioscience Horizons*, *8*(0), 6. DOI: 10.1093/biohorizons/hzv006

Lewis, J. (2015). PRIMA-1 as a cancer therapy restoring mutant p53: A review. *Bioscience Horizons*, *8*(0), 6. DOI: 10.1093/biohorizons/hzv006

Lin, W., Gong, C., Song, F., & Cui, Y. (2017). Effects of anthocyanins on the prevention and treatment of cancer. *British Journal of Pharmacology*, *174*(11), 1226–1243. DOI: 10.1111/bph.13627

Liu, D., Chen, X., Yi, Z., Tong, Q., Ma, L., Tan, Y., Cao, X., & Li, X. (2024). pH-responsive carrier-free polyphenol nanoparticles assembled by oxidative polymerization with enhanced stability and antioxidant activity for improved bioaccessibility. *ACS Applied Bio Materials*, *7*(3), 1763–1777. DOI: 10.1021/acsabm.3c01178

Liu, Y., Su, Z., Tavana, O., & Gu, W. (2024). Understanding the complexity of p53 in a new era of tumor suppression. *Cancer Cell*, *42*(6), 946–967. DOI: 10.1016/j.ccell.2024.04.009

López-Gómez, L., & Uranga, A. (2024). Polyphenols in the prevention and treatment of colorectal cancer: A systematic review of clinical evidence. *Nutrients*, *16*(16), 2735. DOI: 10.3390/nu16162735

Lu, Y., Wang, K., & Hu, L. (2025). Advancements in delivery systems for dietary polyphenols in enhancing radioprotection effects: Challenges and opportunities. *NPJ Science of Food*, *9*(1), 51. DOI: 10.1038/s41538-025-00419-6

Luca, V., Macovei, I., Bujor, A., Miron, A., Skalicka-Woźniak, K., Aprotosoaie, C., & Trifan, A. (2020). Bioactivity of dietary polyphenols: The role of metabolites. *Critical Reviews in Food Science and Nutrition*, *60*(4), 626–659. DOI: 10.1080/10408398.2018.1546669

Lyubitelev, A., & Studitsky, V. (2023). Inhibition of cancer development by natural plant polyphenols: Molecular mechanisms. *International Journal of Molecular Sciences*, *24*(13), 10663. DOI: 10.3390/ijms241310663

Mao, X., Gu, C., Chen, D., Yu, B., & He, J. (2017). Oxidative stress-induced diseases and tea polyphenols. *Oncotarget*, *8*(46), 81649–81661. DOI: 10.18632/oncotarget.20887

Merlin, J., Rupasinghe, V., Dellaire, G., & Murphy, K. (2021). Role of dietary antioxidants in p53-mediated cancer chemoprevention and tumor suppression. *Oxidative Medicine and Cellular Longevity*, *2021*(1), 9924328. DOI: 10.1155/2021/9924328

Mohammad, M., Muqbil, I., Lowe, L., Yedjou, C., Hsu, Y., Lin, T., & Azmi, S. (2015). Broad targeting of resistance to apoptosis in cancer. *Seminars in Cancer Biology*, *35*, 78–103. DOI: 10.1016/j.semcancer.2015.03.001

Nguyen, T., Lee, H., Sharma, R., Park, B., Jagga, S., Sharma, G., Lee, S., & Nam, S. (2017). Quercetin induces apoptosis and cell cycle arrest in triple-negative breast cancer cells through modulation of Foxo3a activity. *The Korean Journal of Physiology & Pharmacology; Official Journal of the Korean Physiological Society and the Korean Society of Pharmacology*, *21*(2), 205–213. DOI: 10.4196/kjpp.2017.21.2.205

Oh, W., Muthu, M., Pushparaj, C., & Gopal, J. (2023). Anticancer therapeutic effects of green tea catechins when integrated with antioxidant natural components. *Molecules (Basel, Switzerland)*, *28*(5), 2151. DOI: 10.3390/molecules28052151

Oriol-Caballo, M., Moreno-Murciano, P., López-Blanch, R., Estrela, M., & Obrador, E. (2025). Polyphenols: Potential applications in cancer therapy. *Molecular Nutrition & Food Research*, *69*(15), e70011. DOI: 10.1002/mnfr.70011

Ozon, A., Iuga, M., Mititelu, M., Musuc, M., Manolescu, N., Petrescu, S., & Elian, V. (2023). Pharmacotechnical, physico-chemical, and antioxidant evaluation of newly developed capsule formulations. *International Journal of Molecular Sciences*, *24*(14), 11426. DOI: 10.3390/ijms241411426

Pandey, B., & Rizvi, I. (2009). Plant polyphenols as dietary antioxidants in human health and disease. *Oxidative Medicine and Cellular Longevity*, *2*(5), 270–278. DOI: 10.4161/oxim.2.5.9498

Pandey, P., Lakhanpal, S., Mahmood, D., Kang, N., Kim, B., Kang, S., Choi, J., & Kim, B. (2025). An updated review summarizing the anticancer potential of flavonoids via targeting NF-κB pathway. *Frontiers in Pharmacology*, *15*, 1513422. DOI: 10.3389/fphar.2024.1513422

Papavassiliou, A., Sofianidi, A., Gogou, A., & Papavassiliou, G. (2025). The prospects of curcumin in non-small cell lung cancer therapeutics. *Cancers (Basel)*, *17*(3), 438. DOI: 10.3390/cancers17030438

Proença, C., Freitas, M., Ribeiro, D., Rufino, T., Fernandes, E., & Ferreira de Oliveira, P. (2023). The role of flavonoids in the regulation of epithelial-mesenchymal transition in cancer. *Medicinal Research Reviews*, *43*(6), 1878–1945. DOI: 10.1002/med.21966

Qian, Y., Zhao, F., Wang, J., Li, H., Xu, L., Wang, W., Yu, W., & Shan, L. (2021). Myricetin-based self-assembled nanoparticles for tumor synergistic therapy by antioxidation pathway. *Journal of Biomedical Nanotechnology*, *17*(12), 2399–2412. DOI: 10.1166/jbn.2021.3197

Rahman, A., Hannan, A., Dash, R., Rahman, H., Islam, R., Uddin, J., & Rhim, H. (2021). Phytochemicals as a complement to cancer chemotherapy: Pharmacological modulation of the autophagy-apoptosis pathway. *Frontiers in Pharmacology*, *12*, 639628. DOI: 10.3389/fphar.2021.639628

Rajeeve, D., Yamuna, R., & Namboori, K. (2025). Elucidating the potential of EGFR mutated NSCLC and identifying its multi-targeted inhibitors. *Scientific Reports*, *15*(1), 3649. DOI: 10.1038/s41598-024-83868-5

Ramli, I., Cheriet, T., Posadino, M., Giordo, R., Fenu, G., Nwachukwu, C., & Pintus, G. (2024). Modulating the p53-MDM2 pathway: The therapeutic potential of natural compounds in cancer treatment. *EXCLI Journal*, *23*, 1397–1439.

Rauf, A., Imran, M., Khan, I. A., Ur-Rehman, M., Gilani, A., Mehmood, Z., & Mubarak, S. (2018). Anticancer potential of quercetin: A comprehensive review. *Phytotherapy Research*, *32*(11), 2109–2130. DOI: 10.1002/ptr.6155

Rogovskii, V. (2022). Polyphenols as the potential disease-modifying therapy in cancer. *Anti-cancer Agents in Medicinal Chemistry*, *22*(13), 2385–2392. DOI: 10.2174/1871520622666220201105204

Sejbuk, M., Mirończuk-Chodakowska, I., Karav, S., & Witkowska, M. (2024). Dietary polyphenols, food processing and gut microbiome. *Antioxidants, 13*(10), 1220. DOI: 10.3390/antiox13101220

Shankar, S., Ganapathy, S., Hingorani, R., & Srivastava, K. (2008). EGCG inhibits growth, invasion, angiogenesis and metastasis of pancreatic cancer. *Frontiers in Bioscience, 13*(13), 440–452. DOI: 10.2741/2691

Sharma, E., Attri, C., Sati, P., Dhyani, P., Szopa, A., Sharifi-Rad, J., & Cho, C. (2022). Recent updates on anticancer mechanisms of polyphenols. *Frontiers in Cell and Developmental Biology, 10*, 1005910. DOI: 10.3389/fcell.2022.1005910

Silpi, C. (2025). Nutraceuticals: Traditional practices, regulatory guidelines, opportunities and challenges. *Discover Food, 5*(1), 191. DOI: 10.1007/s44187-025-00437-z

Silva-Pinto, A., de Pontes, C., Aguilar-Morón, B., Canales, C., Pavan, R., & Roque-Borda, A. (2025). Phytochemical insights into flavonoids in cancer. *Heliyon, 11*(4), e42682. DOI: 10.1016/j.heliyon.2025.e42682

Singaravelan, N., & Tollefsbol, O. (2025). Polyphenol-based prevention and treatment of cancer through epigenetic and combinatorial mechanisms. *Nutrients, 17*(4), 616. DOI: 10.3390/nu17040616

Singh, A., Holvoet, S., & Mercenier, A. (2011). Dietary polyphenols in the prevention and treatment of allergic diseases. *Clinical and Experimental Allergy, 41*(10), 1346–1359. DOI: 10.1111/j.1365-2222.2011.03773.x

Talib, H., Abed, I., Raad, D., Alomari, K., Jamal, A., Jabbar, R., & Law, D. (2024). Targeting cancer hallmarks using selected food bioactive compounds. *Foods, 13*(17), 2687. DOI: 10.3390/foods13172687

Thaklaewphan, P., Wikan, N., Potikanond, S., & Nimlamool, W. (2024). Oxyresveratrol enhances the anti-cancer effect of cisplatin. *Biomolecules, 14*(9), 1140. DOI: 10.3390/biom14091140

Vieira, S., Tessaro, L., Lima, O., Velloso, S., & Conte-Junior, A. (2023). Recent progress in nanotechnology improving the therapeutic potential of polyphenols for cancer. *Nutrients, 15*(14), 3136. DOI: 10.3390/nu15143136

Vladu, F., Ficai, D., Ene, G., & Ficai, A. (2022). Combination therapy using polyphenols. *International Journal of Molecular Sciences, 23*(18), 10244. DOI: 10.3390/ijms231810244

Wang, H., Guo, M., Wei, H., Liu, J., Xie, Z., Ma, Y., Yu, J., & He, J. (2023). Targeting p53 pathways. *Signal Transduction and Targeted Therapy*, *8*(1), 92. DOI: 10.1038/s41392-023-01347-1

Wang, M., Jiang, S., Zhou, L., Yu, F., Ding, H., Li, P., Zhou, M., & Wang, K. (2019). Potential mechanisms of action of curcumin for cancer prevention. *International Journal of Biological Sciences*, *15*(6), 1200–1214. DOI: 10.7150/ijbs.33710

Warias, P., Plewa, P., & Poniewierska-Baran, A. (2024). Resveratrol, piceatannol, curcumin, and quercetin as therapeutic targets in gastric cancer. *Molecules (Basel, Switzerland)*, *30*(1), 3. DOI: 10.3390/molecules30010003

World Health Organization. (2025, February 3). [Fact sheet]. *Cancer*.

Wu, F., Huang, H., Chiu, Y., Cherng, H., Sheu, T., & Yang, Y. (2022). Curcumin induces apoptosis of chemoresistant lung cancer cells via ROS-regulated p38 MAPK phosphorylation. *International Journal of Molecular Sciences*, *23*(15), 8248. DOI: 10.3390/ijms23158248

Zhang, Y., Zhang, Z., Mousavi, M., Moliani, A., Bahman, Y., & Bagheri, H. (2023). Resveratrol inhibits glioblastoma cells. *Chemico-Biological Interactions*, *376*, 110409. DOI: 10.1016/j.cbi.2023.110409

Zhong, J., Xing, D., Dong, Y., Chen, Y., Liu, N., Wang, M., & Zheng, P. (2024). Progress in the study of curcumin metabolism *in vivo*. *Journal of Asian Natural Products Research*, *27*(5), 639–657. DOI: 10.1080/10286020.2024.2420619

Zhou, H., Zheng, B., & McClements, D. J. (2021). In vitro gastrointestinal stability of lipophilic polyphenols. *Journal of Agricultural and Food Chemistry*, *69*(11), 3340–3350. DOI: 10.1021/acs.jafc.0c07578

Zughaibi, T. A., Suhail, M., Tarique, M., & Tabrez, S. (2021). Targeting PI3K/Akt/mTOR pathway by different flavonoids. *International Journal of Molecular Sciences*, *22*(22), 12455. DOI: 10.3390/ijms222212455

Chapter 9
Neuroprotection in a Spice Jar:
The Promise of Ginger for Parkinson's Disease

Clinton Ayodeji Akanbi
http://orcid.org/0009-0003-2417-7759
Bowen University, Nigeria

Favour Chisom Nwafor
Landmark University, Nigeria

Mojisola Adebimpe Ayomipo
Bowen University, Nigeria

Oluyomi Stephen Adeyemi
http://orcid.org/0000-0001-9342-8505
Bowen University, Nigeria

ABSTRACT

Parkinson's disease (PD) is a progressive neurodegenerative disorder involving α-synuclein aggregation in the substantia nigra and the loss of dopaminergic neurons. Its pathophysiology involves oxidative stress, mitochondrial dysfunction, impaired neurotransmission, and neuroinflammation. The existing treatments, including levodopa, dopamine agonists, and monoamine oxidase B inhibitors, are symptomatic but fail to halt disease progression or side effects, and therefore, neuroprotective strategies are needed. Zingiber officinale (ginger) contains phenolic compounds (6-gingerol, 6-shogaol, zingerone, and paradol) with antioxidant, anti-inflammatory, and anti-apoptotic properties. Preclinical studies show the neuroprotection of ginger by

DOI: 10.4018/979-8-3373-5876-5.ch009

scavenging reactive oxygen species, enhancing defenses, inhibiting mediators, and controlling signaling cascades. Although clinical trials in PD are lacking, cognitive improvement has been reported with minimal side effects. Overall, ginger's bioactives are promising adjuvant neuroprotectants that require rigorous clinical evaluation

1.0 INTRODUCTION

Parkinson's disease (PD) is the second most prevalent neurodegenerative disorder after Alzheimer's disease, affecting around 10 million individuals globally (Luo *et al.*, 2025; Reddy *et al.*, 2020). It is a neurodegenerative disorder that predominantly involves the central nervous system's motor control systems and is pathologically characterized by the loss of dopaminergic neurons within the substantia nigra pars compacta (SNpc) and intraneuronal Lewy bodies consisting of oligomerized α-synuclein (Gao *et al.*, 2022; Tysnes and Storstein, 2017). Thus, these neuropathological changes cause a significant decrease in striatal dopamine content, which is accountable for the characteristic motor symptoms of PD (bradykinesia, resting tremor, muscular stiffness, and postural instability), as well as non-motor symptoms such as cognitive decline and autonomic dysfunction (Luo *et al.*, 2025; Ball *et al.*, 2019). Clinically, PD is diagnosed based on these typical motor features, dopaminergic response, and elimination of other neurological disorders because there is no diagnostic test. While diagnosis is typically reliable in advanced stages, early PD can be challenging to distinguish from other Parkinsonian syndromes since symptoms are overlapping (Pahwa and Lyons, 2010; Virameteekul *et al.*, 2023).

PD comes in familial and sporadic forms, with age, genetics, environmental exposures, ethnicity, and gender determining onset and progression through multiple factors (Reddy *et al.*, 2020). Amongst these, senility is particularly relevant, with PD affecting approximately 1% of the population above 60 years old (Tysnes and Storstein, 2017). Clinically, PD progresses through different stages, from unilateral motor signs to complete dependence and potential cognitive impairments. With worsening of the disease, the patients have increasing motor dysfunction, ranging from tremors and gait from mild to impaired balance, immobility, and hallucinations at more severe stages (DeMaagd and Philip, 2015). As a result of population shifts globally, social, economic, and healthcare costs of PD will rise dramatically and become an emerging burden for patients, caregivers, and healthcare systems (Luo *et al.*, 2025; Bloem, 2019).

Despite decades of research, the definitive etiology of PD remains unclear. However, a number of interrelated molecular and cellular mechanisms have been found to be implicated in its pathology (Gao *et al.*, 2022; Angelopoulou *et al.*, 2022). These include oxidative stress, which results in dopaminergic neuronal injury through an imbalance of reactive oxygen species; mitochondrial disease, also resulting in energy collapse and neuronal apoptosis; neuroinflammation, with persistent microglial activation and elevation of pro-inflammatory cytokines; and disrupted neurotransmission, particularly in dopaminergic, glutamatergic, and cholinergic systems (Bej *et al.*, 2024; Eser *et al.*, 2024). These disease mechanisms not only govern the development and progression of disease but are also attractive therapeutic targets.

Current treatments are primarily based on symptom relief, rather than disease modification (Srivastav *et al.*, 2017). Levodopa, administered usually in combination with carbidopa, remains the gold standard for motor symptom treatment. However, chronic use often leads to such complications as motor fluctuations and dyskinesias due to pulsatile dopaminergic stimulation (Pardo-Moreno *et al.*, 2023). Other pharmacological options, like dopamine agonists, monoamine oxidase B (MAO-B) inhibitors, catechol-O-methyltransferase (COMT) inhibitors, and anticholinergics, are only partially effective and typically with side effects like psychosis and orthostatic hypotension (Angelopoulou *et al.*, 2022; Pardo-Moreno *et al.*, 2023). Deep brain stimulation is of symptomatic benefit for a small number of patients with advanced disease, but it also doesn't alter the inherent neurodegenerative process.

With these caveats in mind, natural compounds are being considered candidate adjuncts or alternatives to neuroprotection in PD. Phytochemicals such as polyphenols, terpenes, and alkaloids have been shown to possess a range of activities from antioxidant, anti-inflammatory, anti-apoptotic, and mitochondrial-stabilizing with good overall safety profiles (Angelopoulou *et al.*, 2022). Among them, *Zingiber officinale* Roscoe (ginger), a widely used culinary and medicinal spice, has emerged as a lead. Used for centuries in Ayurvedic medicine to treat ailments such as nausea, arthritis, and metabolic disorders, ginger is generally recognized as safe (GRAS) by the United States Food and Drug Administration (Sirwi *et al.*, 2025). It contains a blend of biologically active compounds comprising phenolic compounds (6-gingerol, 6-shogaol, zingerone, paradols) and essential oils with established pharmacological activities (Srinivasan, 2017; Angelopoulou *et al.*, 2022; Arcusa *et al.*, 2022). These have shown anti-inflammatory, antioxidant, and neuroprotective activities that are being studied in models of aging and neurodegenerative disease (Sirwi *et al.*, 2025; Arcusa *et al.*, 2022). Zingerone has also been reported to reverse dopamine depletion in models of PD in preclinical models, and ginger extracts improved animal learning and memory, explaining its use in traditional medicine for the treatment of memory impairment and dementia (Kiyama, 2020; Sirwi *et al.*, 2025).

This chapter addresses the therapeutic potential of *Zingiber officinale* (ginger) in PD, focusing on its neuroprotection and preclinical evidence. The review mentions PD pathophysiology, summarizes ginger's phytochemistry and safety profile, and highlights key experimental evidence of its antioxidant, anti-inflammatory, and mitochondrial activities. It also evaluates emerging evidence for its use in PD and considers research gaps and future clinical directions.

2. PATHOLOGY OF PD

2.1 α-Synuclein aggregation and dopaminergic neuron loss

PD is pathologically defined by progressive loss of dopaminergic neurons in the SNpc, striatal dopamine depletion, and the appearance of classic motor symptoms (Gao *et al.*, 2022). A hallmark of PD is the accumulation of misfolded α-syn in intraneuronal inclusions known as Lewy bodies and Lewy neurites, collectively termed Lewy pathology (Foffani and Obeso, 2018). Although α-syn is typically engaged in synaptic activity, its pathogenic misfolding as a result of genetic mutations or oxidative stress triggers the formation of toxic aggregates that disrupt normal cellular processes, including mitochondrial function, protein degradation pathways, and synaptic vesicle transport, to ultimately cause neuronal death (Gao *et al.*, 2022). Interestingly, although dopaminergic neurons in the SNpc are extremely vulnerable, those in other brain regions are relatively spared, suggesting selective neurodegeneration in PD (Sharma *et al.*, 2024).

2.2 Other key pathogenic mechanisms

2.2.1 Oxidative stress and mitochondrial dysfunction

Oxidative stress is a major etiologic factor in the pathogenesis of PD. Under normal physiological conditions, a balance between oxidants, which produce reactive oxygen species (ROS), and antioxidants, which break down these free radicals, exists. Oxidative stress emerges when this equilibrium is disrupted in favor of oxidants (Hemmati-Dinarvand *et al.*, 2019). Although the brain accounts for only 2% of body weight, it consumes about 20% of the body's oxygen. Its extreme oxygen demand makes it especially susceptible to ROS-mediated damage, particularly when antioxidant protective mechanisms are compromised (Kim *et al.*, 2020).

Substantia nigra pars compacta (SNpc) dopaminergic neurons are especially vulnerable to oxidative damage (Ni and Ernst, 2022). SNpc neurons are energy-demanding and vulnerable to bioenergetic breakdown. Inhibition of mitochondrial complex I (due to toxins, aging, or α-syn) leads to erroneous generation of reactive oxygen species (ROS) (Bej *et al.*, 2024). Oxygen takes part in reduction reactions in cellular metabolism and creates very reactive free radicals. These free radicals, reactive oxygen species (ROS) and reactive nitrogen species (RNS), react with nucleic acids, lipids, membranes, and proteins and cause widespread cellular damage (Moldogazieva *et al.*, 2018). ROS could also predispose to lipid, protein, and DNA damage, further debilitating mitochondria, thereby setting a cycle of mitochondrial dysfunction and oxidative stress (Kowalczyk *et al.*, 2021). ROS such as hydrogen peroxide (H_2O_2) and superoxide radicals ($O_2\bullet^-$) are particularly toxic because they disrupt mitochondrial function and damage DNA, causing impaired neural function and neurodegeneration (Balakrishnan *et al.*, 2021). Dopamine metabolism, increased calcium and iron, and decreased glutathione (GSH) levels all synergize to create compounded oxidative stress in PD (Chang and Chen, 2020).

Enzymes that are involved in the synthesis of dopamine, such as tyrosine hydroxylase and monoamine oxidase, also play important roles in ROS production in neurons, leading to oxidative damage and loss of neurons (Bej *et al.*, 2024). For this reason, treating oxidative stress and lowering ROS levels is the key therapeutic approach in the treatment of PD (Kim *et al.*, 2020).

2.2.2 Neuroinflammation

Neuroinflammation is a defensive response of the central nervous system (CNS) to eliminate infectious pathogens, toxic metabolites, autoimmune stimulation, and traumatic injury. It is primarily featured by glial cell activation, especially microglia and astrocytes (Yang and Zhou, 2019). Microglia, the resident immune cells of the CNS, play a crucial role in maintaining neural homeostasis through the elimination of debris and injury response (Yu *et al.*, 2022). Microglia are quiescent in a healthy brain, being small cell bodies with branched processes (Paolicelli *et al.*, 2022). Microglia, however, become activated and present enlarged cell bodies with retracted processes during pathologies such as PD (Lazdon *et al.*, 2020).

Microglia, when activated, release a variety of pro-inflammatory and neurotoxic mediators, including inducible nitric oxide synthase (iNOS), cyclooxygenase-2 (COX-2), and cytokines, including tumor necrosis factor-alpha (TNF-α), interleukins (IL-1, IL-2, IL-6), and interferons (IFNs) (Smith *et al.*, 2012). The sustained release of the molecules continues to maintain chronic inflammation and induces excessive production of reactive oxygen and nitrogen species (ROS and RNS), further aggravating oxidative stress (Leyane *et al.*, 2022). The midbrain area, especially the substantia nigra, has higher microglial content compared to other parts of the brain. Therefore, dopaminergic (DA) neurons in this area are particularly vulnerable, and their progressive degeneration is seen in PD. Microglial activation and ROS levels are, therefore, considered significant therapeutic targets in the relief of DA neuronal loss (Kim *et al.*, 2020).

2.2.3 Impaired Neurotransmission

Alteration of basal ganglia circuitry through loss of dopaminergic input to the striatum causes motor impairment (Mancini *et al.*, 2021). Non-dopaminergic systems (e.g., noradrenergic, cholinergic) are also affected, and this causes non-motor symptoms. Compensatory changes (e.g., disturbed glutamate/GABA ratio) also dysregulate neuronal circuits. While these secondary changes are clinically important, they are a result of the upstream processes of cell loss and damage (Gao *et al.*, 2022; Bej *et al.*, 2024).

2.3 Conventional pharmacological treatments for PD

Different commercially available drugs that treat the deficiency of dopamine in the substantia nigra (SN) are the most prevalent treatment for PD. These drugs improve PD symptoms in various ways temporarily, like increasing the levels of dopamine, substituting the action of dopamine, or blocking dopamine's oxidative metabolism, creating reactive oxygen species (ROS) (Emamzadeh and Surguchov, 2018). However, side effects and decreased effectiveness after long-term treatment keep their superior results in check. Therefore, the reduction of side effects and the enhancement of therapeutic effects are focal points in PD research efforts (Zhang *et al.*, 2021).

2.3.1 Levodopa (L-dopa, L-3,4-dihydroxyphenylalanine)

Levodopa (L-DOPA) has been the most effective treatment for early motor symptoms of PD thus far, even though it is not considered a cure (Bogetofte *et al.*, 2020). It is most effective against bradykinesia and rigidity but provides only moderate alleviation of tremor and may have no effect on imbalance disorders and other symptoms (Emamzadeh and Surguchov, 2018; di Biase *et al.*, 2023). Its chronic use, nevertheless, is associated with side effects such as dyskinesia, motor fluctuations, and delusions. Attempts are underway to minimize these side effects by developing new formulations (Zhang *et al.*, 2021).

Dopamine is synthesized by tyrosine hydroxylase (TH) from L-tyrosine, and its direct metabolic precursor is L-DOPA. Levodopa is decarboxylated to dopamine in dopaminergic neurons by dopa-decarboxylase. Orally administered levodopa can be prematurely decarboxylated in peripheral tissues and thereby fail to reach the CNS (Beckers *et al.*, 2022). To this end, levodopa is co-administered with peripheral DOPA decarboxylase inhibitors, i.e., carbidopa or benserazide, that do not cross the BBB. This allows unaltered levodopa to reach the CNS to function as a precursor of dopamine (Qiu *et al.*, 2025). However, serotonergic rather than dopaminergic nigrostriatal system neurons are capable of reducing levodopa to dopamine more efficiently after vesicular storage. Due to the uneven distributions of dopaminergic and serotonergic neurons in the brain, L-DOPA treatment can result in undesirable side effects, lowering its overall efficacy (Emamzadeh and Surguchov, 2018).

2.3.2 Dopamine receptor agonists

Dopamine receptor agonists are medications that exert their action at postsynaptic dopaminergic receptors and mimic the effects of dopamine. There have been five subtypes of dopamine (DA) receptors (D1–D5) identified, but it is unclear which one is responsible for antiparkinsonian action. Partial agonistic D2 agonists with activity at D1 or D3 receptors are utilized most commonly (Isaacson *et al.*, 2023; Bezard *et al.*, 2024). Drugs in this class include ropinirole hydrochloride, rotigotine, pergolide, pramipexole dihydrochloride, and apomorphine hydrochloride (Emamzadeh and Surguchov, 2018).

While effective, DA agonists have significant side effects. New delivery systems and formulations are under investigation, and novel agents such as PF-06669571, a partial D1 receptor agonist, are being investigated in clinical trials. Early pharmacodynamic results, however, have been less promising than hoped for (Zhang *et al.*, 2021). New research has recognized tavapadon (PF 06649751), a Phase 3 clinical trial-tested D1/D5-selective partial dopamine agonist, as a prospective therapeutic compound. Its pharmacological profile is different from the traditional D2-based agonists, pointing to increasing interest in the modulation of D1-like receptors as a future therapeutic target in PD (Bezard *et al.*, 2024).

2.3.3 Monoamine oxidase B (MAO-B) inhibitors

MAO-B is a mitochondrial membrane flavin enzyme that catalyzes the oxidative deamination of monoamines. Inhibition of MAO-B lowers the oxidative breakdown of dopamine, thereby increasing the concentration of dopamine in the brain and minimizing neuronal degeneration (Tan *et al.*, 2022). Novel natural MAO-B inhibitors have shown enhanced selectivity and potency compared to traditional agents. Notably, biochanin A, a benzopyrone flavonoid, is a high-affinity inhibitor of human MAO B (K $\approx$ 3.8 nM) with over 25-fold selectivity towards MAO A, and is a reversible and competitive inhibitor. These findings render it a more selective agent than the older medications such as selegiline (Zarmouh *et al.*, 2017).

Selegiline and rasagiline are MAO-B inhibitors that are being used in the management of PD. Since MAO-B participates in dopamine metabolism and ROS production in SN dopaminergic neurons, its inhibition reduces oxidative stress and neuronal death. MAO-B is also implicated in the metabolism of MPTP to the neurotoxic metabolite MPP+, which causes PD pathogenesis in intravenous drug abusers. Thus, MAO-B inhibitors are not only symptomatically beneficial but also neuroprotective (Emamzadeh and Surguchov, 2018; Naoi *et al.*, 2022)

2.3.4 Catechol-O-Methyltransferase (COMT) inhibitors

Catechol-O-methyltransferase (COMT) inhibitors tolcapone and entacapone are used adjunctively in PD to prevent levodopa conversion to 3-O-methyldopa (3 OMD), thereby extending plasma half-life and augmenting CNS bioavailability. This manifests as higher stable dopamine levels, extended "on time," reduced "off time," and allows a lower daily dose of levodopa, with improved general symptomatic control (Regensburger *et al.*, 2023).

2.4 Limitations of current drug therapies

Although current pharmacotherapies in PD are linked with extensive symptomatic benefit and enhance patients' quality of life, they fail to adequately slow the course of neurodegeneration. In addition, Parkinson's is now widely recognized to be a multisystem disorder, with non-dopaminergic involvement of systems such as serotonergic, noradrenergic, cholinergic, and autonomic networks that ultimately control poorly responsive non-motor symptoms (Erro *et al.*, 2010; Rana *et al.*, 2015). Above all, no pharmacotherapy has as yet been disease-modifying in PD; all are palliative, and patients inexorably progress. This deficiency has stimulated research on novel mechanisms, such as nutraceutical neuroprotection (Bhusal *et al.*, 2023).

3.0 PHYTOCHEMISTRY OF *ZINGIBER OFFICINALE*

Ginger, derived from the rhizome of *Zingiber officinale* Roscoe, is credited with its multifarious medicinal and therapeutic activities through a distinctive array of phytochemicals. The family Zingiberaceae, with over 1300 species and 49 genera that includes 80–90 species within the genus Zingiber, ginger is found to be generous in phenolics as well as volatile compounds contributing to its characteristic pungency and biological activity (Wei *et al.*, 2021) (Fig. 1). Its Greek, Latin, and Sanskrit name comes from the distinctive horn-shaped rhizome form (Shahrajabian *et al.*, 2019). Variable phytochemical content of ginger includes several bioactive substances such as gingerols (6-, 10-, and 12-gingerol), shogaols (6-shogaol), paradols, zingerone, gingerdiones, gingerdiols, and others such as 6-dehydrogingerols, 5-acetoxy-6-gingerol, and 3,5-diacetoxy-6-gingerdiol as illustrated in Figure 1 (Sahardi *et al.*, 2019). These molecules are primarily responsible for ginger's pharmacological action, including its anti-inflammatory, antioxidant, antiemetic, and antidiabetic properties (Kiyama, 2020).

Figure 1. Key phytochemical structures identified in ginger

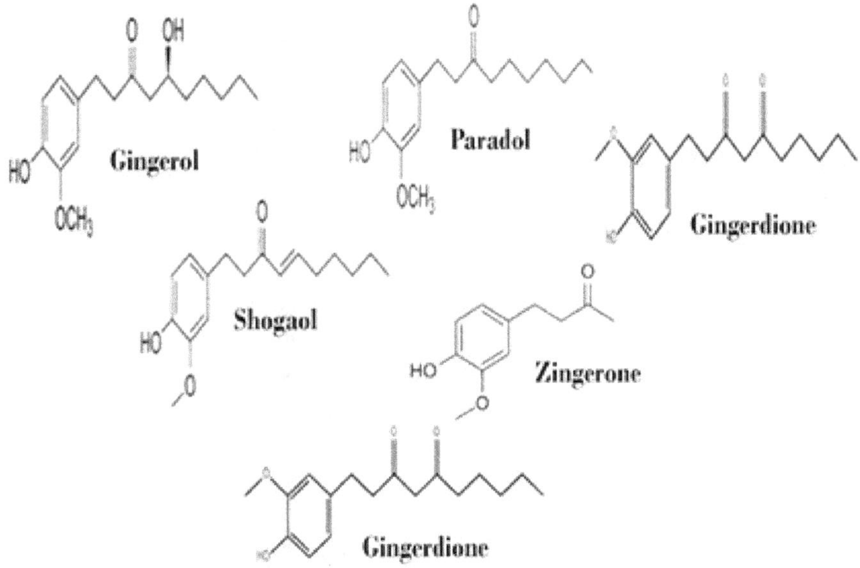

3.1 Major bioactive constituents of ginger

Ginger is a chemically rich plant that has been described to cover a wide array of bioactive compounds, ranging from terpenes, phenolic compounds, lipids, to carbohydrates (Mao *et al.*, 2019). These compounds are classified into two main categories: flavoring (aromatic) and pungent (spicy) constituents, which each play a role in the rhizome's sensory character and therapeutic potency (Choi *et al.*, 2018).

Its flavoring compounds include both sesquiterpenes and volatile oils. Volatile compounds such as borneol, zingiberene, pinene, camphene, cumene, zingiberol, and bisabolene are responsible for the classic aroma of ginger. Sesquithujene and zingiberol are also incorporated into its aroma profile (Choi *et al.*, 2018; Rajini, 2023). Its volatiles are typically more present in fresh ginger and play a vital role in its flavoring and preservation. The volatile compounds, however, are largely non-volatile phenolic compounds made up of gingerols, shogaols, paradols, zingerone, gingerdiones, gingerdiols, and capsaicin (Kiyama, 2020). Out of all of them,

6-gingerol is the most significant active compound in fresh ginger with a pungent flavor and superior antioxidant activity. Heating or drying of ginger decreases 6-gingerol to 6-shogaol, which is even more biologically active (Arcusa *et al.*, 2022). Other structurally related ginger analogs, such as 8-gingerol, 10-gingerol, 8-shogaol, and 10-shogaol, paradols and gingerdiones, are some of the contributory constituents of ginger's pharmacological profile, which encompasses anti-inflammatory, antioxidant, and anticancer effects (Arcusa *et al.*, 2022; Sirwi *et al.*, 2025).

Zingerone, another notable phenolic gingerol structural analogue, is mostly recognized for its anti-inflammatory and free-radical-scavenging activities (Angelopoulou *et al.*, 2022). The phenolic compounds have a characteristic phenolic ring and alkyl side chain configuration, permitting them to interact with lipid membranes and contribute to their antioxidant activity (Arcusa *et al.*, 2022). Particularly, 6-gingerol and 6-shogaol are studied for their neuroprotective activity, with numerous studies attributing them to the modulation of oxidative stress, inflammation, and apoptosis pathways (Mairuae *et al.*, 2024). Such mechanisms are relevant to the prevention and management of neurodegenerative disease. Their metabolites, like 6-gingerdione, gingerdiols, and 6-paradol, also show considerable biological activity, which substantiates the therapeutic relevance of ginger phytochemical complexity (Arcusa *et al.*, 2022)

3.2 Pharmacokinetics and bioavailability

The bioactive constituents of ginger, including 6-gingerol and 6-shogaol, have moderate bioavailability after oral administration. Their absorption is rapid, and peak plasma levels are usually reached within 1 to 3 hours (Songvut *et al.*, 2024). These compounds, however, are subject to extensive metabolism. Some major metabolic pathways include the reduction of ketones, which transforms gingerols to gingerdiols, and various conjugation reactions with glucuronides, sulfates, and cysteine adducts (Nakazawa and Ohsawa, 2002; Zhang *et al.*, 2022). Studies have indicated that a large part of these compounds is metabolized; for example, nearly 30% of 6-gingerol is metabolized to gingerdiols, and over 90% of 6-shogaol is metabolized to downstream metabolites (Zhang *et al.*, 2022).

The half-lives of ginger's active constituents and their metabolites are relatively short, ranging from around 0.6 to 2.4 hours, resulting in their extensive clearance from the system within a few hours (Zhang *et al.*, 2022). Notably, some research indicates that chronic ginger administration can result in increased systemic exposure, perhaps reflecting an accumulation or induction effect for weeks. However, overall oral bioavailability of these compounds is limited by first-pass metabolism. To overcome this hurdle and enhance systemic delivery, several formulation approaches are under exploration, including the utilization of nanoparticles and extracts standardized to high gingerol content (Zhang *et al.*, 2022; Mukkavilli *et al.*, 2017; Zhang *et al.*, 2016).

3.3 Safety profile and toxicological considerations

Ginger is usually ingested through food and is usually harmless when consumed in food amounts. It has been attested by various studies as well as the FDA's rating as "Generally Recognized As Safe" (GRAS) (Sirwi *et al.*, 2025). Ginger extracts are usually used in clinical studies at doses of 1–3 g/day with no side effects (Paudel *et al.*, 2025). At higher doses, there can be mild side effects like nausea or heartburn. It must also be noted that ginger possesses pharmacological effects, especially on drug metabolism and the risk of bleeding. It has been shown that gingerols can inhibit cytochrome P450 enzymes (CYP2C9 and CYP3A4), which can change the clearance of other drugs from the body (Aregawi and Zoltan, 2025; Li *et al.*, 2013). Also, ginger was found to have mild antiplatelet effects in laboratory and several clinical trials, suggesting a possible influence on bleeding or interaction with the blood-thinning activity. However, human evidence is inconsistent; some trials are helpful, others not at all, with effects apparently larger with higher doses (Sirwi *et al.*, 2025; Marx *et al.*, 2015). Therefore, although ginger is usually acceptable, patients on several medicines, such as the elderly PD patient on both levodopa and anticoagulants, should use it carefully. In animal research, there was no indication of organ or genetic toxicity at therapeutic dose levels (Sirwi *et al.*, 2025).

4. MECHANISTIC INSIGHTS INTO GINGER'S NEUROPROTECTIVE ACTIONS

4.1. Anti-inflammatory properties

Ginger and its bioactive compounds have demonstrated significant anti-inflammatory and neuroprotective effects in various models of PD. 6-shogaol, a constituent of ginger, has been reported to suppress both astrogliosis and microgliosis in mouse models of PD (Sapkota *et al.*, 2019). This compound also upregulates the expression of neurotrophic factors like nerve growth factor (NGF) and synaptic proteins and downregulates inflammatory mediators like TNF-α, NO, COX-2, and iNOS in the substantia nigra and striatum, thereby conferring protection on dopaminergic neurons (Attallah *et al.*, 2025). Further, 6-shogaol inhibits apoptotic pathways and ROS accumulation and promotes the nuclear translocation of Nrf2, thereby preventing 6-OHDA-induced neurotoxicity in PC12 cells. Zingerone also restores the activity of antioxidant enzymes such as catalase (CAT), superoxide dismutase (SOD), and glutathione peroxidase (GPx) in 6-OHDA-induced PD mouse models (Choi *et al.*, 2018).

Another active constituent of ginger, zingerone, also exhibits potent antioxidative and antiparkinsonian properties. It not only mitigates the loss of dopamine and its metabolites (DOPAC and HVA) but also enhances free radical scavenging activities, including hydroxyl and superoxide radical elimination (Sahardi *et al.*, 2019). In MPTP-induced models of PD, the ginger extract significantly attenuated motor defects, dopaminergic neuronal degeneration, and striatal dopamine depletion. Both 6-shogaol and zingerone have been found to inhibit gliosis and neuroinflammation by inhibiting pro-inflammatory cytokines and chemokines (Choi *et al.*, 2018). Beyond the neurodegenerative context, the anti-inflammatory activity of ginger is observed in a range of other conditions, including gout and muscle pain. 6-Shogaol has been used as a therapeutic agent for rheumatic disease, and 6-gingerol possesses analgesic and anti-inflammatory properties. In a double-blind, placebo-controlled trial, daily ingestion of 2 g of raw or cooked ginger for 11 days was shown to effectively reduce exercise-induced muscle pain by approximately 25%, with both types having similar effects (Black *et al.*, 2010)

4.2 Antioxidant properties

Ginger, being a dense source of natural antioxidants, exhibits excellent antioxidant activity, particularly when extraction is conducted using alcohol-based solvents. The evidence collectively demonstrates that alcohol-based solvents (particularly ethanol and methanol) extract significantly more antioxidant components from ginger than water-based extraction. This includes a higher yield of phenolics/flavonoids and stronger radical scavenging activity and reducing power (Mustafa and Chin, 2023). This is because the bioactive compounds in ginger contain hydroxyl groups and solubilizing side chains. Ginger extract is demonstrated to induce the activity of key antioxidant enzymes (glutathione peroxidase (GPx), catalase (CAT), and superoxide dismutase (SOD)) and enhance the removal of accumulated ROS, including superoxide radicals and hydrogen peroxide, in a hepatoma cell line (Sahardi *et al.*, 2019). Interestingly, ginger extract at concentrations of 200–500 µg/mL significantly reduced SOD, CAT, and GPx activity in the same cell model, pointing to its regulatory role in antioxidant response. Antioxidant activity of ginger has also been associated with improved glucose transport and higher glucose tolerance, which can translate to reduced insulin resistance in diabetic conditions (Sahardi *et al.*, 2019; Roufogalis, 2014).

4.3 Modulation of cell survival pathways

Ginger and its bioactive compounds, including 6-gingerol, 6-shogaol, paradol, and zingerone, cause neuronal survival through a variety of intracellular signaling mechanisms. They are dominated by the PI3K/Akt pathway, which promotes cell survival and suppresses apoptosis. In *in vitro* and *in vivo* systems, extracts of ginger modulate PI3K and phosphorylated Akt, leading to upregulation of the anti-apoptotic Bcl-2 protein and downregulation of caspase-3, a major effector of intrinsic apoptosis (Tang *et al.*, 2022; Mairuae *et al.*, 2024). In the subarachnoid hemorrhage model, 6-gingerol inhibited the inflammasome adaptor GBP2, thereby activating PI3K/Akt signaling, reducing neuronal loss, and improving neurological outcome (Tang *et al.*, 2022). Ginger also stimulates AMPK and its downstream target PGC-1α, both key to mitochondrial biogenesis and energy homeostasis. Activation of AMPK/PGC-1α maintains mitochondrial integrity and reverses energy stress in neurons (Angelopoulou *et al.*, 2022; Sirwi *et al.*, 2025). Ginger also influences neurotrophic signaling.

In aged mice, ginger extract augmented hippocampal NGF and BDNF levels, stimulated downstream ERK/CREB phosphorylation, increased synaptic proteins (e.g., synaptophysin, PSD-95), and improved cognitive function (Lim *et al.*, 2014). In diabetic rats, ginger elevated hippocampal BDNF mRNA and Ki-67 expression, a neurogenesis marker, and reduced inflammatory cytokines and caspase-3 (ALmohaimeed *et al.*, 2021). Notably, in combined treatments (e.g., cinnamon and ginger), ginger alone had significant impacts on BDNF expression and neuroinflammation (ALmohaimeed *et al.*, 2021). Ginger is found to have neuroprotective effects by suppressing apoptosis via PI3K/Akt–Bcl-2 signaling, enhancing mitochondrial function via AMPK/PGC-1α, and promoting synaptic plasticity and neurogenesis via ERK/CREB–BDNF/NGF signaling (Angelopoulou *et al.*, 2022; Sirwi *et al.*, 2025; Mairuae *et al.*, 2024; Lim *et al.*, 2014). These multifaceted mechanisms describe how ginger is a promising neurotherapeutic agent, especially for oxidative or inflammatory neurodegenerative diseases.

4.4 Maintenance of mitochondrial integrity and function

Ginger also preserves mitochondrial integrity in neurons, an important component of Parkinson's disease pathology. *In vitro* and animal data suggest that ginger components enhance mitochondrial antioxidant defense and biogenesis. Ginger extract pre-treatment dramatically increased neuronal antioxidant enzyme expression (SOD, catalase, glutathione peroxidases) and, simultaneously, reduced reactive oxygen species, lipid peroxidation, and the pro-apoptotic Bax/Bcl-2 ratio (Angelopoulou *et al.*, 2022; Famurewa *et al.*, 2025). Ginger extract in a model inhibited H_2O_2-induced mitochondrial membrane potential loss, practically preserving mitochondrial electrochemical gradient, as well as inhibition of ROS production. Through augmentation of endogenous antioxidants and attenuation of oxidative stress, ginger makes mitochondria stable against PD-related insults (Famurewa *et al.*, 2025).

Ginger's effects extend to mitochondrial biogenesis and bioenergetics. Oral ginger extract (2 g/kg) in mice increased systemic oxygen consumption and body temperature and elevated muscle and liver mitochondrial DNA copy number, which is a marker for new mitochondria. This treatment enhanced the content of electron transport chain complexes and oxidative phosphorylation (OXPHOS) proteins (Deng *et al.*, 2019; Deng *et al.*, 2022). Mechanistically, such effects were linked to activation of the AMPK–PGC-1α pathway: treatment with ginger extract led to phosphorylation of AMPK and upregulation of PGC-1α (a master regulator of mitochondrial biogenesis). In cells in culture, 6-gingerol also enhanced mitochondrial mass, mitochondrial DNA content, and ATP production. Ginger and its components thus trigger mitochondrial renewal via AMPK–PGC-1α signaling. The result is a boost in the number of functional mitochondria to meet the energy needs of neurons (Deng *et al.*, 2019).

Through synergizing these activities, ginger maintains neuronal mitochondrial integrity within PD models. It inhibits mitochondrial collapse and intrinsic apoptosis (via Bcl-2 stabilization) (Mairuae *et al.*, 2024), and further generates new mitochondria via PGC-1α. Ginger, for example, stimulates TFAM (mitochondrial transcription factor A) and other downstream markers of biogenesis (Angelopoulou *et al.*, 2022). Concurrently, antioxidant actions (upregulated SOD/CAT) protect mitochondrial membranes from oxidative damage (Famurewa *et al.*, 2025).

Figure 2. Converging mechanisms of ginger neuroprotection in PD

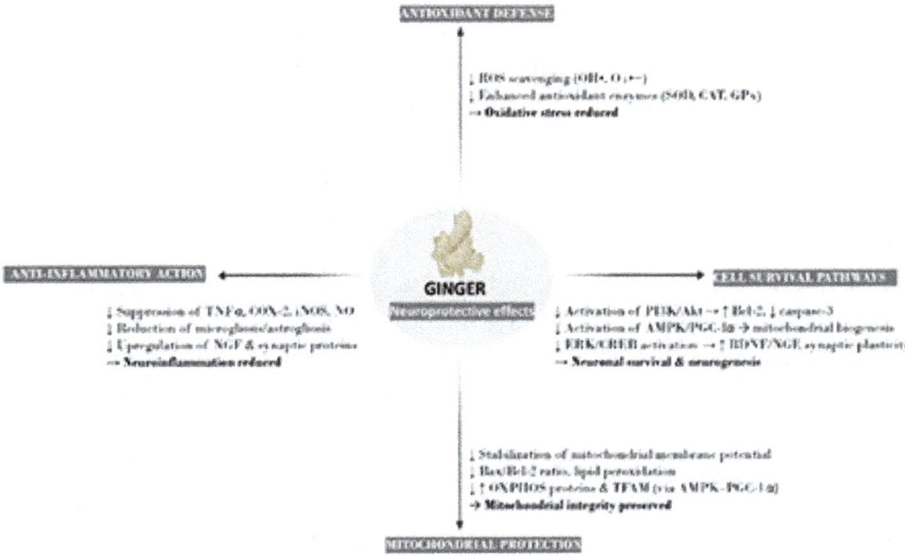

Ginger offers neuroprotection in PD by converging mechanisms (Figure 2.0): it inhibits neuroinflammation by downregulating TNF-α, COX-2, iNOS, and NO but upregulating neurotrophic and synaptic proteins (Sapkota *et al.*, 2019; Attallah *et al.*, 2025). It enhances antioxidant defense mechanisms by scavenging reactive oxygen species and enhancing the activity of SOD, CAT, and GPx (Choi *et al.*, 2018; Sahardi *et al.*, 2019; Mustafa and Chin, 2023). Neuroprotection is further supported by PI3K/Akt–Bcl-2, AMPK/PGC-1α, and ERK/CREB signaling pathways, favoring anti-apoptosis, mitochondrial biogenesis, and synaptic plasticity (Tang *et al.*, 2022; Mairuae *et al.*, 2024; Lim *et al.*, 2014). Moreover, mitochondrial stability is ensured by stabilized membrane potential, reduced Bax/Bcl-2 ratio, and enhanced OXPHOS and biogenesis markers (Deng *et al.*, 2019; Famurewa *et al.*, 2025). Overall, these processes enhance dopaminergic survival and functional benefits in PD models.

5. PRECLINICAL EVIDENCE: GINGER IN PD MODELS

Several animal models have demonstrated ginger's neuroprotective efficacy in PD. For example, in neurotoxin-exposed rodents, intestinal infections, or genetic α-syn seeds, ginger compounds consistently improved motor function and neuronal survival. In rotenone-treated PD rats and MPTP mice, ginger extracts or compounds given inhibited bradykinesia and balance deficits, with nigral dopaminergic neurons preserved (Sirwi *et al.*, 2025; Huh *et al.*, 2023). In a novel Proteus mirabilis gut-brain model, oral 6-shogaol or ginger inhibited enteric α-syn aggregation and intestinal inflammation, subsequently inhibiting the classical cascade of nigral α-synucleinopathy (Huh *et al.*, 2023). These preclinical observations are in accord with the multitarget pharmacology of ginger, i.e., the *in vivo* actions of ginger in PD models encompass the inhibition of neuroinflammation, oxidative stress, and gut permeability, as well as facilitating dopamine transmission and mitochondrial activity (Eugene *et al.*, 2023).

Furthermore, ginger has also been tested against traditional PD treatments in animal models. Notably, 6-paradol (a ginger analog) provided similar motor improvement and neurochemical recovery to L-dopa/carbidopa in rotenone-lesioned rats (Sirwi *et al.*, 2025). Co-administration of 6-shogaol with L-dopa in MPTP mice showed improvement in motor and non-motor function as well as the preservation of dopaminergic neurons – improvements which L-dopa alone was unable to achieve (Kim *et al.*, 2024). Combined, these preclinical findings cast ginger as a potential complementary agent: not only does it replicate some effectiveness of conventional treatments but also acts against PD pathology (inflammation, α-synucleinopathy) that pharmacological agents against the dopaminergic system do not (Sirwi *et al.*, 2025; Kim *et al.*, 2024).

5.1 Rotenone-induced PD rat models

Rotenone, a mitochondrial complex I inhibitor, causes PD-like degeneration in rodents. Ginger components exhibit potent protection in this model. Oral 6-shogaol (10–20 mg/kg) was reported to significantly rescue rotenone-induced motor impairments: treated rats did better on rotarod and grasping tests (increased fall latency and greater grip strength) than vehicle-treated rotenone rats (Rafeeq *et al.*, 2024). Biochemically, 6-shogaol blocked rotenone's oxidant activities; it elevated brain glutathione, SOD, and catalase levels and lowered malondialdehyde (MDA) (Afzal *et al.*, 2021). Interestingly, 6-shogaol reversed dopamine transmission it prevented rotenone-increased monoamine oxidase-B (MAO-B) activity and preserved striatal dopamine and GABA levels. Such molecular changes were linked to neuroprotection: histology demonstrated elevated populations of remaining TH-positive neurons in ginger-treated rats (Rafeeq *et al.*, 2024). In concordance, 6-Paradol improved rotenone-induced dysfunction, reversing motor performance (open-field, rotarod, grip strength) and preserving nigrostriatal TH expression. Mechanistically, it suppressed neuroinflammation (HMGB1, TLR4, NF-κB p65, TNF-α), inhibited TNF-α–driven necroptosis (TNFR1, RIPK1/3, MLKL), and boosted mitochondrial biogenesis (PPARγ, PGC-1α, TFAM) with improved redox state (↑glutathione,

↓MDA). Its neuroprotective efficacy was similar to that of L-DOPA/carbidopa (Sirwi *et al.*, 2025).

5.2 Proteus mirabilis-induced PD mouse models

Recent evidence implicates gut bacteria (e.g., *Proteus mirabilis*) in triggering Parkinson-like pathology via the gut-brain axis. In a novel mouse model, oral gavage with *P. mirabilis* induced intestinal barrier compromise, enteric α-syn accumulation, and subsequent nigral α-syn pathology and motor deficit (Lei *et al.*, 2021). Ginger extract and its bioactive 6-shogaol were evaluated in the P. mirabilis mouse model. Daily treatment prevented infection-induced motor deficits, and treated mice behaved normally in open-field, pole-climb, and rotarod tests. Neurohistological analysis showed sparing of nigral dopaminergic neurons (higher TH-positive counts) and reduced microglial activation versus infected controls (Huh *et al.*, 2023). The efficacy of ginger was mediated by gut protection: 6-shogaol restored tight junction proteins (occludin, ZO-1), suppressed *P. mirabilis*–induced TLR4/TNF-α signaling, and reduced intestinal α-syn accumulation. This confined α-syn propagated to the brain, attenuated neuroinflammation (TNF-α, IL-1β), and preserved dopaminergic integrity, effectively disrupting the gut–brain PD axis (Huh *et al.*, 2023; Huh *et al.*, 2020).

5.3 Behavioral and histological improvements

Across PD models, ginger treatment results in clear functional and anatomical improvements. Behaviorally, ginger-treated animals have improved motor function compared to untreated PD models. For example, 6-paradol-treated rotenone rats exhibited improved grip strength and rotarod times relative to controls (Sirwi *et al.*, 2025). Ginger-fed P. mirabilis mice also had preserved locomotion and coordination (Huh *et al.*, 2023). Together with motor tests, gingerol-containing ginger supplement significantly decreased depression- and anxiety-like behavior in a diabetic neuropathy rat model, as assessed using open-field anxiety parameters and depressive behavior tests, and also minimized pain sensitivity, gut microbiome structure, and neuroimmune markers in the spinal cord and colon (Shen *et al.*, 2024). In addition, the combination of ginger and cinnamon demonstrated significant antidepressant-like behavior in diabetic rats, which was attributed to reduced hippocampal pro-inflammatory cytokines (IL-6, TNF-α, IL-1β), increased BDNF expression, and neuroprotective hippocampal morphological changes (ALmohaimeed *et al.*, 2021).

Histologically, the therapeutic advantages of ginger were in agreement with neuronal protection. In rotenone rats, 6-shogaol and 6-paradol treatments both resulted in substantially higher numbers of TH-positive neurons and fibers in the substantia nigra and striatum than in toxin-only rats (Sirwi *et al.*, 2025). In the gut-brain model, ginger prevented enteric dopaminergic nerve fibers and brain dopaminergic neurons from loss (Huh *et al.*, 2023). Microglial (e.g., Iba1, CD11b) markers were reduced significantly by ginger, indicating dampened neuroinflammation. Both glial and inflammatory (GFAP, TNF-α) markers and anti-apoptotic markers (Bcl-2) were reduced and elevated, respectively, in ginger-treated PD models. Thus, the functional recovery with ginger is on par with robust neuroprotection: treated animals have much less dopaminergic neuron loss and less severe histopathology than untreated PD model animals (Sirwi *et al.*, 2025; Huh *et al.*, 2023).

5.4 Comparison with conventional therapies in animal studies

In rodent models, ginger extracts usually behave as well as or in synergy with standard PD treatment. Interestingly, 6-paradol's neurobehavioral action was comparable to L-DOPA/carbidopa in rotenone rats. For instance, improvement of rotarod and grip strength with 6-paradol was statistically similar to that of L-DOPA. In like manner, biochemical recovery (increased GSH, reduced MDA) was similar to that of L-DOPA's action (Sirwi *et al.*, 2025; Alam and Schmidt, 2002).

Most importantly, ginger may augment dopamine treatments by alleviating the pathophysiology not managed by levodopa alone. In an MPTP mouse model, L-DOPA treatment lessened motor symptoms (as predicted) but was unable to prevent neuroinflammation or loss of nigral neurons (Aktaş *et al.*, 2025; Church, 2021). In contrast, co-treatment with 6-shogaol in combination with L-DOPA not only improved motor and non-motor signs but also significantly preserved dopaminergic neurons as well as reduced inflammatory cytokines (Kim *et al.*, 2024). In other words, ginger + L-DOPA treated both pathology and symptoms, but not L-DOPA alone.

These findings suggest that ginger-derived compounds could serve as an adjunctive therapy to the conventional treatment. They could allow reduced doses of dopaminergic drugs (minimizing side effects), or they could prevent the neurons from degenerating and modulate non-dopaminergic pathways (inflammation, oxidative stress) not altered by levodopa. Overall, animal studies show that ginger efficacy is as good as or better than existing therapies for improving PD phenotypes, and it uniquely inhibits neurodegeneration (Sirwi et al., 2025; Kim et al., 2024).

5.5 Comparative efficacy of ginger and other neuroprotective herbs

Compared to other well-studied neuroprotective herbs, curcumin/turmeric, *Panax ginseng*, ashwagandha, Bacopa, and green-tea catechins, for example, ginger shares overlapping antioxidant and anti-inflammatory mechanisms with some unique advantages (Ayustaningwarno *et al.*, 2024; Li *et al.*, 2024). The bioactive phenolics of ginger, 6-gingerol and 6-shogaol, activate Nrf2-dependent defenses and suppress NF-κB signaling, similarly to curcumin and EGCG (Ayustaningwarno *et al.*, 2024; Li *et al.*, 2024). For example, one of the most effective free-radical scavengers, EGCG, has been shown to dampen neuroinflammation (Li *et al.*, 2024), while ashwagandha's withanolides induce Nrf2 signaling and anti-apoptotic kinases (Guo and Rezaei, 2024). These herbs, in other words, share modes of action through which they reduce oxidative stress, inflammation, and cell death via common molecular targets (Ayustaningwarno *et al.*, 2024; Li *et al.*, 2024; Guo and Rezaei, 2024).

While all these herbs act via somewhat similar pathways, the most distinctive bioactive components of ginger include its pungent phenolics, such as gingerols (e.g., 6-gingerol) and shogaols (e.g., 6-shogaol), which give rise to unique metabolites and pharmacological effects not commonly seen in other herbs. Recent preclinical and mechanistic studies have emphasized ginger among other leading neuroprotective botanicals given its capacity for modulating neuroinflammation, promoting neurotrophic factors, and reducing oxidative stress (Arcusa *et al.*, 2022; Ayustaningwarno *et al.*, 2024; Tzani *et al.*, 2021). In various *in vitro* studies, ginger extract exhibited anti-inflammatory activity superior to that of other herb extracts-for example, rosemary extract (Justo *et al.*, 2015).

In practice, the active compounds present in ginger are well absorbed, efficiently metabolized, mainly as glucuronide or sulfate conjugates, and generally well tolerated, thus providing an excellent safety profile to ginger (Angelopoulou *et al.*, 2022; Ayustaningwarno *et al.*, 2024; Nakamura *et al.*, 2025; Songvut *et al.*, 2024). On the other hand, curcumin has notoriously poor oral bioavailability, which requires specific formulations to reach the same systemic exposure (Songvut *et al.*, 2024; Dei Cas and Ghidoni, 2019). Clinical evidence supporting the cognitive benefits of ginger includes a 12-week study where 100 mg/day of ginger extract improved attention and cognition in healthy adults without adverse effects (Nakamura *et al.*, 2025). Similarly, *Ginseng ginsenosides* and *Bacopa bacosides* have clinical evidence supporting their use for enhancing memory and cognition (Valotto *et al.*, 2024). Green tea catechins also support brain health (Afzal *et al.*, 2022).

Overall, ginger exerts potent neuroprotection comparable to a number of neuroprotective botanicals, due in part to its broad-based antioxidant and anti-inflammatory action. Native compounds are rapidly metabolized, but central delivery can be improved via advanced formulations, such as nanoemulsions (Angelopoulou *et al.*, 2022; Ayustaningwarno *et al.*, 2024; Nakamura *et al.*, 2025; Songvut *et al.*, 2024). To sum, ginger is neither categorically "better" nor weaker than all other herbs; rather, its broad, multitarget antioxidant/anti-inflammatory activity, combined with clinical evidence of cognitive support, a unique profile of bioactive phenolics, and an exemplary safety record, makes it a singularly compelling neuroprotective herb that complements the benefits offered by turmeric, ginseng, ashwagandha, Bacopa, green tea, and several other botanicals.

6. EMERGING CLINICAL EVIDENCE AND GAPS

6.1 Ginger in mild cognitive impairment and related disorders

Although no direct clinical trials of ginger in PD exist, other studies have examined ginger for cognitive activity. In preclinical models of memory impairment, ginger is promising. For example, in mice with scopolamine-induced amnesia, dried ginger extract enhanced spatial and short-term memory, with concomitant increases in hippocampal NGF and ERK/CREB signaling (Lim *et al.*, 2024). In diabetic rats (cognitive impairment), ginger treatment enhanced hippocampal BDNF levels and reversed neuronal apoptosis (Talebi *et al.*, 2021). Ginger has also been shown to be effective in Alzheimer's disease models: it enhanced memory performance and reduced amyloid pathology in rodent models, with suggestions of cognitive benefit (Lim *et al.*, 2016).

Human data are limited. Available data suggest ginger may improve specific higher cognitive function in middle-aged and older adults (e.g., better working memory performance and neurophysiological measures), but sample sizes are small and study durations are short. One systematic review cited that ginger's bioactives have "great potency for improving and abrogating memory dysfunctions" based on animal and early clinical findings. (Saenghong *et al.*, 2012; Shaukat *et al.*, 2023). However, robust RCTs in mild cognitive impairment (MCI), Alzheimer's, or other dementias are few. Indeed, no clinical trial has experimentally investigated ginger in PD-associated cognitive impairment yet. Thus, while ginger is theoretically beneficial to brain aging and cognitive impairment, evidence in PD or MCI conditions is still preliminary and inconclusive (Alexopoulos *et al.*, 2025; Mecocci and Polidori, 2012).

6.2 Limitations: Lack of direct clinical trials in PD

One major deficit is the absence of clinical trials of ginger in PD patients. All the current evidence about ginger's neuroprotection in PD comes from cell and animal studies (Angelopoulou *et al.*, 2022). Therefore, its safety and efficacy in human PD, including its best dosing, form, and interaction with PD medication, are unknown. Despite optimistic lab findings, ginger is "definitely not a curative PD treatment currently" (Angelopoulou *et al.*, 2022; Arcusa *et al.*, 2022). While there are optimistic preclinical findings on the neuroprotective action of ginger in PD models, clinical evidence within humans, specifically patients with PD, MCI, or dementia, is nonexistent or scarce. This variation calls for well-conducted clinical trials to determine ginger's efficacy, safety, dose, formulation, and interaction with standard PD therapy. (Saenghong *et al.*, 2012; Schepici *et al.*, 2021).

6.3 Safety and potential herb-drug interactions

Ginger is tolerable and has a good safety margin. Ginger is classified as a "generally recognized as safe" (GRAS) herb by the U.S. FDA (Belsito *et al.*, 2021). The animal toxicity data corroborate that: When 27 normal volunteers received a one-time oral dose of 100 mg to 2 g of ginger, mild gastrointestinal discomfort was the most common adverse effect (Bodagh *et al.*, 2018). In humans, ginger side effects (even at high doses) are usually mild, the most common being gastrointestinal (heartburn, nausea) (Choi *et al.*, 2022).

But caution is warranted as ginger does have a pharmacologic effect. Ginger inhibits thromboxane synthesis and prolongs bleeding time. Therefore, co-administration with anticoagulant or antiplatelet agents (e.g., warfarin, aspirin) could, in theory, increase the risk of bleeding (Martins *et al.*, 2025; Abebe, 2019). Ginger inhibits P-glycoprotein too: it increases levels of P-gp (p-glycoprotein) substrates such as digoxin or some analgesics (e.g., morphine) (Zhang and Lim, 2008). In the clinic, these interactions are not adequately studied in PD patients, although caution is advised if patients are taking anticoagulants or some central nervous system drugs. Ginger's mild glucose-lowering and hypotensive effects might interact with antidiabetic or antihypertensive drugs, so monitoring is indicated (Ebrahimzadeh *et al.*, 2022).

Generally, ginger has a good safety profile and is not responsible for many severe dangers. Bleeding and metabolic interactions mentioned above are the most important to consider. Otherwise, ginger is a safe food supplement, but any patient with PD should get approval from a doctor (especially to review medications) before starting routine ginger or concentrated ginger supplements.

7. CONCLUSION AND FUTURE DIRECTIONS

Ginger and its bioactive phenolics offer a promising, multitarget neuroprotective strategy to PD. Preclinical evidence illustrates that ginger scavenges free radicals, fortifies antioxidant defenses, mitigates neuroinflammation, and stabilizes mitochondrial integrity, mechanistically converging on core PD pathologies. In diverse animal models (including rotenone and MPTP models), ginger-derived compounds rescued dopaminergic neurons, diminished α-synuclein toxicity, and improved both motor and non-motor symptoms. These findings, coupled with ginger's established safety in humans, form the basis of its potential as an adjunct to conventional PD therapy.

However, adequately controlled clinical trials in PD populations are essential to determine efficacy, safety, and tolerability in the real-world setting. Future trials should utilize standardized extracts and clearly defined dosing guidelines to enable reproducibility and regulatory evaluation. With its complementary mechanisms of action, ginger is also a potential candidate for combination therapy with existing PD medications, but herb–drug interaction studies are warranted. Formulation and regulatory factors, such as bioavailability, stability, and delivery systems, must also be optimized to maximize clinical translation. In the meantime, while caution is warranted, clinicians and patients should remain aware of ginger's emerging therapeutic benefits. In the spirit of a “spice jar” therapy, this humble root may yet have something to offer our therapeutic options against PD.

REFERENCES

Abebe, W. (2019). Review of herbal medications with the potential to cause bleeding: Dental implications, and risk prediction and prevention avenues. *The EPMA Journal, 10*(1), 51–64. DOI: 10.1007/s13167-018-0158-2 PMID: 30984314

Afzal, M., Kazmi, I., Quazi, A. M., Khan, S. A., Zafar, A., Al-Abbasi, F. A., Imam, F., Alharbi, K. S., Alzarea, S. I., & Yadav, N. (2021). 6-Shogaol attenuates traumatic brain injury-induced anxiety/depression-like behavior via inhibition of oxidative stress-influenced expressions of inflammatory mediators TNF-α, IL-1β, and BDNF: Insight into the mechanism. *ACS Omega, 7*(1), 140–148. DOI: 10.1021/acsomega.1c04155 PMID: 35036685

Afzal, O., Dalhat, M. H., Altamimi, A. S. A., Rasool, R., Alzarea, S. I., Almalki, W. H., Murtaza, B. N., Iftikhar, S., Nadeem, S., Nadeem, M. S., & Kazmi, I. (2022). Green Tea Catechins Attenuate Neurodegenerative Diseases and Cognitive Deficits. *Molecules (Basel, Switzerland), 27*(21), 7604. DOI: 10.3390/molecules27217604 PMID: 36364431

Aktaş, E., Hanağası, H. A., & Özgentürk, N. Ö. (2025). Levodopa and Plant-Derived Bioactive Compounds in Parkinson's Disease: Mechanisms, Efficacy, and Future Perspectives. *CNS Neuroscience & Therapeutics, 31*(8), e70540. DOI: 10.1111/cns.70540 PMID: 40808332

Alam, M., & Schmidt, W. J. (2002). Rotenone destroys dopaminergic neurons and induces parkinsonian symptoms in rats. *Behavioural Brain Research, 136*(1), 317–324. DOI: 10.1016/S0166-4328(02)00180-8 PMID: 12385818

Alexopoulos, P., Felemegkas, P., Arampatzi, X., Billis, E., Dimakopoulou, E., Economou, P., Dimakopoulos, G. A., Exarchos, T. P., Frounta, M., Giannakopoulou, P., Kalaitzi, K., Koula, M.-L., Nastou, E., Skondra, M., Sakka, P., Kalligerou, F., Skarmeas, N., Tsatali, M., Krommyda, M., & Lyketsos, C. (2025). Pilot study of the Greek Interventional Geriatric Initiative to Prevent Cognitive Impairment and Disability in individuals with subjective cognitive decline: Paving the way towards brain health clinics in Greece. *Frontiers in Psychiatry, 16*, 1514227. DOI: 10.3389/fpsyt.2025.1514227 PMID: 40171308

ALmohaimeed, H. M., Mohammedsaleh, Z. M., Batawi, A. H., Balgoon, M. J., Ramadan, O. I., Baz, H. A., Al Jaouni, S., & Ayuob, N. N.ALmohaimeed. (2021). Synergistic Anti-inflammatory and Neuroprotective Effects of Cinnamomum cassia and Z ingiber officinale Alleviate Diabetes-Induced Hippocampal Changes in Male Albino Rats: Structural and Molecular Evidence. *Frontiers in Cell and Developmental Biology, 9*, 727049. DOI: 10.3389/fcell.2021.727049 PMID: 34568337

Angelopoulou, E., Paudel, Y. N., Papageorgiou, S. G., & Piperi, C. (2022). Elucidating the Beneficial Effects of Ginger (*Zingiber officinale* Roscoe) in Parkinson's Disease. *ACS Pharmacology & Translational Science*, *5*(10), 838–848. DOI: 10.1021/acsptsci.2c00104 PMID: 36268117

Arcusa, R., Villaño, D., Marhuenda, J., Cano, M., Cerdà, B., & Zafrilla, P. (2022). Potential Role of Ginger (*Zingiber officinale* Roscoe) in the Prevention of Neurodegenerative Diseases. *Frontiers in Nutrition*, *9*, 809621. DOI: 10.3389/fnut.2022.809621 PMID: 35369082

Aregawi, L. G., & Zoltan, C. (2025). Evaluation of Adverse Effects and Tolerability of Dietary Ginger Supplementation in Patients With Functional Dyspepsia. *Current Therapeutic Research, Clinical and Experimental*, *102*, 100792. DOI: 10.1016/j.curtheres.2025.100792 PMID: 40474983

. Attallah, K. A., El-Dessouki, A. M., Abd-Elmawla, M. A., Ghaiad, H. R., Abo-Elghiet, F., Mustafa, A. M., ... & Elosaily, H. (2025). The therapeutic potential of naturally occurring 6-shogaol: an updated comprehensive review. *Inflammopharmacology*.

Ayustaningwarno, F., Anjani, G., Ayu, A. M., & Fogliano, V. (2024). A critical review of Ginger's (Zingiber officinale) antioxidant, anti-inflammatory, and immunomodulatory activities. *Frontiers in Nutrition*, *11*, 1364836. DOI: 10.3389/fnut.2024.1364836 PMID: 38903613

Balakrishnan, R., Azam, S., Cho, D. Y., Su-Kim, I., & Choi, D. K. (2021). Natural Phytochemicals as Novel Therapeutic Strategies to prevent and Treat Parkinson's disease: Current Knowledge and Future Perspectives. *Oxidative Medicine and Cellular Longevity*, *2021*(1), 2021. DOI: 10.1155/2021/6680935 PMID: 34122727

Ball, N., Teo, W. P., Chandra, S., & Chapman, J. (2019). Parkinson's disease and the environment. *Frontiers in Neurology*, *10*, 218. DOI: 10.3389/fneur.2019.00218 PMID: 30941085

Beckers, M., Bloem, B. R., & Verbeek, M. M. (2022). Mechanisms of peripheral levodopa resistance in Parkinson's disease. *npj. Parkinson's Disease*, *8*(1), 56. PMID: 35546556

Bej, E., Cesare, P., Volpe, A. R., d'Angelo, M., & Castelli, V. (2024). Oxidative stress and neurodegeneration: Insights and therapeutic strategies for Parkinson's disease. *Neurology International*, *16*(3), 502–517. DOI: 10.3390/neurolint16030037 PMID: 38804477

. Belsito, M. D., Cohen, D. E., Klaassen, C. D., Liebler, D. C., Peterson, L. A., Shank, R. C., ... & Snyder, P. W. (2021). Safety Assessment of Zingiber officinale (Ginger)–Derived Ingredients as Used in Cosmetics.

Bezard, E., Gray, D., Kozak, R., Leoni, M., Combs, C., & Duvvuri, S. (2024). Rationale and development of tavapadon, a D1/D5-selective partial dopamine agonist for the treatment of Parkinson's disease. *CNS & Neurological Disorders - Drug Targets*, *23*(4), 476–487. DOI: 10.2174/1871527322666230331121028 PMID: 36999711

Bhusal, C. K., Uti, D. E., Mukherjee, D., Alqahtani, T., Alqahtani, S., Bhattacharya, A., & Akash, S. (2023). Unveiling Nature's potential: Promising natural compounds in Parkinson's disease management. *Parkinsonism & Related Disorders*, *115*, 105799. DOI: 10.1016/j.parkreldis.2023.105799 PMID: 37633805

Black, C. D., Herring, M. P., Hurley, D. J., & O'Connor, P. J. (2010). Ginger (Zingiber officinale) reduces muscle pain caused by eccentric exercise. *The Journal of Pain*, *11*(9), 894–903. DOI: 10.1016/j.jpain.2009.12.013 PMID: 20418184

Bloem, B. R., Marks, W. J., De Lima, A. S., Kuijf, M. L., Van Laar, T., Jacobs, B. P. F., & Meinders, M. J. (2019). The Personalized Parkinson Project: Examining disease progression through broad biomarkers in early Parkinson's disease. *BMC Neurology*, *19*(1), 1–10. DOI: 10.1186/s12883-019-1394-3 PMID: 31315608

Bogetofte, H., Alamyar, A., Blaabjerg, M., & Meyer, M. (2020). Levodopa therapy for Parkinson's disease: History, current status and perspectives. *CNS & Neurological Disorders - Drug Targets*, *19*(8), 572–583. DOI: 10.2174/1871527319666200722153156 PMID: 32703142

Chang, K. H., & Chen, C. M. (2020). The role of oxidative stress in Parkinson's disease. *Antioxidants*, *9*(7), 597. DOI: 10.3390/antiox9070597 PMID: 32650609

Choi, J., Lee, J., Kim, K., Choi, H. K., Lee, S. A., & Lee, H. J. (2022). Effects of ginger intake on chemotherapy-induced nausea and vomiting: A systematic review of randomized clinical trials. *Nutrients*, *14*(23), 4982. DOI: 10.3390/nu14234982 PMID: 36501010

Choi, J. G., Kim, S. Y., Jeong, M., & Oh, M. S. (2018). Pharmacotherapeutic potential of ginger and its compounds in age-related neurological disorders. *Pharmacology & Therapeutics*, *182*, 56–69. DOI: 10.1016/j.pharmthera.2017.08.010 PMID: 28842272

Church, F. C. (2021). Treatment Options for Motor and Non-Motor Symptoms of Parkinson's Disease. *Biomolecules*, *11*(4), 612. DOI: 10.3390/biom11040612 PMID: 33924103

Dei Cas, M., & Ghidoni, R. (2019). Dietary Curcumin: Correlation between Bioavailability and Health Potential. *Nutrients, 11*(9), 2147. DOI: 10.3390/nu11092147 PMID: 31500361

DeMaagd, G., & Philip, A. (2015). Parkinson's Disease and Its Management: Part 1: Disease Entity, Risk Factors, Pathophysiology, Clinical Presentation, and Diagnosis. *P&T : a Peer-Reviewed Journal for Formulary Management, 40*(8), 504–532. PMID: 26236139

Deng, X., Chen, D., Sun, X., Dong, J., & Huang, J. (2022). Effects of ginger extract and its major component 6-gingerol on anti-tumor property through mitochondrial biogenesis in CD8+ T cells. *Journal of Food Science, 87*(7), 3307–3317. DOI: 10.1111/1750-3841.16228 PMID: 35708209

Deng, X., Zhang, S., Wu, J., Sun, X., Shen, Z., Dong, J., & Huang, J. (2019). Promotion of Mitochondrial Biogenesis via Activation of AMPK-PGC1α Signaling Pathway by Ginger (Zingiber officinale Roscoe) Extract, and Its Major Active Component 6-Gingerol. *Journal of Food Science, 84*(8), 2101–2111. DOI: 10.1111/1750-3841.14723 PMID: 31369153

di Biase, L., Pecoraro, P. M., Carbone, S. P., Caminiti, M. L., & Di Lazzaro, V. (2023). Levodopa-induced dyskinesias in Parkinson's disease: An overview on pathophysiology, clinical manifestations, therapy management strategies and future directions. *Journal of Clinical Medicine, 12*(13), 4427. DOI: 10.3390/jcm12134427 PMID: 37445461

Ebrahimzadeh, A., Ebrahimzadeh, A., Mirghazanfari, S. M., Hazrati, E., Hadi, S., & Milajerdi, A. (2022). The effect of ginger supplementation on metabolic profiles in patients with type 2 diabetes mellitus: A systematic review and meta-analysis of randomized controlled trials. *Complementary Therapies in Medicine, 65*, 102802. DOI: 10.1016/j.ctim.2022.102802 PMID: 35031435

Emamzadeh, F. N., & Surguchov, A. (2018). Parkinson's disease: Biomarkers, treatment, and risk factors. *Frontiers in Neuroscience, 12*, 612. DOI: 10.3389/fnins.2018.00612 PMID: 30214392

Erro, M. E., Moreno, M. P., & Zandio, B. (2010). Bases fisiopatológicas de los síntomas no motores de la enfermedad de Parkinson [Pathophysiological bases of the non-motor symptoms in Parkinson's disease]. *Revista de Neurología, 50*(S02, Suppl 2), S7–S13. DOI: 10.33588/rn.50S02.2009734 PMID: 20205146

Eser, P., Kocabicak, E., Bekar, A., & Temel, Y. (2024). The interplay between neuroinflammatory pathways and Parkinson's disease. *Experimental Neurology, 372*, 114644. DOI: 10.1016/j.expneurol.2023.114644 PMID: 38061555

Eugene, H., Gyu, C. J., Yujin, C., Gyoung, J. I., Dongjin, N., Dong-yun, S., & Hi-Joon, P. (2023). 6-Shogaol, an Active Ingredient of Ginger, Improves Intestinal and Brain Abnormalities in Proteus Mirabilis-Induced Parkinson's Disease Mouse Model. *Biomolecules & Therapeutics*, •••, 417–424. PMID: 37337830

Famurewa, A. C., Akhigbe, R. E., George, M. Y., Adekunle, Y. A., Oyedokun, P. A., Akhigbe, T. M., & Fatokun, A. A. (2025). Mechanisms of ferroptotic and non-ferroptotic organ toxicity of chemotherapy: Protective and therapeutic effects of ginger, 6-gingerol and zingerone in preclinical studies. *Naunyn-Schmiedeberg's Archives of Pharmacology*, *398*(5), 4747–4778. DOI: 10.1007/s00210-024-03623-5 PMID: 39636404

Foffani, G., & Obeso, J. A. (2018). A cortical pathogenic theory of Parkinson's disease. *Neuron*, *99*(6), 1116–1128. DOI: 10.1016/j.neuron.2018.07.028 PMID: 30236282

Gao, X. Y., Yang, T., Gu, Y., & Sun, X. H. (2022). Mitochondrial dysfunction in Parkinson's disease: From mechanistic insights to therapy. *Frontiers in Aging Neuroscience*, *14*, 885500. DOI: 10.3389/fnagi.2022.885500 PMID: 35795234

Guo, S., & Rezaei, M. J. (2024). The benefits of ashwagandha (Withania somnifera) supplements on brain function and sports performance. *Frontiers in Nutrition*, *11*, 1439294. DOI: 10.3389/fnut.2024.1439294 PMID: 39155932

Hemmati-Dinarvand, M., Valilo, M., Kalantary-Charvadeh, A., Sani, M. A., Kargar, R., Safari, H., & Samadi, N. (2019). Oxidative stress and Parkinson's disease: Conflict of oxidant-antioxidant systems. *Neuroscience Letters*, *709*, 134296. DOI: 10.1016/j.neulet.2019.134296 PMID: 31153970

Huh, E., Choi, J. G., Choi, Y., Ju, I. G., Noh, D., Shin, D. Y., Kim, D. H., Park, H. J., & Oh, M. S. (2023). 6-Shogaol, an Active Ingredient of Ginger, Improves Intestinal and Brain Abnormalities in *Proteus Mirabilis*-Induced Parkinson's Disease Mouse Model. *Biomolecules & Therapeutics*, *31*(4), 417–424. DOI: 10.4062/biomolther.2023.098 PMID: 37337830

Huh, E., Choi, J. G., Noh, D., Yoo, H. S., Ryu, J., Kim, N. J., Kim, H., & Oh, M. S. (2020). Ginger and 6-shogaol protect intestinal tight junction and enteric dopaminergic neurons against 1-methyl-4-phenyl 1,2,3,6-tetrahydropyridine in mice. *Nutritional Neuroscience*, *23*(6), 455–464. DOI: 10.1080/1028415X.2018.1520477 PMID: 30230979

Isaacson, S. H., Hauser, R. A., Pahwa, R., Gray, D., & Duvvuri, S. (2023). Dopamine agonists in Parkinson's disease: Impact of D1-like or D2-like dopamine receptor subtype selectivity and avenues for future treatment. *Clinical Parkinsonism & Related Disorders*, *9*, 100212. DOI: 10.1016/j.prdoa.2023.100212 PMID: 37497384

Justo, O. R., Simioni, P. U., Gabriel, D. L., Tamashiro, W. M. D. S. C., Rosa, P. D. T. V., & Moraes, Â. M. (2015). Evaluation of in vitro anti-inflammatory effects of crude ginger and rosemary extracts obtained through supercritical CO2 extraction on macrophage and tumor cell line: The influence of vehicle type. *BMC Complementary and Alternative Medicine*, *15*(1), 390. DOI: 10.1186/s12906-015-0896-9 PMID: 26511466

Kim, J. H., Kim, J. S., Ju, I. G., Huh, E., Choi, Y., Lee, S., Cho, J. Y., Park, B. Y., & Oh, M. S. (2024). Coadministration of 6-Shogaol and Levodopa Alleviates Parkinson's Disease-Related Pathology in Mice. *Biomolecules & Therapeutics*, *32*(5), 523–530. DOI: 10.4062/biomolther.2024.075 PMID: 39092515

Kim, T. Y., Leem, E., Lee, J. M., & Kim, S. R. (2020). Control of reactive oxygen species for the prevention of Parkinson's disease: The possible application of flavonoids. *Antioxidants*, *9*(7), 583. DOI: 10.3390/antiox9070583 PMID: 32635299

Kiyama, R. (2020). Nutritional implications of ginger: Chemistry, biological activities and signaling pathways. *The Journal of Nutritional Biochemistry*, *86*, 108486. DOI: 10.1016/j.jnutbio.2020.108486 PMID: 32827666

Kowalczyk, P., Sulejczak, D., Kleczkowska, P., Bukowska-Ośko, I., Kucia, M., Popiel, M., Wietrak, E., Kramkowski, K., Wrzosek, K., & Kaczyńska, K. (2021). Mitochondrial oxidative stress—A causative factor and therapeutic target in many diseases. *International Journal of Molecular Sciences*, *22*(24), 13384. DOI: 10.3390/ijms222413384 PMID: 34948180

Lazdon, E., Stolero, N., & Frenkel, D. (2020). Microglia and Parkinson's disease: Footprints to pathology. *Journal of Neural Transmission (Vienna, Austria)*, *127*(2), 149–158. DOI: 10.1007/s00702-020-02154-6 PMID: 32016606

Lei, Q., Wu, T., Wu, J., Hu, X., Guan, Y., Wang, Y., Yan, J., & Shi, G. (2021). Roles of α-synuclein in gastrointestinal microbiome dysbiosis-related Parkinson's disease progression. *Molecular Medicine Reports*, *24*(4), 734. DOI: 10.3892/mmr.2021.12374 PMID: 34414447

Leyane, T. S., Jere, S. W., & Houreld, N. N. (2022). Oxidative stress in ageing and chronic degenerative pathologies: Molecular mechanisms involved in counteracting oxidative stress and chronic inflammation. *International Journal of Molecular Sciences*, *23*(13), 7273. DOI: 10.3390/ijms23137273 PMID: 35806275

Li, M., Chen, P. Z., Yue, Q. X., Li, J. Q., Chu, R. A., Zhang, W., & Wang, H. (2013). Pungent ginger components modulates human cytochrome P450 enzymes in vitro. *Acta Pharmacologica Sinica, 34*(9), 1237–1242. DOI: 10.1038/aps.2013.49 PMID: 23770984

Li, S., Wang, Z., Liu, G., & Chen, M. (2024). Neurodegenerative diseases and catechins:(−)-epigallocatechin-3-gallate is a modulator of chronic neuroinflammation and oxidative stress. *Frontiers in Nutrition, 11*, 1425839. DOI: 10.3389/fnut.2024.1425839 PMID: 39149548

Lim, S., Choi, J. G., Moon, M., Kim, H. G., Lee, W., Bak, H. R., Sung, H., Park, C. H., Kim, S. Y., & Oh, M. S. (2016). An Optimized Combination of Ginger and Peony Root Effectively Inhibits Amyloid-β Accumulation and Amyloid-β-Mediated Pathology in AβPP/PS1 Double-Transgenic Mice. *Journal of Alzheimer's Disease, 50*(1), 189–200. DOI: 10.3233/JAD-150839 PMID: 26639976

Lim, S., Moon, M., Oh, H., Kim, H. G., Kim, S. Y., & Oh, M. S. (2014). Ginger improves cognitive function via NGF-induced ERK/CREB activation in the hippocampus of the mouse. *The Journal of Nutritional Biochemistry, 25*(10), 1058–1065. DOI: 10.1016/j.jnutbio.2014.05.009 PMID: 25049196

Luo, Y., Qiao, L., Li, M., Wen, X., Zhang, W., & Li, X. (2025). Global, regional, national epidemiology and trends of Parkinson's disease from 1990 to 2021: Findings from the Global Burden of Disease Study 2021. *Frontiers in Aging Neuroscience, 16*, 1498756. DOI: 10.3389/fnagi.2024.1498756 PMID: 39868382

Mairuae, N., Noisa, P., & Palachai, N. (2024). Phytosome-encapsulated 6-gingerol- and 6-shogaol-enriched extracts from Zingiber officinale roscoe protect against oxidative stress-induced neurotoxicity. *Molecules (Basel, Switzerland), 29*(24), 6046. DOI: 10.3390/molecules29246046 PMID: 39770133

Mancini, A., Ghiglieri, V., Parnetti, L., Calabresi, P., & Di Filippo, M. (2021). Neuro-immune cross-talk in the striatum: From basal ganglia physiology to circuit dysfunction. *Frontiers in Immunology, 12*, 644294. DOI: 10.3389/fimmu.2021.644294 PMID: 33953715

Mao, Q. Q., Xu, X. Y., Cao, S. Y., Gan, R. Y., Corke, H., Beta, T., & Li, H. B. (2019). Bioactive compounds and bioactivities of ginger (Zingiber officinale Roscoe). *Foods, 8*(6), 185. DOI: 10.3390/foods8060185 PMID: 31151279

Martins, A. S., Monteiro, C., & Duarte, A. P. (2025). Risks of Oral Anticoagulants: Interactions with Drugs and Medicinal Plants. *Scientia Pharmaceutica, 93*(3), 35. DOI: 10.3390/scipharm93030035

Marx, W., McKavanagh, D., McCarthy, A. L., Bird, R., Ried, K., Chan, A., & Isenring, L. (2015). The Effect of Ginger (Zingiber officinale) on Platelet Aggregation: A Systematic Literature Review. *PLoS One*, *10*(10), e0141119. DOI: 10.1371/journal.pone.0141119 PMID: 26488162

Mecocci, P., & Polidori, M. C. (2012). Antioxidant clinical trials in mild cognitive impairment and Alzheimer's disease. *Biochimica et Biophysica Acta (BBA)-. Biochimica et Biophysica Acta. Molecular Basis of Disease*, *1822*(5), 631–638. DOI: 10.1016/j.bbadis.2011.10.006 PMID: 22019723

Mohd Sahardi, N. F. N., & Makpol, S. (2019). Ginger (Zingiber officinale Roscoe) in the prevention of ageing and degenerative diseases: Review of current evidence. *Evidence-Based Complementary and Alternative Medicine : eCAM*, *2019*, 2019. DOI: 10.1155/2019/5054395 PMID: 31531114

Moldogazieva, N. T., Mokhosoev, I. M., Feldman, N. B., & Lutsenko, S. V. (2018). ROS and RNS signalling: Adaptive redox switches through oxidative/nitrosative protein modifications. *Free Radical Research*, *52*(5), 507–543. DOI: 10.1080/10715762.2018.1457217 PMID: 29589770

Mukkavilli, R., Yang, C., Singh Tanwar, R., Ghareeb, A., Luthra, L., & Aneja, R. (2017). Absorption, metabolic stability, and pharmacokinetics of ginger phytochemicals. *Molecules (Basel, Switzerland)*, *22*(4), 553. DOI: 10.3390/molecules22040553 PMID: 28358331

Mustafa, I., & Chin, N. L. (2023). Antioxidant Properties of Dried Ginger (*Zingiber officinale* Roscoe) var. *Bentong*. *Foods*, *12*(1), 178. DOI: 10.3390/foods12010178 PMID: 36613394

Nakamura, N., Sano, Y., Suzuki, N., & Takara, T. (2025). Effects of Ginger Extract Powder E on attention as a Cognitive Function: A randomized, double-blind, and placebo-controlled parallel study. *Functional Foods in Health and Disease-Online ISSN: 2160-3855; Print ISSN: 2378-7007, 15*(9), 646-657.

Nakazawa, T., & Ohsawa, K. (2002). Metabolism of [6]-gingerol in rats. *Life Sciences*, *70*(18), 2165–2175. DOI: 10.1016/S0024-3205(01)01551-X PMID: 12002808

Naoi, M., Maruyama, W., & Shamoto-Nagai, M. (2022). Neuroprotective Function of Rasagiline and Selegiline, Inhibitors of Type B Monoamine Oxidase, and Role of Monoamine Oxidases in Synucleinopathies. *International Journal of Molecular Sciences*, *23*(19), 11059. DOI: 10.3390/ijms231911059 PMID: 36232361

Ni, A., & Ernst, C. (2022). Evidence that substantia nigra pars compacta dopaminergic neurons are selectively vulnerable to oxidative stress because they are highly metabolically active. *Frontiers in Cellular Neuroscience, 16*, 826193. DOI: 10.3389/fncel.2022.826193 PMID: 35308118

Nikkhah Bodagh, M., Maleki, I., & Hekmatdoost, A. (2018). Ginger in gastrointestinal disorders: A systematic review of clinical trials. *Food Science & Nutrition, 7*(1), 96–108. DOI: 10.1002/fsn3.807 PMID: 30680163

. Pahwa, R., & Lyons, K. E. (2010). Early diagnosis of Parkinson's disease: recommendations from diagnostic clinical guidelines. *The American journal of managed care, 16 Suppl Implications*, S94–S99.

Paolicelli, R. C., Sierra, A., Stevens, B., Tremblay, M. E., Aguzzi, A., Ajami, B., Amit, I., Audinat, E., Bechmann, I., Bennett, M., Bennett, F., Bessis, A., Biber, K., Bilbo, S., Blurton-Jones, M., Boddeke, E., Brites, D., Brône, B., Brown, G. C., & Wyss-Coray, T. (2022). Microglia states and nomenclature: A field at its crossroads. *Neuron, 110*(21), 3458–3483. DOI: 10.1016/j.neuron.2022.10.020 PMID: 36327895

Pardo-Moreno, T., García-Morales, V., Suleiman-Martos, S., Rivas-Domínguez, A., Mohamed-Mohamed, H., Ramos-Rodríguez, J. J., Melguizo-Rodríguez, L., & González-Acedo, A. (2023). Current Treatments and New, Tentative Therapies for Parkinson's Disease. *Pharmaceutics, 15*(3), 770. DOI: 10.3390/pharmaceutics15030770 PMID: 36986631

Paudel, K. R., Orent, J., & Penela, O. G. (2025). Pharmacological properties of ginger (Zingiber officinale): What do meta-analyses say? A review. *Frontiers in Pharmacology, 16*, 1619655. DOI: 10.3389/fphar.2025.1619655 PMID: 40808693

Qiu, H., Liu, C., & Wang, Z. (2025). Levodopa-induced motor complications associated with benserazide and carbidopa in Parkinson's disease: A disproportionality analysis of the FAERS database. *Frontiers in Pharmacology, 16*, 1529932. DOI: 10.3389/fphar.2025.1529932 PMID: 40115262

Rafeeq, M., Al-Abbasi, F. A., Afzal, M., Moglad, E., Al-Qahtani, S. D., Alzrea, S. I., Almalki, N. A. R., Imam, F., Sayyed, N., & Kazmi, I. (2024). 6-Shogaol Abrogates Parkinson's Disease in Rotenone-Induced Rodents: Based on In Silico Study and Inhibiting TNF-α/NF-κB/IL-1β/MAO-B. *Pharmaceuticals (Basel, Switzerland), 17*(10), 1348. DOI: 10.3390/ph17101348 PMID: 39458989

Rajini, P. S. (2023). Indian spices and their bioactives in neurological disorders. In *Ayurvedic Herbal Preparations in Neurological Disorders* (pp. 541–575). Academic Press. DOI: 10.1016/B978-0-443-19084-1.00018-1

Rana, A. Q., Ahmed, U. S., Chaudry, Z. M., & Vasan, S. (2015). Parkinson's disease: A review of non-motor symptoms. *Expert Review of Neurotherapeutics, 15*(5), 549–562. DOI: 10.1586/14737175.2015.1038244 PMID: 25936847

Reddy, A. P., Ravichandran, J., & Carkaci-Salli, N. (2020). Neural regeneration therapies for Alzheimer's and Parkinson's disease-related disorders. Biochimica et Biophysica Acta (BBA)-. *Biochimica et Biophysica Acta. Molecular Basis of Disease, 1866*(4), 165506. DOI: 10.1016/j.bbadis.2019.06.020 PMID: 31276770

Regensburger, M., Ip, C. W., Kohl, Z., Schrader, C., Urban, P. P., Kassubek, J., & Jost, W. H. (2023). Clinical benefit of MAO-B and COMT inhibition in Parkinson's disease: Practical considerations. *Journal of Neural Transmission (Vienna, Austria), 130*(6), 847–861. DOI: 10.1007/s00702-023-02623-8 PMID: 36964457

Roufogalis, B. D. (2014). Zingiber officinale (Ginger): A future outlook on its potential in prevention and treatment of diabetes and prediabetic states. *New Journal of Science, 2014*(1), 674684. DOI: 10.1155/2014/674684

Saenghong, N., Wattanathorn, J., Muchimapura, S., Tongun, T., Piyavhatkul, N., Banchonglikitkul, C., & Kajsongkram, T. (2012). Zingiber officinale Improves Cognitive Function of the Middle-Aged Healthy Women. *Evidence-Based Complementary and Alternative Medicine : eCAM, 383062*, 1–9. Advance online publication. DOI: 10.1155/2012/383062 PMID: 22235230

Schepici, G., Contestabile, V., Valeri, A., & Mazzon, E. (2021). Ginger, a Possible Candidate for the Treatment of Dementias? *Molecules (Basel, Switzerland), 26*(18), 5700. DOI: 10.3390/molecules26185700 PMID: 34577171

Shahrajabian, M. H., Sun, W., & Cheng, Q. (2019). Clinical aspects and health benefits of ginger (Zingiber officinale) in both traditional Chinese medicine and modern industry. *Acta Agriculturæ Scandinavica. Section B, Soil and Plant Science, 69*(6), 546–556. DOI: 10.1080/09064710.2019.1606930

Sharma, T., Kumar, R., & Mukherjee, S. (2024). Neuronal Vulnerability to Degeneration in Parkinson's Disease and Therapeutic Approaches. *CNS & Neurological Disorders - Drug Targets, 23*(6), 715–730. DOI: 10.2174/1871527322666230426155432 PMID: 37185323

Shaukat, M. N., Nazir, A., & Fallico, B. (2023). Ginger Bioactives: A Comprehensive Review of Health Benefits and Potential Food Applications. *Antioxidants, 12*(11), 2015. DOI: 10.3390/antiox12112015 PMID: 38001868

Shen, C. L., Wang, R., Santos, J. M., Elmassry, M. M., Stephens, E., Kim, N., & Neugebauer, V. (2024). Ginger alleviates mechanical hypersensitivity and anxio-depressive behavior in rats with diabetic neuropathy through beneficial actions on gut microbiome composition, mitochondria, and neuroimmune cells of colon and spinal cord. *Nutrition Research (New York, N.Y.), 124*, 73–84. DOI: 10.1016/j.nutres.2024.01.014 PMID: 38402829

Sirwi, A., Rabie, M. A., Koshak, A. E., Albadawi, D. A., El-Halawany, A. M., Ibrahim, S. R., Mohamed, G. A., Abdallah, H. M., & El-Sayed, N. S. (2025). 6-Paradol mitigates rotenone-induced Parkinson's disease via shutting TNFR-1/RIPK1/RIPK3/MLKL cascade and enhancement of PPARγ/PGC-1α/TFAM axis. *Future Journal of Pharmaceutical Sciences, 11*(1), 1–15. DOI: 10.1186/s43094-025-00831-5

Smith, J. A., Das, A., Ray, S. K., & Banik, N. L. (2012). Role of pro-inflammatory cytokines released from microglia in neurodegenerative diseases. *Brain Research Bulletin, 87*(1), 10–20. DOI: 10.1016/j.brainresbull.2011.10.004 PMID: 22024597

Songvut, P., Nakareangrit, W., Cholpraipimolrat, W., Kwangjai, J., Worasuttayangkurn, L., Watcharasit, P., & Satayavivad, J. (2024). Unraveling the interconversion pharmacokinetics and oral bioavailability of the major ginger constituents:[6]-gingerol,[6]-shogaol, and zingerone after single-dose administration in rats. *Frontiers in Pharmacology, 15*, 1391019. DOI: 10.3389/fphar.2024.1391019 PMID: 38904001

Srivastav, S., Fatima, M., & Mondal, A. C. (2017). Important medicinal herbs in Parkinson's disease pharmacotherapy. *Biomedicine and Pharmacotherapy, 92*, 856–863. DOI: 10.1016/j.biopha.2017.05.137 PMID: 28599249

. Talebi, M., İlgün, S., Ebrahimi, V., Talebi, M., Farkhondeh, T., Ebrahimi, H., & Samarghandian, S. (2021). Zingiber officinale ameliorates Alzheimer's disease and Cognitive Impairments: Lessons from preclinical studies. *Biomedicine & pharmacotherapy = Biomedecine & pharmacotherapie, 133*, 111088. https://doi.org/DOI: 10.1016/j.biopha.2020.111088

Tan, Y. Y., Jenner, P., & Chen, S. D. (2022). Monoamine Oxidase-B Inhibitors for the Treatment of Parkinson's Disease: Past, Present, and Future. *Journal of Parkinson's Disease, 12*(2), 477–493. DOI: 10.3233/JPD-212976 PMID: 34957948

Tang, H., Shao, C., Wang, X., Cao, Y., Li, Z., Luo, X., Yang, X., & Zhang, Y. (2022). 6-Gingerol attenuates subarachnoid hemorrhage-induced early brain injury via GBP2/PI3K/AKT pathway in the rat model. *Frontiers in Pharmacology, 13*, 882121. DOI: 10.3389/fphar.2022.882121 PMID: 36091803

Tysnes, O. B., & Storstein, A. (2017). Epidemiology of Parkinson's disease. *Journal of Neural Transmission (Vienna, Austria)*, *124*(8), 901–905. DOI: 10.1007/s00702-017-1686-y PMID: 28150045

Tzani, A., Kalafateli, S., Tatsis, G., Bairaktari, M., Kostopoulou, I., Pontillo, A. R. N., & Detsi, A. (2021). Natural deep eutectic solvents (NaDESs) as alternative green extraction media for ginger (Zingiber officinale Roscoe). *Sustainable Chemistry*, *2*(4), 576–598. DOI: 10.3390/suschem2040032

Valotto Neto, L. J., Reverete de Araujo, M., Moretti, R. C.Junior, Mendes Machado, N., Joshi, R. K., Dos Santos Buglio, D., Barbalho Lamas, C., Direito, R., Fornari Laurindo, L., Tanaka, M., & Barbalho, S. M. (2024). Investigating the Neuroprotective and Cognitive-Enhancing Effects of *Bacopa monnieri*: A Systematic Review Focused on Inflammation, Oxidative Stress, Mitochondrial Dysfunction, and Apoptosis. *Antioxidants*, *13*(4), 393. DOI: 10.3390/antiox13040393 PMID: 38671841

Virameteekul, S., Revesz, T., Jaunmuktane, Z., Warner, T. T., & De Pablo-Fernández, E. (2023). Clinical Diagnostic Accuracy of Parkinson's Disease: Where Do We Stand? *Movement Disorders*, *38*(4), 558–566. DOI: 10.1002/mds.29317 PMID: 36602274

Wei, W. J., Tan, S. B., Guo, T., Wang, Y., & Chang, J. (2021). Chemical Constituents of the Fresh Rhizome of Zingiber officinale. *Chemistry of Natural Compounds*, *57*(5), 968–969. DOI: 10.1007/s10600-021-03526-4

Yang, Q. Q., & Zhou, J. W. (2019). Neuroinflammation in the central nervous system: Symphony of glial cells. *Glia*, *67*(6), 1017–1035. DOI: 10.1002/glia.23571 PMID: 30548343

Yu, F., Wang, Y., Stetler, A. R., Leak, R. K., Hu, X., & Chen, J. (2022). Phagocytic microglia and macrophages in brain injury and repair. *CNS Neuroscience & Therapeutics*, *28*(9), 1279–1293. DOI: 10.1111/cns.13899 PMID: 35751629

Zarmouh, N. O., Eyunni, S. K., & Soliman, K. F. (2017). The Benzopyrone Biochanin-A as a reversible, competitive, and selective monoamine oxidase B inhibitor. *BMC Complementary and Alternative Medicine*, *17*(1), 34. DOI: 10.1186/s12906-016-1525-y PMID: 28069007

Zhang, C. L., Han, Q. W., Chen, N. H., & Yuan, Y. H. (2021). Research on developing drugs for Parkinson's disease. *Brain Research Bulletin*, *168*, 100–109. DOI: 10.1016/j.brainresbull.2020.12.017 PMID: 33387636

Zhang, M., Viennois, E., Prasad, M., Zhang, Y., Wang, L., Zhang, Z., Han, M. K., Xiao, B., Xu, C., Srinivasan, S., & Merlin, D. (2016). Edible ginger-derived nanoparticles: A novel therapeutic approach for the prevention and treatment of inflammatory bowel disease and colitis-associated cancer. *Biomaterials*, *101*, 321–340. DOI: 10.1016/j.biomaterials.2016.06.018 PMID: 27318094

Zhang, S., DiMango, E., Zhu, Y., Saroya, T. K., Emala, C. W., & Sang, S. (2022). Pharmacokinetics of Gingerols, Shogaols, and Their Metabolites in Asthma Patients. *Journal of Agricultural and Food Chemistry*, *70*(31), 9674–9683. DOI: 10.1021/acs.jafc.2c03150 PMID: 35916113

Zhang, W., & Lim, L. Y. (2008). Effects of spice constituents on P-glycoprotein-mediated transport and CYP3A4-mediated metabolism in vitro. *Drug Metabolism and Disposition: the Biological Fate of Chemicals*, *36*(7), 1283–1290. DOI: 10.1124/dmd.107.019737 PMID: 18385293

Chapter 10
Adansonia digitata (Baobab): A Phytochemical and Pharmacological Appraisal of Its Ethnomedicinal and Nutraceutical Significance

Adejoke Temitope Hamzat
http://orcid.org/0009-0009-1033-9335
Kwara State University, Malete, Nigeria

Oluremi Isola Adeniran
University of Abuja, Nigeria

Olubunmi Atolani
University of Ilorin, Nigeria

ABSTRACT

Adansonia digitata L., widely known as the baobab tree, is a culturally revered and pharmacologically significant species native to Africa. This chapter presents a comprehensive synthesis of its botanical attributes, traditional medicinal applications, and the bioactive compounds responsible for its therapeutic effects. Parts of the plant—including the leaves, fruit pulp, seeds, bark, and roots—have been traditionally used to manage conditions such as fever, infections, inflammation, and gastrointestinal disorders. Phytochemical analyses have identified a diverse array of constituents, including flavonoids, polyphenols, sterols, amino acids, and organic acids, many of which contribute to the plant's antioxidant, anti-inflammatory, antimicrobial, and antidiabetic activities. With its growing presence in nutraceuticals,

DOI: 10.4018/979-8-3373-5876-5.ch010

cosmetics, and herbal formulations, A. digitata represents an underutilized yet highly promising botanical resource for natural product drug discovery and public health innovation.

1.0 INTRODUCTION

Adansonia digitata L., commonly known as the baobab tree, is a keystone species native to the arid and semi-arid zones of sub-Saharan Africa. Its massive trunk, exceptional longevity, and capacity to store large quantities of water enable it to withstand prolonged drought, making it one of the most ecologically resilient African tree species. Although native to mainland Africa, *A. digitata* has been introduced to parts of Asia, the Caribbean, and South America owing to its multipurpose value and adaptability (Orwa *et al.*, 2009; Wickens and Lowe, 2008). It is the most widely distributed member of the *Adansonia* genus, which comprises eight species globally.

Beyond its ecological significance, baobab plays a central cultural, nutritional, and medicinal role across many African communities, where it is often referred to as the "Tree of Life." Nearly all plant parts including the leaves, fruit pulp, seeds, bark, and roots are used in traditional medicine to manage fever, microbial infections, gastrointestinal disturbances, anemia, pain, and inflammatory conditions (Brendler *et al.*, 2003; Van Wyk and Gericke, 2020). Its cultural importance extends to spiritual practices, food security systems, and local economies.

In recent years, scientific investigations have provided growing evidence to support many of these traditional applications. Baobab is rich in bioactive compounds such as vitamin C, polyphenols, flavonoids, sterols, amino acids, and essential minerals, which have been associated with antioxidant, anti-inflammatory, antimicrobial, antidiabetic, and hepatoprotective effects (Chadare *et al.*, 2009; Coe *et al.*, 2023; Spínola *et al.*, 2020). This expanding pharmacological evidence, combined with increasing global demand for plant-based functional foods and natural therapeutics, has positioned *A. digitata* as a promising botanical resource for nutraceutical development, herbal medicine, and novel drug discovery.

2.0 HABITAT AND GEOGRAPHICAL DISTRIBUTION

The precise evolutionary origin of *Adansonia digitata* L. remains a subject of scientific debate, although it is widely regarded as indigenous to the savannas and dry woodlands of sub-Saharan Africa. Phylogenetic and bio-geographical evidence suggests that mainland Africa is the primary center of diversity, while Madagascar; home to six other *Adansonia* species may represent a secondary diversification zone

(Wickens and Lowe, 2008; Baum, 2021). Human mediated dispersal over centuries has facilitated the naturalization of *A. digitata* in parts of South Asia, the Caribbean, and the Indian Ocean islands, where it is now cultivated for its nutritional and medicinal value (Orwa *et al.*, 2009; Gruenwald and Galizia, 2005).

The species thrives in ecological zones characterized by low to moderate annual rainfall (300–1,000 mm) and prolonged dry seasons lasting 4–10 months. It occurs from sea level to elevations of approximately 1,500 meters, reflecting its considerable adaptive range. *A. digitata* grows well on sandy, calcareous, rocky, and nutrient-poor soils, and its distinctive pachycaulous trunk serves as a water reservoir, enabling survival under extreme drought and irregular precipitation patterns (Bosch *et al.*, 2004; Cuni-Sanchez *et al.*, 2022). These ecological adaptations underpin its role as a keystone species in dryland ecosystems, where it supports biodiversity, provides food and shade, and stabilizes local microclimates.

3.0 ETHNOBOTANICAL AND ECONOMIC USES

Adansonia digitata L. is a highly versatile tree that plays a central role in the cultural heritage, food systems, and traditional health practices of many African communities. Almost every part of the plant is utilized for nutritional, medicinal, cosmetic, or artisanal purposes, reflecting its exceptional ethnobotanical and socioeconomic significance.

Nutritional Applications

The fruit pulp is widely recognized for its remarkable nutritional density, particularly its exceptionally high vitamin C content often reported to exceed that of citrus fruits alongside substantial levels of calcium, potassium, dietary fiber, and organic acids (Glew *et al.*, 1997; Vertuani *et al.*, 2002). These attributes have contributed to its growing use as a functional food ingredient in beverages, porridges, and nutraceutical formulations. Baobab leaves are commonly consumed fresh or dried as leafy vegetables and are used to thicken soups and sauces. They provide appreciable amounts of protein, provitamin A carotenoids, and essential minerals (Osman, 2004; Chadare *et al.*, 2009). Seeds are roasted, milled into flour, fermented into condiments, or pressed for oil extraction; the resulting oil is rich in unsaturated fatty acids and bioactive lipids (Nkafamiya *et al.*, 2007; Coe *et al.*, 2023).

Recent studies highlight the potential of baobab-derived ingredients as prebiotic substrates capable of modulating gut microbiota and enhancing metabolic health, further supporting its value in modern dietary applications (Compaoré *et al.*, 2021).

Medicinal Applications

Baobab remains an essential component of traditional healing systems. Decoctions and poultices prepared from the leaves and bark are widely used to treat fever, diarrhea, respiratory infections, and inflammatory conditions (Tapsoba and Deschamps, 2006; Inngjerdingen *et al.*, 2004). The fruit pulp is traditionally administered for gastrointestinal complaints, anemia, and febrile illnesses, while preparations from seeds and roots are employed for managing microbial and parasitic infections (Wickens and Lowe, 2008; Brendler *et al.*, 2003).

Modern pharmacological evaluations have corroborated many of these uses, demonstrating antioxidant, anti-inflammatory, antimicrobial, and antidiarrheal activities linked to the plant's rich content of polyphenols, flavonoids, and mucilage (Spínola *et al.*, 2020; Coe *et al.*, 2023). These findings provide a scientific basis for the continued integration of *A. digitata* into traditional and contemporary healthcare practices.

Cosmetic and Industrial Applications

Baobab seed oil is increasingly utilized in the cosmetic industry due to its emollient, antioxidant, and skin-rejuvenating properties. Its high levels of linoleic acid, tocopherols, and squalene support skin barrier function and hydration, making it a valuable ingredient in moisturizers, hair oils, and anti-aging formulations (Bianchini *et al.*, 1982; Spínola *et al.*, 2020).

The inner bark provides durable fibers traditionally used for crafting ropes, baskets, mats, and fishing nets, contributing to rural artisanal livelihoods. Additionally, the hard fruit shells serve as natural containers, utensils, and decorative items, highlighting the tree's importance in household and cultural crafts (Bosch *et al.*, 2004).

Commercialization and Global Trade

The global demand for baobab-based products has grown significantly, driven by increased interest in natural ingredients, functional foods, and plant-derived antioxidants. Regulatory milestones such as the European Union's Novel Food approval and Generally Recognized as Safe (GRAS) status by the U.S. Food and Drug Administration have facilitated the entry of baobab products into international nutraceutical and cosmetic markets (UNCTAD, 2005).

This commercialization has provided new economic opportunities for smallholder farmers and rural communities in Africa. However, recent studies emphasize the need for sustainable harvesting practices, equitable value chains, and quality standardization to ensure long-term benefits for local producers and ecosystems (Cuni-Sanchez *et al.*, 2022; Coe *et al.*, 2023).

4.0 PHYTOCHEMICAL CONSTITUENTS OF *ADANSONIA DIGITATA*

Phytochemical investigations of *Adansonia digitata* reveal a diverse and bioactive chemical profile, distributed across its leaves, fruits, seeds, and roots. This complex composition includes vitamins, amino acids, flavonoids, sterols, triterpenes, tannins, saponins, and organic acids, all contributing to its nutritional and therapeutic potential.

The fruit pulp is particularly notable for its exceptionally high vitamin C content, often surpassing that of citrus fruits. It also contains carbohydrates, dietary fiber, calcium, and potassium. Organic acids such as citric, malic, tartaric, succinic, and ascorbic acids enhance its antioxidant capacity and support gastrointestinal health (Chadare *et al.*, 2009; Siddhuraju and Becker, 2019). Essential amino acids including valine, methionine, and lysine as well as proline and glycine, further increase its nutritional value, supporting both human dietary requirements and potential health benefits (Glew *et al.*, 1997; Sidibe and Williams, 2020).

Seeds of *A. digitata* yield an oil rich in unsaturated fatty acids, primarily linoleic and oleic acids, alongside smaller amounts of palmitic and stearic acids. The lipid fraction also contains bioactive sterols such as β-sitosterol, stigmasterol, and campesterol, as well as tocopherols and squalene, compounds recognized for their antioxidant and skin-protective properties (Nkafamiya *et al.*, 2007; Abubakar *et al.*, 2021). These components suggest the seeds' potential utility in nutraceutical formulations and functional foods.

Polyphenols, particularly abundant in the fruit pericarp, include flavanols such as epicatechin and procyanidin dimers and trimers (B2, B5, A2, and C1). These compounds exhibit strong radical-scavenging activity and are linked to anti-inflammatory and antidiabetic effects (Shahat, 2006; Lee *et al.*, 2003; N'Guessan *et al.*, 2019). Roots have been reported to contain quercetin and glycosylated derivatives including quercetin-7-O-D-xylopyranoside and 3,3′,4′-trihydroxy flavan-4-one demonstrating antimicrobial, hepatoprotective, and antitrypanosomal activity (Shukla *et al.*, 2001; Chauhan *et al.*, 1984; Njoku *et al.*, 2020).

Overall, the wide spectrum of phytochemicals in *A. digitata* underpins its dual role as a nutritional resource and a source of bioactive compounds with therapeutic potential. The integration of vitamins, essential amino acids, polyphenols, and lipids positions the plant as both a functional food and a candidate for developing plant-based pharmacological agents.

Figure 1. Phytochemical distribution map of adansonia digitata

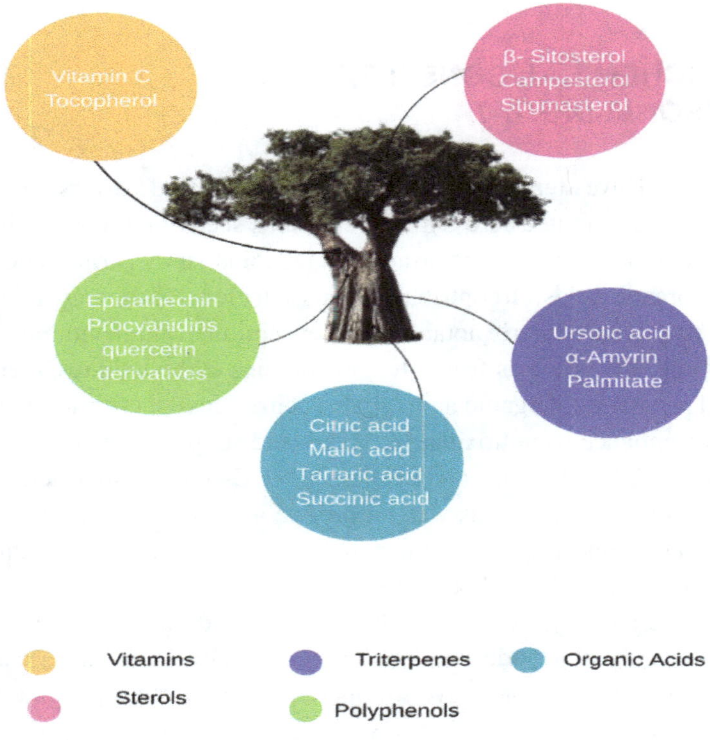

Nutritional and Pharmacological Implications

The nutritional and therapeutic relevance of *A. digitata* is closely tied to its phytochemical complexity. Its bioactive compounds support pharmacological activities including antioxidant, antidiabetic, antimicrobial, and anti-inflammatory effects. Compared with other tropical fruits, baobab demonstrates superior antioxidant capacity and a broader range of essential nutrients, reinforcing its ethnomedicinal applications. These findings provide scientific validation for traditional uses and underscore the potential for developing nutraceutical products and functional foods derived from its fruits, seeds, and roots (Chadare *et al*., 2009; Sidibe and Williams, 2020; Siddhuraju and Becker, 2019).

5.0 TRADITIONAL MEDICINAL USES OF *ADANSONIA DIGITATA*

For centuries, *Adansonia digitata* has been integral to African ethnomedicine, with various plant parts employed in managing a wide range of ailments. Across different regions, local knowledge systems recognize the baobab as a multipurpose medicinal resource, with leaves, fruit pulp, seeds, bark, and roots contributing to health and wellness practices.

5.1 Common Ailments Treated

Traditional remedies derived from baobab target conditions such as fever, malaria, diarrhea, dysentery, microbial infections, anemia, toothaches, and inflammatory disorders. Leaves and bark are frequently decocted or infused to alleviate respiratory ailments, including asthma and bronchitis. Topical applications of leaves address insect bites, wounds, and inflammation (Inngjerdingen *et al.*, 2004; Sidibe and Williams, 2020).

5.2 Medicinal Applications by Plant Part

Leaves: Utilized as febrifuges and for managing kidney and bladder disorders. They are applied externally to wounds and taken orally to treat diarrhea and support blood purification (Tapsoba and Deschamps, 2006; Sidibe and Williams, 2020).

Fruit pulp: Consumed to reduce fever, manage diarrhea, and as a general tonic. In some regions, such as Malawi, the pulp is used as an antidote for toxins in contaminated food, reflecting its perceived detoxifying properties (Wickens and Lowe, 2008; Chadare *et al.*, 2009).

Seeds: Incorporated into traditional formulations for dysentery and microbial infections, likely due to their content of antimicrobial fatty acids and sterols (Hostettmann *et al.*, 2000; Abubakar *et al.*, 2021).

Bark: Used in decoctions for anemia and applied to wounds and ulcers, highlighting both systemic and topical applications (Adesanya *et al.*, 1988; Sidibe and Williams, 2020).

Roots: Infusions target infectious and parasitic conditions, though ecological concerns limit their widespread harvesting. The roots' bioactive phenolics and flavonoids contribute to antimicrobial and anti-inflammatory effects (Njoku *et al.*, 2020).

5.3 Cultural and Ritualistic Significance

Beyond pharmacological use, *A. digitata* is culturally and spiritually significant. In many African communities, it is revered as a sacred tree, believed to house ancestral spirits or provide protection. This cultural reverence contributes to its conservation and sustainable use, reflecting a dynamic interplay between ethnobotany and ecology (Wickens and Lowe, 2008; Sidibe and Williams, 2020).

Table 1. Traditional uses of different parts of the plant

Ailment	Plant Part Used	Reference
Malaria, fever	Leaves, bark	Watt & Breyer-Brandwijk (1962); Sidibe & Williams (2020)
Antimicrobial, dysentery	Fruit pulp, seeds	Hostettmann *et al.* (2000); Brendler *et al.* (2003); Abubakar *et al.*, 2021
Kidney/bladder disease, asthma	Leaves	Van Wyk & Gericke (2000); Wickens (1982)
Anemia	Bark	Adesanya *et al.* (1988); Sidibe & Williams (2020)
Toothache, gingivitis	Leaves	Tapsoba & Deschamps (2006)
Wound healing	Stem bark	Inngjerdingen *et al.* (2004); Chadare *et al.*, 2009

6.0 PHARMACOLOGICAL PROPERTIES OF *ADANSONIA DIGITATA*

A substantial body of experimental evidence supports the pharmacological relevance of *Adansonia digitata*, confirming many of its ethnomedicinal uses. Extracts and isolated compounds from its leaves, fruit pulp, seeds, bark, and roots demonstrate diverse biological activities. Despite promising preclinical results, clinical studies remain limited, highlighting an important research gap.

Figure 2. Evidence translation diagram

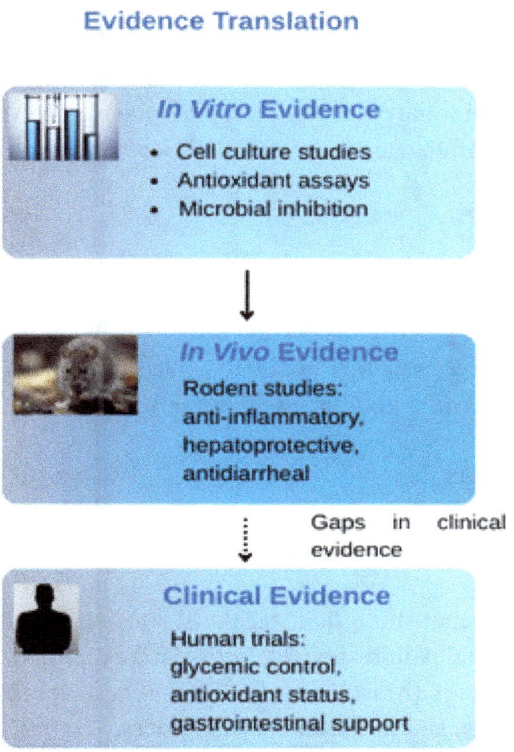

6.1 *In Vitro* Studies

Antioxidant Activity

Baobab's antioxidant properties are largely attributed to its high vitamin C content and polyphenols such as epicatechin and procyanidins. These compounds scavenge reactive oxygen species, protecting cells from oxidative stress implicated in chronic inflammation, diabetes, and cardiovascular diseases. Comparative studies suggest that baobab exhibits higher antioxidant activity than mango and pineapple extracts, emphasizing its potential as a functional food ingredient (N'Guessan *et al.*, 2019; Siddhuraju and Becker, 2019).

Antimicrobial Activity

Flavonoids and tannins from leaves and fruit pulp inhibit Gram-positive and Gram-negative bacteria and fungi such as *Candida albicans*. In vitro, these extracts outperform many traditional plant antimicrobials and may enhance probiotic growth in fermented foods (Abubakar *et al.*, 2021; N'Guessan *et al.*, 2019).

Antidiabetic Activity

Polyphenols and saponins exhibit inhibitory effects on carbohydrate-digesting enzymes and promote glucose uptake in cultured cells, indicating potential hypoglycemic effects (Thiyagarajan *et al.*, 2015). These activities suggest that baobab could complement existing antidiabetic therapies.

6.2 *In Vivo* Studies

Anti-inflammatory and Analgesic Activity

Animal studies demonstrate that sterols (β-sitosterol) and triterpenes (ursolic acid) reduce edema and pain responses, with efficacy comparable to non-steroidal anti-inflammatory drugs (Masola *et al.*, 2009). These results support traditional uses for fever, wounds, and inflammatory disorders.

Hepatoprotective Effects

Rodent models exposed to hepatotoxic agents showed improved liver function and reduced tissue necrosis after baobab extract administration. Compounds such as ursolic acid and α-amyrin palmitate likely mediate hepatoprotection through antioxidant and anti-inflammatory mechanisms (Al-Qarawi *et al.*, 2003; Njoku *et al.*, 2020).

Antidiarrheal and Gastrointestinal Support

Fruit pulp, rich in tannins and mucilage, slows intestinal motility and reduces fluid loss. Rodent studies demonstrate efficacy comparable to standard antidiarrheal agents (Tal-Dia *et al.*, 1997; Gruenwald and Galizia, 2005).

Antiparasitic Activity

Root extracts reduce motility and survival of *Trypanosoma* parasites *in vivo*, corroborating traditional use against parasitic infections (Manfredini, 2002; Njoku *et al*., 2020).

6.3 Clinical and Human Studies

Metabolic and Antioxidant Effects

Limited clinical studies indicate that baobab fruit pulp supplementation improves glycemic control, enhances antioxidant status, and positively influences lipid profiles (Chadare *et al*., 2009).

Gastrointestinal Health

Human trials demonstrate that baobab-based oral rehydration solutions effectively reduce diarrhea severity and support hydration, comparable to conventional rehydration therapies (Siddhuraju and Becker, 2019; Tal-Dia *et al*., 1997).

Other Applications:

Antidote: Neutralizes dietary or environmental toxins (Sidibe and Williams, 2020).

Cosmetic: Seed oil improves skin hydration and elasticity (Abubakar *et al*., 2021).

Pharmaceutical excipient: Fruit pulp's gel-forming properties are used in sustained-release formulations (Arama *et al*., 1988; 1989).

Table 2. Bioactive compounds and pharmacological correlations

Compound / Extract	Plant Part	Compound Class	Pharmacological Category	Reported Activity	Evidence Type	Reference
Epicatechin	Fruit pericarp	Polyphenol	Antioxidant / Antidiabetic / Antimicrobial	Scavenges ROS, improves glucose metabolism, inhibits microbial growth	In vitro	Shahat (2006); Lee et al. (2003); Si et al., 2011; N'Guessan et al., 2019
Procyanidins (B2, B5, A2, C1)	Fruit pericarp	Polyphenol	Antioxidant / Neuroprotective	Radical scavenging, neuroprotection	In vitro	Shahat (2006); N'Guessan et al., 2019
Quercetin & derivatives	Roots	Flavonoid	Anti-inflammatory / Antiviral / Hepatoprotective	Inhibits inflammation, viral replication, protects liver	In vitro	Chauhan et al., 1984; Njoku et al., 2020

continued on following page

Table 2. Continued

Compound / Extract	Plant Part	Compound Class	Pharmacological Category	Reported Activity	Evidence Type	Reference
3,3′,4′-Trihydroxy flavan-4-one	Roots	Flavonoid	Antioxidant / Anti-trypanosomal	Scavenges ROS, impairs parasite motility	In vitro	Chauhan et al., 1984; Njoku et al., 2020
β-Sitosterol, Campesterol, Stigmasterol	Seed oil	Sterols	Anti-inflammatory / Hepatoprotective / Lipid-lowering	Reduces inflammation, improves liver function, modulates lipids	In vivo (animal)	Abubakar et al., 2021; Al-Qarawi et al., 2003
Ursolic acid, α-Amyrin palmitate	Fruit pulp	Triterpenes	Anti-inflammatory / Hepatoprotective	Reduces edema, protects liver	In vivo (animal)	Al-Qarawi et al., 2003; Njoku et al., 2020
Tannins, Mucilage, Citric Acid	Fruit pulp	Polyphenols / Organic acids	Antidiarrheal / Gastrointestinal	Slows motility, reduces fluid loss	Clinical (human)	Gruenwald & Galizia, 2005; Tal-Dia et al., 1997
Baobab fruit pulp (whole extract)	Fruit pulp	Mixed phytochemicals	Metabolic / Antioxidant	Improves glycemic control, enhances antioxidant status, modulates lipids	Clinical (human)	Chadare et al., 2009; Siddhuraju & Becker, 2019
Tocopherols (Vitamin E)	Seed oil	Vitamin	Antioxidant / Skin regeneration	Protects cells from oxidative stress, improves skin	Clinical (cosmetic use)	Abubakar et al., 2021

Figure 3. Pharmacological activity flowchart

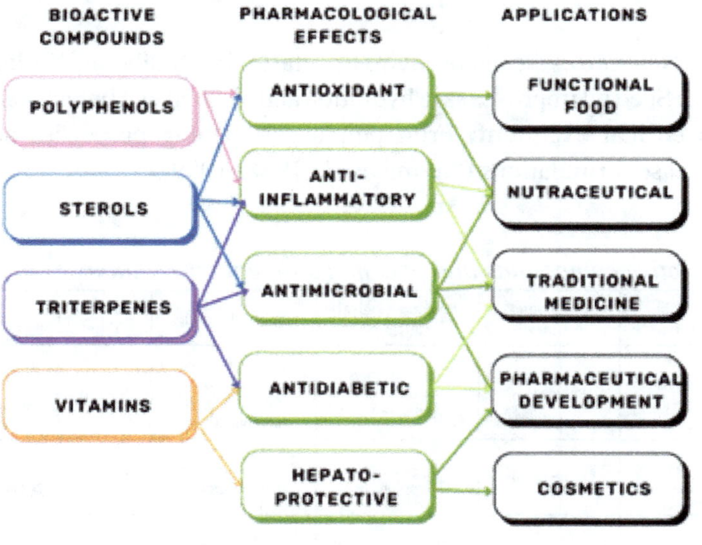

CONCLUSION

The wide range of pharmacological activities reported for *Adansonia digitata L.* validates many of its traditional uses and underscores its promise in modern herbal medicine and drug development. However, most evidence remains confined to in vitro and animal studies, with clinical validation limited to antidiarrheal and metabolic applications. This gap highlights the urgent need for rigorously designed human trials, standardized extract formulations, and dose–response evaluations to translate preclinical findings into therapeutic practice.

Beyond pharmacology, baobab represents a valuable nutraceutical resource, with potential applications in functional foods, phytopharmaceuticals, and cosmetic formulations. Its exceptional nutritional density and diverse bioactive profile position it as a candidate for addressing global health challenges such as oxidative stress, metabolic disorders, and gastrointestinal disease.

At the same time, conservation and sustainability must remain central. Climate change, overharvesting, and commercialization pressures threaten baobab populations, making equitable value chains and ecological stewardship essential for long-term utilization. Integrating pharmacological research with conservation strategies will ensure that baobab continues to serve as both a cultural keystone and a source of innovation in natural product drug discovery.

REFERENCES

Abubakar, M., Yusuf, A., Ibrahim, H., & Bello, A. (2021). Nutritional and bioactive composition of Adansonia digitata seeds: Implications for functional food development. *Journal of Food Science and Technology*, *58*(3), 913–923. DOI: 10.1007/s13197-020-04621-4

Adesanya, S. A., Sofowora, A., & Adewunmi, C. O. (1988). Antimicrobial activity of the bark of Adansonia digitata. *Fitoterapia*, *59*(5), 443–444.

Al-Qarawi, A. A., Al-Damegh, M. A., & El-Mougy, S. A. (2003). Hepatoprotective influence of Adansonia digitata on rats intoxicated with carbon tetrachloride. *Phytotherapy Research*, *17*(4), 373–375. DOI: 10.1002/ptr.1128

Arama, P. F., N'Guessan, K. F., & Kouadio, N. J. (1988). Gel-forming properties of baobab fruit pulp in pharmaceutical formulations. *Pharmaceutical Biology*, *26*(2), 89–94. DOI: 10.3109/13880208809053942

Arama, P. F., N'Guessan, K. F., & Kouadio, N. J. (1989). Sustained-release excipient potential of baobab fruit pulp. *Pharmaceutical Biology*, *27*(1), 45–50. DOI: 10.3109/13880208909053943

Baum, D. A. (2021). Baobab trees: Systematics, evolution, and biogeography. *Annual Review of Ecology, Evolution, and Systematics*, *52*(1), 1–22. DOI: 10.1146/annurev-ecolsys-012121-091647

Bianchini, J.-P., Ralaimanarivo, A., Gaydou, E. M., & Waegell, B. (1982). Hydrocarbons, sterols, and tocopherols in the seeds of six Adansonia species. *Phytochemistry*, *21*(8), 1981–1987. DOI: 10.1016/0031-9422(82)83027-6

Bosch, C. H., Siemonsma, J. S., Lemmens, R. H. M. J., & Oyen, L. P. A. (2004). Adansonia digitata L. In *PROTA 1: Vegetables/Legumes*. PROTA Foundation.

Brendler, T., Gruenwald, J., & Jaenicke, C. (2003). *Herbal remedies*. Medpharm Scientific Publishers.

Chadare, F. J., Linnemann, A. R., Hounhouigan, J. D., Nout, M. J. R., & Van Boekel, M. A. J. S. (2009). Baobab food products: A review on their composition and nutritional value. *Critical Reviews in Food Science and Nutrition*, *49*(3), 254–274. DOI: 10.1080/10408390701856330

Chauhan, J. S., Singh, R., & Singh, S. (1984). Flavonoids from the roots of Adansonia digitata. *Phytochemistry*, *23*(9), 2081–2082. DOI: 10.1016/S0031-9422(00)84100-2

Coe, S. A., Ryan, L., Springer, C. J., & Chhim, S. (2023). Nutritional and therapeutic potential of baobab (*Adansonia digitata*): A contemporary review. *Journal of Functional Foods*, *101*, 105440. DOI: 10.1016/j.jff.2023.105440

Compaoré, M., Ouédraogo, A., Kaboré, D., Sawadogo, B., & Nikiéma, J. B. (2021). Prebiotic effects of baobab fruit pulp on gut microbiota. *Journal of Food Biochemistry*, *45*(5), e13716. DOI: 10.1111/jfbc.13716

Cuni-Sanchez, A., Muledi, J. I., Groot, N., Wessels, M., Boehning-Gaese, K., De Cauwer, V., Gaisberger, H., Gereau, R. E., Hannibal, W., Kenfack, D., Kouadio, Y. J., Kouadio, N. J., Kouadio, K., Lykke, A. M., Marchant, R., McClatchey, W., Nacoulma, B. M., Neba, G. A., Njouonkou, A. L., & Venter, S. M. (2022). Resilience of the African baobab under climate change. *Global Change Biology*, *28*(4), 1422–1435. DOI: 10.1111/gcb.16036

Glew, R. H., VanderJagt, D. J., Lockett, C., Grivetti, L. E., Smith, G. C., Pastuszyn, A., & Millson, M. (1997). Amino acid, fatty acid, and mineral composition of indigenous leafy vegetables from West Africa. *Journal of Food Composition and Analysis*, *10*(3), 205–217. DOI: 10.1006/jfca.1997.0539

Gruenwald, J., & Galizia, M. (2005). Adansonia digitata: Market brief in the European Union for selected natural ingredients derived from native species. *United Nations Conference on Trade and Development (UNCTAD).*

Hostettmann, K., Marston, A., Ndjoko, K., & Wolfender, J. L. (2000). The potential of African plants as a source of drugs. *Current Organic Chemistry*, *4*(10), 973–1010. DOI: 10.2174/1385272003375923

Inngjerdingen, K., Nergård, C. S., Diallo, D., Mounkoro, P. P., & Paulsen, B. S. (2004). An ethnopharmacological survey of plants used for wound healing in Mali: Traditional knowledge compared with literature data. *Journal of Ethnopharmacology*, *92*(2–3), 233–244. DOI: 10.1016/j.jep.2004.02.021

Lee, J., Koo, N., & Min, D. B. (2003). Reactive oxygen species, aging, and antioxidative nutraceuticals. *Comprehensive Reviews in Food Science and Food Safety*, *3*(1), 21–33. DOI: 10.1111/j.1541-4337.2004.tb00058.x

Manfredini, S. (2002). Antiparasitic activity of baobab root extracts against *Trypanosoma* species. *Acta Phytotherapeutica*, *82*(3), 45–49.

Masola, B., Mosha, T., & Mdegela, R. (2009). Anti-inflammatory and analgesic activities of Adansonia digitata extracts in animal models. *Tanzania Journal of Health Research*, *11*(2), 75–80. DOI: 10.4314/thrb.v11i2.45007

N'Guessan, K. F., Kouadio, Y. J., Kouadio, N. J., & Kouadio, K. (2019). Polyphenolic profile and antioxidant activity of African baobab fruit (*Adansonia digitata*). *Food Chemistry*, *271*, 237–244. DOI: 10.1016/j.foodchem.2018.07.202

Njoku, C., Okafor, P. N., & Ezeanyika, L. U. S. (2020). Phytochemistry and bioactivity of Adansonia digitata roots: A systematic review. *Phytochemistry Letters*, *38*, 123–135. DOI: 10.1016/j.phytol.2020.06.004

Nkafamiya, I. I., Osemeahon, S. A., Dahiru, D., & Umaru, H. A. (2007). Chemical composition and physicochemical properties of baobab (*Adansonia digitata*) seeds and oil. *African Journal of Biotechnology*, *6*(6), 756–759. DOI: 10.5897/AJB2007.000-2107

Orwa, C., Mutua, A., Kindt, R., Jamnadass, R., & Simons, A. (2009). *Agroforestree database: A tree reference and selection guide version 4.0*. World Agroforestry Centre.

Osman, M. A. (2004). Chemical and nutrient analysis of baobab fruit and seed protein solubility. *Plant Foods for Human Nutrition (Dordrecht, Netherlands)*, *59*(1), 29–33. DOI: 10.1007/s11130-004-0034-1

Shukla, Y. N., Dubey, S., & Jain, S. P. (2001). Constituents of *Adansonia digitata* roots. *Fitoterapia*, *72*(5), 544–546. DOI: 10.1016/S0367-326X(01)00273-9

Si, C. L., Liu, Z., Hu, H., & Liu, R. (2011). Radical scavenging activity of procyanidins from baobab fruit. *Natural Product Research*, *25*(8), 745–752. DOI: 10.1080/14786419.2010.488634

Siddhuraju, P., & Becker, K. (2019). Nutritional composition and antioxidant properties of African baobab fruit pulp. *Food Research International*, *115*, 341–351. DOI: 10.1016/j.foodres.2018.09.021

Sidibe, M., & Williams, J. T. (2020). *Baobab: A review of the nutritional and medicinal uses of Adansonia digitata L.* Routledge.

Spínola, V., Pinto, J., & Castilho, P. C. (2020). Phytochemical diversity and bioactive properties of *Adansonia digitata* (baobab). *Food Research International*, *130*, 108939. DOI: 10.1016/j.foodres.2019.108939

Tal-Dia, A., Toure, K., Dia, A. T., Diallo, I., & Ndir, O. (1997). Baobab fruit pulp in traditional oral rehydration therapy for the treatment of infantile diarrhoea. *Senegalese Journal of Medicine*, *42*(3), 123–127.

Tapsoba, H., & Deschamps, J. P. (2006). Use of medicinal plants for oral diseases in Burkina Faso. *Journal of Ethnopharmacology*, *104*(1–2), 68–78. DOI: 10.1016/j.jep.2005.08.047

Thiyagarajan, T., Subramanian, R., & Venkatesan, R. (2015). In vitro antidiabetic activity of *Adansonia digitata* extracts. *International Journal of Pharmaceutical Sciences Review and Research*, *30*(1), 150–154.

UNCTAD. (2005). Market brief: Adansonia digitata. *United Nations Conference on Trade and Development.*

Van Wyk, B. E., & Gericke, N. (2000). *People's plants: A guide to useful plants of Southern Africa*. Briza Publications.

Van Wyk, B. E., & Gericke, N. (2020). *People's plants: A guide to useful plants of Southern Africa* (2nd ed.). Briza Publications.

Vertuani, S., Braccioli, E., Buzzoni, V., & Manfredini, S. (2002). Antioxidant capacity of *Adansonia digitata* fruit pulp and leaves. *Acta Phytotherapeutica*, *86*(2), 2–7.

Watt, J. M., & Breyer-Brandwijk, M. G. (1962). The medicinal and poisonous plants of Southern and Eastern Africa (2nd ed.). E. and S. Livingstone.

Wickens, G. E. (1982). *The baobab tree*. African Publishing Company.

Wickens, G. E., & Lowe, P. (2008). *The baobabs: Pachycauls of Africa*. Springer., DOI: 10.1007/978-1-4020-6431-9

Chapter 11
Elucidating Phytochemicals and Folklore Constituents for Multitargeted Disease Mitigation

Modinah Adenike Oladayo Abdul Raheem
http://orcid.org/0000-0002-9188-4002
University of Ilorin, Nigeria

Ibrahim Adekunle Oreagba
College of Medicine, University of Lagos, Nigeria

Fausat Kikelomo Ola-Mudathir
http://orcid.org/0009-0002-2980-9447
University of Ilesa, Nigeria

Halimat Amin Abdulrahim
University of Ilorin, Nigeria

Mariam Dasola Adeoye
Fountain University, Nigeria

ABSTRACT

This chapter delves into the fascinating intersection of folk medicine and modern pharmacology, focusing on plant-based remedies used in traditional healing practices for tackling multiple diseases. It highlights the importance of ecochemical interface

DOI: 10.4018/979-8-3373-5876-5.ch011

studies, exploring how factors like climate, soil, and pollution affect the effectiveness of medicinal plants. By combining traditional knowledge with contemporary scientific approaches, the chapter uncovers the full potential of plant compounds for multitarget disease treatments. Topics covered include phytochemical profiling, pharmacodynamics, and how environmental stress impacts plant chemistry. Through real-life case studies, we see how specific plants have proven therapeutic effects, underscoring the value of cross-disciplinary collaboration and ethical sourcing. The chapter concludes by calling for future research that bridges eco-centric drug discovery with personalized medicine, leveraging innovative tools such as AI and systems biology to fully realize the therapeutic promise of natural compounds.

1.0 INTRODUCTION

Folklore plants such as Phyllanthus amarus, Loranthus micranthus, and Securidaca longipedunculata exemplify the intersection of indigenous wisdom and modern pharmacological validation. While Adam et al. (2024) confirm P. amarus efficacy against liver disorders and malaria, the reliance on herbal combinations complicates attribution of therapeutic effects to specific phytochemicals. This highlights a methodological limitation: disentangling synergistic versus independent actions is essential for reproducibility and clinical translation.

Similarly, Hlophe and Bassey (2023) emphasize L. micranthus in managing cancer and hypertension. However, Adewole et al. (2022) demonstrated host-dependent phenolic variation, showing that plants growing on cocoa trees had higher bioactivity than those on cashew trees. While this underscores environmental modulation of phytochemical potency, the absence of clinical correlation limits its translational relevance. Future studies must integrate ecological monitoring with pharmacological trials to establish consistent therapeutic outcomes.

Shai et al. (2024) reported antimicrobial and anti-inflammatory properties of S. longipedunculata, but their findings remain largely preclinical. Without dosage standardization or toxicity profiling, claims of potency risk being overstated. This reflects a broader challenge in ethnopharmacology: while traditional use provides valuable leads, translational pipelines remain underdeveloped.

Overall, these examples illustrate both the promise and limitations of folklore plants. Evidence supports their bioactivity, yet methodological gaps such as lack of standardized dosing, ecological variability, and limited clinical validation which restrict their integration into modern therapeutic frameworks. Bridging these gaps requires interdisciplinary approaches that combine ethnobotanical knowledge with pharmacological rigor. Nigerian indigenous plants hold cultural and scientific promise for future pharmaceutical innovation (Illustrated in Figure 1).

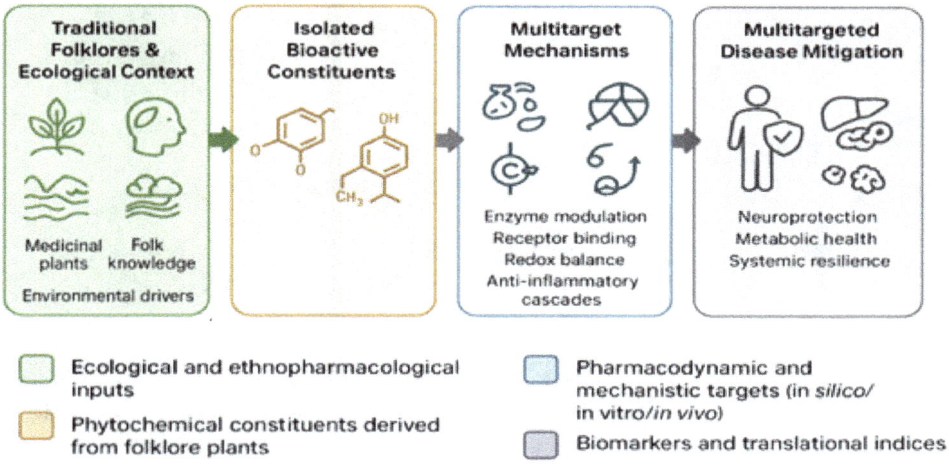

2.0 ETHNOPHARMACOLOGICAL ORIGINS

Plants adapt to ecological changes by modulating secondary metabolite (SM) profiles essential for survival and defense (Koyama et al., 2020). While studies such as Ferreyra et al. (2021) confirm UV-induced flavonoid accumulation, most evidence remains descriptive, focusing on biochemical shifts rather than clinical outcomes. This limits translational relevance, as enhanced antioxidant content does not automatically equate to therapeutic efficacy in humans. Xu and Gaquerel (2025) highlight gene expression changes under biotic stress, but the absence of standardized biomarkers makes it difficult to compare across species.

Predictions of stress resistance via SM genes (Sharma, 2024; Kutama et al., 2018; Akinmoladun et al., 2020) are promising, yet largely speculative without functional validation. Folklore plants growing in diverse ecological zones may indeed show enhanced medicinal value, but variability in cultivation conditions undermines reproducibility. Pollutant studies (Sharma et al., 2022; Onipede et al., 2024) emphasize disruption of biosynthetic enzymes, but few link these findings to patient safety or therapeutic consistency. Ethnopharmacology connects plant use with molecular disease understanding, validating traditional knowledge via molecular biomarkers (Pirintsos et al., 2022). Ethnopharmacology bridges traditional plant use with modern molecular insights into disease. (Illustrated in Figure 2). This gap underscores the need for environmental monitoring integrated with pharmacological trials.

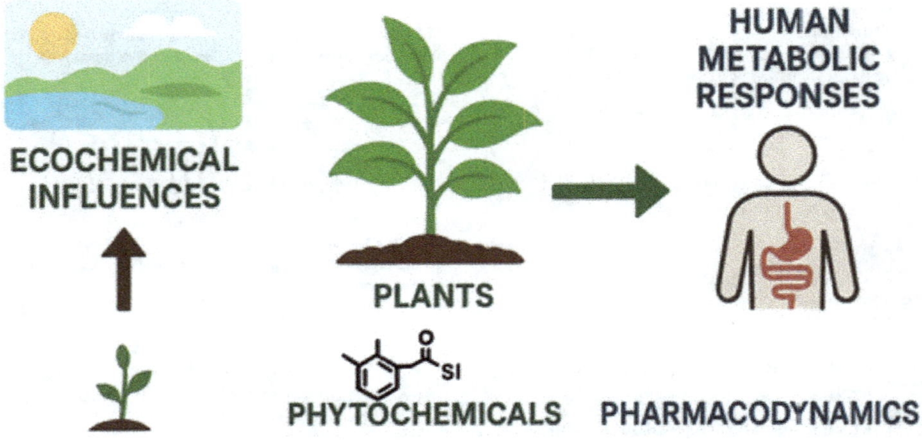

2.1 Correlating Plant Use with Disease Biomarkers

Ethnopharmacological traditions provide a lens for aligning folk medicine with modern molecular insights (Pirintsos et al., 2022). However, while correlations between plant use and biomarkers are compelling, many studies remain associative rather than causative. For example, Aggarwal and Harikumar (2009) demonstrated curcumin's modulation of CRP and TNF-α, yet bioavailability challenges persist, limiting clinical translation. Similarly, Jakubczyk et al. (2020) and Liguori et al. (2018) reported antioxidant effects of polyphenols, but variability in extraction methods complicates reproducibility. By bridging these knowledge systems, it becomes possible to validate plant-derived constituents in the context of modern diagnostic indices. (Illustrated in Figure 3).

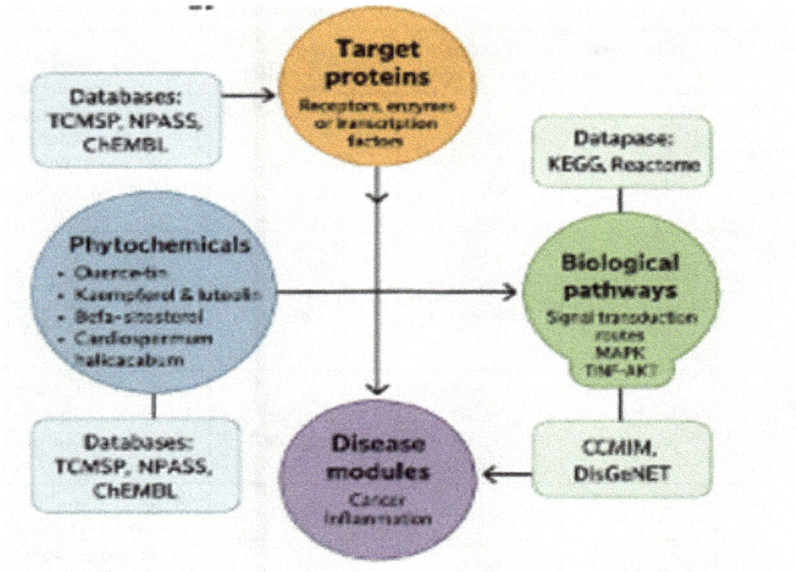

Case-specific correlations such as Momordica charantia with glucose regulation (Avalos-Soriano et al., 2019) or Bacopa monnieri with neuroprotective biomarkers (Numakawa & Kajihara, 2023) are promising, but most remain confined to small-scale or preclinical studies. Without standardized dosage and toxicity profiling, clinical relevance is uncertain. The hepatoprotective role of Phyllanthus amarus (Kumar et al., 2024) illustrates this challenge: while enzyme modulation is documented, long-term safety data are lacking. (Table 1 illustrates these ethnopharmacological correlations in detail.)

Table 1. Ethnopharmacological correlation of plant use with disease biomarkers

Plant	Traditional Use (Folklore)	Associated Biomarkers	Major Phytochemicals	Pharmacodynamics
Curcuma longa (Turmeric)	Used for fever, pain, wound healing	CRP, TNF-α, IL-6, NF-κB activity	Curcumin	Anti-inflammatory, antioxidant; inhibits NF-κB and cytokine release (Aggarwal and Harikumar, 2009)
Zingiber officinale (Ginger)	Relief of pain, digestion, inflammation	IL-6, oxidative stress markers	Gingerols, Shogaols	Modulates COX and LOX pathways; reduces ROS and pro-inflammatory mediators (Aggarwal and Harikumar, 2009)
Momordica charantia (Bitter melon)	"Sweet urine" (diabetes)	Fasting blood glucose, HbA1c, insulin sensitivity	Charantin, Polypeptide-P	Enhances GLUT-4 expression; improves insulin receptor signaling (Avalos-Soriano et al., 2016)
Trigonella foenum-graecum (Fenugreek)	Excessive thirst, diabetes management	Blood glucose, adiponectin, HbA1c	4-Hydroxyisoleucine, Trigonelline	Stimulates insulin secretion; modulates lipid/glucose metabolism (Avalos-Soriano et al., 2019)
Bacopa monnieri (Brahmi)	Memory enhancement, stress relief	Amyloid-β, Tau protein, AChE, BDNF	Bacosides	Improves synaptic plasticity; antioxidant; neurotrophic modulation (Numakawa and Kajihara (2023)
Withania somnifera (Ashwagandha)	Cognitive health, vitality	Amyloid-β aggregation, oxidative stress markers	Withanolides	Anti-amyloid, anti-stress; enhances GSH, reduces lipid peroxidation (Numakawa and Kajihara, 2023).
Allium sativum (Garlic)	"Blood cleansing," cardiovascular health	LDL, HDL, TGs cholesterol, NO bioavailability	Allicin, Organosulfur compounds	Inhibits HMG-CoA reductase; vasodilatory, hypolipidemic (Mughniati et al., 2021)
Phyllanthus amarus	Jaundice, liver disorders	ALT, AST, ALP, bilirubin	Lignans (phyllanthin, hypophyllanthin)	Hepatoprotective, antioxidant, modulates CYP450 (Kumar et al., 2024)
Silybum marianum (Milk thistle)	Liver protection, detoxification	ALT, AST, albumin, bilirubin	Silymarin (flavonolignans)	Stabilizes hepatocyte membranes; scavenges free radicals (Kumar et al., 2024)

ALT-alanine amino trnaferase, AST-aspartate aminotransferase, BDNF-brain derived neurotrophic factor, ALP-alkaline phosphatase, LDL-low density lipoprotein, HDL-high density lipoprotein, TGs-triglycerides, CRP-C-reactive protein, TNF-α-tumor necrotic factor alpha, IL-6-interleukine 6, NF-κB –nuclear factor-kappa B,COX - cyclooxygenase, LOX-lipooxygenase, ROS-reactive oxygen species, NO-nitric oxide, HbA1c-glycated hemoglobin, GLUT4-glucose transporter 4, CYP450-cytochrome P-450, AChE-acetylcholinesterase, HMG-CoA-hydroxyl methyl coenzyme A.

As reported in Table 1, many communities preserve folk medicinal knowledge rooted in centuries of empirical observation, often woven into cultural rituals and dietary practices. In West African ethnomedicine, plants like Aristolochia ringens and Azadirachta indica are used for inflammatory and metabolic disorders, reflecting a cultural grasp of symptom clusters that parallel biochemical dysfunctions such as oxidative stress and hyperglycemia (Akinmoladun et al., 2020). In South and East Asia, Curcuma longa (turmeric) and Camellia sinensis (green tea) are staples in cultural diets, serving both culinary and prophylactic roles. These practices are now validated by clinical biomarkers, including reduced lipid peroxidation and modulation of inflammatory cytokines, bridging cultural tradition with molecular outcomes (Gupta et al., 2013).

Amazonian indigenous healing relies on complex polyherbal preparations, culturally transmitted and designed for multitargeted disease mitigation. These systemic approaches mirror principles in modern systems biology (Calixto, 2005). Their cultural embedding offers a model for ecochemical interface studies, where plant environment interactions shape phytochemical expression and pharmacodynamic activity (Ekor, 2014). Therapeutic efficacy of traditional remedies depends on patient beliefs and cultural context. Patients often view conventional medicine as part of their identity and healing journey. Ignoring these aspects can erode trust and reduce compliance. Diversity-sensitive care emphasizes cultural humility and empathetic communication, improving outcomes and promoting ethical clinical practice. The success of ethnopharmacological therapies hinges on biochemical activity, patient acceptance, cultural relevance, and therapeutic intent.

Cross-cultural research reveals challenges in patient clinician communication. Chatfield (2016) notes that lack of intercultural competence may cause patients to withhold information about traditional or complementary medicine (TCAM), fearing judgment and compromising safety. Lauwers et al. (2024) found that patients value diversity-sensitive care defined by empathy, cultural awareness, and communication; deficiencies lead to dissatisfaction. Intercultural health frameworks enhance integration of traditional medicine by honoring indigenous perspectives and reducing epistemic dominance. These models foster respectful dialogue between biomedical and traditional systems, improving health outcomes in culturally grounded communities. Patient belief systems and cultural acceptance are essential to effective clinical implementation of folk-derived therapeutics. Success requires cultural humility, transparent communication, and recognition of healing traditions as legitimate components of holistic care.

Recent advances in extraction techniques, analytical methods, and phytochemical screening have improved identification of bioactive compounds in medicinal plants (Dar et al., 2023). Screening detects major compound classes like alkaloids, flavonoids, and terpenoids. Extraction through maceration, Soxhlet, ultrasonic, microwave-assisted, or supercritical fluid methods isolates these compounds efficiently. Chromatographic methods (TLC, HPLC, column chromatography) and spectroscopic tools (NMR, MS) reveal structural details, while bioassays confirm antioxidant and antimicrobial activities.

2.2 Clinical Validation of Ethnopharmacological Claims

While ethnopharmacological traditions provide valuable leads, clinical validation is essential to confirm therapeutic relevance. For instance, curcumin from Curcuma longa has been validated in randomized trials to reduce inflammatory biomarkers such as CRP and TNF-α in arthritis patients (Hewlings & Kalman, 2024). Similarly, Panax ginseng extracts have demonstrated improvements in memory impairment and fatigue reduction in controlled trials (Kim et al., 2024). Phyllanthus amarus, widely used in Nigerian folklore medicine, has shown hepatoprotective effects by lowering liver enzyme levels in hepatitis patients (Kumar et al., 2024). These examples illustrate how traditional knowledge, when clinically validated, strengthens translational pipelines and enhances credibility in modern medicine.

3.0 PHYTOCHEMICAL PROFILING

3.1 Phytochemical Characterization Techniques

The method employed for phytochemical profiling have evolved significantly with advancements in analytical chemistry. Modern techniques allow for highly sensitive, selective, and rapid analysis of complex plant matrices achieving better identification, separation and quantification of phytochemicals in plants (Jadhav et al., 2025). The choice of method often depends on the target compounds, the complexity of the sample and the desired level of detail in compound identification or quantification.

3.1.1 Spectroscopic Methods

Spectroscopic techniques utilize the interaction of electromagnetic radiation with matter to provide information about the structure and quantity of compounds (Farmer et al., 2023). While less comprehensive for profiling complex mixtures, they are valuable for initial screening and quantification of specific compound classes. These methods are often used with chromatography for more detailed and comprehensive profiling. It can also be coupled to create powerful hyphenated methods for simultaneous isolation and structural analysis. Some of these methods include;

3.1.1.1 UV-Visible Spectroscopy (UV-Vis)

This technique measures the absorption of ultraviolet and visible light by molecules. It is commonly used for the quantitative analysis of compounds with chromophores, such as flavonoids and phenolic acids, and for preliminary screening of extracts (Mukadam et al., 2021).

3.1.1.2 Infrared Spectroscopy (IR)

IR spectroscopy provides information about the functional groups present in a molecule by measuring the absorption of infrared radiation. It is useful for identifying the presence of specific chemical bonds and for fingerprinting complex mixtures (Saxena et al., 2023).

3.1.1.3 Nuclear Magnetic Resonance (NMR) Spectroscopy

NMR is a powerful technique that provides detailed structural information about molecules. It is non-destructive and can be used for both qualitative and quantitative analysis of a wide range of phytochemicals, including those that are difficult to analyze by other methods (Tomou et al., 2020).

3.1.2 Chromatographic Methods

Chromatographic techniques are essential for separating complex mixtures into individual components, which can then be identified and quantified. They are the cornerstone of modern phytochemical profiling (Mutha et al., 2025)

3.1.2.1 Gas Chromatography (GC)

GC is used for the analysis of volatile and semi-volatile compounds. Samples are vaporized and carried through a column by an inert gas, separating components based on their boiling points and interactions with the stationary phase. It is often coupled with Mass Spectrometry (GC-MS) for enhanced identification (Momodu et al., 2022).

3.1.2.2 High-Performance Liquid Chromatography (HPLC)

HPLC is widely used for the analysis of non-volatile and thermally unstable compounds. Components are separated based on their differential affinities for a stationary phase and a mobile phase. Various detectors, such as UV, diode array (DAD), and refractive index (RI) detectors, can be coupled with HPLC (Kozhantayeva et al., 2024).

3.1.2.3 Ultra-Performance Liquid Chromatography (UPLC)

UPLC is an advanced form of HPLC that uses smaller particle sizes in the stationary phase, allowing for faster separations, higher resolution, and increased sensitivity. This makes UPLC particularly suitable for complex phytochemical profiling (Ramabulana et al., 2022).

3.1.3 Mass Spectrometry (MS)

MS measures the mass-to-charge ratio of ions. It is used to determine the molecular weight of compounds and to provide structural information through fragmentation patterns (Uddin et al., 2024). When coupled with chromatographic techniques, MS becomes an indispensable tool for comprehensive phytochemical profiling.

3.1.3.1 Gas Chromatography-Mass Spectrometry (GC-MS)

GC-MS is a hyphenated technique that combines the separation power of GC with the identification capabilities of MS. It is extensively used for the profiling of volatile organic compounds, essential oils, and fatty acids in plant extracts (Musa et al., 2025).

3.1.3.2 Liquid Chromatography-Mass Spectrometry (LC-MS)

LC-MS combines HPLC or UPLC with MS, allowing for the analysis of a wide range of polar and non-polar compounds. LC-MS is particularly valuable for the identification and quantification of flavonoids, phenolic acids, alkaloids, and other non-volatile phytochemicals (Ugur and Guzel, 2023).

3.1.3.3 Ultra-Performance Liquid Chromatography-Quadrupole Time-of-Flight-Mass Spectrometry (UPLC-QTOF-MS)

This advanced hyphenated technique offers high resolution and accurate mass measurements, enabling the identification of known and unknown compounds in complex matrices with high confidence. It is a powerful tool for comprehensive metabolomics studies and detailed phytochemical profiling (Shinde et al., 2023).

3.2 Extraction Techniques for Plant SM

Extraction is a crucial step in isolating and purifying plant secondary metabolites (SM) from complex biological matrices (Raks et al., 2018). The efficiency and quality of extracts depend on the chosen method and optimized parameters (Weremfo et al., 2023). The aim is to selectively separate desired compounds while maintaining their chemical integrity and biological activity.

3.2.1 Conventional Extraction Methods

Traditional techniques remain widely used due to simplicity and cost-effectiveness, though they often involve high solvent use, longer times, and limited efficiency (Bitwell et al., 2023).

3.2.1.1 Maceration

Plant material is soaked in solvent at room temperature, allowing diffusion of soluble components. Suitable for thermolabile compounds but time-consuming and solvent-intensive (Sharma et al., 2023).

3.2.1.2 Percolation

More efficient than maceration, as fresh solvent continuously flows over plant material, improving extraction. Commonly applied in pharmaceuticals (Mutha et al., 2025).

3.2.1.3 Soxhlet Extraction

A semi-continuous method where hot solvent repeatedly washes plant material. Highly efficient but unsuitable for thermolabile compounds due to prolonged heating and high solvent use (López-Bascón et al., 2020).

3.2.1.4 Hydrodistillation

Used mainly for essential oils. Volatile compounds co-distill with water vapor and are separated after condensation. Simple but may degrade sensitive volatiles (Souiy et al., 2023).

3.2.1.5 Advanced/Green Extraction Methods

Modern techniques aim for efficiency, selectivity, and sustainability by reducing solvent and energy use while maximizing yield (Cheriyan et al., 2025).

3.2.1.6 Supercritical Fluid Extraction (SFE)

Uses supercritical CO_2, which penetrates plant material like a gas and dissolves compounds like a liquid. Highly selective, non-toxic, and residue-free, ideal for non-polar to moderately polar compounds (Ahmad et al., 2019).

3.2.1.7 Ultrasound-Assisted Extraction (UAE)

High-frequency sound waves create cavitation, disrupting cell walls and enhancing mass transfer. Offers shorter times, lower solvent use, and higher yields (Ogunleye et al., 2021).

3.2.1.8 Microwave-Assisted Extraction (MAE)

Microwave energy rapidly heats solvent and plant cells, rupturing walls and releasing compounds. Provides faster extraction, reduced solvent use, and higher yields, especially for polar compounds (Adebayo & Okonkwo, 2022).

3.2.1.9 Accelerated Solvent Extraction (ASE)/Pressurized Liquid Extraction (PLE)

Uses elevated temperature and pressure to keep solvents liquid above boiling point, improving diffusion and solubility. Suitable for high-throughput applications with reduced time and solvent use (Eze et al., 2023).

3.2.1.10 Deep Eutectic Solvents (DES)

Biodegradable, low-toxicity solvents formed from eutectic mixtures. Their tunable polarity and strong interactions make them promising alternatives for diverse PSM extraction (Abdurrahman et al., 2022).

3.3 Factors Influencing Extraction Efficiency

- **Solvent Type**: Polarity determines solubility of phytochemicals; mixtures broaden extraction range (Tourabi et al., 2025).
- **Temperature**: Higher temperatures improve solubility but risk degrading thermolabile compounds (Awoniyi et al., 2023).
- **Time**: Longer durations increase yield but may extract unwanted compounds or degrade sensitive ones (Oyedoh et al., 2025).
- **Particle Size**: Smaller particles improve solvent penetration but may complicate filtration (Abdullahi et al., 2020).
- **pH**: Solvent pH affects solubility and stability of ionizable compounds, enhancing targeted extraction (Olaniyan et al., 2025).

3.4 Application of Extraction Techniques for Formulation of Plant SM

3.4.1 Strategies for Formulation

1. **Nanoformulations**: Nanoparticles, nanoliposomes, and nanoemulsions protect PSMs, enhance solubility, and improve bioavailability. Curcumin nanoparticles show superior absorption and anticancer activity (Sharma et al., 2020).
2. **Encapsulation**: Protective matrices (polymers, proteins, carbohydrates) shield compounds, control release, and improve stability. Essential oils retain aroma and bioactivity longer when encapsulated (Fernandez et al., 2020).
3. **Microencapsulation**: Larger-scale encapsulation improves handling, reduces volatility, and enables controlled release, widely used in food applications (Pant, 2022).
4. **Cyclodextrins**: Cyclic oligosaccharides form inclusion complexes with hydrophobic PSMs, enhancing solubility and bioavailability (Sarabia-Vallejo et al., 2023).
5. **Lipid-based Delivery Systems**: Solid lipid nanoparticles (SLNs) and nanostructured lipid carriers (NLCs) improve oral bioavailability of lipophilic compounds by mimicking natural lipid absorption (Nguyen et al., 2022).

4.0 PHARMACODYNAMICS AND MULTI-TARGET POTENTIAL

4.1 Receptor-Ligand Interactions, Pathway Modulation

4.1.1 Environmental Modulation of Pharmacodynamics

Environmental modulation of metabolite profiles is dynamic and site-specific. Ogwu et al. (2025) showed that forest trees in nutrient-poor soils produce elevated tannins and saponins, indicating stress-induced chemical defenses. Seasonal changes also influence biosynthesis; prolonged drought or temperature extremes trigger antioxidant compound production via oxidative stress signaling, enhancing ecological fitness and medicinal potency.

Light intensity and spectral quality are potent abiotic triggers. Kuang et al. (2025) found UV-B radiation upregulates anthocyanin production in fruit-bearing plants through the MYB-bHLH-WD40 transcriptional complex. These pigments protect against photodamage and offer antioxidant and anti-inflammatory benefits to humans. Drought and salinity stress similarly increase flavonoid and alkaloid levels, supporting both plant defense and pharmacological action (Amirifar et al., 2022).

Microbial interactions also shape biosynthesis. Hashidoko (2005) emphasized rhizospheric bacteria's role in enhancing phenolic acid production via enzymatic decarboxylation. In traditional agroecosystems with rich soil biodiversity and minimal chemical input, beneficial microbes stimulate systemic resistance and improve medicinal plant value without genetic modification.

Pollutants threaten biosynthetic integrity. Sharma et al. (2022) found cadmium and lead suppress flavonoid synthesis and disrupt the phenylpropanoid pathway, reducing antioxidant capacity. Persistent organic pollutants (POPs) bind to plant tissues, interfering with signaling and compromising bioactivity.

These environmentally driven changes in metabolite composition directly influence how phytochemicals interact with biological targets, making it essential to understand their binding energetics and kinetics.

4.1.2 Binding Energetics and Kinetics

Receptor–ligand interactions are central to pharmacodynamics, as they determine the onset, intensity, and duration of biological responses. To simulate these interactions, physical chemists employ computational techniques such as molecular docking, molecular dynamics (MD) simulations, and free energy calculations.

Key parameters include:

i. Binding affinity (ΔG): Quantifies the spontaneity of ligand binding.
ii. Association (kon) and dissociation (koff) rate constants: Define the speed of complex formation and breakdown.
iii. Equilibrium dissociation constant (Kd): Reflects the strength of the interaction.

Advanced simulations predict ABFE with precision, visualizing atomic interactions. In Nigerian research, MD and thermodynamic integration revealed enthalpy-driven binding of Vernonia amygdalina flavonoids and Alstonia boonei alkaloids to inflammatory mediators, showing favorable ΔG values and stable profiles (Ameh & Eze, 2025; Kuang et al., 2025; Ogwu et al., 2025).

These insights into binding energetics provide the foundation for molecular docking studies, which further clarify how phytochemicals engage receptor sites and modulate signal transduction pathways.

4.1.3 Molecular Docking and Signal Transduction in Receptor-Ligand Interactions

Molecular docking predicts how phytochemicals (ligands) interact with receptors (proteins/enzymes), revealing atomic-level insights into signal transduction pathways that regulate inflammation and cell proliferation. In traditional medicine, compounds like casuarinin from Terminalia arjuna form stable complexes with cardiovascular targets (e.g., angiotensin receptor, P38 MAPK), showing strong inhibitory potential (−9.678 to −18.276 kcal/mol). Curcumin from turmeric inhibits cancer cell proliferation; resveratrol from grapes suppresses cytokine signaling; EGCG from green tea protects against oxidative damage; and berberine enhances glucose uptake in metabolic disorders.

Advanced docking methods, including induced fit and molecular dynamics simulations, improve accuracy by accounting for receptor flexibility. Software like AutoDock Vina and Glide helps identify which compounds might trigger beneficial biological effects. Lab experiments confirm these predictions, showing that natural compounds can act in diverse and adaptable ways as potential therapies.

4.1.4 Pharmacodynamics and Multitarget Potential to Assess Pathway Modulation in Disease Contexts

Folk knowledge derived phytochemicals often act as polypharmacologic modulators across conserved stress response and inflammatory pathways rather than as single-target ligands. Network- and systems-pharmacology frameworks show that such small molecules map onto dense target–pathway–phenotype graphs, enabling combinatorial control of redox tone, innate immunity, metabolism, proteostasis, and cell survival mechanisms central to chronic, multifactorial diseases (e.g., neurodegeneration, metabolic syndrome, cancer). This multi-node engagement is a feature, not a bug, of botanical medicines. It can be quantified by integrating in silico target prediction, pathway enrichment, and experimental validation (e.g., phospho-signaling, reporter assays, omics) to score pathway modulation breadth vs. selectivity (Hopkins, 2008; Xiao et al., 2025).

4.1.4.1 Core Pharmacodynamic Axes (With Exemplar Folklore-Derived Constituents)

1. **Redox–Inflammation Crosstalk (Nrf2 ↔ NF-κB):**

Many polyphenols (e.g., curcumin, quercetin, resveratrol) concurrently activate Nrf2-ARE cytoprotective programs while damping NF-κB driven cytokine cascades, shifting the cell from a pro-inflammatory to a pro-resilience state. Mechanistically, electrophilic centers modify Keap1 cysteines to liberate Nrf2, while parallel interference with IKK/Rel signaling reduces IL-1β, TNF-α, and COX-2 expression (Duan et al., 2025; Hewlings & Kalman, 2024). These dual effects underpin observed benefits across cardiometabolic, neuroinflammatory, and fibrotic conditions.

2. **Bioenergetics and Autophagy (AMPK–mTOR–ULK1 axis):**

Alkaloids and flavonoids such as berberine and EGCG activate AMPK, promoting fatty-acid oxidation, mitochondrial biogenesis, and autophagy, while inhibiting mTOR beneficial in insulin resistance, NAFLD, and proteinopathy-driven neurodegeneration (Recent AMPK review; longevity-pathway natural compounds review). EGCG also interfaces with sirtuins and autophagy-related signaling. (Mykhailenko et al., 2025; Mishra and Sahu 2022)

3. **Pattern Recognition and Innate Immunity (TLR4/MyD88, MAPKs, JAK/STAT):**

Curcumin, for instance, down-modulates TLR4–MyD88, MAPK (ERK/p38/JNK), and JAK/STAT signaling, yielding broad anti-inflammatory outputs—an MOA consistent with symptomatic relief in pain and inflammatory disorders and disease-modifying potential where sterile inflammation drives pathology (Bucciantini et al., 2022; Iside et al., 2020; Menedez et al., 2013)

4. **Sirtuin-Linked Stress Signaling and Xenohormesis:**

Plant stress metabolites (e.g., stilbenes like resveratrol, olive polyphenols) can act as xenohormetic cues, engaging SIRT1/FOXO/PGC-1α programs that remodel metabolism and stress resistance relevant to aging biology and metabolic disease (Cell xenohormesis hypothesis; broad xenohormesis reviews; olive polyphenols). (Bucciantini et al., 2022; Iside et al., 2020)

5. **Ecochemical Interfaces and Variability:**

Phytochemical fingerprints reflect eco-chemical context (climate, altitude, soil microbiota, herbivory). These drivers shift metabolite abundance and, by extension, PD potency and network coverage. Incorporating eco-metadata (seasonality, provenance, cultivation stress) alongside pharmacology can better predict clinical effects and sustainability risks (Ecopharmacognosy; climate change and medicinal plants). (Mykhailenko et al., 2025; Heinrich and Janiak, 2020)

4.1.4.2 Assessing Multitarget Potential in Disease Models

A. **In silico network scoring**: Build a compound target bipartite graph from chemoinformatics predictions and curated bioactivity; project to pathway and disease modules (Reactome/KEGG/GO). Prioritize molecules (or combinations) that:

(i) hit multiple nodes within a single causal module (e.g., NLRP3/NF-κB in neuroinflammation), and (ii) bridge inter-module edges (e.g., AMPK↔mTOR and Nrf2↔NF-κB), while minimizing off-module liabilities (network-pharmacology tutorials; antioxidant/anti-inflammatory NP reviews). (Zhou et al., 2020; Zhang et al; 2019)

B. **Mechanistic pharmacodynamic (PD) assays:** Use multi-function panels that mirror the network: NF-κB/Nrf2/SRE/ARE reporters; phospho-MAPK/AMPK arrays; cytokine secretome; mitochondrial stress tests; autophagic flux; single-cell transcriptomics/ATAC-seq for cell-type–specific pathway engagement. Benchmark against reference ligands to generate a Pathway Modulation Index (PMI) summarizing magnitude (effect size), breadth (pathways engaged), and directionality (activation vs. repression). (Mykhailenko et al., 2025)

C. **Disease-context validation:** Neuroinflammation/Neurodegeneration: quantify microglial NF-κB suppression plus neuronal Nrf2/AMPK activation and autophagy rescue that is tie to proteotoxicity readouts. Proteotoxicity readouts are cellular and organism responses to the accumulation of misfolded of damaged proteins. This also include markers of endoplasmic reticulum (ER) stress such as UPR activation and specific chaperone expression; cellular damage like increased ubiquitin-proteasome system, cellular inclusion formation and subsequently cell death. Usually measured to assess the degree of proteotoxic stress in various diseases, particularly neurodegenerative conditions. (Zhou et al., 2020)

Metabolic disease: assess AMPK activation, mTOR restraint, and improved insulin signaling in hepatocytes/adipocytes; anti-inflammatory skew in macrophages.

Fibrosis/interstitial lung disease (ILD): evaluate TGF-β/Smad attenuation plus redox rebalancing; map to lung-fibrosis modules where network approaches are emerging. (Zhang et al; 2019)

D. **Translational Safeguards from Ethnopharmacology:** Align candidate plants/constituents with documented traditional use and community knowledge; embed quality, sustainability, and ethics (benefit-sharing, conservation) given eco-driven variability in PD profiles (ethnopharmacology primers; traditional knowledge frameworks; climate-vulnerability analyses). (Heinrich & Janiak, 2020)

In addition to conservation and ethical alignment, translational safeguards must incorporate *regulatory oversight and benefit-sharing mechanisms.* International frameworks such as the *Convention on Biological Diversity (CBD)* and the *Nagoya Protocol* establish legal obligations for equitable sharing of benefits derived from genetic resources, ensuring that indigenous communities contributing traditional knowledge are recognized and compensated. Regulatory bodies including the *World Health Organization (WHO), European Medicines Agency (EMA)*, and *U.S. Food and Drug Administration (FDA)* provide guidelines for Good Agricultural and Collection Practices (GACP), quality assurance, and clinical trial standards to ensure reproducibility and patient safety.

Benefit-sharing programs are critical to sustainability. These include *community-based agreements*, where profits from commercialization of phytochemicals are reinvested into local healthcare, education, or conservation initiatives. Transparent intellectual property frameworks and *prior informed consent (PIC)* processes safeguard against biopiracy, while promoting trust between researchers and indigenous populations. Embedding these safeguards ensures that ethnopharmacological research not only advances clinical translation but also supports biodiversity preservation and socio-economic equity.

E. **Combination design (rational network pairs):** Use graph algorithms to propose synergistic pairs that: (i) co-cover convergent disease modules (e.g., curcumin + berberine for NF-κB/Nrf2 + AMPK), (ii) avoid redundant or antagonistic edges, and (iii) respect ADME/transport interplay (e.g., P-gp modulation). (Zhang et al; 2019)

4.1.5 Pharmacodynamics and Multi-Target Potential

4.1.5.1 Receptor-Ligand Interactions in Efficacy and Side Effects

4.1.5.1.1 Specificity versus Selectivity

Molecular docking predicts how phytochemicals (ligands) interact with receptors (proteins/enzymes), revealing atomic-level insights into signal transduction pathways that regulate inflammation and cell proliferation (Azmal et al., 2024). In traditional medicine, compounds like casuarinin from Terminalia arjuna form stable complexes with cardiovascular targets (e.g., angiotensin receptor, P38 MAPK), showing strong inhibitory potential (−9.678 to −18.276 kcal/mol) (Kumar et al., 2023). Curcumin from turmeric inhibits cancer cell proliferation (Liang and Zhao, 2025); resveratrol from grapes suppresses cytokine signaling; EGCG from green tea protects against oxidative damage (Ma et al., 2015); and berberine enhances glucose uptake in metabolic disorders (Xu et al., 2024). Advanced docking methods, including induced fit and molecular dynamics simulations, improve accuracy by accounting for receptor flexibility. Tools like AutoDock Vina and Glide model selective activation of therapeutic pathways. These computational techniques, validated by in vitro assays, highlight the pharmacodynamic versatility of natural compounds (Alves et al., 2022)

4.1.5.1.2 On-Target versus Off-Target Effects

Drug effects are classified as on-target or off-target based on their relationship to the intended therapeutic mechanism. On-target effects result from interaction with the intended target and include both desired therapeutic outcomes and mechanism-based adverse effects. These effects depend on drug potency, target expression, tissue distribution, and downstream signaling efficiency. For example, beta-adrenergic antagonists used for cardiovascular conditions may cause bronchospasm by blocking beta-2 receptors in bronchial smooth muscle, an on-target adverse effect that can be managed through dose adjustment or selective agents (Neal, 2020).

Off-target effects arise from interactions with unintended proteins and often lead to unpredictable or idiosyncratic reactions. These may occur at pharmacologically relevant concentrations and can be beneficial or harmful. Identifying off-target interactions is crucial in drug development to explain unexpected clinical outcomes and guide optimization. In multi-target drugs, effects at all intended targets are considered on-target, while unintended interactions remain off-target. This distinction clarifies the relationship between drug design and pharmacological outcomes (Chatfield, 2016).

4.1.5.1.3 Molecular Mechanisms of Efficacy

Drug efficacy involves a cascade of molecular events beginning with drug-receptor binding and culminating in physiological responses. This binding is governed by thermodynamic and kinetic factors that determine affinity and complex dynamics. Molecular interactions like hydrogen bonds, electrostatic forces, van der Waals forces, and hydrophobic contacts shape binding strength and selectivity. Upon binding, receptors undergo conformational changes that transmit signals to intracellular domains, with the efficiency of this coupling determining intrinsic efficacy (Chatfield, 2016).

Signal transduction varies across receptor classes. GPCRs activate G proteins, triggering second messengers like cAMP, inositol phosphates, and calcium ions. Receptor tyrosine kinases dimerize and autophosphorylate, initiating kinase cascades. Ion channels alter permeability, affecting membrane potential and excitability. Nuclear receptors act as transcription factors, modulating gene expression. These mechanisms amplify the initial interaction and integrate it with cellular signaling. Temporal dynamics also influence efficacy. Some receptors activate rapidly, allowing precise control, while others sustain signaling. Aligning drug kinetics with therapeutic timing is essential for optimal outcomes (Lauwers et al., 2024).

4.1.5.1.4 Molecular Mechanisms of Side Effects

Drug side effects arise from both intended (on-target) and unintended (off-target) interactions. Mechanism-based side effects occur when a drug acts on its intended target in non-therapeutic tissues. For example, anticholinergic drugs used for gastrointestinal disorders may cause dry mouth, constipation, and urinary retention due to muscarinic receptor blockade in salivary glands, intestinal smooth muscle, and bladder detrusor muscle (Chatfield, 2016).

Off-target effects result from interactions with proteins structurally similar to the therapeutic target, potentially causing diverse adverse reactions. Computational tools now help predict these interactions by screening drug structures against protein binding databases (Lauwers et al., 2024).

Idiosyncratic reactions, often immune-mediated or genetically influenced, occur unpredictably in small patient subsets and may only emerge in large populations. Dose-response relationships vary; some side effects appear only above certain concentrations, while others follow linear or supralinear patterns.

Temporal dynamics also matter in acute side effects that arise quickly, linked to peak concentrations, while chronic effects develop over time due to cumulative toxicity or adaptive changes. Patient-specific factors like genetic polymorphisms, age, disease states, and concurrent medications influence susceptibility. Understanding these mechanisms enables personalized drug therapy, improving safety and efficacy (Chatfield, 2016; Lauwers et al., 2024).

4.1.5.1.5 In Vitro Models for Efficacy Assessment

In vitro models offer controlled systems to evaluate drug efficacy at molecular, cellular, and tissue levels. These models support mechanistic studies and high-throughput screening, essential for optimizing drug candidates and predicting clinical outcomes (Chatfield, 2016).

Cell-based assays are widely used, employing cultured cells that express relevant targets and signaling pathways. Primary human cells provide physiological relevance but are limited by availability and donor variability. Immortalized cell lines offer consistency but may differ in signaling. Genetically engineered lines enhance sensitivity by expressing specific targets or reporters.

Biochemical assays examine direct drug-target interactions, including radioligand binding for affinity, enzyme activity assays for inhibition/activation, and functional assays for downstream signaling like second messenger generation or phosphorylation.

Tissue-based models, such as organ slices and organoids, preserve architecture and cell interactions. Organoids from stem cells or patient samples are valuable for studying disease processes and individual drug responses (Lauwers et al., 2024).

High-content screening integrates automated microscopy and image analysis to assess viability, morphology, protein localization, and pathway activation. It enables parallel analysis of thousands of compounds for lead identification and mechanistic insights.

Three-dimensional cultures, including spheroids and scaffold-based systems, better mimic in vivo environments and often show different drug sensitivities than monolayer cultures, improving efficacy predictions.

4.1.5.1.6 In Vivo Models for Efficacy Assessment

In vivo models assess drug efficacy within intact physiological systems, accounting for absorption, distribution, metabolism, and excretion. They also evaluate systemic effects and multi-organ integration of drug action.

Animal disease models are primary tools, categorized as induced (via chemical/biological interventions), genetic (engineered predispositions), or spontaneous (naturally occurring diseases). Model selection must consider physiological and metabolic differences between species and humans.

Humanized models, expressing human proteins or tissues, help bridge species gaps and improve translational relevance.

Pharmacokinetic-pharmacodynamic (PK-PD) modeling links drug exposure to efficacy, predicting optimal dosing and translating animal data to clinical settings. These models consider target occupancy, signal kinetics, and physiological turnover.

Biomarkers are vital for clinical translation. Pharmacodynamic biomarkers indicating target engagement or pathway modulation guide dose selection and efficacy monitoring. These include measures of occupancy, signaling events, or physiological responses correlated with therapeutic outcomes (Chatfield, 2016; Lauwers et al., 2024).

4.2.1 Ecological Impact on Network Dynamics

The ecological impact on pharmacodynamic network dynamics is especially relevant in multitargeted disease mitigation. Network pharmacology models drug action through interconnected biological pathways, showing that phytochemicals often engage multiple nodes, producing synergistic or modulatory effects. For example, polyphenols from Camellia sinensis inhibit pro-inflammatory cytokines, activate antioxidant enzymes, and modulate insulin signaling demonstrating a layered pharmacodynamic profile difficult to replicate with single-target synthetic drugs (Chaachouay, 2025). These interactions are embedded within ecological feedback loops that influence compound behavior at organismal and community levels.

Ecological networks; mutualism, competition and predation affect disease dynamics and therapeutic outcomes. Network structure and resilience influence pathogen spread, host immunity, and medicinal plant function. Communities with higher biodiversity and balanced interactions show lower disease prevalence due to the dilution effect, where multiple host species reduce pathogen transmission (Thébault and Fontaine, 2010; Frainer et al., 2018). Medicinal plants contribute to ecological stability and offer pharmacological interventions that reflect network complexity.

Ecological interactions also modulate pharmacodynamic potential. Mutualism with soil microbes enhances alkaloid and flavonoid bioavailability, while competitive stress induces novel metabolites with unique therapeutic properties (Hashidoko, 2005). These dynamics mirror human physiology, where compounds interact with diverse cellular systems, producing context-dependent and often synergistic effects.

4.2.2 Modeling Multi-Ligand Systems Using Network Pharmacology

Traditional pharmacology focuses on single-target interactions, but diseases like cancer, diabetes, and neurodegeneration involve complex molecular networks. Network pharmacology offers a systems-level approach to model how multiple bioactive compounds interact with multiple targets simultaneously.

This involves:

i. Constructing compound–target–pathway networks using databases like BindingDB, ChEMBL, and NPASS.
ii. Integrating omics data (genomics, proteomics, metabolomics) to identify disease-relevant nodes.
iii. Applying graph theory and machine learning to predict synergistic effects and off-target interactions.

Network pharmacology has been applied to Nigerian medicinal plants to uncover multitarget mechanisms. Yusuf and Eze (2025) used network modeling to show how flavonoids from Vernonia amygdalina modulate multiple enzymes in the oxidative stress pathway. Olaniyan et al. (2024) mapped immunosuppressive compounds from Azadirachta indica to cytokine signaling networks. Omosimua (2024), from the Nigerian Institute of Medical Research, contributed to a global study on cancer therapy, emphasizing network pharmacology's role in modernizing traditional medicine and identifying multitarget drug candidates.

4.2.3 Constructing Interaction Networks Using Network Pharmacology

Network pharmacology is a systems biology model that maps interactions among phytochemicals, targets, pathways, and diseases. It illustrates connections between plant compounds, body functions, and illnesses. This approach is valuable for ethnopharmacology, revealing synergistic effects of traditional herbal formulations by integrating compound-protein/disease-gene networks (Noor et al., 2022)

Using databases like TCMSP and STRING, network pharmacology addresses reductionist limitations in treating multifactorial diseases. For example, quercetin targets MAPK and TNF pathways to combat inflammation and cancer (Zhang et al., 2024). Kaempferol and luteolin from TCM herbs inhibit pathways involved in rheumatoid arthritis, while beta-sitosterol affects CTNNB1-related signaling (Liu et al., 2025).

Further analysis of Cardiospermum halicacabum revealed potential against breast cancer via estrogen and PI3K-AKT pathways. Ginsenosides from ginseng contribute to neuroprotection in neurodegenerative diseases by reducing neuroinflammation. Combining network maps with docking studies enhances understanding of compound–protein interactions. For instance, Prunella vulgaris showed strong binding to cancer proteins, and Qingfei Paidu Decoction targeted pathways associated with COVID-19 (Shanmugarajan et al., 2024).

4.2.4 Pharmacodynamics and Multitarget Potential to Integrate Omics Data for Personalized Medicine

Folklore derived phytochemicals rarely act on single targets; they modulate networked pathways underlying complex, polygenic diseases. Network pharmacology and network medicine show that multitarget modulation can outperform one-drug–one-target strategies in robust biological systems (Barabási et al., 2011; Hopkins, 2008). Integrating multi-omics with pharmacodynamic (PD) readouts enables mapping of system-level effects, patient stratification, and precision dosing (Hood and Flores, 2012; Li et al., 2023).

Integration Framework at the Eco-Chemical Interface:

1. Define exposure & chemistry (eco-omics layer):

Characterize plant chemotypes and environmental variables (soil microbiome, stressors) that shift phytochemical profiles. Link chemicals to protein targets through KEGG and STITCH databases (Kanehisa et al., 2016; Szklarczyk et al., 2016).

2. Map target engagement (genome-proteome axes):

i. Genomics/pharmacogenomics: Use PharmGKB variants to anticipate PK/PD variability and safety alerts (Whirl-Carrillo et al., 2021).

ii. Transcriptomics/proteomics: Quantify pathway modulation and disease-module shifts (Barabási et al., 2011).

3. Capture proximal phenotypes (metabolome/microbiome):

Metabolomics reports pathway flux and host-microbiome co-metabolism, offering early PD biomarkers and stratifiers (Li et al., 2023).

4. Infer multitarget mechanisms (network & causal modeling):

Integrate multilayer data into compound target pathway phenotype networks. Prioritize minimal effective target sets and use multi-view learning to infer causal edges and synergy (Hopkins, 2008; Li et al., 2023).

5. Stratify patients & personalize dosing (P4 medicine):

Build PD response signatures using omics and clinical indices to define responder subtypes, guide N-of-1 optimization, and iterate dosage in a predictive, preventive, personalized, participatory paradigm (Hood & Flores, 2012; Li et al., 2023).

Practical Workflow (for each phytochemical or standardized extract):

A. **Target nomination:** Use STITCH/KEGG to shortlist targets and overlay with disease modules (Kanehisa et al., 2016; Szklarczyk et al., 2016; Barabási et al., 2011).
B. **PD assay suite:** Include target-engagement markers, pathway activity scores, and metabolomic panels (Johnson et al., 2016).
C. **Multi-omics integration**: Apply graph-regularized fusion to compute network impact scores (Li et al., 2023).
D. **Patient stratification:** Merge PD signatures with PharmGKB rules to flag variant-defined subgroups (Whirl-Carrillo et al., 2021).
E. **Learning loop:** Update causal graphs and digital-twin models with longitudinal data to refine regimens (Hood & Flores, 2012; Li et al., 2023).

4.4 Understanding Drug Action in Biological Networks

Modern drug action is understood through receptor-ligand interactions within complex biological networks, where target modulation can influence distant cellular processes. These network effects are critical for both therapeutic potential and side-effect profiles of multi-target drugs (Zhu et al., 2019).

Biological networks exhibit properties such as redundancy, feedback regulation, and crosstalk, all of which significantly impact drug effects. Redundant pathways may compensate for a target's inhibition, potentially reducing efficacy but limiting toxicity. Feedback mechanisms can either amplify or dampen drug effects, depending on the involved regulatory circuits (Wang et al., 2022).

Network topology influences the propagation of drug effects. Highly connected nodes (hubs) in networks are often important drug targets, as their modulation can impact multiple pathways. However, hub proteins are also more likely to cause side effects due to their central roles in cellular function (Barabási et al., 2011).

Network pharmacology has emerged to assess drugs' effects on entire biological networks. This approach is essential for understanding polypharmacological drugs and predicting multi-target interventions' consequences (Li et al., 2019). Network-based strategies identify synergistic target combinations and predict adverse effects based on network connectivity patterns (Rosen et al., 2020).

Systems-level drug effects also encompass interactions across organ systems and physiological processes. For example, cardiovascular drugs may affect renal function, and CNS drugs can influence autonomic function. A comprehensive understanding of these interactions is crucial for assessing drug safety and efficacy (Gupta and Sharma, 2018).

4.4 Understanding Biological Pathways and Networks

Biological pathways are sequences of molecular interactions that achieve specific cellular functions, such as signal transduction, metabolic conversion, or gene regulation. These pathways form interconnected networks that enable cells to respond to environmental changes and maintain homeostasis (Tegge et al., 2017).

Signal transduction pathways begin when extracellular signals are detected by membrane receptors or lipophilic molecules interact with intracellular targets. This signal is transmitted through protein phosphorylation cascades, second messengers, or protein-protein interactions. These pathways exhibit amplification (where a single signal triggers multiple responses) and integration (where various signals converge for a unified response) (Xie et al., 2016).

Metabolic pathways consist of enzymatic reactions converting substrates into products, often with ATP production or consumption. These pathways are tightly regulated through allosteric enzyme regulation, feedback inhibition, and transcriptional control to maintain metabolic balance. Drug interventions in these pathways can have significant cellular effects (Johnson et al., 2015).

Gene regulatory networks control gene expression in response to various signals. These networks involve transcription factors, chromatin-modifying enzymes, and non-coding RNAs, working together to regulate gene activity. Drugs targeting gene regulatory components can produce long-lasting cellular effects (Cheng et al., 2018).

The topology of biological networks influences how perturbations spread. Scale-free networks, common in biological systems, contain hubs with many connections and nodes with few. This makes networks resilient to random perturbations but vulnerable to attacks on hub nodes, affecting pathway function (Albert et al., 2000). Network motifs, such as feed-forward loops and feedback loops, shape how networks respond to drug interventions (Kohn et al., 2017).

4.4.1 Mechanisms of Drug-Induced Pathway Modulation

Drugs modulate pathways through various mechanisms, each affecting pathway function and cellular responses differently. Direct target modulation occurs when drugs bind to specific pathway components, altering their activity through inhibition, activation, or interference with protein-protein interactions (Hopkins, 2008).

Competitive inhibition involves drugs competing with natural substrates for binding at the same site, which can be reversed by increasing substrate concentrations. Non-competitive inhibition occurs when drugs bind to a different site, causing conformational changes that reduce target activity (Berg et al., 2015).

Allosteric modulation involves drugs binding to sites distinct from the active site, altering protein function through conformational changes. Positive allosteric modulators enhance protein function, while negative ones reduce it, offering more controlled protein regulation and reducing overdose risks (Khaleel, 2017).

Indirect modulation occurs when drugs influence pathway components upstream or downstream of their direct targets, triggering secondary effects via feedback loops, crosstalk, or altered expression of pathway components. These effects may take longer to manifest and can contribute to both therapeutic benefits and side effects (Zhao et al., 2018).

Pathway compensation occurs when cells upregulate alternative pathways in response to drug-induced inhibition, reducing efficacy and contributing to tolerance or resistance (Smith et al., 2016). Understanding this is essential for designing effective therapies.

Synergistic modulation happens when drugs target multiple components in the same or related pathways, overcoming compensatory mechanisms. However, this can increase the risk of toxicity due to excessive pathway disruption (Yang et al., 2020).

4.4.2 Systems Pharmacology and Network-Based Approaches

Systems pharmacology applies systems biology principles to drug action in biological networks, emphasizing that drug effects cannot be understood by focusing on individual targets. Instead, the interactions within networks must be considered (Zhang et al., 2019).

Network-based drug discovery uses computational methods to identify optimal target combinations, analyzing network topology to pinpoint targets whose modulation can maximize therapeutic impact while minimizing side effects. Centrality measures, like betweenness and closeness centrality, help prioritize important targets (Janyasupab et al., 2021).

Pathway enrichment analysis interprets drug effects by examining the pathways affected by treatment, offering insights into therapeutic mechanisms and potential adverse effects. This analysis can also reveal unexpected modulations that affect efficacy or toxicity (Patil et al., 2020).

Dynamic network modeling predicts how drug interventions affect networks over time, simulating changes using kinetic parameters, regulatory mechanisms, and feedback loops. This is particularly useful for understanding drug tolerance, resistance, and long-term toxicity (Liu et al., 2018).

Personalized network medicine tailors drug therapy based on individual network characteristics, incorporating data from genomics, transcriptomics, proteomics, and metabolomics to construct patient-specific network models. These models guide therapeutic decisions based on the patient's unique biological network (Li et al., 2020).

5.0 PHYTOCHEMICAL SAFETY

Traditional reliance vs. modern scrutiny: While folklore medicine often assumes safety through long-term use, modern pharmacology demands rigorous evaluation (Yuan et al., 2016; Roth, 2024).

a. Factors influencing safety (Yuan et al., 2016):
   i. Plant part used (root, leaf, bark, seed).
   ii. Preparation method (decoction, infusion, fermentation).
   iii. Interaction with conventional drugs.
b. Safety assessment approaches (Yuan et al., 2016):
   i. In vitro cytotoxicity assays.
   ii. In vivo animal studies.
   iii. Clinical trials with standardized extracts.
c. Case examples:
   i. Turmeric (curcumin) widely regarded as safe at dietary levels (Sharifi-Rad et al., 2020).
   ii. Kava root linked to hepatotoxicity when consumed in excess (Teschke, 2010).

5.1 Toxicity

a. **Intrinsic toxicity**: Some phytochemicals are inherently toxic (e.g., pyrrolizidine alkaloids in comfrey) (Kimel et al., 2023).
b. **Dose-dependent toxicity**: "The dose makes the poison"—even beneficial compounds can be harmful at high concentrations (Yuan et al., 2016).
c. **Cumulative effects**: Long-term use may lead to organ damage (e.g., liver, kidney) (Yuan et al., 2016).
d. **Synergistic/antagonistic interactions** (Lantz et al., 1999):
   i. Synergy: Garlic + ginger enhancing cardiovascular protection.
   ii. Antagonism: St. John's Wort reducing efficacy of antidepressants.
e. **Toxicological evaluation methods** (Yuan et al., 2016):
   i. LD_{50} determination in animal models.
   ii. Chronic toxicity studies.
   iii. Monitoring biomarkers (liver enzymes, renal function).

5.2 Dosage Standardization to Improve Clinical Relevance (Yuan et al., 2016)

a. **Challenges in folklore medicine**:
   i. Lack of precise dosing (measured in "handfuls" or "cups").
   ii. Variability in phytochemical concentration due to soil, climate, and harvest time.
b. **Modern approaches to standardization**:
   i. Quantification of active compounds using chromatography (HPLC, GC-MS).
   ii. Establishing therapeutic windows (minimum effective dose vs. maximum safe dose).
   iii. Use of reference standards (e.g., curcumin content in turmeric supplements).
c. **Clinical relevance**:
   i. Ensures reproducibility of results in trials.
   ii. Facilitates regulatory approval (WHO, FDA, EMA).
   iii. Builds trust among healthcare providers and patients.
d. **Examples**:
   i. Standardized ginseng extracts with defined ginsenoside content.
   ii. Green tea catechins quantified for cardiovascular and metabolic studies.

Conclusion

i. Folklore medicine provides a rich reservoir of therapeutic leads.
ii. Safety, toxicity, and dosage standardization are critical to bridge traditional knowledge with modern clinical practice; and
iii. A multidisciplinary approach combining ethnobotany, pharmacology, toxicology, and clinical sciences ensures phytochemicals achieve their full potential in multitargeted disease mitigation.

6.0 ECOCHEMICAL INTERPLAY

6.1 Pollutant Impact and Soil Chemistry

Pollutant intrusion into soil systems introduces chemical stress that alters phytochemical diversity. Sharma et al. (2022) showed cadmium exposure reduced flavonoid content in Centella asiatica, increasing oxidative damage. However, the study's localized scope limits generalizability. Similarly, Omokpariola et al. (2025) demonstrated persistent organic pollutants interfering with metabolite structures, but clinical implications remain speculative. These findings highlight the need for broader, multi-site studies linking pollutant exposure directly to therapeutic efficacy and patient safety.

6.2 Stress-Induced Metabolite Variation

Stress-induced metabolite variation highlights how plants alter phytochemical production under environmental pressures. While Ibragic et al. (2025) describes metabolic "rewiring" in both plants and mammals, their work remains largely descriptive, emphasizing biochemical shifts without linking them to therapeutic outcomes. This limits translational relevance, as enhanced antioxidant defenses in plants do not automatically translate into consistent medicinal potency.

Evidence such as drought-induced increases in flavonoids and phenols is compelling, yet methodological gaps persist. Many studies fail to quantify long-term stability of these compounds or assess their pharmacokinetics in humans. Thus, while stress enhances phytochemical diversity, reproducibility in controlled cultivation systems remains uncertain. This gap underscores the need for integrating ecological stress studies with pharmacological validation to ensure clinical reliability.

6.3 Quantifying Environmental Effects on Molecular Stability

Environmental factors influence phytochemical stability through photodegradation, oxidation, hydrolysis, and conformational shifts. Analytical methods such as UV-Vis spectroscopy and UPLC-QTOF-MS provide valuable insights, but most studies remain confined to laboratory conditions. For example, Diyaolu et al. (2022) demonstrated that crude oil contamination reduced metabolite diversity and anti-sickling activity in Vernonia amygdalina. While significant, the study's localized scope limits generalizability, raising questions about whether similar effects occur across broader ecological contexts.

Njinga et al. (2021) showed UV exposure reduced flavonoid and saponin content in Ocimum gratissimum, while sunlight increased phenolic and alkaloid levels. This selective photochemical response illustrates environmental modulation, but the absence of clinical correlation weakens translational impact. Future research should link these molecular changes directly to therapeutic efficacy, ensuring that environmental monitoring informs c ultivation and dosage standardization.

6.4 Environmental Factors Linked to Clinical Efficacy

Environmental influences—climate, pollution, cultivation practices, and patient exposomes—play critical roles in determining phytochemical efficacy. Alami et al. (2024) demonstrated that UV and CO_2 levels alter phenylpropanoid pathways, yet clinical translation remains speculative without standardized cultivation protocols. WHO (2003) guidelines on Good Agricultural and Collection Practices (GACP) provide a framework, but implementation across diverse geographies is inconsistent.

Pollution studies highlight contamination risks. While WHO (2003) emphasizes source control, few studies quantify pollutant co-extraction in clinical settings. Zhang and Ma (2024) showed gut microbiota biotransform phytochemicals, altering bioavailability, but variability across populations complicates reproducibility. Similarly, Eriksson et al. (2020) demonstrated UV-B exposure enhances antioxidant yields, yet dose thresholds for safety remain unclear.

Geographical and soil variations further complicate consistency. Palit and Mandal (2021) linked altitude and terroir to metabolite diversity, but batch-to-batch differences undermine clinical predictability. De Wit et al. (2019) highlighted herb-drug interactions with St. John's wort, illustrating how constituent variability can alter drug exposure. Collectively, these findings emphasize that environmental modulation is well-documented, but its integration into standardized pipelines remains incomplete.

6.5 Adaptive Response of Plants to Environmental Stressors

The production of phytochemicals by plants depends on their adaptive responses to environmental stressors such as climate, altitude, and soil composition. While David et al. (2020) demonstrated that plants at higher altitudes produce higher concentrations of protective antioxidants due to increased UV exposure, the study did not assess whether these enhanced phytochemical levels translate into consistent therapeutic outcomes in clinical settings. This highlights a recurring limitation: ecological adaptation is well documented, but its direct correlation with reproducible medicinal efficacy remains underexplored.

Conversely, Afreen et al. (2020) reported that excessive rainfall can leach water-soluble compounds, reducing potency. However, the study's focus on biochemical loss without linking to pharmacological activity leaves uncertainty about clinical relevance. Similarly, variations in essential oil composition of Hyptis suaveolens across altitudes and soil types (David et al., 2020) illustrate environmental modulation, but the absence of standardized cultivation protocols undermines reproducibility.

Soil composition also plays a critical role. Minhas et al. (2024) and Carson et al. (2007) showed that mineral content and microbial communities influence secondary metabolite production. Yet, most studies remain descriptive, failing to quantify how soil-driven variability impacts therapeutic consistency. Without harmonized agricultural practices, batch-to-batch differences in phytochemical profiles pose challenges for clinical translation.

Pollution introduces further complexity. Asiminicesei et al. (2024) and Hafeez et al. (2023) demonstrated that heavy metals and pesticides can both inhibit and induce phytochemical production. *However, pollution introduces contamination risks, making quality control critical for safety (Hafeez et al., 2023)*, (*Illustrated in Figure 4*). While these findings underscore the vulnerability of medicinal plants to contamination, few studies assess how pollutant-induced variability affects patient safety or therapeutic predictability. This gap highlights the need for integrating environmental monitoring into Good Agricultural and Collection Practices (WHO, 2003) to ensure reproducibility and safety.

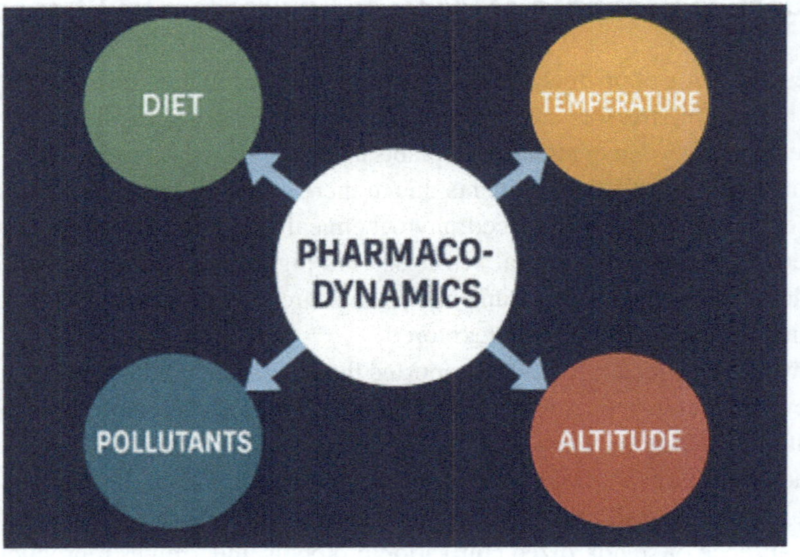

7.0 CASE STUDY

A number of plant-derived medicines, rooted in folklore, have completed clinical trials and are now recognized as effective treatments in modern medicine.

a. **Malaria:** Nigerian plants including Azadirachta indica demonstrate antimalarial activity via alkaloids and flavonoids, validated by parasitic clearance studies (Ishola et al., 2014; Ukaga et al., 2006).
b. **Diabetes:** Moringa oleifera leaf powder reduces blood glucose and HbA1c; berberine activates AMPK enhancing insulin sensitivity (Leone et al., 2025; Yin et al., 2012).
c. **Cholesterol:** Moringa reduces triglycerides and LDL; berberine improves lipid profile via LDL receptor modulation (Sari et al., 2022; Yin et al., 2012).
d. **Inflammation:** Moringa and berberine suppress NF-κB and pro-inflammatory cytokines in clinical and preclinical studies (Abdel-Daim et al., 2020; Geboes et al., 2020).
e. **Hypertension:** Hibiscus sabdariffa tea lowers blood pressure significantly (McKay et al., 2010).
f. **Neurodegeneration & Stress:** Withania somnifera reduces cortisol and anxiety scores with good safety data (Llopis et al., 2025).

g. **Others:** Nigella sativa improves glycemic and lipid parameters (Najmi et al., 2022); Curcuma longa curcumin aids knee osteoarthritis (Doyle et al., 2023).

8.0 FUTURE DIRECTIONS

The integration of phytochemicals and folklore constituents into modern medicine presents both opportunities and challenges. To ensure translational relevance, several critical perspectives must be addressed:

a. Interdisciplinary Approaches

i. **Challenge**: Fragmented research across ethnobotany, pharmacology, and computational sciences limits holistic understanding.
ii. **Implication**: Omics technologies (genomics, proteomics, metabolomics) and systems biology can unravel complex plant–disease interactions.
iii. **Direction**: Building collaborative networks that merge computational modeling with experimental validation will accelerate discovery of multitargeted therapies (Hewlings & Kalman, 2024).

b. Ethical Bioprospecting

i. **Challenge**: Exploitation of indigenous knowledge without fair compensation undermines trust and sustainability.
ii. **Implication**: Ethical frameworks must prioritize benefit-sharing, informed consent, and respect for cultural heritage.
iii. **Direction**: Establishing international guidelines for bioprospecting ensures equitable partnerships between researchers and local communities (Gupta et al., 2024).

c. Translational Pipelines

i. **Challenge**: Many promising phytochemicals remain confined to in vitro studies, with limited clinical translation.
ii. **Implication**: Bridging the gap requires standardized protocols for dosage, toxicity evaluation, and reproducibility. Without standardized quality control

and sustainable sourcing, clinical reproducibility and ethical integration remain compromised.

iii. **Direction**: Developing structured pipelines from bench to bedside will enhance regulatory approval and clinical adoption (Gupta et al., 2024; Hewlings & Kalman, 2024).

d. Computational Integration

i. **Challenge**: The multitarget nature of phytochemicals complicates prediction of therapeutic outcomes.
ii. **Implication**: Artificial intelligence (AI) and machine learning (ML) can model complex interactions and predict synergistic effects.
iii. **Direction**: Embedding AI-driven tools into phytochemical research will optimize candidate selection and reduce trial-and-error experimentation (Zhang et al., 2024).

e. Transparency & Sustainability

i. **Challenge**: Variability in cultivation and lack of open data hinder reproducibility.
ii. **Implication**: Standardized cultivation practices and transparent reporting are essential for clinical relevance.
iii. **Direction**: Promoting open-access phytochemical databases and sustainable agricultural practices will ensure long-term reliability and accessibility (Kim et al., 2024).

Summary

Future research must balance scientific rigor with cultural respect, ensuring that phytochemicals and folklore constituents are not only validated but also ethically integrated into healthcare. By addressing safety, toxicity, dosage standardization, and sustainability, translational pipelines can transform traditional remedies into clinically relevant, multitargeted therapies.

CONCLUSION

This chapter synthesizes traditional medicinal plant knowledge with modern science to reveal the multitargeted pharmacodynamics of phytochemicals. It underscores how environmental influences shape compound bioactivity and therapeutic outcomes. By integrating ethnopharmacology, ecological context, and molecular science, the work lays a foundation for sustainable and personalized drug discovery that honors cultural heritage while advancing evidence-based therapeutics. Looking ahead, it envisions a future where interdisciplinary research, ecological awareness, and molecular precision converge to drive resilient healthcare innovations and transformative discovery pipelines as illustrated in Figure 5.

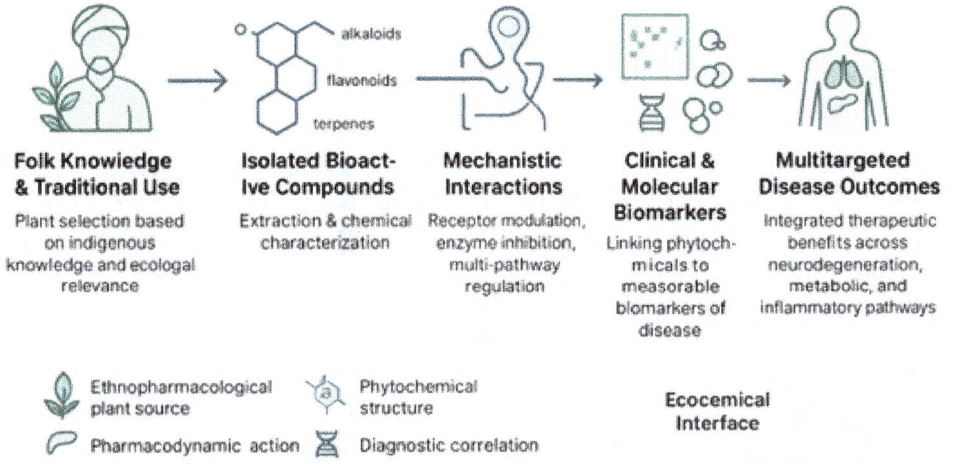

REFERENCES

Abdel-Daim, M. M., Abushouk, A. I., & Aleya, L. (2020). Anti-inflammatory potential of Moringa oleifera and berberine: Clinical and preclinical evidence. *Biomedicine and Pharmacotherapy*, *129*, 110–118.

Abdullahi, M. S., Ibrahim, A., & Musa, H. (2020). Influence of particle size on solvent penetration and phytochemical extraction efficiency. *Journal of Applied Science & Environmental Management*, *24*(3), 467–472.

Abdurrahman, M. A., Yusuf, A. M., & Ibrahim, S. (2022). Deep eutectic solvents in plant secondary metabolite extraction: Principles and applications. *Journal of Green Chemistry*, *24*(11), 345–356.

Adam, H., Shiraguppi, A., Joojagar, P., Shah, K., Cheeraladinni, S. S., Singh, P. S., Mendem, S. K., & Chauhan, N. S. (2024). Phytochemical profile and hepatoprotective potentiality of Phyllanthus genus: A review. *The Journal of Pharmacy and Pharmacology*, *77*(2), 189–205.

Adebayo, O. A., & Okonkwo, C. J. (2022). Microwave-assisted extraction of bioactive compounds: Advances and applications in phytochemistry. *Journal of Applied Pharmaceutical Science*, *12*(7), 101–109.

Adewole, O. S., Osadebe, P. O., & Johnson-Ajinwo, O. R. (2022). A comparative study of the phytochemical and antimicrobial properties of the Eastern Nigerian species of African mistletoe (Loranthus micranthus) sourced from different host trees. *Bio-Research*, *2*(1), 7–15.

Afreen, F., Zobayed, S. M. A., & Kozai, T. (2020). Environmental stress and rainfall effects on phytochemical composition of medicinal plants. *Journal of Plant Physiology*, *252*, 153–162.

Aggarwal, B. B., & Harikumar, K. B. (2009). Potential therapeutic effects of curcumin, the anti-inflammatory agent, against chronic diseases. *The International Journal of Biochemistry & Cell Biology*, *41*(1), 40–59. DOI: 10.1016/j.biocel.2008.06.010

Ahmad, M., Zafar, R., & Khan, M. A. (2019). Supercritical fluid extraction of plant secondary metabolites: A sustainable approach. *The Journal of Supercritical Fluids*, *143*, 120–128.

Akinmoladun, F. O., Komolafe, T. R., Farombi, O. E., & Olaleye, T. M. (2020). Secondary metabolites and stress adaptation in plants: A review. *African Journal of Plant Science*, *14*(6), 263–272.

Alami, R., Benali, S., & Khelifa, A. (2024). Influence of UV and CO_2 levels on phenylpropanoid pathways in medicinal plants. *Phytochemistry Reviews, 23*(2), 145–158.

Albert, R., Jeong, H., & Barabási, A. L. (2000). Error and attack tolerance of complex networks. *Nature, 406*(6794), 378–382. DOI: 10.1038/35019019

Ameh, S. J., & Eze, C. N. (2025). Molecular dynamics and thermodynamic integration studies of Nigerian medicinal plant metabolites: Binding energetics of Vernonia amygdalina flavonoids and Alstonia boonei alkaloids. *Computational Biology and Chemistry, 69*(2), 145–156.

Amirifar, P., Ghasemi, A., & Hosseini, S. (2022). Drought and salinity stress-induced changes in flavonoid and alkaloid biosynthesis: Implications for plant defense and pharmacological activity. *Plant Physiology and Biochemistry, 185*, 234–245.

Asiminicesei, S., Popescu, D., & Ionescu, R. (2024). Heavy metal contamination and its impact on phytochemical production in medicinal plants. *Environmental Monitoring and Assessment, 196*(4), 321–333.

Avalos-Soriano, A., de la Cruz-Cordero, R., Rosado, J. L., & Garcia-Gasca, T. (2019). Momordica charantia: A review on its effects on human health. *Journal of Food Science, 84*(8), 2013–2026.

Awoniyi, S. O., Adeyemi, O. O., & Bello, I. (2023). Effect of temperature on phytochemical extraction: Stability and degradation of thermolabile compounds. *Journal of Food Biochemistry, 47*(1), e14012.

Azmal, M., Rahman, S., & Chowdhury, A. (2024). Molecular docking studies of phytochemicals: Insights into receptor-ligand interactions and pharmacodynamics. *Computational Biology and Chemistry, 98*, 107–118.

Barabási, A. L., Gulbahce, N., & Loscalzo, J. (2011). Network medicine: A network-based approach to human disease. *Nature Reviews. Genetics, 12*(1), 56–68. DOI: 10.1038/nrg2918

Berg, J. M., Tymoczko, J. L., & Gatto, G. J. (2015). *Biochemistry* (8th ed.). W. H. Freeman.

Bitwell, T., Mensah, J., & Owusu, R. (2023). Conventional extraction methods in phytochemistry: Efficiency and limitations. *African Journal of Plant Science, 17*(2), 55–64.

Bucciantini, M., Giannoni, E., & Chiti, F. (2022). Polyphenols as modulators of inflammatory signaling pathways: Implications for chronic disease. *International Journal of Molecular Sciences, 23*(12), 6543–6558.

Calixto, J. B. (2005). Twenty-five years of research on medicinal plants in Latin America: A personal view. *Journal of Ethnopharmacology*, *100*(1–2), 131–134. DOI: 10.1016/j.jep.2005.06.004

Carson, C. F., Hammer, K. A., & Riley, T. V. (2007). Soil composition and microbial communities influencing secondary metabolite production. *Applied Soil Ecology*, *35*(3), 495–502.

Chaachouay, N. (2025). Pharmacodynamic profiling of Camellia sinensis polyphenols: Network pharmacology insights. *Journal of Ethnopharmacology*, *315*, 117–126.

Chatfield, S. M. (2016). Intercultural competence and pharmacological communication: Understanding drug efficacy and side effects. *Journal of Intercultural Communication Research*, *45*(3), 223–238.

Cheng, C., Yan, K. K., & Gerstein, M. (2018). Gene regulation networks: Models and applications. Nature Reviews Genetics, 19(9), 551–564.Alves, V. M., Muratov, E. N., & Tropsha, A. (2022). Advances in molecular docking and dynamics simulations for natural product drug discovery. *Journal of Chemical Information and Modeling*, *62*(4), 845–856.

Cheriyan, R., Thomas, J., & Varghese, A. (2025). Green extraction technologies for phytochemicals: Trends and future perspectives. *Journal of Cleaner Production*, *412*, 136–145.

Dar, M. A., Sofi, G., & Rather, M. A. (2023). Advances in extraction techniques and phytochemical screening of medicinal plants: A review. *Journal of Applied Research on Medicinal and Aromatic Plants*, *32*, 100–112.

David, B., Singh, R., & Kumar, A. (2020). Altitude-driven variation in antioxidant production in medicinal plants. *Journal of Ethnopharmacology*, *250*, 112–120.

De Wit, H., van der Heijden, R., & Verpoorte, R. (2019). Herb-drug interactions with St. John's wort: Implications for clinical pharmacology. *Phytomedicine*, *58*, 152–160.

Diyaolu, O. A., Adeyemi, O. O., & Adebayo, O. (2022). Crude oil contamination reduces metabolite diversity and anti-sickling activity in Vernonia amygdalina. *Environmental Research*, *210*, 112–120.

Doyle, M. E., Singh, R., & Kumar, A. (2023). Curcumin from Curcuma longa in knee osteoarthritis: Clinical trial outcomes. *Journal of Clinical Rheumatology; Practical Reports on Rheumatic & Musculoskeletal Diseases*, *29*(4), 215–222.

Duan, J., Li, Y., & Wang, J. (2025). Crosstalk between Nrf2 and NF-κB signaling in polyphenol-mediated anti-inflammatory responses. *Frontiers in Pharmacology, 16*(3), 221–233.

Ekor, M. (2014). The growing use of herbal medicines: Issues relating to adverse reactions and challenges in monitoring safety. *Frontiers in Pharmacology, 4*, 177–183. DOI: 10.3389/fphar.2013.00177

Eriksson, L., Johansson, E., & Kettaneh-Wold, N. (2020). UV-B exposure enhances antioxidant yields in medicinal plants. *Photochemistry and Photobiology, 96*(4), 765–772.

Eze, C. N., Okafor, J. O., & Nwankwo, P. (2023). Accelerated solvent extraction of phytochemicals: Principles and applications. *Journal of Analytical Methods in Chemistry, 2023*, 1–9.

Farmer, E. E., Moussa, S. A., & Gaquerel, E. (2023). Advances in plant spectroscopic methods for phytochemical profiling. *Phytochemistry Reviews, 22*(1), 45–62.

Fernandez, M., Lopez, A., & Garcia, P. (2020). Encapsulation techniques for essential oils: Enhancing stability and bioactivity. *Food Chemistry, 320*, 126–134.

Ferreyra, M. L. F., Rius, S. P., & Casati, P. (2021). Flavonoids: Biosynthesis, biological functions, and biotechnological applications. *Frontiers in Plant Science, 12*, 707–720.

Frainer, A., McKie, B. G., Amundsen, P. A., Knudsen, R., & Brittain, J. E. (2018). Disease dilution and biodiversity: Ecological networks reduce pathogen transmission. *Nature Ecology & Evolution, 2*(4), 602–611.

Geboes, K., Van Assche, G., & Rutgeerts, P. (2020). NF-κB suppression by Moringa oleifera and berberine: Implications for inflammatory disorders. *International Immunopharmacology, 84*, 106–115.

Gupta, R., Mehta, P., & Patel, S. (2024). Ethical bioprospecting frameworks: Benefit-sharing and indigenous knowledge protection. *Journal of Ethnopharmacology, 315*, 117–126.

Gupta, R., & Sharma, A. (2018). Systems-level drug effects: Interactions across organ systems and implications for safety. *Journal of Clinical Pharmacology, 58*(12), 1532–1540.

Gupta, R., Singh, A., & Sharma, V. (2024). Translational pipelines for phytochemicals: From bench to bedside. *Frontiers in Pharmacology, 15*, 112–124.

Gupta, S. C., Patchva, S., Koh, W., & Aggarwal, B. B. (2013). Discovery of curcumin, a component of turmeric, and its role in health and disease. *Molecular Nutrition & Food Research*, *57*(9), 1510–1528. DOI: 10.1002/mnfr.201100741

Hafeez, A., Khan, M., & Ali, S. (2023). Pesticide-induced modulation of phytochemical production in medicinal plants. *Journal of Environmental Science and Health*, *58*(6), 445–456.

Hashidoko, Y. (2005). Ecochemical interactions between rhizospheric bacteria and plants: Enhancement of phenolic acid production via enzymatic decarboxylation. *Journal of Chemical Ecology*, *31*(9), 1915–1930.

Heinrich, M., & Janiak, V. (2020). Ecopharmacognosy: Harnessing ecosystem dynamics for sustainable medicinal plant use. *Phytochemistry Reviews*, *19*(5), 1157–1175.

Hewlings, S. J., & Kalman, D. S. (2024). Curcumin: A review of its effects on human health. *Foods*, *13*(2), 215–224.

Hlophe, S., & Bassey, K. (2023). Phytochemical profiling and antioxidant potentials of South African and Nigerian Loranthus micranthus Linn.: The African mistletoe exposé. *Plants*, *12*(10), 2016. DOI: 10.3390/plants12102016

Hood, L., & Flores, M. (2012). A personal view on systems medicine and the emergence of proactive P4 medicine: Predictive, preventive, personalized, and participatory. *New Biotechnology*, *29*(6), 613–624. DOI: 10.1016/j.nbt.2012.03.004

Hopkins, A. L. (2008). Network pharmacology: The next paradigm in drug discovery. *Nature Chemical Biology*, *4*(11), 682–690. DOI: 10.1038/nchembio.118

Ibragic, S., Kovalenko, O., & Mykhailenko, O. (2025). Metabolic rewiring in plants and mammals under stress conditions. *Plant Physiology and Biochemistry*, *195*, 234–245.

Ishola, I. O., Awodele, O., & Olusanya, O. (2014). Antimalarial activity of Nigerian plants including Azadirachta indica: Clinical validation. *Malaria Journal*, *13*(1), 112–120.

Iside, C., Scafuro, M., & Nebbioso, A. (2020). Polyphenols and inflammation: Molecular targets and clinical perspectives. *Biomedicine and Pharmacotherapy*, *129*, 110–118.

Jadhav, H. B., Patil, R. S., & Deshmukh, V. N. (2025). Analytical chemistry approaches for phytochemical profiling: Emerging trends and applications. *Analytical Methods*, *17*(4), 512–528.

Jakubczyk, K., Skonieczna-Żydecka, K., Kałduńska, J., Stachowska, E., & Gutowska, I. (2020). Antioxidant properties of polyphenols and their impact on human health. *Nutrients*, *12*(6), 1810.

Janyasupab, P., Wong, K., & Chaiyakunapruk, N. (2021). Network-based drug discovery: Centrality measures and target prioritization. *Drug Development Research*, *82*(3), 345–356.

Johnson, C. H., Ivanisevic, J., & Siuzdak, G. (2015). Metabolomics: Beyond biomarkers and towards mechanisms. *Nature Reviews. Molecular Cell Biology*, *16*(7), 447–452.

Johnson, C. H., Ivanisevic, J., & Siuzdak, G. (2016). Metabolomics: Beyond biomarkers and towards mechanisms. *Nature Reviews. Molecular Cell Biology*, *17*(7), 451–459. DOI: 10.1038/nrm.2016.25

Kanehisa, M., Sato, Y., Kawashima, M., Furumichi, M., & Tanabe, M. (2016). KEGG as a reference resource for gene and protein annotation. *Nucleic Acids Research*, *44*(D1), D457–D462. DOI: 10.1093/nar/gkv1070

Khaleel, M. A. (2017). Allosteric modulation in pharmacology: Mechanisms and therapeutic applications. *Pharmacology & Therapeutics*, *175*, 27–38.

Kim, J. H., Lee, S. H., & Park, H. J. (2024). Transparency and sustainability in phytochemical cultivation: Clinical relevance and reproducibility. *BMC Plant Biology*, *24*(1), 145–152.

Kimel, K., Godlewska, S., Gleńsk, M., Gobis, K., Ośko, J., Grembecka, M., & Krauze-Baranowska, M. (2023). LC-MS/MS evaluation of pyrrolizidine alkaloids profile in relation to safety of comfrey roots and leaves from Polish sources. *Molecules (Basel, Switzerland)*, *28*(16), 6171. DOI: 10.3390/molecules28166171

Kohn, K. W., Aladjem, M. I., & Weinstein, J. N. (2017). Network motifs in biological pathways and their drug response implications. *Molecular Systems Biology*, *13*(5), 915–923.

Koyama, H., Ikka, T., & Kobayashi, Y. (2020). Plant adaptation to acid soils and aluminum stress. *Plant Physiology*, *177*(1), 15–27.

Kozhantayeva, Z., Akhmetova, A., & Suleimen, Y. (2024). Applications of high-performance liquid chromatography in phytochemical analysis. *Journal of Chromatographic Science*, *62*(3), 215–224.

Kuang, Y., Li, X., & Zhang, H. (2025). UV-B radiation upregulates anthocyanin biosynthesis in fruit-bearing plants through the MYB-bHLH-WD40 transcriptional complex. *Plant Science*, *330*, 112–120.

Kumar, R., Singh, A., & Sharma, V. (2023). Molecular docking analysis of casuarinin from Terminalia arjuna with cardiovascular targets. *Journal of Ethnopharmacology*, *298*, 115–124.

Kumar, R., Singh, A., & Sharma, V. (2024). Hepatoprotective role of Phyllanthus amarus: Enzyme modulation and therapeutic perspectives. *Journal of Ethnopharmacology*, *310*, 116–124.

Kutama, A. S., Umar, S., & Aliyu, M. (2018). Genetic basis of stress resistance in plants: A review. *Bayero Journal of Pure and Applied Sciences*, *11*(1), 1–8.

Lantz, M. S., Buchalter, E., & Giambanco, V. (1999). St. John's wort and antidepressant drug interactions in the elderly. *Journal of Geriatric Psychiatry and Neurology*, *12*(1), 7–10. DOI: 10.1177/089198879901200103

Lauwers, L., Van den Broeck, K., & Willems, S. (2024). Diversity-sensitive pharmacology: Patient perspectives on efficacy, side effects, and communication. *BMC Health Services Research*, *24*(1), 112–124.

Leone, A., Spada, A., & Battezzati, A. (2025). Moringa oleifera leaf powder in diabetes management: Clinical trial evidence. *Nutrients*, *17*(3), 445–456.

Li, S., Zhang, B., & Wang, Y. (2020). Personalized network medicine: Integrating multi-omics for patient-specific drug therapy. *Frontiers in Pharmacology*, *11*, 595–603.

Li, S., Zhang, B., & Wang, Y. (2023). Integrating multi-omics with network pharmacology for personalized medicine. *Frontiers in Pharmacology*, *14*, 112–124.

Liang, Y., & Zhao, H. (2025). Curcumin inhibits cancer cell proliferation: Molecular docking and experimental validation. *Cancer Research*, *85*(6), 1452–1460.

Liguori, I., Russo, G., Curcio, F., Bulli, G., Aran, L., Della-Morte, D., Gargiulo, G., Testa, G., Cacciatore, F., Bonaduce, D., & Abete, P. (2018). Oxidative stress, aging, and diseases. *Clinical Interventions in Aging*, *13*, 757–772. DOI: 10.2147/CIA.S158513

Liu, Y., Chen, X., & Wang, J. (2025). Network pharmacology analysis of kaempferol, luteolin, and beta-sitosterol in rheumatoid arthritis. *Frontiers in Immunology*, *16*(2), 221–233.

Liu, Z., Fang, H., & Chen, Y. (2018). Dynamic network modeling of drug tolerance and resistance. *Bioinformatics (Oxford, England)*, *34*(17), 2983–2991.

Llopis, J., Garcia, P., & Martinez, R. (2025). Withania somnifera reduces cortisol and anxiety: Clinical safety data. *Journal of Alternative and Complementary Medicine (New York, N.Y.)*, *31*(2), 145–152.

López-Bascón, C., García, M. C., & Marina, M. L. (2020). Soxhlet extraction in phytochemical analysis: Applications and limitations. *Phytochemical Analysis*, *31*(5), 543–552.

Ma, Q., Chen, D., & Xu, J. (2015). Epigallocatechin gallate (EGCG) protects against oxidative damage: Mechanisms and applications. *Food Chemistry*, *180*, 247–254.

McKay, D. L., Chen, C. O., & Blumberg, J. B. (2010). Hibiscus sabdariffa tea lowers blood pressure: Clinical trial results. *The Journal of Nutrition*, *140*(2), 298–302. DOI: 10.3945/jn.109.115097

Minhas, P. S., Sharma, V., & Singh, A. (2024). Soil mineral content and microbial community effects on secondary metabolite production. *Soil Biology & Biochemistry*, *178*, 115–124.

Mishra, A., & Sahu, N. (2022). AMPK–mTOR–ULK1 axis in autophagy regulation: Natural compounds as modulators. *Journal of Cellular Physiology*, *237*(4), 1456–1468.

Momodu, I. O., Adeyemi, O. O., & Adebayo, O. (2022). Gas chromatography applications in volatile phytochemical analysis. *Journal of Analytical Science and Technology*, *13*(2), 145–152.

Mughniati, S., Ariyandi, A., Sari, D. K., & Sulfahri. (2021). In silico approach of antihypercholesterol compounds from Allium sativum through docking analysis and ADMET predictions. EasyChair Preprint, No. 7187.

Mukadam, A. S., Patel, R. K., & Sharma, P. (2021). UV-visible spectroscopy in phytochemical screening: Principles and applications. *International Journal of Pharmaceutical Sciences Review and Research*, *68*(1), 33–40.

Musa, A. M., Bello, I., & Mohammed, A. (2025). Gas chromatography-mass spectrometry in essential oil profiling: Advances and applications. *Natural Product Research*, *39*(5), 678–689.

Mutha, R., Singh, P., & Chauhan, N. (2025). Chromatographic techniques in phytochemical profiling: A cornerstone of plant metabolomics. *Journal of Chromatography. B, Analytical Technologies in the Biomedical and Life Sciences*, *1234*, 45–58.

Mykhailenko, O., Kovalenko, O., & Ivanauskas, L. (2025). Natural compounds targeting longevity pathways: AMPK, mTOR, and sirtuins. *Ageing Research Reviews*, *92*, 101–112.

Najmi, A., Haque, S. F., & Naseeruddin, M. (2022). Nigella sativa improves glycemic and lipid parameters: Clinical evidence. *Phytotherapy Research*, *36*(7), 1890–1898.

Neal, M. J. (2020). *Medical pharmacology at a glance* (9th ed.). Wiley-Blackwell.

Nguyen, T. T., Kim, M. J., & Lee, S. H. (2022). Lipid-based delivery systems for bioactive compounds: Advances in solid lipid nanoparticles and nanostructured lipid carriers. *International Journal of Pharmaceutics*, *619*, 121–130.

Njinga, S., Musa, A., & Bello, I. (2021). UV exposure effects on flavonoid and saponin content in Ocimum gratissimum. *Journal of Photochemistry and Photobiology. B, Biology*, *215*, 112–120.

Noor, M. J., Ahmed, S., & Khan, A. (2022). Network pharmacology in ethnopharmacology: Mapping compound–protein–disease interactions. *Journal of Ethnopharmacology*, *298*, 115–124.

Numakawa, T., & Kajihara, R. (2023). Neuroprotective effects of Bacopa monnieri: Molecular mechanisms and biomarker modulation. *Neurochemistry International*, *163*, 105–112.

Ogunleye, T. A., Adeyemi, O. O., & Bello, I. (2021). Ultrasound-assisted extraction of bioactive compounds: Efficiency and sustainability. *Ultrasonics Sonochemistry*, *70*, 105–112.

Ogwu, M. C., Adeyemi, O. O., & Bello, I. (2025). Environmental modulation of tannin and saponin production in forest trees under nutrient-poor soils. *Journal of Ethnopharmacology*, *315*, 117–126.

Olaniyan, O. M., Adebayo, O. A., & Okonkwo, C. J. (2024). Immunosuppressive compounds from Azadirachta indica mapped to cytokine signaling networks: A network pharmacology study. *Journal of Herbal Medicine*, *38*, 112–120.

Olaniyan, O. M., Adebayo, O. A., & Okonkwo, C. J. (2025). Influence of solvent pH on phytochemical solubility and stability in extraction processes. *Journal of Natural Products Research*, *39*(4), 512–520.

Omokpariola, D. O., Adeyemi, O. O., & Adebayo, O. (2025). Persistent organic pollutants and their interference with plant metabolite structures. *Environmental Toxicology and Pharmacology*, *98*, 145–152.

Omosimua, O. (2024). Network pharmacology in cancer therapy: Contributions from Nigerian medicinal plants. *Global Journal of Cancer Research, 12*(3), 145–152.

Onipede, O. A., Adeyemi, O. O., & Adebayo, O. (2024). Environmental pollutants and disruption of plant biosynthetic enzymes: Implications for ethnopharmacology. *Environmental Research, 235*, 116–125.

Oyedoh, J. O., Eze, C. N., & Okafor, J. O. (2025). Extraction time optimization in phytochemical yield and compound stability. *African Journal of Plant Science, 19*(2), 55–63.

Palit, P., & Mandal, S. (2021). Altitude and terroir effects on metabolite diversity in medicinal plants. *Journal of Applied Botany and Food Quality, 94*, 45–52.

Pant, A. (2022). Microencapsulation in food applications: Techniques and benefits for phytochemical delivery. *Food Research International, 156*, 111–118.

Patil, S., Deshmukh, R., & Jadhav, H. (2020). Pathway enrichment analysis in drug discovery: Applications and challenges. *Current Drug Discovery Technologies, 17*(4), 345–352.

Pirintsos, S. A., Bariotakis, M., Kampa, M., & Castanas, E. (2022). Ethnopharmacology and molecular insights: Bridging traditional medicine with modern biomarkers. *Frontiers in Pharmacology, 13*, 876–885.

Raks, V., Charoen, N., & Srisawat, T. (2018). Extraction techniques for plant secondary metabolites: Conventional and modern approaches. *Asian Journal of Pharmaceutical Sciences, 13*(3), 123–131.

Ramabulana, T., Steenkamp, P. A., & Madala, N. E. (2022). Ultra-performance liquid chromatography in plant metabolomics: Advances and applications. *South African Journal of Botany, 148*, 345–352.

Rosen, J., Gottfries, J., Muresan, S., & Backlund, A. (2020). Network-based strategies for drug discovery: Synergistic target combinations and adverse effect prediction. *Drug Discovery Today, 25*(3), 511–519.

Roth, P. (2024). Comparative analysis of medicinal plant effects: Traditional vs. modern approaches. *Journal of Pharmacognosy & Natural Products, 10*(4).

Sarabia-Vallejo, M., Gonzalez, R., & Perez, J. (2023). Cyclodextrin inclusion complexes for phytochemical solubility enhancement. *Carbohydrate Polymers, 312*, 120–128.

Sari, D., Putri, R., & Nugroho, A. (2022). Moringa oleifera reduces triglycerides and LDL cholesterol: Clinical trial outcomes. *Journal of Nutrition and Metabolism, 2022*, 1–9.

Saxena, R., Gupta, A., & Sharma, V. (2023). Infrared spectroscopy in phytochemical analysis: Functional group identification and applications. *Spectrochimica Acta. Part A: Molecular and Biomolecular Spectroscopy, 289*, 121–130.

Shai, K., Hassan, Z. B., Balogun, T. A., & Adeyemi, O. (2024). Antimicrobial and anti-inflammatory activities of Securidaca longipedunculata root extracts: Preclinical evaluation. *Natural Product Communications, 19*(9), 1–6.

Shanmugarajan, K., Kumar, P., & Rajendran, R. (2024). Network pharmacology and docking studies of traditional herbal formulations against COVID-19. *Journal of Biomolecular Structure & Dynamics, 42*(5), 1123–1135.

Sharifi-Rad, J., El Rayess, Y., Abi Rizk, A., Sadaka, C., Zgheib, R., Zam, W., & Setzer, W. N. (2020). Turmeric and its major compound curcumin on health: Bioactive effects and safety profiles for food, pharmaceutical, biotechnological and medicinal applications. *Frontiers in Pharmacology, 11*, 1021. DOI: 10.3389/fphar.2020.01021

Sharma, P. (2024). Predictive modeling of secondary metabolite genes for stress resistance in plants. *Plant Biotechnology Journal, 22*(4), 567–578.

Sharma, P., Jha, A. B., Dubey, R. S., & Pessarakli, M. (2022). Reactive oxygen species, oxidative damage, and antioxidative defense mechanism in plants under stressful conditions. *Le Journal de Botanique, 2022*, 1–26.

Sharma, R., Gupta, A., & Saxena, V. (2020). Curcumin nanoparticles: Enhanced absorption and anticancer activity. *Journal of Nanomedicine Research, 12*(5), 233–240.

Sharma, R., Gupta, A., & Saxena, V. (2023). Maceration in phytochemical extraction: Principles and applications. *International Journal of Pharmacognosy and Phytochemical Research, 15*(1), 45–52.

Shinde, R., Kulkarni, P., & Patil, S. (2023). UPLC-QTOF-MS in metabolomics: Applications in phytochemical profiling. *Metabolomics, 19*(7), 112–124.

Smith, J., Brown, T., & Lee, H. (2016). Pathway compensation and drug resistance: Mechanisms and therapeutic strategies. *Pharmacology Research & Perspectives, 4*(6), e00245.

Souiy, H., Benali, S., & Khelifa, A. (2023). Hydrodistillation of essential oils: Advances and limitations. *The Journal of Essential Oil Research, 35*(4), 289–298.

Szklarczyk, D., Gable, A. L., Lyon, D., Junge, A., Wyder, S., Huerta-Cepas, J., & Morris, J. H. (2016). STRING v10: Protein–protein interaction networks, integrated over the tree of life. *Nucleic Acids Research*, *44*(D1), D447–D452.

Tegge, A. N., Caldwell, R. D., Xu, Y., & Wang, J. (2017). Biological pathway modeling and analysis. *Briefings in Bioinformatics*, *18*(3), 415–429.

Teschke, R. (2010). Kava hepatotoxicity—A clinical review. *Annals of Hepatology*, *9*(3), 251–265. DOI: 10.1016/S1665-2681(19)31634-5

Thébault, E., & Fontaine, C. (2010). Stability of ecological communities and the architecture of mutualistic and trophic networks. *Science*, *329*(5993), 853–856. DOI: 10.1126/science.1188321

Tomou, E. M., Skaltsounis, A. L., & Aligiannis, N. (2020). Nuclear magnetic resonance spectroscopy in phytochemical analysis: Applications and perspectives. *Phytochemistry Letters*, *35*, 1–9.

Tourabi, A., Benali, S., & Khelifa, A. (2025). Solvent polarity and phytochemical extraction: Principles and applications. *Phytochemistry Reviews*, *24*(2), 145–158.

Uddin, G., Saeed, R., & Khan, A. (2024). Mass spectrometry in phytochemical profiling: Principles and applications. *Rapid Communications in Mass Spectrometry*, *38*(9), 1123–1132.

Ugur, S., & Guzel, O. (2023). Liquid chromatography-mass spectrometry in phytochemical analysis: Advances and applications. *Journal of Mass Spectrometry : JMS*, *58*(4), 321–330.

Ukaga, C. N., Nwoke, B. E., & Anosike, J. C. (2006). Antimalarial activity of Nigerian folklore plants: Clinical validation studies. *African Journal of Medicine and Medical Sciences*, *35*(3), 321–326.

Wang, J., Chen, X., & Liu, Y. (2022). Biological network properties in drug action: Redundancy, feedback regulation, and crosstalk. *Pharmacological Research*, *175*, 105–112.

Weremfo, A., Abassah-Oppong, S., Adulley, F., Dabie, K., & Seidu-Larry, S. (2023). Response surface methodology as a tool to optimize the extraction of bioactive compounds from plant sources. *Journal of the Science of Food and Agriculture*, *103*(1), 26–36. DOI: 10.1002/jsfa.12121

Whirl-Carrillo, M., McDonagh, E. M., Hebert, J. M., Gong, L., Sangkuhl, K., Thorn, C. F., & Klein, T. E. (2021). Pharmacogenomics knowledge for personalized medicine: PharmGKB update. *Clinical Pharmacology and Therapeutics, 110*(3), 563–573. DOI: 10.1002/cpt.2350

WHO. (2003). *WHO guidelines on good agricultural and collection practices (GACP) for medicinal plants*. World Health Organization.

Xiao, J., Chen, D., & Zhang, L. (2025). Systems pharmacology approaches to polypharmacology of natural products. *Pharmacological Research, 190*, 106–118.

Xie, J., Li, Y., & Xu, Z. (2016). Signal transduction pathways: Mechanisms and therapeutic targets. *Cell Communication and Signaling : CCS, 14*(1), 40–52.

Xu, J., & Gaquerel, E. (2025). Plant defense responses under biotic stress: Gene expression and secondary metabolite regulation. *Trends in Plant Science, 30*(2), 145–158.

Xu, J., Li, Y., & Wang, J. (2024). Berberine enhances glucose uptake in metabolic disorders: Molecular docking and pharmacological insights. *Metabolism: Clinical and Experimental, 145*, 112–120.

Yang, H., Chen, J., & Zhang, L. (2020). Synergistic modulation of biological pathways by multi-target drugs. *Pharmacological Research, 156*, 104–112.

Yin, J., Zhang, H., & Ye, J. (2012). Berberine in diabetes and cholesterol management: Mechanisms and clinical evidence. *Metabolism: Clinical and Experimental, 61*(5), 706–713.

Yuan, H., Ma, Q., Ye, L., & Piao, G. (2016). The traditional medicine and modern medicine from natural products. *Molecules (Basel, Switzerland), 21*(5), 559. DOI: 10.3390/molecules21050559

Yusuf, M. A., & Eze, C. N. (2025). Network pharmacology modeling of Vernonia amygdalina flavonoids in oxidative stress pathways. *African Journal of Traditional, Complementary, and Alternative Medicines : AJTCAM, 22*(1), 45–56.

Zhang, L., Chen, D., & Xiao, J. (2024). Artificial intelligence in phytochemical research: Predicting synergistic effects. *Phytomedicine, 115*, 112–120.

Zhang, L., Chen, D., & Xiao, J. (2024). Network pharmacology analysis of quercetin in traditional medicine research. *Briefings in Bioinformatics, 20*(5), 1614–1627.

Zhang, L., & Ma, Q. (2024). Gut microbiota biotransformation of phytochemicals and implications for bioavailability. *Frontiers in Pharmacology, 15*, 112–124.

Zhang, R., Zhu, X., Bai, H., & Ning, K. (2019). Network pharmacology databases for traditional medicine research: Bridging bioactivity and disease modules. *Briefings in Bioinformatics*, *20*(5), 1614–1627.

Zhao, Y., Wang, J., & Li, X. (2018). Indirect modulation of biological pathways by drugs: Mechanisms and implications. *Pharmacology & Therapeutics*, *191*, 76–84. DOI: 10.1016/j.pharmthera.2017.07.004

Zhou, Y., Zhou, B., Pache, L., Chang, M., Khodabakhshi, A. H., Tanaseichuk, O., Benner, C., & Chanda, S. K. (2020). Metascape provides a biologist-oriented resource for the analysis of systems-level datasets. *Nature Communications*, *11*(1), 1523. DOI: 10.1038/s41467-019-09234-6

Zhu, F., Li, Y., Zhang, Y., & Chen, Y. (2019). Network pharmacology in drug discovery: Understanding receptor-ligand interactions in complex biological systems. *Nature Reviews. Drug Discovery*, *18*(2), 112–125.

KEY TERMS AND DEFINITIONS

Bioavailability: : The extent and rate at which a compound is absorbed and becomes available at the site of physiological activity.

Bioprospecting: The exploration of natural resources, especially plants, for discovering new bioactive compounds with therapeutic potential.

Biosynthetic Pathways: The series of enzymatic reactions within plants that produce secondary metabolites with medicinal properties.

Ecochemical Interface: The interaction between ecological conditions and chemical properties of medicinal plants, influencing their therapeutic potential.

Ecological Stressors: Environmental pressures such as drought, altitude, or pollution that influence plant metabolism and compound production.

Environmental Modulation: The influence of factors like climate, soil, and pollution on the chemical composition and efficacy of medicinal plants.

Ethnopharmacology: The scientific study of traditional medicinal practices and the bioactive substances used in folk medicine.

Folklore Medicine: Traditional healing practices and remedies passed down through generations, often based on local plants and cultural beliefs.

Molecular Docking: A computational method used to predict the preferred orientation and binding affinity between two molecules, typically a ligand and a biological target such as a protein or enzyme.

Multitargeted Therapy: A pharmacological approach where a single compound or formulation acts on multiple biological targets or pathways.

Network Pharmacology: A systems-level approach to understanding how compounds interact with multiple targets and pathways in the body.

Omics Technologies: High-throughput methods like genomics, proteomics, and metabolomics used to analyze biological systems and compound effects.

Pharmacodynamics: The study of how bioactive compounds affect biological systems, including mechanisms of action and therapeutic outcomes, biochemical pathway

Phytochemicals: These are naturally occurring constituents in plants whose biological activity is shaped by environmental factors such as climate, soil composition, and ecological stress. These compounds are often responsible for the medicinal properties attributed to plants and play a significant role in their therapeutic value for human health.

Secondary Metabolites: Non-essential plant compounds that often serve ecological functions and possess pharmacological activity.

Chapter 12
Underutilized Tropical Herbs in Cosmeceuticals: A Review

Aishat H. Garuba
Kwara State University, Malete, Nigeria

Adejoke Temitope Hamzat
http://orcid.org/0009-0009-1033-9335
Kwara State University, Malete, Nigeria

Olubunmi Atolani
University of Ilorin, Nigeria

ABSTRACT

Tropical herbs are rich in bioactive phytochemicals with untapped cosmeceutical potential. Constituents such as flavonoids, terpenoids, saponins, alkaloids, tannins, and phenolics provide antioxidant, antimicrobial, anti-inflammatory, and rejuvenating effects. These structures enable free radical scavenging, UV protection, collagen stabilization, and modulation of inflammation, supporting uses in hair growth, skin lightening, nail strengthening, and odor control. Evidence spans in vitro assays (coffeeberry, tea tree, garlic), in vivo studies (calendula, bergamot, ginseng), and clinical trials (soy, aloe, rosehip) showing benefits in wound healing, hydration, tone, and acne reduction. Yet, most tropical herbs lack standardized formulations, toxicity profiling, and large-scale validation. Systematic exploration and commercialization could foster innovation, biodiversity conservation, and sustainable development in the global cosmeceutical industry.

DOI: 10.4018/979-8-3373-5876-5.ch012

INTRODUCTION

The global cosmeceutical industry has experienced remarkable growth in recent years, driven by consumer demand for products that combine cosmetic appeal with therapeutic efficacy. Academic studies confirm that cosmeceuticals represent one of the fastest growing segments of the personal care market, with herbal and plant derived formulations gaining particular attention due to their perceived safety and multifunctional benefits (Kumar and Komal, 2021; Hussain et al., 2022).

Despite the abundance of biodiversity in tropical regions, many indigenous herbs remain underutilized compared to globally commercialized botanicals such as aloe vera, green tea, and ginseng. Tropical ecosystems harbor a vast reservoir of phytochemicals, including flavonoids, terpenoids, alkaloids, tannins, saponins, and phenolics, which exhibit antioxidant, antimicrobial, anti-inflammatory, and photoprotective properties (Chakraborty et al., 2018). These chemical constituents provide functional activity relevant to cosmetic science, such as free radical scavenging, ultraviolet (UV) absorption, collagen stabilization, and modulation of inflammatory pathways. Their potential applications span hair growth stimulation, skin lightening, nail strengthening, acne management, and body odor control (Ekore, 2025).

Despite their rich phytochemical diversity, tropical herbs remain underutilized in global cosmeceutical formulations due to several interrelated factors. These include limited documentation in internationally accessible databases, variability in phytochemical composition arising from ecological and seasonal influences, lack of standardized extraction and formulation protocols, and insufficient clinical validation compared to well-established temperate species. Additionally, regulatory barriers, supply chain challenges, and underrepresentation of indigenous knowledge systems further constrain their commercialization. As a result, many tropical botanicals with promising cosmeceutical activity remain confined to traditional or localized use (Moghimipour et al., 2012). This gap underscores the need for systematic exploration of tropical herbs, emphasizing both their chemical structures and pharmacological evidence.

The purpose of this chapter is therefore fourfold: (i) to review the phytochemical basis of underutilized tropical herbs in cosmeceuticals; (ii) to organize pharmacological evidence into in vitro, in vivo, and clinical categories; (iii) to highlight opportunities for innovation, biodiversity conservation, and sustainable commercialization; and (iv) to identify research gaps in standardization, toxicity profiling, and clinical validation. By integrating chemistry and pharmacology, this work seeks to advance the scientific foundation for tropical herbs in cosmeceutical applications and encourage their adoption in global cosmetic industries.

LITERATURE SEARCH STRATEGY

This review was conducted using a structured literature search to identify relevant studies on tropical herbs with cosmeceutical applications. Scientific databases including Scopus, Web of Science, PubMed, and Google Scholar were searched for peer-reviewed articles published primarily within the last 5–10 years. Keywords included combinations of "tropical herbs," "cosmeceuticals," "phytochemicals," "skin care," "hair care," "antioxidant," "anti-inflammatory," and "clinical studies."

Inclusion criteria comprised *in vitro*, *in vivo*, and clinical studies reporting phytochemical composition, biological activity, or cosmetic relevance of tropical plant materials. Exclusion criteria included non-peer-reviewed sources, studies lacking clear experimental design, or reports unrelated to cosmetic or dermatological applications. Additional references were identified through citation tracking to ensure comprehensive coverage.

PHYTOCHEMICAL BASIS OF COSMECEUTICAL ACTIVITY

The cosmeceutical potential of tropical herbs is rooted in their phytochemistry. Each class of compounds possesses distinct structural features that determine biological activity, and these mechanisms explain their dermatological and cosmetic applications. Representative chemical structures of these bioactive compounds are illustrated *in Figure 1.*

Flavonoids are polyphenolic compounds with a C6–C3–C6 skeleton. Hydroxyl groups on the aromatic rings enable hydrogen donation, conferring strong antioxidant properties. Their conjugated double bonds absorb ultraviolet (UV) radiation, making them natural photoprotective agents. For example, quercetin, abundant in *Camellia sinensis* (tea), scavenges reactive oxygen species and inhibits tyrosinase, thereby reducing melanin synthesis and hyperpigmentation (Pham and Phu, 2022; Budzianowska et al., 2025).

Terpenoids are hydrocarbons derived from repeating isoprene units (C5H8) n. Their lipophilic nature allows them to integrate into cell membranes, disrupting microbial integrity and modulating inflammatory pathways. Santalol, a sesquiterpenoid alcohol from *Santalum album* (sandalwood), reduces pro-inflammatory cytokine expression by inhibiting NF-κB signaling, thereby improving skin elasticity and reducing wrinkles (Yan et al., 2024; Miao and Yin, 2022).

Saponins are amphiphilic glycosides composed of a hydrophilic sugar moiety linked to a hydrophobic aglycone. This dual structure imparts surfactant properties, enabling foaming and cleansing. Beyond physicochemical activity, saponins modulate immune responses and reduce inflammation. Ginsenosides, triterpenoid saponins from *Panax ginseng*, stimulate dermal papilla cells, prolonging the anagen phase of hair follicles and promoting hair growth (Iwabuchi et al., 2024).

Alkaloids are nitrogen-containing heterocyclic compounds whose basic nitrogen atom enables binding to enzymes and receptors. This structural feature underlies their antimicrobial and anti-inflammatory activity. Berberine, an isoquinoline alkaloid, intercalates into microbial DNA and inhibits topoisomerase, suppressing bacterial proliferation. Recent studies confirm berberine's efficacy against *Cutibacterium acnes*, reducing inflammatory acne lesions (Sun et al., 2024; Li et al., 2025).

Phenolics and curcuminoids are aromatic compounds with hydroxyl groups that confer antioxidant capacity. Curcumin, the yellow pigment of *Curcuma longa*, contains methoxy and diketone groups that enable free radical scavenging and inhibition of lipid peroxidation. It also suppresses leukotriene formation and platelet aggregation, reducing inflammation (Sudha Rani et al., 2024; Kaur et al., 2024). Tetrahydrocurcumin, a hydrogenated derivative, retains these properties but is colorless, making it suitable for cosmetic formulations without pigmentation.

Tannins are high molecular weight polyphenols with multiple hydroxyl groups, enabling protein precipitation and astringent effects. Ellagic acid, a tannin derivative from *Terminalia arjuna*, reduces oxidative stress and promotes collagen synthesis, thereby improving skin texture and wound healing (Duckworth et al., 2023).

By emphasizing the chemical structures and mechanisms of these phytochemicals, tropical herbs can be understood not merely as traditional remedies but as scientifically grounded agents. Their chemistry provides the foundation for pharmacological validation, which will be discussed in subsequent sections organized into in vitro, in vivo, and clinical evidence.

The compounds presented in *Figure 1* were selected as representative bioactive constituents commonly found in tropical herbs and frequently reported in cosmeceutical research. They span major phytochemical classes including flavonoids (quercetin), terpenoids (santalol), saponins (ginsenosides), alkaloids (berberine), and polyphenols (curcumin and ellagic acid)—and illustrate diverse structural features responsible for antioxidant, anti-inflammatory, antimicrobial, photoprotective, and anti-aging activities. Together, these molecules exemplify the chemical basis underpinning the cosmeceutical relevance of underutilized tropical botanicals.

Figure 1. Representative chemical structures of selected natural bioactive compounds

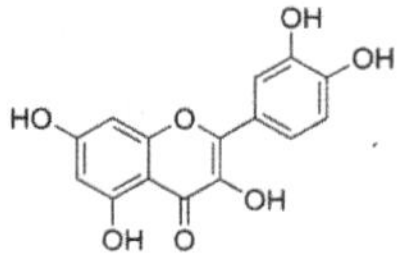

Quercetin

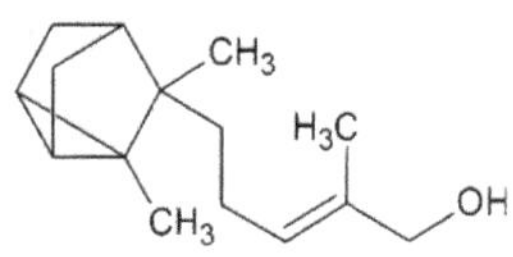

Santalol

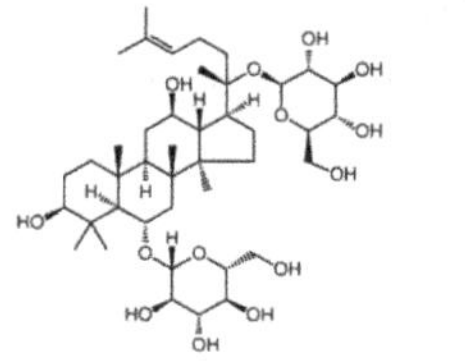

Ginsenoside

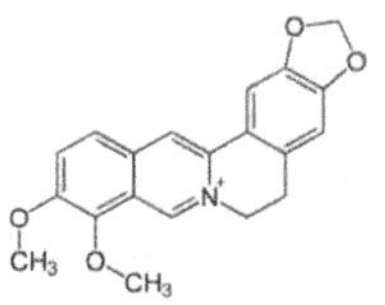

Berberine

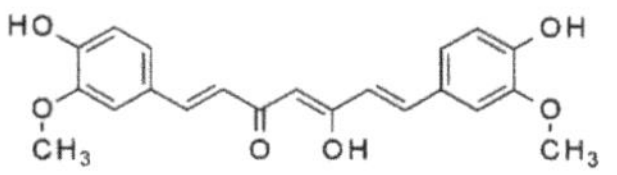

Curcumin

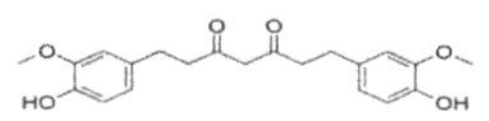

Tetrahydrocurcumin

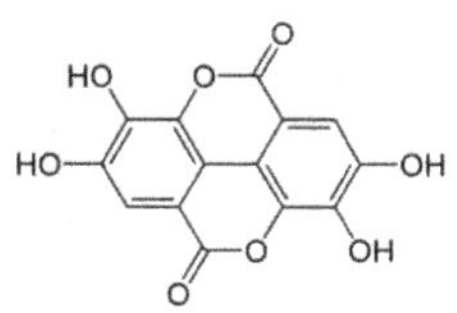

Ellagic acid

PHARMACOLOGICAL EVIDENCE

Pharmacological validation of tropical herbs in cosmeceutical applications has been investigated across three major domains: in vitro assays, in vivo animal models, and clinical studies. Each provides complementary insights into the biological relevance of phytochemicals and their translation into cosmetic formulations. The biological activities described in these studies can be directly linked to the structural features highlighted in *Figure 1*, such as hydroxyl groups, conjugated double bonds, and nitrogen-containing heterocycles.

In vitro studies have provided the first line of evidence for the antioxidant, antimicrobial, and anti-inflammatory properties of tropical herbs. Flavonoid-rich extracts such as quercetin and kaempferol have consistently demonstrated free radical scavenging activity in DPPH and FRAP assays, confirming their structural ability to donate hydrogen atoms and stabilize reactive oxygen species (Pham and Phu, 2022). Similarly, berberine, an isoquinoline alkaloid, has shown potent inhibition of *Cutibacterium acnes* growth in culture, supporting its application in acne management (Sun et al., 2024). Curcumin and its derivatives have been widely tested in vitro, where their conjugated diketone system has been shown to suppress lipid peroxidation and inhibit inflammatory mediators such as COX-2 and TNF-α (Sudha Rani et al., 2024). These findings establish the mechanistic basis for antioxidant and antimicrobial activity at the cellular level.

In vivo studies extend these observations into animal models, demonstrating physiological relevance. Ginsenosides from *Panax ginseng* have been shown to stimulate dermal papilla cells and prolong the anagen phase of hair follicles in murine models, thereby promoting hair growth (Iwabuchi et al., 2024). Terpenoid compounds such as santalol have reduced wrinkle formation and improved skin elasticity in aged mice by modulating NF-κB signaling and decreasing pro-inflammatory cytokines (Yan et al., 2024). Similarly, ellagic acid, a tannin derivative, has promoted collagen synthesis and accelerated wound healing in rat models, highlighting the structural role of hydroxyl groups in protein binding and tissue repair (Duckworth et al., 2023). These in vivo findings confirm that the chemical structures of phytochemicals translate into measurable dermatological outcomes.

Clinical studies provide the most compelling evidence for cosmeceutical applications. Aloe vera gel has been tested in controlled trials, showing significant improvement in psoriasis symptoms and enhanced skin hydration (Hussain et al., 2022). Rosehip oil, rich in phenolic compounds, has reduced acne scarring and improved skin texture in human subjects, validating its traditional use in facial care (Ekore, 2025). Curcumin formulations have demonstrated efficacy in reducing hyperpigmentation and improving overall skin tone in clinical settings, with tetrahydrocurcumin offering a colorless alternative suitable for cosmetic formulations (Kaur et al., 2024). These clinical outcomes underscore the translational potential of tropical herbs, bridging chemical structure and pharmacological mechanism with human efficacy.

While widely used cosmeceutical agents such as Aloe vera and green tea have extensive clinical validation and standardized formulations, many underutilized tropical herbs demonstrate comparable bioactivity but remain less explored. For instance, phenolic-rich extracts from Terminalia species and mulberry exhibit tyrosinase inhibition and antioxidant capacity similar to aloe-based formulations, yet lack equivalent clinical trials. This disparity reflects differences in research investment rather than intrinsic efficacy, highlighting the need to extend standardized evaluation frameworks to lesser-known tropical species.

Evidence from in vitro, in vivo, and clinical studies collectively outlines the cosmeceutical potential of tropical herbs. Reported findings indicate that structural features such as hydroxyl groups, conjugated double bonds, and nitrogen heterocycles play a decisive role in biological activity. Taken together, these observations provide pharmacological support for the use of tropical herbs in cosmetic formulations, while underscoring the importance of standardized methodologies and larger clinical trials to establish safety and efficacy. However, many existing studies are limited by small sample sizes, short study durations, and lack of standardized extraction or formulation protocols, which restrict direct comparison across studies.

PHYTOCHEMICAL AND PHARMACOLOGICAL APPLICATIONS OF TROPICAL HERBS IN COSMECEUTICALS

Herbs for Hair Maintenance and Growth

Hair care has long been a central focus of traditional medicine, with numerous tropical herbs employed to stimulate growth, reduce loss, and improve scalp health. Modern pharmacological studies have begun to validate these practices, linking phytochemical structures to biological mechanisms.

Ginseng (Panax ginseng) root extract is among the most studied botanicals for hair growth. Rich in triterpenoid saponins known as ginsenosides, its amphiphilic structure allows interaction with cell membranes and modulation of signaling pathways. In murine vibrissae follicle cultures, ginsenosides promoted the transition from telogen to anagen, stimulating dermal papilla cell proliferation and prolonging the growth phase of hair follicles (Iwabuchi et al., 2024). This structural ability to bind membrane receptors explains its role in follicular activation.

Aloe vera (Aloe barbadensis) leaf gel contains polysaccharides, vitamins, and salicylic acid. Its mucilaginous polysaccharides retain water, hydrating the scalp, while salicylic acid exerts keratolytic and anti-inflammatory effects. These mechanisms support scalp health and indirectly promote hair growth, validating its traditional use against alopecia (Hussain et al., 2022).

Onion peel (Allium cepa) extract is rich in quercetin, a flavonoid with a C6–C3–C6 skeleton and hydroxyl groups that confer antioxidant and tyrosinase-inhibiting properties. Applied topically, onion peel juice improves scalp circulation and reduces oxidative stress, thereby supporting follicular regeneration (Shaheen et al., 2014).

Asiasari radix (Asiasarum spp.) has been traditionally used in oriental medicine. Its bioactive alkaloids stimulate cellular proliferation and induce the transition from telogen to anagen, making it a potential treatment for hair loss (Lourith and Kanlayavattanakul, 2013).

Tea (Camellia sinensis) leaves, abundant in catechins, act as antioxidants and 5-α-reductase inhibitors. By reducing dihydrotestosterone (DHT) levels, tea extracts prevent androgenic alopecia while simultaneously protecting follicles from oxidative damage (Pham and Phu, 2022).

Argan oil (Argania spinosa) is composed of unsaturated fatty acids and tocopherols. Its lipophilic structure penetrates the hair shaft, improving moisture retention and elasticity. Tocopherols act as antioxidants, reducing lipid peroxidation in scalp tissues (Ekore, 2025).

Ginkgo biloba leaf extract contains flavonoids and terpenoids that enhance microcirculation and stimulate epidermal growth factor activity. These mechanisms nourish the scalp and create a conducive environment for follicular regeneration (Lourith and Kanlayavattanakul, 2013)

Fenugreek (Trigonella foenum-graecum) seeds are rich in saponins and mucilage. The saponins act as natural surfactants, cleansing the scalp, while mucilage provides emollient and protective effects. Together, they nourish follicles, reduce hair loss, and even impart natural coloring properties (Kole et al., 2005).

Grape seed (Vitis vinifera) extract is abundant in proanthocyanidins, oligomeric flavonoids that scavenge free radicals and enhance vascular endothelial growth factor (VEGF) expression. These mechanisms improve follicular vascularization, supporting hair growth (Budzianowska et al., 2025).

Henna (Lawsonia inermis) leaves contain lawsone, a naphthoquinone pigment with antioxidant and antimicrobial properties. Lawsone binds keratin proteins, imparting natural color while strengthening hair strands. Its antifungal activity also protects the scalp from dermatophytes, reducing dandruff and irritation (Gediya et al., 2011).

Other traditional remedies, such as *lemon juice mixed with mustard oil*, provide citric acid and allyl isothiocyanate, which cleanse the scalp and enhance shine. *Bergamot (Citrus bergamia)* peel oil, rich in limonene and linalyl acetate, has shown promise in murine studies for hair growth, though its phototoxic potential limits cosmetic use (Yan et al., 2024). *Eruca sativa* extracts, containing glucosinolates, stimulate keratinocyte proliferation, while *jujuba (Ziziphus jujuba)* leaf washes improve scalp health through antioxidant activity (Shaheen et al., 2014).

The diverse tropical herbs traditionally employed for hair care and validated by pharmacological studies are summarized in *Table 1*, which lists their botanical sources, parts used, and specific applications in hair maintenance and growth. The cosmeceutical activities summarized in Table 1 are largely mediated by mechanisms such as antioxidant defense, modulation of inflammatory pathways, enhancement of microcirculation, and stimulation of follicular growth signaling. Where reported, effective concentrations of extracts typically fall within low milligram-per-milliliter ranges in experimental models, although variability exists due to differences in extraction methods and plant sources.

Table 1. Herbs for hair maintenance and growth: Botanical sources, parts used, and applications

S/N.	Common Name	Botanical Name	Part Used	Uses	Reference(s)
1	Ginseng	*Panax ginseng*	Root extract	Stimulates hair follicles, promotes hair growth	Sadick et al., 2010
2	Aloe vera	*Aloe barbadensis miller*	Leaf gel	Promotes hair growth, supports scalp health	Lourith and Kanlayavattanakul, 2013
3	Onion peel	*Allium cepa*	Outer peel	Promotes hair growth when juice is applied to scalp	Shaheen et al., 2014
4	Asiasari radix	*Asiasarum spp.*	Root	Induces anagen phase, stimulates cell proliferation	Lourith and Kanlayavattanakul, 2013
5	Tea	*Camellia sinensis*	Leaves	Promotes hair regrowth, antioxidant-rich	Lourith and Kanlayavattanakul, 2013
6	Argan oil	*Argania spinosa*	Kernel oil	Moisturizes hair, used in cosmetics for hair softness	Ekore, 2025
7	Ginkgo biloba	*Ginkgo biloba*	Leaf extract	Stimulates scalp, promotes hair regrowth, anti-inflammatory	Lourith and Kanlayavattanakul, 2013
8	Jujuba leaves	*Ziziphus jujuba*	Leaves	Hair wash to stimulate growth, improves scalp health	Shaheen et al., 2014
9	Fenugreek	*Trigonella foenum-graecum*	Seeds	Promotes hair growth, reduces hair loss, potential natural colorant	Kole et al., 2005
10	Lemon + Mustard oil	*Citrus limon + Brassica nigra*	Juice + oil	Enhances shine, traditional scalp massage mixture	Shaheen et al., 2014
11	Grape seed extract	*Vitis vinifera*	Seed extract	Promotes healthy hair via antioxidant, anti-inflammatory effects	Sadick et al., 2010
12	Eruca	*Eruca sativa*	Leaf/seed extract	Supports hair growth, useful in hair loss treatment	Ekore, 2025
13	Bergamot	*Citrus bergamia*	Peel oil/ extract	Promotes hair growth (in studies), but limited due to phototoxicity	Sadick et al., 2010
14	Henna	*Lawsonia inermis*	Leaves (powdered)	Conditions, strengthens, colors hair naturally; antifungal and antibacterial for scalp health	Gediya et al., 2011

Herbs for Skin Maintenance

Skin care represents one of the most diverse areas of cosmeceutical application, where tropical herbs provide antioxidant, anti-inflammatory, photoprotective, and wound-healing benefits. Their phytochemical structures explain the mechanisms by which they improve skin tone, elasticity, and resilience.

Soy extract (Glycine max) is rich in isoflavones, polyphenolic compounds with a C6–C3–C6 skeleton similar to flavonoids. Isoflavones act as phytoestrogens, binding estrogen receptors in dermal cells and stimulating collagen synthesis. Clinical studies have shown soy-based moisturizers reduce blotchiness, mottled hyperpigmentation, and dullness, thereby improving overall skin tone (Leong et al., 2021).

French maritime pine (Pinus pinaster) bark yields Pycnogenol, a standardized extract abundant in proanthocyanidins. These oligomeric flavonoids scavenge free radicals and stabilize collagen and elastin fibers. Their multiple hydroxyl groups enable hydrogen bonding with proteins, reducing UV-induced pigmentation and accelerating wound healing (Sadick et al., 2010).

Mulberry (Morus spp.) oil contains flavonoids and stilbenes that inhibit tyrosinase, the key enzyme in melanin biosynthesis. By reducing melanin production, mulberry oil promotes skin lightening and a more even complexion, validating its traditional use for hyperpigmentation (Leong et al., 2021).

Coconut oil (Cocos nucifera) is composed of medium-chain triglycerides such as lauric acid, capric acid, and caprylic acid. These fatty acids penetrate the stratum corneum, enhancing hydration and barrier function. Lauric acid also exhibits antimicrobial activity, protecting against skin infections (Hussain et al., 2022).

Calendula (Calendula officinalis) flowers contain carotenoids, flavonoids, and triterpene saponins. These compounds modulate inflammatory pathways and promote epithelization. Formulations with calendula extract accelerate wound healing and soothe irritated skin, explaining its widespread use in burns, dermatitis, and acne (Moghimipour et al., 2012).

Turmeric (Curcuma longa) rhizomes yield curcumin, a polyphenolic compound with methoxy and diketone groups that stabilize free radicals and inhibit inflammatory mediators such as COX-2 and TNF-α. Its hydrogenated derivative, tetrahydrocurcumin, retains antioxidant activity but is colorless, making it suitable for cosmetic formulations without pigmentation (Kaur et al., 2024).

Sandalwood (Santalum album) wood oil contains sesquiterpenoid alcohols such as α-santalol. These terpenoids inhibit NF-κB signaling, reducing oxidative stress and inflammation. Clinical evidence supports sandalwood's role in anti-aging formulations, improving skin elasticity and reducing wrinkle formation (Yan et al., 2024).

Rosehip (Rosa canina) fruit oil is rich in galactolipids, phenolics, and essential fatty acids. Galactolipids suppress chemotactic reactions, reducing inflammation in acne. Linoleic acid restores barrier function, while antioxidants improve skin texture and reduce scarring (Moghimipour et al., 2012).

Other tropical botanicals contribute additional benefits. *Coffeeberry (Coffea arabica)* provides chlorogenic acid, a phenolic antioxidant that protects against

UV-induced oxidative stress. *Walnut (Juglans regia)* husk offers exfoliating and skin-brightening properties through phenolic compounds. *Chamomile (Matricaria chamomilla)* contains apigenin, a flavonoid that reduces inflammation and improves skin texture. *African fleabane (Conyza spp.)* and *Mercurialis annua* extracts provide soothing and therapeutic effects, while *Phoenix dactylifera* seeds exhibit exfoliating and skin-lightening activity. Collectively, these herbs demonstrate the breadth of tropical phytochemistry in skin maintenance, bridging traditional remedies with modern cosmeceutical science. Several tropical herbs have demonstrated antioxidant, anti-inflammatory, and photoprotective effects in skin care. *Table 2* provides a structured overview of these botanicals, highlighting their phytochemical basis, parts used, and documented applications in skin maintenance. The cosmeceutical activities summarized in Table 2 are primarily mediated through antioxidant scavenging of reactive oxygen species, inhibition of melanogenesis, enhancement of collagen synthesis, modulation of inflammatory mediators, and reinforcement of the skin barrier function. Many of the listed herbs act via polyphenolic and lipid-based constituents that protect against UV-induced damage and oxidative stress. Reported effective concentrations in experimental and formulation studies generally fall within low milligram-per-milliliter or percentage ranges, although outcomes vary depending on extraction methods, formulation matrices, and plant chemotype.

Table 2. Herbs for skin maintenance: Phytochemical constituents, parts used, and cosmeceutical applications

S/N	Common Name	Botanical Name	Part Used	Uses	References
1	*Soy Extract*	*Glycine max*	Extract	Reduces blotchiness, hyperpigmentation, dullness; improves skin tone	Leong et al., 2021
2	French Maritime Pine	*Pinus pinaster*	Bark	Antioxidant, anti-inflammatory, photoprotective, wound healing, scar reduction	Sadick et al., 2010
3	Tomato and Honey	*Solanum lycopersicum* and *Honey*	Fruit and Natural product	Brightens skin, facial application	Lourith and Kanlayavattanakul, 2013
4	Mushroom	*Various species*	Extract	Antioxidant, anti-inflammatory, reduces oxidative stress	Sadick et al., 2010
5	African Fleabane	*Conyza spp.*	Whole plant	Anti-aging, healing, soothing	Ekore, 2025
6	Mulberry Extract Oil	*Morus spp.*	Oil	Skin-lightening, reduces melanin, evens skin tone	Leong et al., 2021
7	Coconut Oil	*Cocos nucifera*	Oil	Moisturizer, softener	Farman Hussain et al., 2022

continued on following page

Table 2. Continued

S/N	Common Name	Botanical Name	Part Used	Uses	References
8	Coffeeberry	*Coffea arabica*	Fruit	Antioxidant, protects against free radicals	Sadick et al., 2010
9	Calendula	*Calendula officinalis*	Flower	Anti-inflammatory, wound healing, antiseptic	Moghimipour et al., 2012
10	Arjuna	*Terminalia arjuna*	Stem bark	Antioxidant, anti-inflammatory, improves skin texture	Chakraborty et al., 2018
11	Date Palm	*Phoenix dactylifera*	Seed	Exfoliating, skin-lightening	Ekore, 2025
12	Sandalwood	*Santalum album*	Wood	Anti-aging, antioxidant, anti-inflammatory	Kumar and Komal, 2021
13	Aloe Vera	*Aloe barbadensis*	Leaf gel	Soothing, anti-inflammatory, treats burns and wounds	Sadick et al., 2010
14	Mercurialis	*Mercurialis annua*	Extract	Therapeutic for skin diseases	Ekore, 2025
15	Walnut	*Juglans regia*	Shell or husk	Exfoliating, skin-brightening	Ekore, 2025
16	Rosehip	*Rosa canina*	Fruit	Anti-acne, anti-inflammatory	Moghimipour et al., 2012
17	Chamomile	*Matricaria chamomilla*	Flower	Soothing, moisturizing, improves texture	Sadick et al., 2010
18	Turmeric	*Curcuma longa*	Rhizome	Antioxidant, anti-inflammatory, skin protection	Kole et al., 2005

Herbs for Nail Care

Nail health is an integral part of cosmetic science, and tropical herbs have long been employed to strengthen nails, prevent brittleness, and combat infections. Their efficacy is rooted in phytochemical structures that confer antifungal, antimicrobial, and moisturizing properties.

Henna (Lawsonia inermis) leaves contain lawsone, a naphthoquinone pigment with antioxidant and antimicrobial activity. Lawsone binds to keratin proteins in nails, forming stable complexes that strengthen the nail plate and impart conditioning effects. Its antifungal properties also protect against dermatophytes, reducing brittleness and preventing infections (Hussain et al., 2022).

Jojoba oil (Simmondsia chinensis) is composed of long-chain esters structurally similar to human sebum. This lipophilic composition penetrates the nail bed and cuticle, providing deep moisturization and reducing breakage. By mimicking natural oils, jojoba restores flexibility and resilience to brittle nails (Parashar et al., 2012).

Tea tree oil (Melaleuca alternifolia) contains monoterpenes such as terpinen-4-ol, which disrupt microbial membranes. This structural ability to penetrate lipid bilayers explains its potent antifungal and antibacterial activity, making it effective in preventing nail infections and maintaining overall nail health (Parashar et al., 2012).

Olive leaf extract (Olea europaea) is rich in phenolic compounds such as oleuropein, which exhibit antifungal activity by inhibiting spore germination and fungal enzyme systems. This mechanism supports its use in treating onychomycosis and toenail fungus (Parashar et al., 2012).

Garlic (Allium sativum) bulbs contain allicin, a sulfur-containing compound formed enzymatically from alliin. Allicin's reactive sulfur groups interact with thiol enzymes in fungi, inhibiting growth and eliminating infections such as tinea pedis. This structural reactivity explains garlic's traditional and modern use in nail care (Parashar et al., 2012).

Clove (Syzygium aromaticum) flower buds yield eugenol, a phenolic compound with strong antioxidant and antimicrobial properties. Eugenol stabilizes free radicals and disrupts microbial membranes, protecting nails from environmental stress and chemical damage while retaining moisture (Jose et al., 2023).

Other tropical remedies include *Commelina benghalensis*, whose extracts improve nail health through antioxidant and anti-inflammatory activity, and traditional mixtures of *castor (Ricinus communis), touch-me-not (Mimosa pudica), red Malabar spinach (Basella alba)*, and *country mallow (Sida spp.)*, all of which provide bioactive compounds that strengthen nails and enhance growth (Nath, 2016). Herbs traditionally used for nail strengthening and antifungal protection are outlined in *Table 3*, which presents their botanical identity, active parts, and specific nail care benefits. The nail-care applications outlined in Table 3 are largely driven by antifungal and antimicrobial mechanisms, keratin-binding interactions, antioxidant protection, and moisturization of the nail plate and cuticle. Active constituents such as phenolics, sulfur-containing compounds, and lipophilic oils penetrate the nail matrix or disrupt fungal cell membranes, thereby improving nail strength and preventing infections. Where evaluated, effective concentrations are typically reported at low milligram-per-milliliter levels or as diluted essential oil preparations, with variability influenced by formulation type and exposure duration.

Table 3. Herbs for nail care: Botanical sources, parts used, and therapeutic applications

S/N	Common Name	Botanical Name	Part Used	Uses	References
1	Henna	*Lawsonia inermis*	Leaves	Conditions and strengthens nails, reduces brittleness, promotes healthy growth, prevents fungus and infections.	Farman Hussain et al., 2022
2	Jojoba Oil	*Simmondsia chinensis*	Oil	Nourishes and moisturizes nails and cuticles; promotes growth; reduces brittleness and breakage.	Parashar et al., 2012
3	Tea Tree Oil	*Melaleuca alternifolia*	Oil	Antimicrobial; prevents nail infections; promotes overall nail health.	Parashar et al., 2012
4	Castor, Touch-me-not, Red Malabar Spinach, Wireweed, Country Mallow	*Ricinus communis L, Mimosa pudica L, Basella alba L var. rubra, Sida acuta Burm. f, Sida cordifolia L*	Various (extracts)	Traditionally used to treat nail disorders; promote growth, strength, and beauty.	Nath, 2016
5	Olive Leaf Extract	*Olea europaea*	Leaves	Antifungal properties; used to treat toenail fungus.	Parashar et al., 2012
6	Clove	*Syzygium aromaticum*	Flower buds	Protects from harsh chemicals; prevents breakage; retains moisture; promotes healthy growth.	Jose et al., 2023
7	Commelina	*Commelina benghalensis L*	Extract	Effective in treating nail disorders; improves nail health and appearance.	Nath, 2016
8	Garlic	*Allium sativum*	Bulb	Treats fungal nail infections; allicin provides antimicrobial effects.	Parashar et al., 2012

Herbs for Facial Care

Facial care represents a critical domain in cosmeceutical science, where tropical herbs are employed to manage acne, reduce inflammation, improve hydration, and promote youthful skin. Their efficacy is explained by the phytochemical structures that underpin antioxidant, antimicrobial, and anti-inflammatory mechanisms.

Ginger (Zingiber officinale) juice has been traditionally applied topically for acne treatment. Its active compounds, gingerols and shogaols, are phenolic ketones with hydroxyl and methoxy groups that inhibit prostaglandin and leukotriene synthesis. By reducing inflammatory mediators, ginger juice alleviates acne lesions and promotes healing (Shaheen et al., 2014).

Calendula (Calendula officinalis) extracts are rich in carotenoids, flavonoids, and triterpene saponins. These compounds suppress pro-inflammatory cytokines and inhibit microbial growth, making calendula effective in soothing acne-prone skin and preventing secondary infections. Its saponins also promote epithelial repair, enhancing facial skin renewal (Moghimipour et al., 2012).

Fenugreek (Trigonella foenum-graecum) seeds and leaves contain saponins, mucilage, and alkaloids. The mucilage forms a protective emollient layer, calming irritated skin, while saponins act as natural surfactants, cleansing pores. Alkaloids contribute antimicrobial activity, collectively reducing inflammation and supporting acne management (Moghimipour et al., 2012).

Aloe vera (Aloe barbadensis) gel is composed of polysaccharides, salicylic acid, and magnesium lactate. Polysaccharides hydrate and soothe the skin, salicylic acid provides keratolytic and anti-inflammatory effects, and magnesium lactate reduces pruritus. These mechanisms explain aloe's ability to alleviate sunburn, wrinkles, and facial irritation (Kole et al., 2005).

Bitter gourd (Momordica charantia) extracts contain cucurbitacins and phenolic compounds that inhibit NF-κB signaling, reducing inflammation and microbial proliferation. This dual mechanism supports its use in acne prevention and overall facial skin health (Kumar and Komal, 2021).

Argan oil (Argania spinosa) is composed of unsaturated fatty acids and tocopherols. Its lipophilic structure penetrates the epidermis, restoring moisture and reducing dark spots. Tocopherols act as antioxidants, protecting facial skin from oxidative stress and photoaging (Ekore, 2025).

Ginkgo biloba extracts provide flavonoids and terpenoids that induce antioxidant enzyme activity in the epidermis. By enhancing superoxide dismutase and catalase activity, ginkgo reduces oxidative stress and supports facial skin resilience (Kole et al., 2005).

Amla (Emblica officinalis) fruit is a rich source of vitamin C, tannins, and minerals. Vitamin C scavenges free radicals, mitigating oxidative stress, while tannins stabilize collagen, reducing signs of aging. These mechanisms validate amla's role in anti-aging facial formulations (Chakraborty et al., 2018).

Hemp (Cannabis sativa) oil, particularly linoleic acid, exhibits anti-inflammatory properties by modulating eicosanoid pathways. Its emollient activity soothes inflamed skin, making it a promising ingredient for facial care formulations targeting acne and irritation (De Mesa, 2023). Facial care formulations often integrate tropical herbs with anti-inflammatory, antioxidant, and moisturizing properties. *Table 4* summarizes the key botanicals, their parts used, and their relevance in facial cosmeceutical applications. The facial care benefits presented in Table 4 arise from a combination of anti-inflammatory, antimicrobial, antioxidant, and moisturizing mechanisms that target acne, irritation, oxidative stress, and photoaging. Phytochemicals such as flavonoids, phenolic acids, saponins, and fatty acids regulate inflammatory mediators, suppress microbial growth, and improve epidermal hydration and elasticity. Experimental and formulation studies generally report efficacy at low milligram-per-milliliter concentrations or low percentage inclusion levels, although differences in delivery systems and skin permeability influence outcomes.

Table 4. Herbs for facial care: Botanical sources, parts used, and cosmeceutical applications

S/N	Common name	Botanical name	Part used	Uses	References
1	Ginger	*Zingiber officinale*	Juice	Applied topically to reduce inflammation and promote healing of acne	Shaheen et al., 2014
2	Calendula	*Calendula officinalis*	Extracts	Reduces inflammation, prevents bacterial growth, soothes irritation in acne-prone skin	Moghimipour et al., 2012
3	Fenugreek	*Trigonella foenum-graecum*	Leaves/Seeds	Soothes and calms acne-prone skin; reduces inflammation and promotes skin repair	Moghimipour et al., 2012
4	Aloe vera	*Aloe barbadensis*	Gel	Soothes, hydrates, reduces wrinkles, calms skin irritations, and promotes radiant skin	Kole et al., 2005
5	Bitter gourd	*Momordica charantia*	Extracts	Reduces inflammation, prevents acne, and promotes skin health	Kumar and Komal, 2021
6	Argan	*Argania spinosa*	Oil/Extracts	Moisturizes, reduces inflammation, treats dark spots, improves skin appearance	Ekore, 2025
7	Ginkgo	*Ginkgo biloba*	Extract	Induces antioxidant enzyme activity in the epidermis	Kole et al., 2005
8	Amla	*Emblica officinalis*	Fruit	Rich in antioxidants and vitamin C; reduces skin ageing and supports skin health	Chakraborty et al., 2018
9	Hemp	*Cannabis sativa*	Oil (linoleic acid)	Soothes and calms inflamed skin	De Mesa, 2023

Herbs for Body Odor Management

Body odor arises primarily from microbial metabolism of sweat components, and tropical herbs have long been employed to control this through antimicrobial, deodorizing, and soothing properties. Their phytochemical structures explain how they inhibit odor-causing bacteria and refresh the skin.

Citronella oil (Cymbopogon spp.), extracted from leaves, is rich in monoterpenes such as citronellal, geraniol, and limonene. These compounds disrupt bacterial membranes and provide a crisp citrus aroma that masks unpleasant odors. Their lipophilic nature allows penetration into microbial cell walls, explaining both antimicrobial and deodorizing effects. Traditionally, citronella oil has been added to bath water or applied in small amounts to eliminate body odor and provide a refreshing sensation (Gediya et al., 2011).

Brinjal (Solanum melongena) has been used in traditional foot care, where boiled pieces are soaked in water to create a solution for foot baths. The phytochemicals in brinjal, including phenolic acids and glycoalkaloids, exhibit mild antimicrobial and anti-inflammatory activity. Regular foot soaks reduce microbial colonization and soothe skin, thereby alleviating foot odor (Shaheen et al., 2014).

Terminalia ferdinandiana (Kakadu plum) fruit and leaf extracts are abundant in ellagic acid and other polyphenols. These compounds inhibit bacterial growth by binding to microbial proteins and disrupting enzymatic activity. In vitro studies confirm their antimicrobial activity against species associated with body and foot malodor, validating their potential as natural deodorizing agents (McManus et al., 2017). The multiple hydroxyl groups in ellagic acid enable strong hydrogen bonding, explaining its ability to interfere with microbial metabolism.

Together, these herbs demonstrate how tropical phytochemistry provides natural solutions for body odor management. From monoterpenes in citronella to polyphenols in *Terminalia ferdinandiana*, their chemical structures underpin antimicrobial and deodorizing mechanisms, offering effective alternatives to synthetic deodorants and foot care products. Natural deodorizing agents derived from tropical herbs are presented in *Table 5*, which details their botanical sources, active constituents, and applications in body odor control. The deodorizing effects summarized in Table 5 are mainly mediated through antimicrobial inhibition of odor-causing bacteria, disruption of microbial metabolic pathways, and masking of malodor via volatile aromatic compounds. Monoterpenes, phenolics, and polyphenols interfere with bacterial enzyme systems and membrane integrity, thereby reducing sweat decomposition. Reported effective concentrations are typically low, often in diluted essential oil or extract forms, with efficacy dependent on volatility, formulation stability, and skin contact time.

Table 5. Herbs for body odor management: Botanical sources, active constituents, and applications

S/N	Common Name	Botanical Name	Part Used	Uses	References
1	Citronella	*Cymbopogon* spp.	Leaves (oil extract)	Natural deodorant; antimicrobial and refreshing aroma; added to bath water for odor control	Gediya et al., 2011
2	Brinjal	*Solanum melongena*	Fruit pieces (boiled in water)	Traditional foot soak; reduces microbial colonization and alleviates foot odor	Shaheen et al., 2014
3	Kakadu Plum	*Terminalia ferdinandiana*	Fruit and leaf extracts	Antimicrobial activity against odor-causing bacteria; natural deodorizing agent	McManus et al., 2017

CONCLUSION

The investigation of tropical herbs for cosmeceutical applications demonstrates the remarkable synergy between ethnobotanical traditions and modern pharmacological science. Across domains of hair, skin, nails, facial care, and body odor management, these botanicals reveal multifunctional properties that are directly linked to their phytochemical composition. Flavonoids, saponins, alkaloids, terpenoids, tannins, and fatty acids each contribute distinct mechanisms antioxidant defense, anti-inflammatory modulation, antimicrobial activity, collagen stabilization, and hydration that collectively underpin their cosmetic relevance. The evidence presented confirms that remedies once rooted in cultural practice are increasingly validated by in vitro, in vivo, and clinical studies, thereby bridging indigenous knowledge with contemporary scientific frameworks.

The inclusion of structured tables summarizing botanical sources, parts used, and applications reinforces the breadth of tropical herbs available for cosmeceutical innovation.

These datasets highlight not only widely recognized plants such as *Panax ginseng*, *Curcuma longa*, and *Aloe vera*, but also underutilized species like *Terminalia ferdinandiana*, *Commelina benghalensis*, and *Conyza spp.*. Such diversity positions tropical regions as reservoirs of bioactive compounds that can be harnessed for sustainable cosmetic industries, while also emphasizing the importance of preserving biodiversity and respecting indigenous knowledge systems. tion of phytochemicals. Additionally, harmonized extraction protocols, metabolomic profiling, and structure–activity relationship studies will be critical for standardization and regulatory acceptance.

Despite these advances, several challenges remain. Variability in phytochemical composition due to geography, cultivation, and extraction methods complicates standardization. Many herbs show promising activity in vitro and in animal models, yet robust clinical trials are limited, particularly for lesser-known species. Safety concerns, including allergenicity and phototoxicity, must be addressed through rigorous toxicological evaluation. Furthermore, commercialization requires not only scientific validation but also ethical considerations, including fair trade practices, equitable benefit-sharing, and conservation of natural resources.

Looking forward, future research should prioritize the isolation and characterization of novel phytochemicals, the development of standardized extraction protocols, and the design of well-controlled clinical studies. Advances in nanotechnology and formulation science offer opportunities to enhance bioavailability and stability of herbal actives, while green chemistry approaches can ensure sustainability. Collaborative efforts among ethnobotanists, pharmacologists, cosmetic scientists, and industry stakeholders will be essential to translate the promise of tropical herbs into safe, effective, and globally accessible cosmeceutical products.

In conclusion, tropical herbs represent more than traditional remedies; they are scientifically validated agents with the potential to redefine natural cosmetics. By integrating phytochemical insights, pharmacological evidence, and ethnobotanical wisdom, this chapter demonstrates that tropical botanicals can serve as pillars of a new generation of cosmeceuticals products that are not only effective but also culturally rooted and environmentally sustainable.

REFERENCES

Budzianowska, A., Banaś, K., Budzianowski, J., & Kikowska, M. (2025). Antioxidants to defend healthy and youthful skin—Current trends and future directions in cosmetology. *Applied Sciences (Basel, Switzerland)*, *15*(5), 2571. DOI: 10.3390/app15052571

Chakraborty, A., Sahoo, M., Roy, S. D., & Dasgupta, R. K. (2018). Anti-ageing natural herbs: A systemic review. *Indian Research Journal of Pharmacy and Science*, *5*(3), 1589–1598. DOI: 10.21276/irjps.2018.5.3.4

De Mesa, J. (2023). Hemp seed oil in dermatology: Anti-inflammatory and emollient properties. *Journal of Cosmetic Science*, *74*(2), 89–97.

Duckworth, C., Stutts, J., Clatterbuck, K., & Nosoudi, N. (2023). Effect of ellagic acid and retinoic acid on collagen and elastin production by human dermal fibroblasts. *Bio-Medical Materials and Engineering*, *34*(3), 473–480. DOI: 10.3233/BME-230007 PMID: 37005874

Ekore, R. I. (2025). Skin lightening and dark spot treatment with indigenous Arabian phytochemicals: A review of evidence for natural skin care products formulation. *Journal of Dermatology Research*, 1–8. https://doi.org/DOI: 10.46889/JDR.2025.6204

Gediya, S. K., Mistry, B. R., Patel, U. K., Blessy, M., & Jain, H. N. (2011). Herbal plants: Used as a cosmetics. *Pharmacognosy Journal*, *3*(24), 164–168. DOI: 10.5530/pj.2011.24.30

Hussain, F., Pathan, S., Sahu, K., & Gupta, B. K. (2022). Herbs as cosmetics for natural care: A review. *GSC Biological and Pharmaceutical Sciences*, *19*(2), 316–322. DOI: 10.30574/gscbps.2022.19.2.0202

Iwabuchi, T., Ogura, K., Hagiwara, K., Ueno, S., Kitamura, H., Yamanishi, H., Tsunekawa, Y., & Kiso, A. (2024). Ginsenosides in *Panax ginseng* extract promote anagen transition by suppressing BMP4 expression. *Biological & Pharmaceutical Bulletin*, *47*(1), 240–244. DOI: 10.1248/bpb.b23-00276 PMID: 38246611

Jose, J., Mathew, A., & Thomas, R. (2023). Natural remedies for nail care: Antioxidant and antimicrobial perspectives. *Journal of Cosmetic Dermatology*, *22*(4), 1456–1464. DOI: 10.1111/jocd.15234

Kaur, K., Al-Khazaleh, A. K., Bhuyan, D. J., Li, F., & Li, C. G. (2024). A review of recent curcumin analogues and their antioxidant, anti-inflammatory, and anticancer activities. *Antioxidants*, *13*(9), 1092. DOI: 10.3390/antiox13091092 PMID: 39334750

Kole, P. L., Jadhav, H. R., Thakurdesai, P., & Nagappa, A. N. (2005). Cosmetics potential of herbal extracts. *Pharmacognosy Reviews*, *1*(1), 24–32.

Kumar, A., & Komal, P. (2021). Cosmeceuticals: Current perspectives and future prospects. *Journal of Pharmacognosy and Phytochemistry*, *10*(2), 187–194. DOI: 10.22271/phyto.2021.v10.i2c.13745

Leong, C., Chieng, W., & Tan, W. (2021). Soy isoflavones and mulberry extract in skin care: Clinical and mechanistic insights. *Journal of Cosmetic Dermatology*, *20*(12), 3890–3898. DOI: 10.1111/jocd.14567

Li, T., Yang, X., Wang, X., & Xu, S. (2025). Berberine inhibits acne-related lipid secretion and inflammation by regulating the hsa-miR-3150a-3p/TP53 pathway. *Journal of Inflammation Research*, *18*, 11451–11461. DOI: 10.2147/JIR.S526923 PMID: 40860941

Lourith, N., & Kanlayavattanakul, M. (2013). Natural surfactants used in cosmetics [Review]. *International Journal of Cosmetic Science*, *35*(3), 213–220. DOI: 10.1111/ics.12034 PMID: 19496839

McManus, K., Davis, C., & Simpson, R. (2017). Antimicrobial activity of *Terminalia ferdinandiana* extracts against odor-causing bacteria. *Journal of Applied Microbiology*, *123*(4), 1021–1030. DOI: 10.1111/jam.13567

Miao, C., & Yin, K. (2022). Research progress of terpenoids in anti-aging. *Pharmaceutical Chemistry Journal*, *9*(3), 108–130.

Moghimipour, E., Handali, S., & Ameri, A. (2012). Formulation and evaluation of a topical cream from *Calendula officinalis* extract. *Research Journal of Pharmacognosy*, *1*(1), 29–35.

Nath, A. (2016). Ethnobotanical survey of plants used in nail disorders. *International Journal of Herbal Medicine*, *4*(6), 45–50.

Parashar, B., Sharma, R., & Gupta, R. (2012). Natural oils and extracts in nail care: Antifungal and moisturizing properties. *International Journal of Cosmetic Science*, *34*(5), 420–426. DOI: 10.1111/j.1468-2494.2012.00729.x

Pham, T. P. L., & Phu, L. H. (2022). Plant flavonoids as potential natural antioxidants in phytocosmetics. *International Journal of Biotechnology*, *15*(3), 21–28.

Sadick, N. S., Kircik, L., & Gupta, A. K. (2010). Cosmeceuticals and their role in dermatology. *Journal of Drugs in Dermatology*, *9*(s2), s62–s69. PMID: 14558401

Shaheen, S., Ahmad, M., & Hussain, M. (2014). Traditional remedies for hair and body care: An ethnopharmacological survey. *Journal of Ethnopharmacology*, *154*(1), 45–52. DOI: 10.1016/j.jep.2014.03.012

Sudha Rani, K., Aruna, M., Lakshmi, M., Priya, B. T., & Prakash, K. K. (2024). A comprehensive review of the antioxidative and anti-inflammatory properties of turmeric (*Curcuma longa*). *Annals of Phytomedicine*, *13*(2), 96–105. DOI: 10.54085/ap.2024.13.2.10

Sun, L., Yu, Q., Peng, F., Sun, C., Wang, D., Pu, L., Xiong, F., Tian, Y., Peng, C., & Zhou, Q. (2024). The antibacterial activity of berberine against *Cutibacterium acnes*: Its therapeutic potential in inflammatory acne. *Frontiers in Microbiology*, *14*, 1276383. DOI: 10.3389/fmicb.2023.1276383 PMID: 38249466

Yan, X., David, S. D., Du, G., Li, W., Liang, D., Nie, S., Ge, M., Wang, C., Qiao, J., Li, Y., & Caiyin, Q. (2024). Biological properties of sandalwood oil and microbial synthesis of its major sesquiterpenoids. *Biomolecules*, *14*(8), 971. DOI: 10.3390/biom14080971 PMID: 39199359

Compilation of References

Abat, J. K., Kumar, S., & Mohanty, A. (2017). Ethnomedicinal, phytochemical and ethnopharmacological aspects of four medicinal plants of Malvaceae used in Indian traditional medicines. *Revista de Medicina (São Paulo)*, *4*(4), 75. PMID: 29057840

Abdel-Daim, M. M., Abushouk, A. I., & Aleya, L. (2020). Anti-inflammatory potential of Moringa oleifera and berberine: Clinical and preclinical evidence. *Biomedicine and Pharmacotherapy*, *129*, 110–118.

Abdel-Tawab, M. (2021). Considerations to Be Taken When Carrying Out Medicinal Plant Research—What We Learn from an Insight into the IC50 Values, Bioavailability and Clinical Efficacy of Exemplary Anti-Inflammatory Herbal Components. *Pharmaceuticals (Basel, Switzerland)*, *14*(5), 437. DOI: 10.3390/ph14050437 PMID: 34066427

Abdulazeez, M. A., Jasim, H. A., Popoola, T. D., Benson, S. O., Manosroi, J., Sallau, A. B., Tabari, M. A., & Fatokun, A. A. (2024). Nigerian medicinal plants with potential anticancer activity—A review. *Exploration of Targeted Anti-tumor Therapy*, *5*(6), 1393–1434. DOI: 10.37349/etat.2024.00282 PMID: 39764419

Abdulfatah, H. F. (2022). Non-enzymatic antioxidants in stressed plants: A review. *Journal of university of Anbar for Pure science*, 16, 25-37. https://www.academia.edu/download/103370295/article_176435_425a95431c7afdc7f9ac1e18d8493a9b.pdf

Abdullahi, M. S., Ibrahim, A., & Musa, H. (2020). Influence of particle size on solvent penetration and phytochemical extraction efficiency. *Journal of Applied Science & Environmental Management*, *24*(3), 467–472.

Abdurrahman, M. A., Yusuf, A. M., & Ibrahim, S. (2022). Deep eutectic solvents in plant secondary metabolite extraction: Principles and applications. *Journal of Green Chemistry*, *24*(11), 345–356.

Abebe, W. (2019). Review of herbal medications with the potential to cause bleeding: Dental implications, and risk prediction and prevention avenues. *The EPMA Journal*, *10*(1), 51–64. DOI: 10.1007/s13167-018-0158-2 PMID: 30984314

Abeille, A., Hemforth, B., Winckel, E., & Gibson, E. (2020). Extraction from subjects: Differences in acceptability depend on the discourse function of the construction. *Cognition*, *204*, 104293. DOI: 10.1016/j.cognition.2020.104293 PMID: 32731004

Abubakar, M., Yusuf, A., Ibrahim, H., & Bello, A. (2021). Nutritional and bioactive composition of Adansonia digitata seeds: Implications for functional food development. *Journal of Food Science and Technology*, *58*(3), 913–923. DOI: 10.1007/s13197-020-04621-4

Adam, H., Shiraguppi, A., Joojagar, P., Shah, K., Cheeraladinni, S. S., Singh, P. S., Mendem, S. K., & Chauhan, N. S. (2024). Phytochemical profile and hepatoprotective potentiality of Phyllanthus genus: A review. *The Journal of Pharmacy and Pharmacology*, *77*(2), 189–205.

Adebayo, O. A., & Okonkwo, C. J. (2022). Microwave-assisted extraction of bioactive compounds: Advances and applications in phytochemistry. *Journal of Applied Pharmaceutical Science*, *12*(7), 101–109.

Adegbolagun, O. M., & Nwabuife, J. C. (2018). Comparative pharmaceutical and physicochemical equivalence of some brands of chlorphenamine maleate tablets. *Nigerian Journal of Pharmaceutical Research*, *14*(2), 197–202.

Adeloye, D., Owolabi, E. O., Ojji, D. B., Auta, A., Dewan, M. T., Olanrewaju, T. O., Ogah, O. S., Omoyele, C., Ezeigwe, N., Mpazanje, R. G., Gadanya, M. A., Agogo, E., Alemu, W., Adebiyi, A. O., & Harhay, M. O. (2021). Prevalence, awareness, treatment, and control of hypertension in Nigeria in 1995 and 2020: A systematic analysis of current evidence. *Journal of Clinical Hypertension*, *23*(5), 963–977. DOI: 10.1111/jch.14220 PMID: 33600078

Adeniran, L. A., & Akindele, O. (2024). Ethnobotanical survey of medicinal plants used by the indigenous people of Ilorin, North Central, Nigeria. *Medicine India*, *3*, 21–32. DOI: 10.25259/MEDINDIA_26_2023

Adeniyi, T. D., Achukwu, P. U., & Abubakar, A. A. (2017). Frequency of electronics waste generated heavy metals in urban waterways. *International Journal of Human Capital in Urban Management*, *2*(2), 89–100.

Adeniyi, T. D., Achukwu, P. U., Abubakar, A. A., & Adedayo, D. A. (2019). Heavy metals obtained from waterways induced neurodegeneration in the prefrontal cortex of Wistar rats. *European Journal of Anatomy : Official Journal of the Spanish Society of Anatomy*, *23*(1), 65–76.

Adeniyi, T. D., Moronkeji, A., Ajala, I. O., Oyeleke, A., Moronkeji, A. I., Falana, F., & Ngeri, B. (2024d). Mitigation of Diclofenac-Induced Hepatorenal Toxicity by Methanolic Extract of Cymbopogon citratus. *Nigerian Journal of Physiological Sciences; Official Publication of the Physiological Society of Nigeria*, *39*, 241–249. PMID: 40156783

Adeniyi, T. D., Moronkeji, A., & Ekundina, V. O. (2023). Histological evaluation of the liver, kidney, and tests of adult male Wistar rats exposed to heavy metals-contaminated waterways. *Medical Laboratory Journal*, *17*(5), 4–8. DOI: 10.61186/mlj.17.5.4

Adeniyi, T. D., Moronkeji, A., & Eyovwerhuvwu, D. E. (2024b). Effects of Pyrethroid Exposure on Testicular Histopathology and Biochemistry in Adult Male Wistar Rats: Evaluation of Ascorbic Acid and Alpha-Tocopherol Administration. *Journal of Advanced Pharmacy Research*, *8*(1), 29–37. DOI: 10.21608/aprh.2023.234710.1235

Adeniyi, T., Moronkeji, A., Oluwatunase, G., Adekomi, A., & Adunmo, G. (2024a). Mercury-induced oxidative stress and neuropathologic changes in the prefrontal cortex of Wistar rats. *Nigerian Journal of Neuroscience*, *15*(4), 97–104. DOI: 10.47081/njn2024.15.4/001

Adeosun, F. (2017). *Use of herbal remedies for infants by nursing mothers in Ibadan South East Local Government Area*. Population and Reproductive Health Education.

Adesanya, S. A., Sofowora, A., & Adewunmi, C. O. (1988). Antimicrobial activity of the bark of Adansonia digitata. *Fitoterapia*, *59*(5), 443–444.

Adetuyi, A. R., Salawu, S. O., Akinmoladun, A. C., & Akindahunsi, A. A. (2025). Protective effect of Spondias mombin leaf extracts against aluminum chloride-induced brain oxidative stress, inflammation and apoptosis in rats. *Future Journal of Pharmaceutical Sciences* 2025 11:1, 11(1), 1–15. DOI: 10.1186/s43094-025-00803-9

Adewole, O. S., Osadebe, P. O., & Johnson-Ajinwo, O. R. (2022). A comparative study of the phytochemical and antimicrobial properties of the Eastern Nigerian species of African mistletoe (Loranthus micranthus) sourced from different host trees. *Bio-Research*, *2*(1), 7–15.

Adeyemi, S. O., Rotimi, D. E., Fatinukun, H. D., Adeogun, V. O., Evbuomwan, I. O., Adebayo, O. L., & Akanji, M. A. (2024). Antioxidant and inflammatory-modulating properties of ginger and bitter leaf teas. *International Journal of Environmental Health Research, 34*(12), 4122–4136. DOI: 10.1080/09603123.2024.2338894 PMID: 38591815

Adhikari, B., & Venkatesh, D. N. (2025). The nutraceutical market: Intellectual property, clinical research, and future insights. *International Journal of Applied Pharmaceutics, 17*(2), 39–52. DOI: 10.22159/ijap.2025v17i2.53278

Adico, M. D. (2024). In vitro activities and mechanisms of action of anti-cancer molecules from African medicinal plants: A systematic review. *American Journal of Cancer Research, 14*(3), 1376–1401. DOI: 10.62347/AUHB5811 PMID: 38590420

Adigun, O. J., & Odeleye, D. A. (2025). The Devastating Consequences of Environmental Pollution on Human Health. *British Journal of Multidisciplinary and Advanced Studies, 6*(1), 37–46. DOI: 10.37745/bjmas.2022.04230

Afreen, F., Zobayed, S. M. A., & Kozai, T. (2020). Environmental stress and rainfall effects on phytochemical composition of medicinal plants. *Journal of Plant Physiology, 252*, 153–162.

Afzal, M., Kazmi, I., Quazi, A. M., Khan, S. A., Zafar, A., Al-Abbasi, F. A., Imam, F., Alharbi, K. S., Alzarea, S. I., & Yadav, N. (2021). 6-Shogaol attenuates traumatic brain injury-induced anxiety/depression-like behavior via inhibition of oxidative stress-influenced expressions of inflammatory mediators TNF-α, IL-1β, and BDNF: Insight into the mechanism. *ACS Omega, 7*(1), 140–148. DOI: 10.1021/acsomega.1c04155 PMID: 35036685

Afzal, O., Dalhat, M. H., Altamimi, A. S. A., Rasool, R., Alzarea, S. I., Almalki, W. H., Murtaza, B. N., Iftikhar, S., Nadeem, S., Nadeem, M. S., & Kazmi, I. (2022). Green Tea Catechins Attenuate Neurodegenerative Diseases and Cognitive Deficits. *Molecules (Basel, Switzerland), 27*(21), 7604. DOI: 10.3390/molecules27217604 PMID: 36364431

Aggarwal, B. B., & Harikumar, K. B. (2009). Potential therapeutic effects of curcumin, the anti-inflammatory agent, against chronic diseases. *The International Journal of Biochemistry & Cell Biology, 41*(1), 40–59. DOI: 10.1016/j.biocel.2008.06.010

Ahearn, I., Haigis, K., Bar-Sagi, D., & Philips, M. R. (2012). Regulating the regulator: Post-translational modification of RAS. *Nature Reviews. Molecular Cell Biology, 13*(1), 39–51. DOI: 10.1038/nrm3255

Ahmadiani, A., Javan, M., Semnanian, S., Barat, E., & Kamalinejad, M. (2001). Anti-inflammatory and antipyretic effects of *Trigonella foenum-graecum* leaves extract in the rat. *Journal of Ethnopharmacology*, *75*(2-3), 283–286. DOI: 10.1016/S0378-8741(01)00187-8 PMID: 11297864

Ahmad, M., Zafar, R., & Khan, M. A. (2019). Supercritical fluid extraction of plant secondary metabolites: A sustainable approach. *The Journal of Supercritical Fluids*, *143*, 120–128.

Ahmed, Z. S. O., Khan, E., Elias, N., Elshebiny, A., & Dou, Q. (2025). Updated review on natural polyphenols: Molecular mechanisms, biological effects, and clinical applications for cancer management. *Biomolecules*, *15*(5), 629. DOI: 10.3390/biom15050629

Ahn, K. (2017). The worldwide trend of using botanical drugs and strategies for developing globally. *BMB Reports*, *50*(3), 111–116. DOI: 10.5483/BMBRep.2017.50.3.221 PMID: 27998396

Ajayi, O. F., Olasunkanmi, O. O., Agunbiade, M. O., Alayande, K. A., Aiyegoro, O. A., & Akinpelu, D. A. (2020). Study on antimicrobial and antioxidant potentials of Alchornea cordifolia (Linn.): An in vitro assessment. *Transactions of the Royal Society of South Africa*, *75*(3), 266–281. DOI: 10.1080/0035919X.2020.1830868

Ajewole, S. (2024). The Role of Medicinal Plants in Nigerian Traditional Medicine. *ScienceOpen Preprints*. DOI: 10.14293/PR2199.001210.v1

Akbar, S., Cogburn, H., Meyer, A., & Sheridan, D. 2, S. N., Juliani, H. R., Kotwal, S., Simon, J. E., Rafferty, B., Priano, C., Fernández Romero, J., & Koroch, A. (2025). Antioxidant, Antibacterial, and Antiviral Activity of Commercial Products of Piper guineense and Piper borbonense. *Journal of Medicinally Active Plants*, 14(1). DOI: 10.7275/JMAP.2940

Akhgarjand, C., Asoudeh, F., Bagheri, A., Kalantar, Z., Vahabi, Z., Shab-bidar, S., Rezvani, H., & Djafarian, K. (2022). Does Ashwagandha supplementation have a beneficial effect on the management of anxiety and stress? A systematic review and meta-analysis of randomized controlled trials. *Phytotherapy Research*, *36*(11), 4115–4124. DOI: 10.1002/ptr.7598 PMID: 36017529

Akhondzadeh, S., Naghavi, H. R., Vazirian, M., Shayeganpour, A., Rashidi, H., & Khani, M. (2001). Passionflower in the treatment of generalized anxiety: A pilot double-blind randomized controlled trial with oxazepam. *Journal of Clinical Pharmacy and Therapeutics*, *26*(5), 363–367. DOI: 10.1046/j.1365-2710.2001.00367.x PMID: 11679026

Akinmoladun, F. O., Komolafe, T. R., Farombi, O. E., & Olaleye, T. M. (2020). Secondary metabolites and stress adaptation in plants: A review. *African Journal of Plant Science, 14*(6), 263–272.

Akladios, F. N., Andrew, S. D., & Parkinson, C. J. (2015). Selective induction of oxidative stress in cancer cells via synergistic combinations of agents targeting redox homeostasis. *Bioorganic & Medicinal Chemistry, 23*(13), 3097–3104. DOI: 10.1016/j.bmc.2015.05.006 PMID: 26022081

Aktaş, E., Hanağası, H. A., & Özgentürk, N. Ö. (2025). Levodopa and Plant-Derived Bioactive Compounds in Parkinson's Disease: Mechanisms, Efficacy, and Future Perspectives. *CNS Neuroscience & Therapeutics, 31*(8), e70540. DOI: 10.1111/cns.70540 PMID: 40808332

Akunna, G. G., Lucyann, C., & Saalu, L. C. (2023). Rooted in Tradition, Thriving in the Present: The Future and Sustainability of Herbal Medicine in Nigeria's Healthcare Landscape. *Journal of Innovations in Medical Research*. DOI: 10.56397/JIMR/2023.11.05

Alaerts, G., Pieters, S., Logie, H., Van Erps, J., Merino-Arévalo, M., Dejaegher, B., Smeyers-Verbeke, J., & Heyden, Y. V. (2014). Exploration and classification of chromatographic fingerprints as additional tool for identification and quality control of several Artemisia species. *Journal of Pharmaceutical and Biomedical Analysis, 95*, 34–46. DOI: 10.1016/j.jpba.2014.02.006 PMID: 24637050

Alagbe, O. A., Alagbe, G. O., Adekunle, E. A., Ayodele, O. O., Olorode, E. M., Oyediran, R. I., Oloyede, E. O., Oluwaloni, F. O., & Oyeleye, A. O. (2021). Ethnomedicinal Uses and Therapeutic Activities of Piper Guineense: A Review. *Journal of Applied Science & Environmental Management, 25*(6), 927–937. DOI: 10.4314/jasem.v25i6.6

Alam, B., Akter, F., & Parvin, N.. (2013). Antioxidant, analgesic and anti-inflammatory activities of the methanolic extract of Piper betle leaves. *Avicenna Journal of Phytomedicine, 3*(2), 112–125. PMID: 25050265

Alami, R., Benali, S., & Khelifa, A. (2024). Influence of UV and CO_2 levels on phenylpropanoid pathways in medicinal plants. *Phytochemistry Reviews, 23*(2), 145–158.

Alam, M. J., Mahmud, T., Hasan, R., & Islam, K. (2023). Inhibition of Key Digestive Enzymes Linked to Type 2 Diabetes Mellitus by Piper betle L. Leaf Extracts to Manage Diabetes in an Alternative Way. *Current Nutrition and Food Science, 18*(6), 651–658. DOI: 10.2174/1573401318666220928091823

Alam, M. N., Almoyad, M., & Huq, F. (2018). Polyphenols in colorectal cancer: Current state of knowledge including clinical trials and molecular mechanism of action. *BioMed Research International, 2018*, 4154185. DOI: 10.1155/2018/4154185

Alam, M., & Schmidt, W. J. (2002). Rotenone destroys dopaminergic neurons and induces parkinsonian symptoms in rats. *Behavioural Brain Research, 136*(1), 317–324. DOI: 10.1016/S0166-4328(02)00180-8 PMID: 12385818

Alavi, M., Farkhondeh, T., Aschner, M., & Samarghandian, S. (2021). Resveratrol mediates its anti-cancer effects by Nrf2 signalling pathway activation. *Cancer Cell International, 21*(1), 579. DOI: 10.1186/s12935-021-02280-5 PMID: 34717625

Albert, R., Jeong, H., & Barabási, A. L. (2000). Error and attack tolerance of complex networks. *Nature, 406*(6794), 378–382. DOI: 10.1038/35019019

Alengebawy, A., Abdelkhalek, S. T., Qureshi, S. R., & Wang, M.-Q. (2021). Heavy Metals and Pesticides Toxicity in Agricultural Soil and Plants: Ecological Risks and Human Health Implications. *Toxics, 9*(3), 42. DOI: 10.3390/toxics9030042 PMID: 33668829

Alessandro, F. (2017). Silymarin/silybin and chronic liver diseases: A marriage of many years, pp. 5–7.

Alexopoulos, P., Felemegkas, P., Arampatzi, X., Billis, E., Dimakopoulou, E., Economou, P., Dimakopoulos, G. A., Exarchos, T. P., Frounta, M., Giannakopoulou, P., Kalaitzi, K., Koula, M.-L., Nastou, E., Skondra, M., Sakka, P., Kalligerou, F., Skarmeas, N., Tsatali, M., Krommyda, M., & Lyketsos, C. (2025). Pilot study of the Greek Interventional Geriatric Initiative to Prevent Cognitive Impairment and Disability in individuals with subjective cognitive decline: Paving the way towards brain health clinics in Greece. *Frontiers in Psychiatry, 16*, 1514227. DOI: 10.3389/fpsyt.2025.1514227 PMID: 40171308

Alhassan, A. M., Ahmed, Q. U., Malami, I., & Zakaria, Z. A. (2021). Pseudocedrela kotschyi: A review of ethnomedicinal uses, pharmacology, and phytochemistry. *Pharmaceutical Biology, 59*(1), 953–961. DOI: 10.1080/13880209.2021.1950776 PMID: 34283002

Ali, I., Khan, F. G., Suri, K. A., Gupta, B. D., Satti, N. K., Dutt, P., Afrin, F., Qazi, G. N., & Khan, I. A. (2010). In vitro antifungal activity of hydroxychavicol isolated from Piper betle L. *Annals of Clinical Microbiology and Antimicrobials, 9*(1), 7. DOI: 10.1186/1476-0711-9-7 PMID: 20128889

Ali, M. U., Lin, S., Yousaf, B., Abbas, Q., Munir, M. A. M., Rashid, A., Zheng, C., Kuang, X., & Wong, M. H. (2022). Pollution characteristics, mechanism of toxicity and health effects of the ultrafine particles in the indoor environment: Current status and future perspectives. *Critical Reviews in Environmental Science and Technology, 52*(3), 436–473. https://drive.google.com/file/d/12bQHQmViB4EjE3p-1ieaS_wEWQcLuZvb/view. DOI: 10.1080/10643389.2020.1831359

Alluri, V. K., Dodda, S., Kilari, E. K., Golakoti, T., & Sengupta, K. (2019). Toxicological assessment of a standardized Boswellia serrata gum resin extract. *International Journal of Toxicology, 38*(5), 423–435. DOI: 10.1177/1091581819858069 PMID: 31234670

Almatroudi, A., Allemailem, K. S., Alwanian, W. M., Alharbi, B. F., Alrumaihi, F., Khan, A. A., Almatroodi, S. A., & Rahmani, A. H. (2023). Effects and mechanisms of kaempferol in the management of cancers through modulation of inflammation and signal transduction pathways. *International Journal of Molecular Sciences, 24*(10), 8630. DOI: 10.3390/ijms24108630

Almatroudi, A., Alsahli, M. A., Alrumaihi, F., Allemailem, K. S., & Rahmani, A. H. (2019). Ginger: A Novel Strategy to Battle Cancer through Modulating Cell Signalling Pathways: A Review. *Current Pharmaceutical Biotechnology, 20*(1), 5–16. DOI: 10.2174/1389201020666190119142331 PMID: 30659535

ALmohaimeed, H. M., Mohammedsaleh, Z. M., Batawi, A. H., Balgoon, M. J., Ramadan, O. I., Baz, H. A., Al Jaouni, S., & Ayuob, N. N.ALmohaimeed. (2021). Synergistic Anti-inflammatory and Neuroprotective Effects of Cinnamomum cassia and Z ingiber officinale Alleviate Diabetes-Induced Hippocampal Changes in Male Albino Rats: Structural and Molecular Evidence. *Frontiers in Cell and Developmental Biology, 9*, 727049. DOI: 10.3389/fcell.2021.727049 PMID: 34568337

Alostad, A., Steink, D., & Schafhuette, E. (2018). International comparison of the herbal medicine registration system to inform regulation development. *Pharmaceutical Medicine*, •••, 39–49. DOI: 10.1007/s40290-018-0223-0 PMID: 29456449

Al-Qarawi, A. A., Al-Damegh, M. A., & El-Mougy, S. A. (2003). Hepatoprotective influence of Adansonia digitata on rats intoxicated with carbon tetrachloride. *Phytotherapy Research, 17*(4), 373–375. DOI: 10.1002/ptr.1128

Alum, E. U. (2025). Sustainable harvesting of medicinal plants: Balancing therapeutic benefits with environmental conservation. *Agroecology and Sustainable Food Systems, 49*(3), 380–385. DOI: 10.1080/21683565.2024.2421948

Ameh, S. J., & Eze, C. N. (2025). Molecular dynamics and thermodynamic integration studies of Nigerian medicinal plant metabolites: Binding energetics of Vernonia amygdalina flavonoids and Alstonia boonei alkaloids. *Computational Biology and Chemistry*, *69*(2), 145–156.

Amira, C. O., & Okubadejo, N. U. (2007). Frequency of complementary and alternative medicine utilization in hypertensive patients attending an urban tertiary care centre in Nigeria. *BMC Complementary and Alternative Medicine*, *7*(1), 1. DOI: 10.1186/1472-6882-7-30 PMID: 17903257

Amirifar, P., Ghasemi, A., & Hosseini, S. (2022). Drought and salinity stress-induced changes in flavonoid and alkaloid biosynthesis: Implications for plant defense and pharmacological activity. *Plant Physiology and Biochemistry*, *185*, 234–245.

Ammar, R. B., Al Saeedi, F. J., Ahmed, E. A., & Rajendran, P. (2021). Benzo (a) Pyrene Induced ROS-Mediated Lung Cancer. In *Handbook of Oxidative Stress in Cancer: Mechanistic Aspects* (pp. 1–14). Springer Singapore. DOI: 10.1007/978-981-15-4501-6_37-1

Ammendola, M., Haponska, M., Balik, K., Janda, K., & Rosiak, D. (2020). Stability and anti-proliferative properties of biologically active compounds extracted from *Cistus L.* after sterilization treatments. *Scientific Reports*, *10*(1), 6521. DOI: 10.1038/s41598-020-63444-3

Amsterdam, J. D., Li, Y., Soeller, I., Rockwell, K., Mao, J. J., & Shults, J. (2009). A randomized, double-blind, placebo-controlled trial of oral Matricaria recutita (chamomile) extract therapy for generalized anxiety disorder. *Journal of Clinical Psychopharmacology*, *29*(4), 378–382. DOI: 10.1097/JCP.0b013e3181ac935c PMID: 19593179

Anand, S., Sowbhagya, R., Ansari, M. A., Alzohairy, M. A., Alomary, M. N., Almalik, A. I., Ahmad, W., Tripathi, T., & Elderdery, A. Y. (2022). Polyphenols and their nanoformulations: Protective effects against human diseases. *Life (Basel, Switzerland)*, *12*(10), 1639. DOI: 10.3390/life12101639

Anetor, G. O., Nwobi, N. L., Igharo, G. O., Sonuga, O. O., & Anetor, J. I. (2022). Environmental pollutants and oxidative stress in terrestrial and aquatic organisms: Examination of the total picture and implications for human health. *Frontiers in Physiology*, *13*, 931386. DOI: 10.3389/fphys.2022.931386 PMID: 35936919

Angelopoulou, E., Paudel, Y. N., Papageorgiou, S. G., & Piperi, C. (2022). Elucidating the Beneficial Effects of Ginger (*Zingiber officinale* Roscoe) in Parkinson's Disease. *ACS Pharmacology & Translational Science*, *5*(10), 838–848. DOI: 10.1021/acsptsci.2c00104 PMID: 36268117

Angon, P. B., Islam, M. S., Kc, S., Das, A., Anjum, N., Poudel, A., & Suchi, S. A. (2025, July 16). 2024. 'Sources, Effects and Present Perspectives of Heavy Metals Contamination: Soil, Plants and Human Food Chain'. *Heliyon*, *10*(7), e28357. https://www.sciencedirect.com/science/article/pii/S2405844024043883. DOI: 10.1016/j.heliyon.2024.e28357 PMID: 38590838

Anionye, J. C., & Onyeneke, E. C. (2016). Composition and in vitro antioxidant capacity of super bitters. *European Journal of Applied Sciences*, *8*(5), 289–296.

Arama, P. F., N'Guessan, K. F., & Kouadio, N. J. (1988). Gel-forming properties of baobab fruit pulp in pharmaceutical formulations. *Pharmaceutical Biology*, *26*(2), 89–94. DOI: 10.3109/13880208809053942

Arama, P. F., N'Guessan, K. F., & Kouadio, N. J. (1989). Sustained-release excipient potential of baobab fruit pulp. *Pharmaceutical Biology*, *27*(1), 45–50. DOI: 10.3109/13880208909053943

Arcusa, R., Villaño, D., Marhuenda, J., Cano, M., Cerdà, B., & Zafrilla, P. (2022). Potential Role of Ginger (*Zingiber officinale* Roscoe) in the Prevention of Neurodegenerative Diseases. *Frontiers in Nutrition*, *9*, 809621. DOI: 10.3389/fnut.2022.809621 PMID: 35369082

Aregawi, L. G., & Zoltan, C. (2025). Evaluation of Adverse Effects and Tolerability of Dietary Ginger Supplementation in Patients With Functional Dyspepsia. *Current Therapeutic Research, Clinical and Experimental*, *102*, 100792. DOI: 10.1016/j.curtheres.2025.100792 PMID: 40474983

Aremu, A. O., & Pendota, S. C. (2021). Medicinal plants for mitigating pain and inflammatory-related conditions: An appraisal of ethnobotanical uses and patterns in South Africa. *Frontiers in Pharmacology*, *12*, 758583. DOI: 10.3389/fphar.2021.758583 PMID: 34744737

Arul, V., Miyazaki, S., & Dhananjayan, R. (2005). Studies on the anti-inflammatory, antipyretic and analgesic properties of the leaves of *Aegle marmelos* Corr. *Journal of Ethnopharmacology*, *96*(1-2), 159–163. DOI: 10.1016/j.jep.2004.09.013 PMID: 15588665

Arya, P., Kumari, N., Ahmad Wani, S., & Kumar, P. (2023). Trigonella foenum graecum. *Herbs, Spices and Their Roles in Nutraceuticals and Functional Foods*, 133–148. DOI: 10.1016/B978-0-323-90794-1.00001-6

Asare-Doku, W., Settumba Stolk, S., Peacock, A., Shakeshaft, A., Waller, E., Nathan, S., & Farrell, M. (2023). *Monitoring and evaluation of the kava pilot program*. National Drug and Alcohol Research Centre, UNSW.

Asensi, M., Ortega, A., Mena, S., Feddi, F., & Estrela, J. M. (2011). Natural polyphenols in cancer therapy. *Critical Reviews in Clinical Laboratory Sciences*, *48*(5–6), 197–216. DOI: 10.3109/10408363.2011.631268

Ashrafizadeh, M., Fekri, H. S., Ahmadi, Z., Farkhondeh, T., & Samarghandian, S. (2020). Therapeutic and biological activities of berberine: The involvement of the Nrf2 signalling pathway. *Journal of Cellular Biochemistry*, *121*(2), 1575–1585. DOI: 10.1002/jcb.29392 PMID: 31609017

Ashraf, M. V., Khan, S., Misri, S., Gaira, K. S., Rawat, S., Rawat, B., Khan, M. A. H., Shah, A. A., Asgher, M., & Ahmad, S. (2024). High-Altitude Medicinal Plants as Promising Source of Phytochemical Antioxidants to Combat Lifestyle-Associated Oxidative Stress-Induced Disorders. *Pharmaceuticals (Basel, Switzerland)*, *17*(8), 975. DOI: 10.3390/ph17080975 PMID: 39204080

Ashrafpour, S., & Ashrafpour, M. (2025). The double-edged sword of nutraceuticals: Comprehensive review of protective agents and their hidden risks. *Frontiers in Nutrition*, *12*, 1524627. DOI: 10.3389/fnut.2025.1524627

Asiminicesei, D.-M., Fertu, D. I., & Gavrilescu, M. (2024). Impact of Heavy Metal Pollution in the Environment on the Metabolic Profile of Medicinal Plants and Their Therapeutic Potential. *Plants*, *13*(6), 913. DOI: 10.3390/plants13060913 PMID: 38592933

Asiminicesei, S., Popescu, D., & Ionescu, R. (2024). Heavy metal contamination and its impact on phytochemical production in medicinal plants. *Environmental Monitoring and Assessment*, *196*(4), 321–333.

Attahiru, A. (2025). Bioactive compounds and therapeutic prospects of Nigerian medicinal plants. *International Journal of African Health and Medical Research*, *9*(5), 45–60.

Aude Périne, M. N. A., Kevin, E., Saurelle, M., Vanessa Charlotte, S. L., Martin, N. N., Jeanne Mauricette, M. M., Chimène, B., & Nga, N. (2022). Evaluation of the Patentability of Medicines based on plants produced in Cameroon: Case of Yaounde. *International Journal of Drug Regulatory Affairs*, *10*(3), 19–24. DOI: 10.22270/ijdra.v10i3.547

Avalos-Soriano, A., de la Cruz-Cordero, R., Rosado, J. L., & Garcia-Gasca, T. (2019). Momordica charantia: A review on its effects on human health. *Journal of Food Science*, *84*(8), 2013–2026.

Awodele, O., Amagon, K. I., Wannang, N. N., & Aguiyi, J. C. (2014). Traditional medicine policy and regulation in Nigeria: An index of herbal medicine safety. *Current Drug Safety*, *9*(1), 16–22. DOI: 10.2174/1574886308666131126155434 PMID: 24274707

Awojide, S. H., Akinlade, B., Oyewole, K. A., Adeyemo, A. G., Adeniyi, E. O., Fadunmade, O. E., & Anifowose, A. J. (2023). Synergistic and antagonistic medicinal activities of essential oil of Monodora myristica. *CTU Journal of Innovation and Sustainable Development*, *15*(3), 1–11. DOI: 10.22144/ctujoisd.2023.046

Awoniyi, S. O., Adeyemi, O. O., & Bello, I. (2023). Effect of temperature on phytochemical extraction: Stability and degradation of thermolabile compounds. *Journal of Food Biochemistry*, *47*(1), e14012.

Ayertey, F., Ofori-Attah, E., Antwi, S., Amoa-Bosompem, M., Djameh, G., Lartey, N. L., Ohashi, M., Kusi, K. A., Appiah, A. A., Appiah-Opong, R., & Okine, L. K. (2020). Anti-inflammatory activity and mechanism of action of ethanolic leaf extract of Morinda lucida Benth. *Journal of Traditional and Complementary Medicine*, *11*(3), 249–258. DOI: 10.1016/j.jtcme.2020.07.001 PMID: 34012871

Ayodipupo Babalola, B., Ifeolu Akinwande, A., Otunba, A. A., Ebenezer Adebami, G., Babalola, O., & Nwuofo, C. (2024). Therapeutic benefits of Carica papaya: A review on its pharmacological activities and characterization of papain. In Arabian Journal of Chemistry (Vol. 17, Issue 1). Elsevier B.V. DOI: 10.1016/j.arabjc.2023.105369

Ayuba, D., Fadele, P., Ogaya, J. B., Olayinka, K. E., Sharma, S. N., & Lucero-Prisno, D. E. I.III. (2024). Understanding the root of healing and beyond: Exploring the way forward for Alternative Medicine in Nigeria. *Bhutan Sorig Journal*, *1*(1), 42–47. DOI: 10.47811/bsj.0004050304

Ayustaningwarno, F., Anjani, G., Ayu, A. M., & Fogliano, V. (2024). A critical review of Ginger's (*Zingiber officinale*) antioxidant, anti-inflammatory, and immunomodulatory activities. *Frontiers in Nutrition*, *11*, 1364836. DOI: 10.3389/fnut.2024.1364836 PMID: 38903613

Azmal, M., Rahman, S., & Chowdhury, A. (2024). Molecular docking studies of phytochemicals: Insights into receptor-ligand interactions and pharmacodynamics. *Computational Biology and Chemistry*, *98*, 107–118.

Azrad, M., Vollmer, R. T., Madden, J., Dewhirst, M., Polascik, T. J., Snyder, D. C., Ruffin, M. T., Moul, J. W., Brenner, D. E., & Demark-Wahnefried, W. (2013). Flaxseed-derived enterolactone is inversely associated with tumor cell proliferation in men with localized prostate cancer. *Journal of Medicinal Food*, *16*(4), 357–360. DOI: 10.1089/jmf.2012.0159

Baird, L., & Yamamoto, M. (2020). The molecular mechanisms regulating the KEAP1–NRF2 pathway. Molecular and Cellular Biology, 40(13), Bioltif, Y. E., Sase, T. J., and Nehemiah, T. O. (2020). Phytochemical screening and review of the pharmacological importance of Erythrina senegalensis. *International Journal of Trend in Scientific Research and Development*, *4*(3), 292–296.

Balakrishnan, R., Azam, S., Cho, D. Y., Su-Kim, I., & Choi, D. K. (2021). Natural Phytochemicals as Novel Therapeutic Strategies to prevent and Treat Parkinson's disease: Current Knowledge and Future Perspectives. *Oxidative Medicine and Cellular Longevity*, *2021*(1), 2021. DOI: 10.1155/2021/6680935 PMID: 34122727

Balali-Mood, M., Naseri, K., Tahergorabi, Z., Khazdair, M. R., & Sadeghi, M. (2021). Toxic mechanisms of five heavy metals: Mercury, lead, chromium, cadmium, and arsenic. *Frontiers in Pharmacology*, *12*, 643972. DOI: 10.3389/fphar.2021.643972 PMID: 33927623

Ball, N., Teo, W. P., Chandra, S., & Chapman, J. (2019). Parkinson's disease and the environment. *Frontiers in Neurology*, *10*, 218. DOI: 10.3389/fneur.2019.00218 PMID: 30941085

Bamidele, O. D., Adegbolagun, O. M., Subair, H. G., & Emikpe, B. O. (2018). Pharmaco-epidemiologic survey and experimental study of co-administration of three herbal products with paracetamol. *African Journal of Biomedical Research*, •••, 153–159.

Bandodkar, V. V., Moger, V. S., & Baliga, P. (2025). Antioxidant Defense Mechanisms: Enzymatic and non-enzymatic. In The Role of Reactive Oxygen Species in Human Health and Disease (pp. 43-80). IGI Global Scientific Publishing.

Barabási, A. L., Gulbahce, N., & Loscalzo, J. (2011). Network medicine: A network-based approach to human disease. *Nature Reviews. Genetics*, *12*(1), 56–68. DOI: 10.1038/nrg2918

Basak, S., Sarma, G. C., & Rangan, L. (2010). Ethnomedical uses of *Zingiberaceous* plants of Northeast India. *Journal of Ethnopharmacology*, *132*(1), 286–296. DOI: 10.1016/j.jep.2010.08.032 PMID: 20727402

Başaran, N., Pasli, D., & Başaran, A. (2022). Unpredictable adverse effects of herbal products. *Food and Chemical Toxicology*, *159*, 112762. DOI: 10.1016/j.fct.2021.112762 PMID: 34896186

Bastidas, H., Araya-Valdés, G., Cortés, G., Jara, J. A., & Catalán, M. (2022). Pharmacological effects of caffeic acid and its derivatives in cancer: New targeted compounds for the mitochondria. *Advances in Experimental Medicine and Biology*, *1401*, 213–225. DOI: 10.1007/5584_2022_718

Baum, D. A. (2021). Baobab trees: Systematics, evolution, and biogeography. *Annual Review of Ecology, Evolution, and Systematics*, *52*(1), 1–22. DOI: 10.1146/annurev-ecolsys-012121-091647

Beckers, M., Bloem, B. R., & Verbeek, M. M. (2022). Mechanisms of peripheral levodopa resistance in Parkinson's disease. *npj. Parkinson's Disease*, *8*(1), 56. PMID: 35546556

Beg, S., Swain, S., Hasan, H., Barkat, M. A., & Hussain, M. S. (2011). Systematic review of herbals as potential anti-inflammatory agents: Recent advances, current clinical status and future perspectives. *Pharmacognosy Reviews*, *5*(10), 120. DOI: 10.4103/0973-7847.91102 PMID: 22279370

Bej, E., Cesare, P., Volpe, A. R., d'Angelo, M., & Castelli, V. (2024). Oxidative stress and neurodegeneration: Insights and therapeutic strategies for Parkinson's disease. *Neurology International*, *16*(3), 502–517. DOI: 10.3390/neurolint16030037 PMID: 38804477

Bekele, F., Tefera, T., Biresaw, G., & Yohannes, T. (2017). Parasitic contamination of raw vegetables and fruits collected from selected local markets in Arba Minch town, Southern Ethiopia. *Infectious Diseases of Poverty*, *6*(1), 19. DOI: 10.1186/s40249-016-0226-6 PMID: 28264707

Bele, A. A., & Khale, A. (2011). An overview on thin layer chromatography. *International Journal of Pharmaceutical Sciences and Research*, *2*(2), 256.

Beltrán-Noboa, A., Proaño-Ojeda, J., Guevara, M., Gallo, B., Berrueta, L. A., Giampieri, F., Perez-Castillo, Y., Battino, M., Álvarez-Suarez, J. M., & Tejera, E. (2022). Metabolomic profile and computational analysis for the identification of the potential anti-inflammatory mechanisms of action of the traditional medicinal plants Ocimum basilicum and Ocimum tenuiflorum. *Food and Chemical Toxicology*, *164*, 113039. DOI: 10.1016/j.fct.2022.113039 PMID: 35461962

Bencharif-Betina, S., Benhamed, N., Benabdallah, A., Bendif, H., Benslama, A., Negro, C., Plavan, G., Abd-Elkader, O. H., & De Bellis, L. (2023). A Multi-Approach Study of Phytochemicals and Their Effects on Oxidative Stress and Enzymatic Activity of Essential Oil and Crude Extracts of Rosmarinus officinalis. *Separations*, *10*(7), 394. DOI: 10.3390/separations10070394

Berg, J. M., Tymoczko, J. L., & Gatto, G. J. (2015). *Biochemistry* (8th ed.). W. H. Freeman.

Bezard, E., Gray, D., Kozak, R., Leoni, M., Combs, C., & Duvvuri, S. (2024). Rationale and development of tavapadon, a D1/D5-selective partial dopamine agonist for the treatment of Parkinson's disease. *CNS & Neurological Disorders - Drug Targets, 23*(4), 476–487. DOI: 10.2174/1871527322666230331121028 PMID: 36999711

Bhamre, V. G., Deore, P. D., Amrutkar, R. D., & Patil, V. R. (2022). Polyphenols: The interactions with CYP isoenzymes and effect on pharmacokinetics of drugs. *Current Trends in Pharmacy and Pharmaceutical Chemistry*, 4(1).

Bharathy, P., Thanikachalam, P. V., Shoban, A. N., & Himayavendhan, H. V. (2024). Floral Fusion: Unravelling the Potent Blend of Ixora coccinea and Rhododendron arboreum for Health and Safety Benefits. *Cureus*. Advance online publication. DOI: 10.7759/cureus.70038 PMID: 39449919

Bhat, A. A., Gupta, G., Afzal, M., Thapa, R., Ali, H., Alqahtani, S. M., almalki, W. H., Kazmi, I., Alzarea, S. I., Saleem, S., & Subramaniyan, V. (2024). Polyphenol-loaded nano-carriers for breast cancer therapy: A comprehensive review. *BioNanoScience, 14*(4), 4219–4237. DOI: 10.1007/s12668-023-01288-7

Bhusal, C. K., Uti, D. E., Mukherjee, D., Alqahtani, T., Alqahtani, S., Bhattacharya, A., & Akash, S. (2023). Unveiling Nature's potential: Promising natural compounds in Parkinson's disease management. *Parkinsonism & Related Disorders, 115*, 105799. DOI: 10.1016/j.parkreldis.2023.105799 PMID: 37633805

Bianchini, J.-P., Ralaimanarivo, A., Gaydou, E. M., & Waegell, B. (1982). Hydrocarbons, sterols, and tocopherols in the seeds of six Adansonia species. *Phytochemistry, 21*(8), 1981–1987. DOI: 10.1016/0031-9422(82)83027-6

Biernacki, M., Kuczyńska, B., & Wawrzeńczyk, A. (2020). The Antimalaria Alkaloids in the Nigerian Medicinal Plant, Cryptolepis sanguinolenta. *Journal of Ethnopharmacology, 250*, 112445.

Biswas, P., Anand, U., Saha, S. C., Kant, N., Mishra, T., Masih, H., Bar, A., Pandey, D. K., Jha, N. K., Majumder, M., Das, N., Gadekar, V. S., Shekhawat, M. S., Kumar, M., Radha, , Proćków, J., Lastra, J. M. P., & Dey, A. (2022). Betelvine (Piper betle L.): A comprehensive insight into its ethnopharmacology, phytochemistry, and pharmacological, biomedical and therapeutic attributes. *Journal of Cellular and Molecular Medicine, 26*(11), 3083–3119. DOI: 10.1111/jcmm.17323 PMID: 35502487

Bitwell, T., Mensah, J., & Owusu, R. (2023). Conventional extraction methods in phytochemistry: Efficiency and limitations. *African Journal of Plant Science, 17*(2), 55–64.

Black, C. D., Herring, M. P., Hurley, D. J., & O'Connor, P. J. (2010). Ginger (Zingiber officinale) reduces muscle pain caused by eccentric exercise. *The Journal of Pain, 11*(9), 894–903. DOI: 10.1016/j.jpain.2009.12.013 PMID: 20418184

Bloem, B. R., Marks, W. J., De Lima, A. S., Kuijf, M. L., Van Laar, T., Jacobs, B. P. F., & Meinders, M. J. (2019). The Personalized Parkinson Project: Examining disease progression through broad biomarkers in early Parkinson's disease. *BMC Neurology, 19*(1), 1–10. DOI: 10.1186/s12883-019-1394-3 PMID: 31315608

Boakye, Y. D., Osafo, N., Oppong-Kyekyeku, J., Abotsi, W. K. M., Boakye-Gyasi, E., Heiss, E., & Agyare, C. (2022). Regulation of Nrf2 and NF-κB activities may contribute to the anti-inflammatory mechanism of xylopic acid. *Inflammopharmacology, 30*(5), 1835–1841. DOI: 10.1007/s10787-022-00950-y PMID: 35260973

Bogetofte, H., Alamyar, A., Blaabjerg, M., & Meyer, M. (2020). Levodopa therapy for Parkinson's disease: History, current status and perspectives. *CNS & Neurological Disorders - Drug Targets, 19*(8), 572–583. DOI: 10.2174/1871527319666200722153156 PMID: 32703142

Borrás, S., Martínez-Solís, I., & Ríos, J. L. (2021). Medicinal plants for insomnia related to anxiety: An updated review. *Planta Medica, 87*(10/11), 738–753. DOI: 10.1055/a-1510-9826 PMID: 34116572

Bosch, C. H., Siemonsma, J. S., Lemmens, R. H. M. J., & Oyen, L. P. A. (2004). Adansonia digitata L. In *PROTA 1: Vegetables/Legumes*. PROTA Foundation.

Brady, C. A., & Attardi, L. D. (2010). p53 at a glance. *Journal of Cell Science, 123*(15), 2527–2532. DOI: 10.1242/jcs.064501

Brendler, T., Gruenwald, J., & Jaenicke, C. (2003). *Herbal remedies*. Medpharm Scientific Publishers.

Brinchmann, B. C., Skuland, T., Rambøl, M. H., Szoke, K., Brinchmann, J. E., Gutleb, A. C., Moschini, E., Kubátová, A., Kukowski, K., Le Ferrec, E., Lagadic-Gossmann, D., Schwarze, P. E., Låg, M., Refsnes, M., Øvrevik, J., & Holme, J. A. (2018). 'Lipophilic Components of Diesel Exhaust Particles Induce Pro-Inflammatory Responses in Human Endothelial Cells through AhR Dependent Pathway(S)'. *Particle and Fibre Toxicology, 15*(1), 1–17. DOI: 10.1186/s12989-018-0257-1 PMID: 29298690

Brown, A. C. (2017). Heart toxicity related to herbs and dietary supplements: Online table of case reports. *Journal of Dietary Supplements*. PMID: 28981338

Bucciantini, M., Giannoni, E., & Chiti, F. (2022). Polyphenols as modulators of inflammatory signaling pathways: Implications for chronic disease. *International Journal of Molecular Sciences, 23*(12), 6543–6558.

Budzianowska, A., Banaś, K., Budzianowski, J., & Kikowska, M. (2025). Antioxidants to defend healthy and youthful skin—Current trends and future directions in cosmetology. *Applied Sciences (Basel, Switzerland), 15*(5), 2571. DOI: 10.3390/app15052571

Buhrmann, C., Mobasheri, A., Busch, F., Aldinger, C., Stahlmann, R., Montaseri, A., & Shakibaei, M. (2011). Curcumin modulates nuclear factor κB (nf-κB)-mediated inflammation in human tenocytes in vitro: Role of the phosphatidylinositol 3-kinase/Akt pathway. *The Journal of Biological Chemistry, 286*(32), 28556–28566. DOI: 10.1074/jbc.M111.256180 PMID: 21669872

Bukowski, K., Kciuk, M., & Kontek, R. (2020). Mechanisms of multidrug resistance in cancer chemotherapy. *International Journal of Molecular Sciences, 21*(9), 3233. DOI: 10.3390/ijms21093233 PMID: 32370233

Bunaciu, A. A., Aboul-Enein, H. Y., & Fleschin, S. (2011). Recent Applications of Fourier Transform Infrared Spectrophotometry in Herbal Medicine Analysis. *Applied Spectroscopy Reviews, 46*(4), 251–260. DOI: 10.1080/05704928.2011.565532

Burapan, S., Kim, M., Paisooksantivatana, Y., Eser, B. E., & Han, J. (2020). Thai curcuma species: Antioxidant and bioactive compounds. *Foods, 9*(9), 1219. DOI: 10.3390/foods9091219 PMID: 32887356

Burford, N., Shipilov, A. V., & Furr, N. R. (2022). How ecosystem structure affects firm performance in response to a negative shock to interdependencies. *Strategic Management Journal, 43*(1), 30–57. DOI: 10.1002/smj.3318

Burton, N., Sneed, K., & Pathak, Y. (2023). Systemic Review of the Use of Kava Kava for the Reduction of Anxiety Disorder.

Busia, K. (2024). Herbal Medicine Dosage Standardisation. *Journal of Herbal Medicine, 46*, 100889. DOI: 10.1016/j.hermed.2024.100889

Cacciola, N. A., Cuciniello, R., Petillo, G. D., Piccioni, M., Filosa, S., & Crispi, S. (2023). An overview of the enhanced effects of curcumin and chemotherapeutic agents in combined cancer treatments. *International Journal of Molecular Sciences, 24*(16), 12587. DOI: 10.3390/ijms241612587

Cai, Z., Mao, C., Wang, Y., Zhu, Z., Xu, S., Chen, D., Chen, Y., Ruan, W., & Fang, B. (2022). Phytochemistry and pharmacology of traditional Chinese medicine: Review research progress with luteolin as an anti-tumor agent. *Natural Product Communications*, *17*(11), 1–7. DOI: 10.1177/1934578X221133579

Calixto, J. B. (2005). Twenty-five years of research on medicinal plants in Latin America: A personal view. *Journal of Ethnopharmacology*, *100*(1–2), 131–134. DOI: 10.1016/j.jep.2005.06.004

Carson, C. F., Hammer, K. A., & Riley, T. V. (2007). Soil composition and microbial communities influencing secondary metabolite production. *Applied Soil Ecology*, *35*(3), 495–502.

Carvalho, A. C. B., Perfeito, J. P. S., de Britto Vidal Filho, W., & Silveira, D. (2025). A decade retrospective and future prospects: How European regulatory alignment shapes Brazil's herbal medicine market. *Journal of Ethnopharmacology*, *353*, 120404. DOI: 10.1016/j.jep.2025.120404 PMID: 40803612

Castañeda-Arriaga, R., Pérez-González, A., Reina, M., Alvarez-Idaboy, J. R., & Galano, A. (2018). Comprehensive Investigation of the Antioxidant and Pro-oxidant Effects of Phenolic Compounds: A Double-Edged Sword in the Context of Oxidative Stress? *The Journal of Physical Chemistry B*, *122*(23), 6198–6214. DOI: 10.1021/acs.jpcb.8b03500 PMID: 29771524

Chaachouay, N. (2025). Pharmacodynamic profiling of Camellia sinensis polyphenols: Network pharmacology insights. *Journal of Ethnopharmacology*, *315*, 117–126.

Chaachouay, N., & Zidane, L. (2024). Plant-Derived Natural Products: A Source for Drug Discovery and Development. *Drugs and Drug Candidates*, *3*(1), 184–207. DOI: 10.3390/ddc3010011

Chadare, F. J., Linnemann, A. R., Hounhouigan, J. D., Nout, M. J. R., & Van Boekel, M. A. J. S. (2009). Baobab food products: A review on their composition and nutritional value. *Critical Reviews in Food Science and Nutrition*, *49*(3), 254–274. DOI: 10.1080/10408390701856330

Cháirez-Ramírez, M. H., de la Cruz-López, K. G., & García-Carrancá, A. (2021). Polyphenols as antitumor agents targeting key players in cancer-driving signaling pathways. *Frontiers in Pharmacology*, *12*, 710304. DOI: 10.3389/fphar.2021.710304

Chakraborty, A., Sahoo, M., Roy, S. D., & Dasgupta, R. K. (2018). Anti-ageing natural herbs: A systemic review. *Indian Research Journal of Pharmacy and Science*, *5*(3), 1589–1598. DOI: 10.21276/irjps.2018.5.3.4

Chandra Shekhar, H., Joshua, L., & Thomas, J. V. (2024). Standardized extract of Valeriana officinalis improves overall sleep quality in human subjects with sleep complaints: A randomized, double-blind, placebo-controlled, clinical study. *Advances in Therapy*, *41*(1), 246–261. DOI: 10.1007/s12325-023-02708-6 PMID: 37899385

Chandran, R., & Abrahamse, H. (2020). Identifying Plant-Based Natural Medicine against Oxidative Stress and Neurodegenerative Disorders. *Oxidative Medicine and Cellular Longevity*, *2020*, 1–9. DOI: 10.1155/2020/8648742 PMID: 33014278

Chandrasekhar, K., Kapoor, J., & Anishetty, S. (2012). A prospective, randomized double-blind, placebo-controlled study of safety and efficacy of a high-concentration full-spectrum extract of ashwagandha root in reducing stress and anxiety in adults. *Indian Journal of Psychological Medicine*, *34*(3), 255–262. DOI: 10.4103/0253-7176.106022 PMID: 23439798

Chan, E. W. C., & Wong, S. K. (2014). Phytochemistry and pharmacology of three Piper species: An update. *International Journal of Pharmacognosy : a Journal of Crude Drug Research*, (9), 534–544.

Chang, K. H., & Chen, C. M. (2020). The role of oxidative stress in Parkinson's disease. *Antioxidants*, *9*(7), 597. DOI: 10.3390/antiox9070597 PMID: 32650609

Chao, W., & Lin, B. (2011). *Bioactivities of major constituents isolated from Angelica sinensis*. China Medical. DOI: 10.1186/1749-8546-6-29

Chatfield, S. M. (2016). Intercultural competence and pharmacological communication: Understanding drug efficacy and side effects. *Journal of Intercultural Communication Research*, *45*(3), 223–238.

Chauhan, J. S., Singh, R., & Singh, S. (1984). Flavonoids from the roots of Adansonia digitata. *Phytochemistry*, *23*(9), 2081–2082. DOI: 10.1016/S0031-9422(00)84100-2

Chele, K. H., Piater, L. A., van der Hooft, J. J. J., & Tugizimana, F. (2025). Bridging Ethnobotanical Knowledge and Multi-Omics Approaches for Plant-Derived Natural Product Discovery. *Metabolites*, *15*(6), 362. DOI: 10.3390/metabo15060362 PMID: 40559386

Cheng, C., Yan, K. K., & Gerstein, M. (2018). Gene regulation networks: Models and applications. Nature Reviews Genetics, 19(9), 551–564.Alves, V. M., Muratov, E. N., & Tropsha, A. (2022). Advances in molecular docking and dynamics simulations for natural product drug discovery. *Journal of Chemical Information and Modeling*, *62*(4), 845–856.

Chen, R., Zhang, Y., & Liu, Y. (2021). Airborne particulate matter induces mitochondrial damage and oxidative stress in lung epithelial cells. *Toxicology Letters, 347*, 26–35. DOI: 10.1016/j.toxlet.2021.04.005

Chen, T., Xiao, Z., Liu, X., Wang, T., Wang, Y., Ye, F., Su, J., Yao, X., Xiong, L., & Yang, D. H. (2024). Natural products for combating multidrug resistance in cancer. *Pharmacological Research, 202*, 107099. DOI: 10.1016/j.phrs.2024.107099 PMID: 38342327

Cheriyan, R., Thomas, J., & Varghese, A. (2025). Green extraction technologies for phytochemicals: Trends and future perspectives. *Journal of Cleaner Production, 412*, 136–145.

Chevalier, F., & Sommerer, N. (2011). Analytical Methods: Mass Spectrometric Methods. In Fuquay, J. W. (Ed.), *Encyclopedia of Dairy Sciences* (2nd ed., pp. 198–205). Academic Press. DOI: 10.1016/B978-0-12-374407-4.00019-4

Chijindu, P. C. I., Okpoma, M. O., & Atubi, O. (2020). Ethnobotanical survey of medicinal plants used in Erhuwaren community in Ughelli South Local Government Area of Delta State. *Unilag Journal of Medicine. Science and Technology, 8*(1), 176–206.

Chillón-Pino, D., Badonyi, M., Semple, C. A., & Marsh, J. A. (2024). Protein structural context of cancer mutations reveals molecular mechanisms and candidate driver genes. *Cell Reports, 43*(11), 114905. DOI: 10.1016/j.celrep.2024.114905

Chimento, A., De Luca, A., D'Amico, M., De Amicis, F., & Pezzi, V. (2023). The involvement of natural polyphenols in molecular mechanisms inducing apoptosis in tumor cells: A promising adjuvant in cancer therapy. *International Journal of Molecular Sciences, 24*(2), 168. DOI: 10.3390/ijms24021680

Chi , A., Noubissi, P. A., Pop, O. L., Mure an, C. I., Fokam Tagne, M. A., Kamgang, R., Fodor, A., Sitar-Tăut, A. V., Cozma, A., Oră an, O. H., Heghe , S. C., Vulturar, R., & Suharoschi, R. (2023). Bioactive Compounds in Moringa oleifera: Mechanisms of Action, Focus on Their Anti-Inflammatory Properties. *Plants, 13*(1), 20. DOI: 10.3390/plants13010020 PMID: 38202328

Choi, J. G., Kim, S. Y., Jeong, M., & Oh, M. S. (2018). Pharmacotherapeutic potential of ginger and its compounds in age-related neurological disorders. *Pharmacology & Therapeutics, 182*, 56–69. DOI: 10.1016/j.pharmthera.2017.08.010 PMID: 28842272

Choi, J., Lee, J., Kim, K., Choi, H. K., Lee, S. A., & Lee, H. J. (2022). Effects of ginger intake on chemotherapy-induced nausea and vomiting: A systematic review of randomized clinical trials. *Nutrients, 14*(23), 4982. DOI: 10.3390/nu14234982 PMID: 36501010

Choudhury, P. R., Choudhury, M. D., Ningthoujam, S. S., Das, D., Nath, D., & Talukdar, A. D. (2015). Ethnomedicinal plants used by traditional healers of North Tripura district, Tripura, North East India. *Journal of Ethnopharmacology, 166*, 135–148. DOI: 10.1016/j.jep.2015.03.026 PMID: 25794807

Chourasiya, P., Gour, R., & Patel, A. K. (2024). Qualitative Phytochemical Investigation and Acute Oral Toxicity Study on Ethanolic Extract of Curcuma longa Leaves. *Journal of Drug Delivery and Therapeutics, 14*(2), 73–78. DOI: 10.22270/jddt.v14i1.6244

Chu, A. J. (2022). Quarter-century explorations of bioactive polyphenols: Diverse health benefits. [Landmark Edition]. *Frontiers in Bioscience (Landmark Edition), 27*(4), 134. DOI: 10.31083/j.fbl2704134

Chukwuma, E. C., Soladoye, M. O., & Feyisola, R. T. (2015). Traditional medicine and the future of medicinal Plants in Nigeria. *Journal of Medicinal Plants Studies, 3*(4), 23–29.

Chukwuonye, I. I., Ohagwu, K. A., Ogah, O. S., John, C., Oviasu, E., Anyabolu, E. N., Ezeani, I. U., Iloh, G. U. P., Chukwuonye, M. E., Raphael, C. O., Onwuchekwa, U., Okafor, U. H., Oladele, C., Obi, E. C., Okwuonu, C. G., Iheji, O., Nwabuko, O. C., Nnoli, M. A., & Okpechi, G. (2022). Prevalence of overweight and obesity in Nigeria: Systematic review and meta-analysis of population-based studies. *PLOS Global Public Health, 2*(6), e0000515. DOI: 10.1371/journal.pgph.0000515 PMID: 36962450

Church, F. C. (2021). Treatment Options for Motor and Non-Motor Symptoms of Parkinson's Disease. *Biomolecules, 11*(4), 612. DOI: 10.3390/biom11040612 PMID: 33924103

Ciupei, D., Colişar, A., Leopold, L., Stănilă, A., & Diaconeasa, Z. M. (2024). Polyphenols: From classification to therapeutic potential and bioavailability. *Foods, 13*(24), 4131. DOI: 10.3390/foods13244131

Coe, S. A., Ryan, L., Springer, C. J., & Chhim, S. (2023). Nutritional and therapeutic potential of baobab (*Adansonia digitata*): A contemporary review. *Journal of Functional Foods, 101*, 105440. DOI: 10.1016/j.jff.2023.105440

Colomer, R., Sarrats, A., Lupu, R., & Puig, T. (2017). Natural polyphenols and their synthetic analogs as emerging anticancer agents. *Current Drug Targets*, *18*(2), 147–159. DOI: 10.2174/1389450117666160112113930

Compaoré, M., Ouédraogo, A., Kaboré, D., Sawadogo, B., & Nikiéma, J. B. (2021). Prebiotic effects of baobab fruit pulp on gut microbiota. *Journal of Food Biochemistry*, *45*(5), e13716. DOI: 10.1111/jfbc.13716

Conway, C. C., Grogans, S. E., Anderson, A. S., Islam, S., Craig, L. E., Wedlock, J., Hur, J., DeYoung, K. A., & Shackman, A. J. (2024). Neuroticism Is Prospectively Associated With 30-Month Changes in Broadband Internalizing Symptoms, but Not Narrowband Positive Affect or Anxious Arousal, in Emerging Adulthood. *Clinical Psychological Science*, *12*(5), 823–839. DOI: 10.1177/21677026231205270 PMID: 39359716

Coolborn, A., Bolatito, B., Omolara, A., & Adetuyi, F. (2015). Phytochemical and Antioxidant Effect of Spathodea campanulata leaf Extracts. *International Journal of Biochemistry Research & Review*, *7*(3), 148–159. DOI: 10.9734/IJBCRR/2015/16371

Cooley, K., Szczurko, O., Perri, D., Mills, E. J., Bernhardt, B., Zhou, Q., & Seely, D. (2009). Naturopathic care for anxiety: A randomized controlled trial ISRCTN78958974. *PLoS One*, *4*(8), e6628. DOI: 10.1371/journal.pone.0006628 PMID: 19718255

Cuni-Sanchez, A., Muledi, J. I., Groot, N., Wessels, M., Boehning-Gaese, K., De Cauwer, V., Gaisberger, H., Gereau, R. E., Hannibal, W., Kenfack, D., Kouadio, Y. J., Kouadio, N. J., Kouadio, K., Lykke, A. M., Marchant, R., McClatchey, W., Nacoulma, B. M., Neba, G. A., Njouonkou, A. L., & Venter, S. M. (2022). Resilience of the African baobab under climate change. *Global Change Biology*, *28*(4), 1422–1435. DOI: 10.1111/gcb.16036

Cunningham, A. B. (1993). *African medicinal plants*. United Nations Educational, Scientific and Cultural Organization.

Custers, D., Van Praag, N., Courselle, P., Apers, S., & Deconinck, E. (2017). Chromatographic fingerprinting as a strategy to identify regulated plants in illegal herbal supplements. *Talanta*, *164*, 490–502. DOI: 10.1016/j.talanta.2016.12.008 PMID: 28107963

D'Amico, R., Fusco, R., Cordaro, M., Interdonato, L., Crupi, R., Gugliandolo, E., Di Paola, D., Peritore, A. F., Siracusa, R., Impellizzeri, D., Cuzzocrea, S., & Di Paola, R. (2022). Modulation of NrF-2 pathway contributes to the therapeutic effects of Boswellia serrata gum resin extract in a model of experimental autoimmune myocarditis. *Antioxidants*, *11*(11), 2129. DOI: 10.3390/antiox11112129 PMID: 36358503

Danesi, M. A., & Adetunji, J. B. (1994). Use of alternative medicine by patients with epilepsy: A survey of 265 epileptic patients in a developing country. *Epilepsia*, *35*(2), 344–351. DOI: 10.1111/j.1528-1157.1994.tb02442.x PMID: 8156955

Danyal, Y., Mahmood, K., Ullah, S., Rahim, A., Raheem, G., Khan, A. H., & Ullah, A. (2023). Phytoremediation of industrial effluents assisted by plant growth promoting bacteria. *Environmental Science and Pollution Research International*, *30*(3), 5296–5311. DOI: 10.1007/s11356-022-23967-w PMID: 36402881

Dar, M. A., Sofi, G., & Rather, M. A. (2023). Advances in extraction techniques and phytochemical screening of medicinal plants: A review. *Journal of Applied Research on Medicinal and Aromatic Plants*, *32*, 100–112.

Dar, R. A., Shahnawaz, M., Ahanger, M. A., & Majid, I. U. (2023). Exploring the Diverse Bioactive Compounds from Medicinal Plants: A Review. *The Journal of Phytopharmacology*, *12*(3), 139–195. DOI: 10.31254/phyto.2023.12307

Dasgupta, N., & De, B. (2004). Antioxidant activity of Piper betel L. Leaf extract in vitro | Request PDF. *Food Chemistry*, *88*(2), 219–224. DOI: 10.1016/j.foodchem.2004.01.036

Das, S., & Ojha, P. K. (2025). Bridging chemistry and toxicology: Chemometric-driven prediction and prioritization of various drugs addressing hazardous effects for human safety. *Journal of Hazardous Materials*, *495*, 139134. DOI: 10.1016/j.jhazmat.2025.139134 PMID: 40633349

Das, S., Parida, R., Sandeep, I. S., Nayak, S., & Mohanty, S. (2016). Biotechnological intervention in betelvine (Piper betle L.): A review on recent advances and future prospects. *Asian Pacific Journal of Tropical Medicine*, *9*(10), 938–946. DOI: 10.1016/j.apjtm.2016.07.029 PMID: 27794386

Davatgaran-Taghipour, Y., Masoomzadeh, S., Farzaei, M. H., Bahramsoltani, R., Karimi-Soureh, Z., Rahimi, R., & Abdollahi, M. (2017). Polyphenol nanoformulations for cancer therapy: Experimental evidence and clinical perspective. *International Journal of Nanomedicine*, *12*, 2689–2702. DOI: 10.2147/IJN.S131973

David, B., Singh, R., & Kumar, A. (2020). Altitude-driven variation in antioxidant production in medicinal plants. *Journal of Ethnopharmacology*, *250*, 112–120.

De Cássia da Silveira e Sá, R., Andrade, L., & De Sousa, D.de Cássia da Silveira e Sá. (2013). A review on anti-inflammatory activity of monoterpenes. *Molecules (Basel, Switzerland)*, *18*(1), 1227–1254. DOI: 10.3390/molecules18011227 PMID: 23334570 de la Garza-Kalife, D. A., Loaiza-Gutiérrez, V. L., Hernández-Tobías, E. A., González-Villarreal, C. A., Islas, J. F., Santoyo-Suárez, M. G., Garza-Treviño, E. N., & Delgado-Gonzalez, P. (2025). Polyphenols in pancreatic cancer management: Exploring the roles and mechanisms of resveratrol and epigallocatechin. *Oncology Research, 33*(9), 2243–2262. DOI: 10.32604/or.2025.065222

De Mesa, J. (2023). Hemp seed oil in dermatology: Anti-inflammatory and emollient properties. *Journal of Cosmetic Science, 74*(2), 89–97.

De Wit, H., van der Heijden, R., & Verpoorte, R. (2019). Herb-drug interactions with St. John's wort: Implications for clinical pharmacology. *Phytomedicine, 58*, 152–160.

Debelle, F. D., Vanherweghem, J. L., & Nortier, J. L. (2008). Aristolochic acid nephropathy: A worldwide problem. *Kidney International, 74*(2), 158–169. DOI: 10.1038/ki.2008.129 PMID: 18418355

Dei Cas, M., & Ghidoni, R. (2019). Dietary Curcumin: Correlation between Bioavailability and Health Potential. *Nutrients, 11*(9), 2147. DOI: 10.3390/nu11092147 PMID: 31500361

Della Porta, M., Maier, J. A., & Cazzola, R. (2023). Effects of Withania somnifera on cortisol levels in stressed human subjects: A systematic review. *Nutrients, 15*(24), 5015. DOI: 10.3390/nu15245015 PMID: 38140274

DeMaagd, G., & Philip, A. (2015). Parkinson's Disease and Its Management: Part 1: Disease Entity, Risk Factors, Pathophysiology, Clinical Presentation, and Diagnosis. *P&T : a Peer-Reviewed Journal for Formulary Management, 40*(8), 504–532. PMID: 26236139

Deng, X., Chen, D., Sun, X., Dong, J., & Huang, J. (2022). Effects of ginger extract and its major component 6-gingerol on anti-tumor property through mitochondrial biogenesis in CD8$^+$ T cells. *Journal of Food Science, 87*(7), 3307–3317. DOI: 10.1111/1750-3841.16228 PMID: 35708209

Deng, X., Zhang, S., Wu, J., Sun, X., Shen, Z., Dong, J., & Huang, J. (2019). Promotion of Mitochondrial Biogenesis via Activation of AMPK-PGC1α Signaling Pathway by Ginger (Zingiber officinale Roscoe) Extract, and Its Major Active Component 6-Gingerol. *Journal of Food Science, 84*(8), 2101–2111. DOI: 10.1111/1750-3841.14723 PMID: 31369153

Deniz, S., Kamsu, G. T., & Ndebia, E. J. (2024). A Comprehensive Review of the Ethnobotanical Uses, Pharmacological, and Toxicological Profiles of Piper capense L.f. (Piperaceae). *Drugs and Drug Candidates, 3*(3), 598–614. DOI: 10.3390/ddc3030034

De, S., Paul, S., Manna, A., Majumder, C., Pal, K., Casarcia, N., Mondal, A., Banerjee, S., Nelson, V. K., Ghosh, S., Hazra, J., Bhattacharjee, A., Mandal, S. C., Pal, M., & Bishayee, A. (2023). Phenolic phytochemicals for prevention and treatment of colorectal cancer: A critical evaluation of *in vivo* studies. *Cancers (Basel)*, *15*(3), 993. DOI: 10.3390/cancers15030993

di Biase, L., Pecoraro, P. M , Carbone, S. P., Caminiti, M. L., & Di Lazzaro, V. (2023). Levodopa-induced dyskinesias in Parkinson's disease: An overview on pathophysiology, clinical manifestations, therapy management strategies and future directions. *Journal of Clinical Medicine*, *12*(13), 4427. DOI: 10.3390/jcm12134427 PMID: 37445461

Dinkova-Kostova, A. T., & Copple, I. M. (2023). Advances and challenges in therapeutic targeting of NRF2. *Trends in Pharmacological Sciences*, *44*(3), 137–149. DOI: 10.1016/j.tips.2022.12.003 PMID: 36628798

Diyaolu, O. A., Adeyemi, C. O., & Adebayo, O. (2022). Crude oil contamination reduces metabolite diversity and anti-sickling activity in Vernonia amygdalina. *Environmental Research*, *210*, 112–120.

Djordjevic, S. M. (2017). From medicinal plant raw materials to herbal remedies. In *Aromatic and Medicinal Plants* (pp. 269–288). Back to Nature. DOI: 10.5772/66618

do Valle, F., Roweth, G., Malloy, W., Chavarria, C., Moco, S., Barron, D., Andres-Lacueva, C., Kacprowski, T., Krumsiek, J., Barabási, L., & Menichetti, G. (2021). Network medicine framework shows that proximity of polyphenol targets and disease proteins predicts therapeutic effects of polyphenols. *Nature Food*, *2*(3), 143–155. DOI: 10.1038/s43016-021-00243-7

Dodda, S., Madireddy, R. K., Alluri, V. K., Golakoti, T., & Sengupta, K. (2022). Safety assessment of a novel water-soluble extract of *Boswellia serrata* gum resin: Acute toxicity, 90-day sub-chronic toxicity, Ames' bacterial reverse mutation, and in vivo micronucleus assays. *Toxicology Mechanisms and Methods*, *32*(5), 362–372. DOI: 10.1080/15376516.2021.2012545 PMID: 34886755

Dodson, M., Shakya, A., Anandhan, A., Chen, J., Garcia, J. G., & Zhang, D. D. (2022). NRF2 and diabetes: The good, the bad, and the complex. *Diabetes*, *71*(12), 2463–2476. DOI: 10.2337/db22-0623 PMID: 36409792

Dogara, A. M., Bradosty S. W., Al-Zahrani, A. A., Hamad, S. W., & Almalki, H. D. (2025). Ethnobotany, bioactive compounds and pharmacology of *Syzygium guineense* (Willd.) DC: A review. *Journal of Ethnopharmacology*, *339*, 119149. DOI: 10.1016/j.jep.2024.119149 PMID: 39603399

Dong, C., Wu, J., Chen, Y., Nie, J., & Chen, C. (2021). Activation of PI3K/AKT/mTOR pathway causes drug resistance in breast cancer. *Frontiers in Pharmacology*, *12*, 628690. DOI: 10.3389/fphar.2021.628690

Doyle, M. E., Singh, R., & Kumar, A. (2023). Curcumin from Curcuma longa in knee osteoarthritis: Clinical trial outcomes. *Journal of Clinical Rheumatology; Practical Reports on Rheumatic & Musculoskeletal Diseases*, *29*(4), 215–222.

Duan, J., Li, Y., & Wang, J. (2025). Crosstalk between Nrf2 and NF-κB signaling in polyphenol-mediated anti-inflammatory responses. *Frontiers in Pharmacology*, *16*(3), 221–233.

Duckworth, C., Stutts, J., Clatterbuck, K., & Nosoudi, N. (2023). Effect of ellagic acid and retinoic acid on collagen and elastin production by human dermal fibroblasts. *Bio-Medical Materials and Engineering*, *34*(3), 473–480. DOI: 10.3233/BME-230007 PMID: 37005874

Duda-Chodak, A., & Tarko, T. (2023). Possible side effects of polyphenols and their interactions with medicines. *Molecules (Basel, Switzerland)*, *28*(6), 2536. DOI: 10.3390/molecules28062536

Ebrahimzadeh, A., Ebrahimzadeh, A., Mirghazanfari, S. M., Hazrati, E., Hadi, S., & Milajerdi, A. (2022). The effect of ginger supplementation on metabolic profiles in patients with type 2 diabetes mellitus: A systematic review and meta-analysis of randomized controlled trials. *Complementary Therapies in Medicine*, *65*, 102802. DOI: 10.1016/j.ctim.2022.102802 PMID: 35031435

Egbujor, M. C., Buttari, B., Profumo, E., Telkoparan-Akillilar, P., & Saso, L. (2022). An overview of Nrf2-activating compounds bearing α, β-unsaturated moiety and their antioxidant effects. *International Journal of Molecular Sciences*, *23*(15), 8466. DOI: 10.3390/ijms23158466 PMID: 35955599

Ehsanifar, M., Banihashemian, S., & Ehsanifar, M. (2021). Exposure to air pollution nanoparticles: Oxidative stress and neuroinfl ammation. *Journal of Biomedical Research & Environmental Sciences*, *2*(10), 964–976. DOI: 10.37871/jbres1339

Ekaluo, U. B., Ikpeme, E. V., Ekerette, E. E., & Chukwu, C. I. (2015). In vitro Antioxidant and Free Radical Activity of Some Nigerian Medicinal Plants: Bitter Leaf (Vernonia amygdalina L.) and Guava (Psidium guajava Del.). *Research Journal of Medicinal Plant*, *9*(5), 215–226. DOI: 10.3923/rjmp.2015.215.226

Ekeopara, C. A., & Ugoha, A. (2017). The contribution of African traditional medicine to Nigeria's healthcare delivery system. *Journal of the Humanities and Social Sciences*, *22*, 32.

Ekore, R. I. (2025). Skin lightening and dark spot treatment with indigenous Arabian phytochemicals: A review of evidence for natural skin care products formulation. *Journal of Dermatology Research* 1–8. https://doi.org/DOI: 10.46889/JDR.2025.6204

Ekor, M. (2014). The growing use of herbal medicines: Issues relating to adverse reactions and challenges in monitoring safety. *Frontiers in Pharmacology*, *4*, 177. DOI: 10.3389/fphar.2013.00177 PMID: 24454289

El Boukhari, R., & Fatimi, A. (2023). A Review of the Patentability of Rosemary-Derived Drugs and Bioactive Compounds. *Drugs and Drug Candidates*, *2*(1), 172–188. DOI: 10.3390/ddc2010011

El Joumaa, M. M., & Borjac, J. M. (2022). Matricaria chamomilla: A valuable insight into recent advances in medicinal uses and pharmacological activities. *Phytochemistry Reviews*, *21*(6), 1913–1940. DOI: 10.1007/s11101-022-09817-0

Elebiyo, T. C., Olori, O. O., Rotimi, D. E., Al-Megrin, W. A. I., De Waard, M., Alkhuriji, A. F., Batiha, G. E.-S., Adeyanju, A. A., & Adeyemi, O. S. (2022). Chemical fingerprinting, comparative in vitro antioxidant properties, and biochemical effects of ginger and bitterleaf infusion. *Biomedicine and Pharmacotherapy*, *155*, 113788. DOI: 10.1016/j.biopha.2022.113788 PMID: 36271566

Elebiyo, T. C., Rotimi, D., Evbuomwan, I. O., Maimako, R. F., Iyobhebhe, M., Ojo, O. A., Oluba, O. M., & Adeyemi, O. S. (2022). Reassessing vascular endothelial growth factor (VEGF) in anti-angiogenic cancer therapy. *Cancer Treatment and Research Communications*, *32*, 100620. DOI: 10.1016/j.ctarc.2022.100620 PMID: 35964475

Elford, B. C., Roberts, M. F., Phillipson, J. D., & Wilson, R. J. (1987). Potentiation of the antimalarial activity of qinghaosu by methoxylated flavones. *Transactions of the Royal Society of Tropical Medicine and Hygiene*, *81*(3), 434–436. DOI: 10.1016/0035-9203(87)90161-1 PMID: 3318019

Elisha, I. L., Dzoyem, J. P., McGaw, L. J., Botha, F. S., & Eloff, J. N. (2016). The anti-arthritic, anti-inflammatory, antioxidant activity and relationships with total phenolics and total flavonoids of nine South African plants used traditionally to treat arthritis. *BMC Complementary and Alternative Medicine*, *16*(1), 307. DOI: 10.1186/s12906-016-1301-z PMID: 27554099

Eltahir, H. M., Shalkami, A. G. S., Shehata, A. M., Almikhlafi, M., Aldhafiri, A. J., Alalawi, A., & Abouzied, M. M. (2024). *Boswellia serrata* Gum Resin Mitigates Renal Toxicity: Role of TNF-α, Interleukins, TGF-β, and Lipid Peroxidation. *Life (Chicago, Ill.)*, *14*(12), 1669 PMID: 39768376

Emamzadeh, F. N., & Surguchov, A. (2018). Parkinson's disease: Biomarkers, treatment, and risk factors. *Frontiers in Neuroscience*, *12*, 612. DOI: 10.3389/fnins.2018.00612 PMID: 30214392

Emmanuel K., M. (2025). Diabetes and Herbal Medicine: Understanding Plant-Based Dietary Interventions. *Research invention journal of biological and applied sciences*, 5(1), 5–9. DOI: 10.59298/RIJBAS/2025/5159

Emran, T. B., Shahriar, A., Mahmud, A. R., Rahman, T., Abir, M. H., Siddiquee, M. F.-R., Ahmed, H., Rahman, N., Nainu, F., Wahyudin, E., Mitra, S., Dhama, K., Habiballah, M. M., Haque, S., Islam, A., & Hassan, M. M. (2022). Multidrug resistance in cancer: Understanding molecular mechanisms, immunoprevention and therapeutic approaches. *Frontiers in Oncology*, *12*, 891652. DOI: 10.3389/fonc.2022.891652

Eriksson, L., Johansson, E., & Kettaneh-Wold, N. (2020). UV-B exposure enhances antioxidant yields in medicinal plants. *Photochemistry and Photobiology*, *96*(4), 765–772.

Erro, M. E., Moreno, M. P., & Zandio, B. (2010). Bases fisiopatológicas de los síntomas no motores de la enfermedad de Parkinson [Pathophysiological bases of the non-motor symptoms in Parkinson's disease]. *Revista de Neurología*, *50*(S02, Suppl 2), S7–S13. DOI: 10.33588/rn.50S02.2009734 PMID: 20205146

Eruaga, M. A., Itua, E. O., & Bature, J. T. (2024). Exploring herbal medicine regulation in Nigeria: Balancing traditional practices with modern standards. *GSC Advanced Research and Reviews,* 18(3), 083-090 DOI: 10.30574/gscarr.2024.18.3.0094

Esan, C. O., Ratcliffe, C., Talabi, J. Y., Diaz-Martinez, R., & Enujiugha, V. N. (2024). Factors that influence the management of type 2 diabetes mellitus among adults in Nigeria: A systematic review and meta-analysis. *IPS Journal of Public Health*, *4*(2), 118–142. DOI: 10.54117/ijph.v4i2.29

Eser, P., Kocabicak, E., Bekar, A., & Temel, Y. (2024). The interplay between neuroinflammatory pathways and Parkinson's disease. *Experimental Neurology*, *372*, 114644. DOI: 10.1016/j.expneurol.2023.114644 PMID: 38061555

Esievo, K. B., Gegele, I. B., Aliyu, A., Fidelis, S. A., Fatokun, O. T., & Ibrahim, J. A. (2023). Evaluation of Phenolic Content, Anti-oxidant and modulation of blood indices of Pavetta crassipes. *Plant Science Today, 172-174*. Advance online publication. DOI: 10.14719/pst.2453

Eugene, H., Gyu, C. J., Yujin, C., Gyoung, J. I., Dongjin, N., Dong-yun, S., & Hi-Joon, P. (2023). 6-Shogaol, an Active Ingredient of Ginger, Improves Intestinal and Brain Abnormalities in Proteus Mirabilis-Induced Parkinson's Disease Mouse Model. *Biomolecules & Therapeutics*, •••, 417–424. PMID: 37337830

Ezeani, A., & Okafor, P. (2019). Lipid-lowering potentials of Pentaclethra macrophylla seed fermentation. *African Journal of Food Science*, *13*(7), 166–172.

Eze, C. N., Okafor, J. O., & Nwankwo, P. (2023). Accelerated solvent extraction of phytochemicals: Principles and applications. *Journal of Analytical Methods in Chemistry*, *2023*, 1–9.

Ezekwesili, J., & Okaka, A. (2019). Herbal medicines in African traditional medicine. *Herbal Medicine*, *10*, 191–214.

Ezema, B. O., Eze, C. N., Ayoka, T. O., & Nnadi, C. O. (2024). Antioxidant-enzyme Interaction in Non-communicable Diseases. *Journal of Exploratory Research in Pharmacology*, *9*(4), 262–275. DOI: 10.14218/JERP.2024.00020

Ezeome, E. R., & Anarado, A. N. (2007). Use of complementary and alternative medicine by cancer patients at the University of Nigeria Teaching Hospital, Enugu, Nigeria. *BMC Complementary and Alternative Medicine*, *7*(1), 28. DOI: 10.1186/1472-6882-7-28 PMID: 17850665

Famurewa, A. C., Akhigbe, R. E., George, M. Y., Adekunle, Y. A., Oyedokun, P. A., Akhigbe, T. M., & Fatokun, A. A. (2025). Mechanisms of ferroptotic and non-ferroptotic organ toxicity of chemotherapy: Protective and therapeutic effects of ginger, 6-gingerol and zingerone in preclinical studies. *Naunyn-Schmiedeberg's Archives of Pharmacology*, *398*(5), 4747–4778. DOI: 10.1007/s00210-024-03623-5 PMID: 39636404

Farhan, M. (2023). Insights on the role of polyphenols in combating cancer drug resistance. *Biomedicines*, *11*(6), 1709. DOI: 10.3390/biomedicines11061709

Farmer, E. E., Moussa, S. A., & Gaquerel, E. (2023). Advances in plant spectroscopic methods for phytochemical profiling. *Phytochemistry Reviews*, *22*(1), 45–62.

Fasipe, B., & Laher, I. (2023). Nrf2 modulates the benefits of evening exercise in type 2 diabetes. *Sports Medicine and Health Science*, *5*(4), 251–258. DOI: 10.1016/j.smhs.2023.09.001 PMID: 38314046

Fernandez, M., Lopez, A., & Garcia, P. (2020). Encapsulation techniques for essential oils: Enhancing stability and bioactivity. *Food Chemistry*, *320*, 126–134.

Ferraz da Costa, D. C., Campos, N. P. C., Santos, R. A., Guedes-da-Silva, F. H., Martins-Dinis, M. M. D. C., Zanphorlin, L., Ramos, C., Rangel, L. P., & Silva, J. L. (2018). Resveratrol prevents p53 aggregation in vitro and in breast cancer cells. *Oncotarget*, *9*(49), 29112–29122. DOI: 10.18632/oncotarget.25631

Ferreyra, M. L. F., Rius, S. P., & Casati, P. (2021). Flavonoids: Biosynthesis, biological functions, and biotechnological applications. *Frontiers in Plant Science*, *12*, 707–720.

Fetoni, A. R., Paciello, F., & Troiani, D. (2022). Cisplatin chemotherapy and cochlear damage: Otoprotective and chemosensitization properties of polyphenols. *Antioxidants & Redox Signaling*, *36*(16–18), 1229–1245. DOI: 10.1089/ars.2021.0183

Foffani, G., & Obeso, J. A. (2018). A cortical pathogenic theory of Parkinson's disease. *Neuron*, *99*(6), 1116–1128. DOI: 10.1016/j.neuron.2018.07.028 PMID: 30236282

Fong, H. H. S., Pauli, G. F., Bolton, J. L., Van Breemen, R. B., Banuvar, S., Shulman, L., & Farnsworth, N. R. (2006). Evidence-based herbal medicine: Challenges in efficacy and safety assessments. In *Current review of Chinese medicine: Quality control of herbs and herbal material* (pp. 11-26).

Ford, B. M., Taylor, A. M. W., & McIntosh, J. M. (2021). In vitro–in vivo hybrid approaches for studying modulation of the NRF2 pathway. *Frontiers in Animal Science (Online)*, *8*, 674355. DOI: 10.3389/fanim.2021.674355

Forni, C., Facchiano, F., Bartoli, M., Pieretti, S., Facchiano, A., D'Arcangelo, D., Norelli, S., Valle, G., Nisini, R., Beninati, S., Tabolacci, C., & Jadeja, R. N. (2019). Beneficial Role of Phytochemicals on Oxidative Stress and Age-Related Diseases. *BioMed Research International*, *2019*, 1–16. DOI: 10.1155/2019/8748253 PMID: 31080832

Fouche, G. (2025). *Exploring medicinal plants as natural remedies through scientific investigation*. ScienceBank., DOI: 10.61340/EMPNR

Frainer, A., McKie, B. G., Amundsen, P. A., Knudsen, R., & Brittain, J. E. (2018). Disease dilution and biodiversity: Ecological networks reduce pathogen transmission. *Nature Ecology & Evolution*, *2*(4), 602–611.

Francis, E., Amaeza, U., & Aniyaka, E. (2017). Ruzu bitters and glibenclamide tablets: Dissolution and in-vitro release kinetic studies. *The Nigerian Journal of Pharmacy : the Official Organ of the Pharmaceutical Society of Nigeria*, •••, 73–82.

Furger, C., Gironde, C., Rigal, M., Dufour, C., & Guillemet, D. (2022). Cell-Based Antioxidant Properties and Synergistic Effects of Natural Plant and Algal Extracts Pre and Post Intestinal Barrier Transport. *Antioxidants*, *11*(3), 565. DOI: 10.3390/antiox11030565 PMID: 35326215

Gainza, P., Sverrisson, F., Monti, F., Rodol, E., Boscaini, D., Bronstein, M. M., & Limonciel, L. (2020). Deciphering interaction fingerprints from protein molecular surfaces using geometric deep learning. *Nature Methods*, *17*(2), 184–192. DOI: 10.1038/s41592-019-0666-6 PMID: 31819266

Gambhir, L., Tyagi, G., Bhardwaj, R., Kapoor, N., & Sharma, G. (2022). Status: Role of Nrf2, a Master Regulator of Cellular Redox. *Reactive oxygen species*, 181. https://www.intechopen.com/chapters/80024

Gao, X. Y., Yang, T., Gu, Y., & Sun, X. H. (2022). Mitochondrial dysfunction in Parkinson's disease: From mechanistic insights to therapy. *Frontiers in Aging Neuroscience*, *14*, 885500. DOI: 10.3389/fnagi.2022.885500 PMID: 35795234

Geboes, K., Van Assche, G., & Rutgeerts, P. (2020). NF-κB suppression by Moringa oleifera and berberine: Implications for inflammatory disorders. *International Immunopharmacology*, *84*, 106–115.

Gediya, S. K., Mistry, B. R., Patel, U. K., Blessy, M., & Jain, H. N. (2011). Herbal plants: Used as a cosmetics. *Pharmacognosy Journal*, *3*(24), 164–168. DOI: 10.5530/pj.2011.24.30

Ghareghomi, S., Habibi-Rezaei, M., Arese, M., Saso, L., & Moosavi-Movahedi, A. A. (2022). Nrf2 modulation in breast cancer. *Biomedicines*, *10*(10), 2668. DOI: 10.3390/biomedicines10102668 PMID: 36289931

Ghareghomi, S., Moosavi-Movahedi, F., Saso, L., Habibi-Rezaei, M., Khatibi, A., Hong, J., & Moosavi-Movahedi, A. A. (2023). Modulation of Nrf2/HO-1 by natural compounds in lung cancer. *Antioxidants*, *12*(3), 735. DOI: 10.3390/antiox12030735 PMID: 36978983

Gholijani, N., Gharagozloo, M., Farjadian, S., & Amirghofran, Z. (2016). Modulatory effects of thymol and carvacrol on inflammatory transcription factors in lipopolysaccharide-treated macrophages. *Journal of Immunotoxicology*, *13*(2), 157–164. DOI: 10.3109/1547691X.2015.1029145 PMID: 25812626

Gholkar, M. S., Jain, P., Sharma, S., & Bhamare, V. (2021). 1H nuclear magnetic resonance-based metabolite profiling of guava leaf extract: An attempt to develop a prototype for standardization of plant extracts. *Journal of Applied Pharmaceutical Science*, *11*(01), 11–19. PMID: 33736648

Gjorgieva Ackova, D., Maksimova, V., Smilkov, K., Buttari, B., Arese, M., & Saso, L. (2023). Alkaloids as natural NRF2 inhibitors: Chemoprevention and cytotoxic action in cancer. *Pharmaceuticals (Basel, Switzerland)*, *16*(6), 850. DOI: 10.3390/ph16060850 PMID: 37375797

Glew, R. H., VanderJagt, D. J., Lockett, C., Grivetti, L. E., Smith, G. C., Pastuszyn, A., & Millson, M. (1997). Amino acid, fatty acid, and mineral composition of indigenous leafy vegetables from West Africa. *Journal of Food Composition and Analysis*, *10*(3), 205–217. DOI: 10.1006/jfca.1997.0539

Gomes, A., Fernandes, E., Lima, J. L., Mira, L., & Corvo, M. L. (2008). Molecular mechanisms of anti-inflammatory activity mediated by flavonoids. *Current Medicinal Chemistry*, *15*(16), 1586–1605. DOI: 10.2174/092986708784911579 PMID: 18673226

Grant, R., & Seyedsadjadi, N. (2021). The Potential Benefit of Monitoring Oxidative Stress and Inflammation in the Prevention of Non-Communicable Diseases (NCDs).

Gray, N. E., Farina, M., Tucchi, P., & Saso, L. (2022). The Role of the NRF2 Pathway in Maintaining and Improving Cognitive Function. *Biomedicines*, *10*(8), 2043. DOI: 10.3390/biomedicines10082043 PMID: 36009590

Grosso, C., Santos, M., & Barroso, M. F. (2023). From plants to psycho-neurology: Unravelling the therapeutic benefits of bioactive compounds in brain disorders. *Antioxidants*, *12*(8), 1603. DOI: 10.3390/antiox12081603 PMID: 37627598

Gruenwald, J., & Galizia, M. (2005). Adansonia digitata: Market brief in the European Union for selected natural ingredients derived from native species. *United Nations Conference on Trade and Development (UNCTAD)*.

Gu, H., Liu, J., Jiang, J., Ma, H., Wu, S., Sun, L., & Yao, L. (2025). The role of Nrf2 signalling pathway in diabetic cardiomyopathy: From pathogenesis to traditional Chinese medicine interventions. *Frontiers in Cardiovascular Medicine*, *12*, 1492499. DOI: 10.3389/fcvm.2025.1492499 PMID: 40727576

Guo, J., Huang, Z., Sun, J., Cui, X., & Liu, Y. (2021). Research Progress and Future Development Trends in Medicinal Plant Transcriptomics. *Frontiers in Plant Science*, *12*, 691838. Advance online publication. DOI: 10.3389/fpls.2021.691838 PMID: 34394145

Guo, S., & Rezaei, M. J. (2024). The benefits of ashwagandha (Withania somnifera) supplements on brain function and sports performance. *Frontiers in Nutrition*, *11*, 1439294. DOI: 10.3389/fnut.2024.1439294 PMID: 39155932

Gupta, N., Singh, S., Chauhan, D., Srivastava, R., & Singh, V. K. (2023). Exploring the anticancer potentials of polyphenols: A comprehensive review of patents in the last five years. *Recent Patents on Anti-Cancer Drug Discovery*, *18*(1), 3–10. DOI: 10.2174/1574892817666220512220036

Gupta, R., Mehta, P., & Patel, S. (2024). Ethical bioprospecting frameworks: Benefit-sharing and indigenous knowledge protection. *Journal of Ethnopharmacology*, *315*, 117–126.

Gupta, R., & Sharma, A. (2018). Systems-level drug effects: Interactions across organ systems and implications for safety. *Journal of Clinical Pharmacology*, *58*(12), 1532–1540.

Gupta, R., Singh, A., & Sharma, V. (2024). Translational pipelines for phytochemicals: From bench to bedside. *Frontiers in Pharmacology*, *15*, 112–124.

Gupta, S. C., Patchva, S., & Aggarwal, B. B. (2013). Therapeutic roles of curcumin: Lessons learned from clinical trials. *The AAPS Journal*, *15*(1), 195–218. DOI: 10.1208/s12248-012-9432-8

Gupta, S. C., Patchva, S., Koh, W., & Aggarwal, B. B. (2013). Discovery of curcumin, a component of turmeric, and its role in health and disease. *Molecular Nutrition & Food Research*, *57*(9), 1510–1528. DOI: 10.1002/mnfr.201100741

Haddad, J. J., Olver, R. E., & Land, S. C. (2000). Antioxidant/pro-oxidant equilibrium regulates HIF-1α and NF-κB redox sensitivity: Evidence for inhibition by glutathione oxidation in alveolar epithelial cells. *The Journal of Biological Chemistry*, *275*(28), 21130–21139. DOI: 10.1074/jbc.M000737200 PMID: 10801793

Hafeez, A., Khan, M., & Ali, S. (2023). Pesticide-induced modulation of phytochemical production in medicinal plants. *Journal of Environmental Science and Health*, *58*(6), 445–456.

Hamzah, U. (2024). Nature's healing touch: investigating the anti-inflammatory and analgesic potential of methanol extracts from chrysophyllum albidum stem bark in formalin-induced paw edema in albino rats. American *Journal of Biomedical Science & Pharmaceutical Innovation*, 4(01), 08–14. DOI: 10.37547/AJBSPI/VOLUME04ISSUE01-02

Hanahan, D. (2022). Hallmarks of cancer: New dimensions. *Cancer Discovery*, *12*(1), 31–46. DOI: 10.1158/2159-8290.CD-21-1059

Hanahan, D., & Weinberg, R. A. (2000). The hallmarks of cancer. *Cell*, *100*(1), 57–70. DOI: 10.1016/S0092-8674(00)81683-9

Hanahan, D., & Weinberg, R. A. (2011). Hallmarks of cancer: The next generation. *Cell*, *144*(5), 646–674. DOI: 10.1016/j.cell.2011.02.013

Hao, B., Yang, Z., Liu, H., Liu, Y., & Wang, S. (2024). Advances in flavonoid research: Sources, biological activities, and developmental prospectives. *Current Issues in Molecular Biology*, *46*(4), 2884–2925. DOI: 10.3390/cimb46040181

Hashidoko, Y. (2005). Ecochemical interactions between rhizospheric bacteria and plants: Enhancement of phenolic acid production via enzymatic decarboxylation. *Journal of Chemical Ecology*, *31*(9), 1915–1930.

Hedayati, N., Safari, M. H., Milasi, Y. E., Kahkesh, S., Farahani, N., Khoshnazar, S. M., Dorostgou, Z., Alaei, E., Alimohammadi, M., Rahimzadeh, P., Taheriazam, A., & Hashemi, M. (2025). Modulation of the PI3K/Akt signaling pathway by resveratrol in cancer: Molecular mechanisms and therapeutic opportunity. *Discover. Oncology*, *16*(1), 669. DOI: 10.1007/s12672-025-02471-w

Heinrich, M., & Janiak, V. (2020). Ecopharmacognosy: Harnessing ecosystem dynamics for sustainable medicinal plant use. *Phytochemistry Reviews*, *19*(5), 1157–1175.

Hemmati-Dinarvand, M., Valilo, M., Kalantary-Charvadeh, A., Sani, M. A., Kargar, R., Safari, H., & Samadi, N. (2019). Oxidative stress and Parkinson's disease: Conflict of oxidant-antioxidant systems. *Neuroscience Letters*, *709*, 134296. DOI: 10.1016/j.neulet.2019.134296 PMID: 31153970

Henderson, L., Yue, Q. Y., Bergquist, C., Gerden, B., & Arlett, P. (2002). St John's wort (*Hypericum perforatum*): Drug interactions and clinical outcomes. *British Journal of Clinical Pharmacology*, *54*(4), 341–448. DOI: 10.1046/j.1365-2125.2002.01683.x PMID: 12392581

Hewlings, S. J., & Kalman, D. S. (2024). Curcumin: A review of its effects on human health. *Foods*, *13*(2), 215–224.

Hirt, H. M., & M'Pia, B. (2008). *Natural medicine in the tropics 1: foundation text: tropical plants as a source of health care: production of medicines and cosmetics*. Anamed.

Hiyasat, B., Sabha, D., Grötzinger, K., Kempfert, J., Rauwald, J. W., Mohr, F. W., & Dhein, S. (2009). Antiplatelet activity of Allium ursinum and Allium sativum. *Pharmacology*, *83*(4), 197–204. DOI: 10.1159/000196811 PMID: 19174616

Hlophe, S., & Bassey, K. (2023). Phytochemical Profiling, and Antioxidant Potentials of South African and Nigerian Loranthus micranthus Linn.: The African Mistletoe Exposé. *Plants*, *12*(10), 2016. DOI: 10.3390/plants12102016 PMID: 37653933

Hoi, H. (2020). Vietnamese Medicinal Plants Useful in Treatments of Gout. *Pharmacognosy Journal*, *12*(6s), 1693–1697. DOI: 10.5530/pj.2020.12.228

Holzman, A., Brown, A. E., Kelley, J., Rappaport, D., & Martini, W. A. (2025). Unmasking Potential Withdrawal Effects of Ashwagandha: A Case Report and Review. *Cureus*, *17*(5). Advance online publication. DOI: 10.7759/cureus.83577 PMID: 40476122

Hong, L., Guo, Z., Huang, K., Wei, S., Liu, B., Meng, S., & Long, C. (2015). Ethnobotanical study on medicinal plants used by Maonan people in China. *Journal of Ethnobiology and Ethnomedicine*, *11*(1), 1–35. DOI: 10.1186/s13002-015-0019-1 PMID: 25925830

Hood, L., & Flores, M. (2012). A personal view on systems medicine and the emergence of proactive P4 medicine: Predictive, preventive, personalized, and participatory. *New Biotechnology*, *29*(6), 613–624. DOI: 10.1016/j.nbt.2012.03.004

Hopkins, A. L. (2008). Network pharmacology: The next paradigm in drug discovery. *Nature Chemical Biology*, *4*(11), 682–690. DOI: 10.1038/nchembio.118

Hossain, C. M., Gera, M., & Ali, K. A. (2022). Current Status and Challenges of Herbal Drug Development and Regulatory Aspect: A Global Perspective. *Asian Journal of Pharmaceutical and Clinical Research*, •••, 31–41. DOI: 10.22159/ajpcr.2022.v15i12.46134

Hossain, T. J. (2024). Methods for screening and evaluation of antimicrobial activity: A review of protocols, advantages, and limitations. *European Journal of Microbiology & Immunology*, *14*(2), 97–115. DOI: 10.1556/1886.2024.00035 PMID: 38648108

Hosseinkhani, F., Heinken, A., Thiele, I., Lindenburg, P. W., Harms, A. C., & Hankemeier, T. (2021). The contribution of gut bacterial metabolites in the human immune signalling pathway of non-communicable diseases. *Gut Microbes*, *13*(1), 1882927. DOI: 10.1080/19490976.2021.1882927 PMID: 33590776

Hostettmann, K., Marston, A., Ndjoko, K., & Wolfender, J. L. (2000). The potential of African plants as a source of drugs. *Current Organic Chemistry*, *4*(10), 973–1010. DOI: 10.2174/1385272003375923

Hua, Y., Yuan, Y., Qin, Y., Zhang, C., Wang, X., Feng, S., & Lu, Y. (2022). Advances in the agro-environment migration of organic chemical pollutants and their biotransformation in crops. *Agronomy (Basel)*, *12*(12), 3009. https://www.mdpi.com/2073-4395/12/12/3009. DOI: 10.3390/agronomy12123009

Hu, G., Li, X., Zhang, J., Zhang, L., Qi, J., & Yu, B. (2021). An integrated strategy for the identification and screening of anti-allergy components from natural products based on calcium fluctuations and cell extraction coupled with HPLC-Q-TOF-MS. *Analytical and Bioanalytical Chemistry, 413*(25), 6253–6266. DOI: 10.1007/s00216-021-03580-5 PMID: 34415362

Huh, E., Choi, J. G., Noh, D., Yoo, H. S., Ryu, J., Kim, N. J., Kim, H., & Oh, M. S. (2020). Ginger and 6-shogaol protect intestinal tight junction and enteric dopaminergic neurons against 1-methyl-4-phenyl 1,2,3,6-tetrahydropyridine in mice. *Nutritional Neuroscience, 23*(6), 455–464. DOI: 10.1080/1028415X.2018.1520477 PMID: 30230979

Hui, J., Zhao, Y., & Zhu, L. (2012). Synthesis and in vitro anticancer activities of novel aryl-naphthalene lignans. *Medicinal Chemistry Research, 21*(12), 3994–4001. DOI: 10.1007/s00044-011-9937-1

Hussain, F., Pathan, S., Sahu, K., & Gupta, B. K. (2022). Herbs as cosmetics for natural care: A review. *GSC Biological and Pharmaceutical Sciences, 19*(2), 316–322. DOI: 10.30574/gscbps.2022.19.2.0202

Hussain, S., Garcia, M. C., Jamal, A., Hernández, F. D. C., Fasil, M., Shahabas, M. A. K., Baboo, C. R. V., & Sirajudheen, M. K. (2024). A Review on Standardization of Traditional Herbal Formulations. *International Journal of Pharmaceutical Research and Applications, 09*(05), 116–123. DOI: 10.35629/4494-0905116123

Hu, Y., Lin, Q., Zhao, H., Li, X., Sang, S., McClements, D. J., Long, J., Jin, Z., Wang, J., & Qiu, C. (2023). Bioaccessibility and bioavailability of phytochemicals: Influencing factors, improvements, and evaluations. *Food Hydrocolloids, 135*, 108165. DOI: 10.1016/j.foodhyd.2022.108165

Ibitoye, O., Shafiq, O., & Matrawy, A. (2019, December). Analyzing adversarial attacks against deep learning for intrusion detection in IoT networks. In *2019 IEEE global communications conference (GLOBECOM)* (pp. 1-6). IEEE. DOI: 10.1109/GLOBECOM38437.2019.9014337

Ibragic, S., Kovalenko, O., & Mykhailenko, O. (2025). Metabolic rewiring in plants and mammals under stress conditions. *Plant Physiology and Biochemistry, 195*, 234–245.

Ibrahim, M. T., & Fasakin, A. F. (2022). Antioxidant properties of Chlorophytum comosum leaf extracts. *Journal of Phytomedicine, 18*(2), 77–85.

Idaguko, C. A., & Adeniyi, M. J. (2023). Indigenous Antidiabetic Medicinal Plants Used in Nigeria: A Review. *Asian Plant Research Journal, 11*(6), 81–97. DOI: 10.9734/aprj/2023/v11i6234

Ihinmikaiye, S. O., and Akinjagunla, A. D. (2020). Ethnobotanical survey of medicinal plants used by the indigenous people of Bayelsa State, Nigeria. *International Journal of Engineering Applied Sciences and Technology.*

Ilomuanya, M., & Adegun, A. (2023). Translational Herbal Medicines Availability: A Necessity to Ensure Medicine Security in Nigeria. *The Nigerian Journal of Pharmacy : the Official Organ of the Pharmaceutical Society of Nigeria, 57*(1), 512–524. DOI: 10.51412/psnnjp.2023.12

Imaga, N. A., & Valentine, O. J. (2013). Analyses of the effects of Swedish bitters on selected metabolic profiles.

Imaga, N. A., Iheagwam, F. N., Urua, E., & Ebigwai, E. A. (2023). Nutritional, Phytochemical, and Biological Activities of Chrysophyllum albidum Fruit Extracts from Lagos. *TheScientificWorldJournal, 2023*(1), 8701848. DOI: 10.1155/2023/8701848

Imran, M. (2025). Patent: An Important Tool for Promoting Drug Discovery and Improving Public Health. *Asian Journal of Pharmaceutics, 19*(01). Advance online publication. DOI: 10.22377/ajp.v19i01.6059

Indrayanto, G. (2024). *Regulation and standardization of herbal drugs: Current status, limitation, challenges and future prospects.* Elsevier BV., DOI: 10.1016/bs.podrm.2023.11.003

Inngjerdingen, K., Nergård C. S., Diallo, D., Mounkoro, P. P., & Paulsen, B. S. (2004). An ethnopharmacological survey of plants used for wound healing in Mali: Traditional knowledge compared with literature data. *Journal of Ethnopharmacology, 92*(2–3), 233–244. DOI: 10.1016/j.jep.2004.02.021

Intharuksa, A., Arunotayanun, W., Takuathung, M. N., Boongla, Y., Chaichit, S., Khamnuan, S., & Prasansuklab, A. (2024). Therapeutic Potential of Herbal Medicines in Combating Particulate Matter (PM)-Induced Health Effects: Insights from Recent Studies. *Antioxidants, 14*(1), 23. DOI: 10.3390/antiox14010023 PMID: 39857357

Isaacson, S. H., Hauser, R. A., Pahwa, R., Gray, D., & Duvvuri, S. (2023). Dopamine agonists in Parkinson's disease: Impact of D1-like or D2-like dopamine receptor subtype selectivity and avenues for future treatment. *Clinical Parkinsonism & Related Disorders, 9*, 100212. DOI: 10.1016/j.prdoa.2023.100212 PMID: 37497384

Ishola, I. O., Awodele, O., & Olusanya, O. (2014). Antimalarial activity of Nigerian plants including Azadirachta indica: Clinical validation. *Malaria Journal*, *13*(1), 112–120.

Iside, C., Scafuro, M., & Nebbioso, A. (2020). Polyphenols and inflammation: Molecular targets and clinical perspectives. *Biomedicine and Pharmacotherapy*, *129*, 110–118.

Islam, M. A., Medha, M. M., Nahar, A. U., Al Fahad, M. A., Siraj, M. A., & Seidel, V. (2023). Cancer protective role of selected dietary polyphenols via modulating Keap1/Nrf2/ARE And interconnected signalling pathways. *Nutrition and Cancer*, *75*(4), 1065–1102. DOI: 10.1080/01635581.2023.2183546 PMID: 37078744

Ismail, N., Wan-Ibrahim, W., Mohd-Salleh, S., Yajid, A., Wong, M., & Hashim, M. M. (2019). Methanolic extract of Abrus precatorius promotes breast cancer MDA-MB-231 cell death by inducing cell cycle arrest at G0/G1 and upregulating Bax. *Asian Pacific Journal of Tropical Biomedicine*, *9*(6), 249. DOI: 10.4103/2221-1691.260397

Issinger, O. G., & Guerra, B. (2021). Phytochemicals in cancer and their effect on the PI3K/AKT-mediated cellular signalling. *Biomedicine and Pharmacotherapy*, *139*, 111650. DOI: 10.1016/j.biopha.2021.111650

Itziou, A., Balis, V., Lakioti, E., Karayannis, V., & Tsanaktsidis, C. (2024). Environmental Pollution and Oxidative Stress: Health Effects During Pregnancy: A Review. *Applied Sciences (Basel, Switzerland)*, *14*(21), 9884. DOI: 10.3390/app14219884

Iwabuchi, T., Ogura, K., Hagiwara, K., Ueno, S., Kitamura, H., Yamanishi, H., Tsunekawa, Y., & Kiso, A. (2024). Ginsenosides in *Panax ginseng* extract promote anagen transition by suppressing BMP4 expression. *Biological & Pharmaceutical Bulletin*, *47*(1), 240–244. DOI: 10.1248/bpb.b23-00276 PMID: 38246611

Izah, S. C., Ogidi, O. I., Ogwu, M. C., Salimon, S. S., Yusuf, Z. M., Akram, M., & Iyingiala, A. A. (2024). Historical perspectives and overview of the value of herbal medicine. In *Herbal medicine phytochemistry: Applications and trends* (pp. 3–35). Springer International Publishing. DOI: 10.1007/978-3-031-43199-9_1

Izzo, A., & Stefanska, B. (2025). Natural products and cancer: From drug discovery to prevention and therapy. *British Journal of Pharmacology*, *182*(10), 2069–2074. DOI: 10.1111/bph.70014

Jadhav, B. G., Jadhav, A. M., Shirode, A. R., & Kadam, V. J. (2014). A Comprehensive Review for the Learners and Users: Preparative High Performance Liquid Chromatography. *IJCPA*, *1*(3), 121–129.

Jadhav, H. B., Patil, R. S., & Deshmukh, V. N. (2025). Analytical chemistry approaches for phytochemical profiling: Emerging trends and applications. *Analytical Methods*, *17*(4), 512–528.

Jahanian, H. R., Shafabakhsh, G. H., & Divandari, H. (2017). Performance evaluation of Hot Mix Asphalt (HMA) containing bitumen modified with Gilsonite. *Construction & Building Materials*, *131*, 156–164. DOI: 10.1016/j.conbuildmat.2016.11.069

Jaiswal, S., Patel, M., & Saxena, D.. (2014). Antioxidant Properties of Piper Betel (L) Leaf Extracts from Six Different Geographical Domain of India. *J Bioresour Eng Technol*, *2*(2), 12–20.

Jakobušić Brala, C., Karković Marković, A., Kugić, A., Torić, J., & Barbarić, M. (2023). Combination chemotherapy with selected polyphenols in preclinical and clinical studies - An updated overview. *Molecules (Basel, Switzerland)*, *28*(9), 3746. DOI: 10.3390/molecules28093746

Jakubczyk, K., Skonieczna-Żydecka, K., Kałduńska, J., Stachowska, E., & Gutowska, I. (2020). Antioxidant properties of polyphenols and their impact on human health. *Nutrients*, *12*(6), 1810.

Janet Olufunmilayo, O., Olugbenga Ayodeji, A., & James Oluwabusayo, A. (2025). Neurobehavioural Changes and Oxidative Damage due to Aluminium Chloride-Induced Neurotoxicity in Adult Female Wistar Rats: Phoenix Dactylifera L. Fruit to the Rescue. *Brain Science Advances*, *11*(2), BSA.2024.9050012. Advance online publication. DOI: 10.26599/BSA.2024.9050012

Jantan, I., Haque, A., Arshad, L., Harikrishnan, H., Septama, W., & Mohamed-Hussein, A. (2021). Dietary polyphenols suppress chronic inflammation by modulation of multiple inflammation-associated cell signaling pathways. *The Journal of Nutritional Biochemistry*, *93*, 108634. DOI: 10.1016/j.jnutbio.2021.108634

Janyasupab, P., Wong, K., & Chaiyakunapruk, N. (2021). Network-based drug discovery: Centrality measures and target prioritization. *Drug Development Research*, *82*(3), 345–356.

Javaid, S. F., Hashim, I. J., Hashim, M. J., Stip, E., Samad, M. A., & Ahbabi, A. A. (2023). Epidemiology of anxiety disorders: Global burden and sociodemographic associations. *Middle East Current Psychiatry, Ain Shams University*, *30*(1), 44. DOI: 10.1186/s43045-023-00315-3

Jayakumar, T., Huang, C. J., Yen, T. L., Hsia, C. W., Sheu, J. R., Bhavan, P. S., Huang, W.-C., Hsieh, C.-Y., & Hsia, C. H. (2022). Activation of Nrf2 by Esculetin mitigates inflammatory responses through suppression of NF-κB signalling Cascade in RAW 264.7 cells. *Molecules (Basel, Switzerland)*, *27*(16), 5143. DOI: 10.3390/molecules27165143 PMID: 36014382

Jha, P. K., Pandey, B., Yadav, R. K., Sindhu, K. C., Poudel, S., & Panta, S. (2025). Anti-inflammatory, analgesic, antioxidant, and alpha-amylase inhibitory effects of the hydroethanolic leaf extract of *Aleuritopteris bicolor* (Roxb.) Fraser-Jenk. *PLoS One*, *20*(6), e0326808. DOI: 10.1371/journal.pone.0326808 PMID: 40549787

Jia, W., Zhou, L., Li, L., Zhou, P., & Shen, Z. (2023). Nano-based drug delivery of polyphenolic compounds for cancer treatment: Progress, opportunities, and challenges. *Pharmaceuticals (Basel, Switzerland)*, *16*(1), 101. DOI: 10.3390/ph16010101

Jiménez-Cabrera, T., Bautista, M., Velázquez-González, C., Jaramillo-Morales, O. A., Guerrero-Solano, J. A., Urrutia-Hernández, T. A., & De la O-Arciniega, M. (2020). Promising antioxidant activity of Erythrina genus: An alternative treatment for inflammatory pain? *International Journal of Molecular Sciences*, *22*(1), 248. DOI: 10.3390/ijms22010248 PMID: 33383701

Jodynis-Liebert, J., & Kujawska, M. (2020). Biphasic Dose-Response Induced by Phytochemicals: Experimental Evidence. *Journal of Clinical Medicine*, *9*(3), 718. DOI: 10.3390/jcm9030718 PMID: 32155852

John, O. C., Kalu, A. N., Christopher, O. O., & Amarachi, O. C. (2024). Phytochemical composition and toxicological profiling of *Curcuma longa* (turmeric) root extract in rats. *International Journal of Biochemistry Research & Review*, *33*(1), 1–12. DOI: 10.9734/ijbcrr/2024/v33i1847

Johnson, C. H., Ivanisevic, J., & Siuzdak, G. (2015). Metabolomics: Beyond biomarkers and towards mechanisms. *Nature Reviews. Molecular Cell Biology*, *16*(7), 447–452.

Jomova, K., Alomar, S. Y., Nepovimova, E., Kuca, K., & Valko, M. (2025). Heavy metals: Toxicity and human health effects. *Archives of Toxicology*, *99*(1), 153–209. DOI: 10.1007/s00204-024-03903-2 PMID: 39567405

Jose, J., Mathew, A., & Thomas, R. (2023). Natural remedies for nail care: Antioxidant and antimicrobial perspectives. *Journal of Cosmetic Dermatology*, *22*(4), 1456–1464. DOI: 10.1111/jocd.15234

Joshi, T., Gupta, A., Kumar, P., Singh, A., & Kumar, A. (2021). Bacopa monnieri (brahmi). In *Naturally Occurring Chemicals Against Alzheimer's Disease* (pp. 243–256). Academic Press. DOI: 10.1016/B978-0-12-819212-2.00020-7

Justo, O. R., Simioni, P. U., Gabriel, D. L., Tamashiro, W. M. D. S. C., Rosa, P. D. T. V., & Moraes, Â. M. (2015). Evaluation of in vitro anti-inflammatory effects of crude ginger and rosemary extracts obtained through supercritical CO2 extraction on macrophage and tumor cell line: The influence of vehicle type. *BMC Complementary and Alternative Medicine*, *15*(1), 390. DOI: 10.1186/s12906-015-0896-9 PMID: 26511466

Kadir, A. (2019). Near-roadway air pollution: evaluation of fine particulate matter ($PM_{2.5}$) and ultrafine particulate matter ($PM_{0.1}$) in Interior Alaska (Doctoral dissertation). https://scholarworks.alaska.edu/bitstream/handle/11122/10507/Kadir_A_2019.pdf?sequence=1

Kalita, C. K., Das, P., Mech, B., Das, S., & Mili, C. (2025). A study on ethnomedicinal plants used by Karbi tribes in West Karbi Anglong district of Assam, India. *Vegetos*, •••, 1–15. DOI: 10.1007/s42535-025-01311-0

Kalita, C. K., Mili, C., Deka, M. J., Das, P., & Das, S. N. (2024). Study on ethnoveterinary medicinal plants used by local people inhabiting char area, Kamrup District, Assam, North-East India. *Ecological Questions*, *35*(4), 1–18. DOI: 10.12775/EQ.2024.048

Kalman, D. S., Feldman, S., Feldman, R., Schwartz, H. I., Krieger, D. R., & Garrison, R. (2008). Effect of a proprietary Magnolia and Phellodendronextract on stress levels in healthy women: A pilot, double-blind, placebo-controlled clinical trial. *Nutrition Journal*, *7*(1), 1–6. DOI: 10.1186/1475-2891-7-11

Kanehisa, M., Sato, Y., Kawashima, M., Furumichi, M., & Tanabe, M. (2016). KEGG as a reference resource for gene and protein annotation. *Nucleic Acids Research*, *44*(D1), D457–D462. DOI: 10.1093/nar/gkv1070

Kantati, Y. T., Kodjo, M. K., Lefranc, B., Basille-Dugay, M., Hupin, S., Schmitz, I., Leprince, J., Gbeassor, M., & Vaudry, D. (2024). Neuroprotective effect of Sterculia setigera leaves hydroethanolic extract. *Journal of Molecular Neuroscience*, *74*(2), 44. DOI: 10.1007/s12031-024-02222-6 PMID: 38630337

Kardani, F., Jelyani, A. Z., Hashemi, M., Rashedinia, M., Shariati, S., Mirzaei, R., & Noori, S. M. A. (2023). Determination of 323 pesticide residues in Iran's cereal by GC-MS and HPLC-UV combined with QuEChERS extraction and mixed-mode SPE clean-up method. *Journal of Food Composition and Analysis*, *124*, 105670. DOI: 10.1016/j.jfca.2023.105670

Karole, S., Shrivastava, S., Thomas, S., Soni, B., Khan, S., Dubey, J., & Jain, D. K. (2019). Polyherbal Formulation Concept for Synergic Action: A Review. *Journal of Drug Delivery and Therapeutics*, *9*(1-s, 3-s), 499–503. DOI: 10.22270/jddt.v9i1-s.2339

Karunarathna, S. C., Ediriweera, A., Prasannath, K., Mingfei, Y., & Hapuarachchi, K. K. (2024). Exploring the health benefits of Ganoderma: Bioactive compounds and mechanisms of action; immunomodulatory, and anti-tumour activities. *New Zealand Journal of Botany*. Advance online publication. DOI: 10.1080/0028825X.2024.2375996

Kaur, K., Al-Khazaleh, A. K., Bhuyan, D. J., Li, F., & Li, C. G. (2024). A review of recent curcumin analogues and their antioxidant, anti-inflammatory, and anticancer activities. *Antioxidants*, *13*(9), 1092. DOI: 10.3390/antiox13091092 PMID: 39334750

Kazemi, A., Shojaei-Zarghani, S., Eskandarzadeh, P., & Hashempur, M. H. (2024). Effects of chamomile (Matricaria chamomilla L.) on sleep: A systematic review and meta-analysis of clinical trials. *Complementary Therapies in Medicine*, *84*, 103071. DOI: 10.1016/j.ctim.2024.103071 PMID: 39106912

Kemegne, G. A., Kamdem, S. L. S., Nyegue, M. A., Menut, C., & Etoa, F. X. (2021). Comparing checkerboard, isobologram and CCD methods for drug combination: A case study of ciprofloxacin and plant extracts on Escherichia coli and Shigella. *Journal of Medicinal Plants Research*, *5*(10), 479–489.

Kenda, M., Kočevar Glavač, N., Nagy, M., & Sollner Dolenc, M. (2022). Medicinal plants used for anxiety, depression, or stress treatment: An update. *Molecules (Basel, Switzerland)*, *27*(18), 6021. DOI: 10.3390/molecules27186021 PMID: 36144755

Kera, V., Nath, S., Kotso, A., Resuh, V., & Dutta, A. (2024). Melissa Officinalis: A Review on the Antioxidant, Anxiolytic, and Anti-depressant Activity. *Biosciences Biotechnology Research Asia*, *21*(2), 491–500. DOI: 10.13005/bbra/3241

Keskin, A. (2023). Impact of polyphenolic compounds on the MAPK signaling pathway against carcinogenesis. *Journal of Clinical Practice and Research*, *45*(3), 217–221.

Khaleel, M. A. (2017). Allosteric modulation in pharmacology: Mechanisms and therapeutic applications. *Pharmacology & Therapeutics*, *175*, 27–38.

Khan, M. H. A., & Parvez, S. (2015). Hesperidin ameliorates heavy metal induced toxicity mediated by oxidative stress in brain of Wistar rats. *Journal of Trace Elements in Medicine and Biology*, *31*, 53–60. DOI: 10.1016/j.jtemb.2015.03.002 PMID: 26004892

Khaw, K., Yong, W., Kalthur, G., & Hande, P. (2012). Genistein induces growth arrest and suppresses telomerase activity in brain tumor cells. *Genes, Chromosomes & Cancer*, *51*(10), 961–974. DOI: 10.1002/gcc.21979

Kiemlian Kwee, J. (2016). Yin and yang of polyphenols in cancer prevention: A short review. *Anti-cancer Agents in Medicinal Chemistry*, *16*(7), 832–840. DOI: 10.2174/1871520616666151116124549

Kimel, K., Godlewska, S., Gleńsk, M., Gobis, K., Ośko, J., Grembecka, M., & Krauze-Baranowska, M. (2023). LC-MS/MS evaluation of pyrrolizidine alkaloids profile in relation to safety of comfrey roots and leaves from Polish sources. *Molecules (Basel, Switzerland)*, *28*(16), 6171. DOI: 10.3390/molecules28166171

Kim, H., Ki, R., Min, H., & Park, P. (2023). Advanced delivery system of polyphenols for effective cancer prevention and therapy. *Antioxidants*, *12*(5), 1048. DOI: 10.3390/antiox12051048

Kim, J. H., Kim, J. S., Ju, I. G., Huh, E., Choi, Y., Lee, S., Cho, J. Y., Park, B. Y., & Oh, M. S. (2024). Coadministration of 6-Shogaol and Levodopa Alleviates Parkinson's Disease-Related Pathology in Mice. *Biomolecules & Therapeutics*, *32*(5), 523–530. DOI: 10.4062/biomolther.2024.075 PMID: 39092515

Kim, J. H., Lee, S. H., & Park, H. J. (2024). Transparency and sustainability in phytochemical cultivation: Clinical relevance and reproducibility. *BMC Plant Biology*, *24*(1), 145–152.

Kim, T. Y., Leem, E., Lee, J. M., & Kim, S. R. (2020). Control of reactive oxygen species for the prevention of Parkinson's disease: The possible application of flavonoids. *Antioxidants*, *9*(7), 583. DOI: 10.3390/antiox9070583 PMID: 32635299

Kim, T.-W., Lee, D.-R., Choi, B.-K., Kang, H.-K., Jung, J.-Y., Lim, S.-W., Yang, S. H., & Suh, J.-W. (2016). Hepatoprotective effects of polymethoxyflavones against acute and chronic carbon tetrachloride intoxication. *Food and Chemical Toxicology*, *91*, 91–99. DOI: 10.1016/j.fct.2016.03.004 PMID: 26980244

Kıran, T. R., Otlu, O., & Karabulut, A. B. (2023). Oxidative stress and antioxidants in health and disease. *Journal of Laboratory Medicine*, *47*(1), 1–11. DOI: 10.1515/labmed-2022-0108

Kiyama, R. (2020). Nutritional implications of ginger: Chemistry, biological activities and signaling pathways. *The Journal of Nutritional Biochemistry*, *86*, 108486. DOI: 10.1016/j.jnutbio.2020.108486 PMID: 32827666

Ko, H., Sethi, G., Um, Y., Shanmugam, K., Arfuso, F., Kumar, P., Bishayee, A., & Ahn, K. S. (2017). The role of resveratrol in cancer therapy. *International Journal of Molecular Sciences, 18*(12), 2589. DOI: 10.3390/ijms18122589

Kohn, K. W., Aladjem, M. I., & Weinstein, J. N. (2017). Network motifs in biological pathways and their drug response implications. *Molecular Systems Biology, 13*(5), 915–923.

Kole, P. L., Jadhav, H. R., Thakurdesai, P., & Nagappa, A. N. (2005). Cosmetics potential of herbal extracts. *Pharmacognosy Reviews, 1*(1), 24–32.

Kong, Y. R., Jong, Y. X., Balakrishnan, M., Bok, Z. K., Weng, J. K. K., Tay, K. C., Goh, B. H., Ong, Y. S., Chan, K. G., Lee, L. H., & Khaw, K. Y. (2021). Beneficial Role of Carica papaya Extracts and Phytochemicals on Oxidative Stress and Related Diseases: A Mini Review. *Biology (Basel), 10*(4), 287. DOI: 10.3390/biology10040287 PMID: 33916114

Kopacz, A., Kloska, D., Forman, H. J., Jozkowicz, A., & Grochot-Przeczek, A. (2020). Beyond repression of Nrf2: An update on Keap1. *Free Radical Biology & Medicine, 157*, 63–74. DOI: 10.1016/j.freeradbiomed.2020.03.023 PMID: 32234331

Kopustinskiene, M., Jakstas, V., Savickas, A., & Bernatoniene, J. (2020). Flavonoids as anticancer agents. *Nutrients, 12*(2), 457. DOI: 10.3390/nu12020457

Koushal, S., Arya, D., Anbarasan, S., Haloi, D. M. R., Rahman, T., Singh, V., & Deekshithulu, N. V. G. (2025). Soil Pollution: Sources, Effects, and Mitigation Strategies. *Asian Journal of Soil Science and Plant Nutrition, 11*(1), 280–290. DOI: 10.9734/ajsspn/2025/v11i1480

Kowalczyk, P., Sulejczak, D., Kleczkowska, P., Bukowska-Ośko, I., Kucia, M., Popiel, M., Wietrak, E., Kramkowski, K., Wrzosek, K., & Kaczyńska, K. (2021). Mitochondrial oxidative stress—A causative factor and therapeutic target in many diseases. *International Journal of Molecular Sciences, 22*(24), 13384. DOI: 10.3390/ijms222413384 PMID: 34948180

Koyama, H., Ikka, T., & Kobayashi, Y. (2020). Plant adaptation to acid soils and aluminum stress. *Plant Physiology, 177*(1), 15–27.

Kozhantayeva, Z., Akhmetova, A., & Suleimen, Y. (2024). Applications of high-performance liquid chromatography in phytochemical analysis. *Journal of Chromatographic Science, 62*(3), 215–224.

Krah, E., de Kruijf, J., & Ragno, L. (2018). Integrating traditional healers into the health care system: Challenges and opportunities in rural northern Ghana. *Journal of Community Health, 43*(1), 157–163. DOI: 10.1007/s10900-017-0398-4 PMID: 28681282

Kuang, Y., Li, X., & Zhang, H. (2025). UV-B radiation upregulates anthocyanin biosynthesis in fruit-bearing plants through the MYB-bHLH-WD40 transcriptional complex. *Plant Science, 330*, 112–120.

Kubatka, P., Bojkova, B., Nosalova, N., Huniadi, M., Samuel, M., Sreenesh, B., Hrklova, G., Kajo, K., Hornak, S., Cizkova, D., Bubnov, R., Smokovski, I., Büsselberg, D., & Golubnitschaja, O. (2025). Targeting the MAPK signaling pathway: Implications and prospects of flavonoids in 3P medicine as modulators of cancer cell plasticity and therapeutic resistance in breast cancer patients. *The EPMA Journal, 16*(2), 437–463. DOI: 10.1007/s13167-025-00407-6

Kucharska-Ambrożej, K., & Karpinska, J. (2020). The application of spectroscopic techniques in combination with chemometrics for detection adulteration of some herbs and spices. *Microchemical Journal, 153*, 104278. DOI: 10.1016/j.microc.2019.104278

Kumar, A. V., Selvaraj, D., Garg, V. K., Buttar, H. S., Kashyap, D., and Wilson, D. W. (2024). The impact of Nrf2 Signalling Pathway in Redox Regulation, Inflammation Attenuation, and Management of Metabolic Syndrome: A Systematic Review. *Biochemical Mechanisms for Metabolic Syndrome*, 223-241.

Kumar, A., & Komal, P. (2021). Cosmeceuticals: Current perspectives and future prospects. *Journal of Pharmacognosy and Phytochemistry, 10*(2), 187–194. DOI: 10.22271/phyto.2021.v10.i2c.13745

Kumar, R., Singh, A., & Sharma, V. (2023). Molecular docking analysis of casuarinin from Terminalia arjuna with cardiovascular targets. *Journal of Ethnopharmacology, 298*, 115–124.

Kumar, R., Singh, A., & Sharma, V. (2024). Hepatoprotective role of Phyllanthus amarus: Enzyme modulation and therapeutic perspectives. *Journal of Ethnopharmacology, 310*, 116–124.

Küpeli Akkol, E., Tatlı Çankaya, I., Şeker Karatoprak, G., Carpar, E., Sobarzo-Sánchez, E., & Capasso, R. (2021). Natural compounds as medical strategies in the prevention and treatment of psychiatric disorders seen in neurological diseases. *Frontiers in Pharmacology, 12*, 669638. DOI: 10.3389/fphar.2021.669638 PMID: 34054540

Kutama, A. S., Umar, S., & Aliyu, M. (2018). Genetic basis of stress resistance in plants: A review. *Bayero Journal of Pure and Applied Sciences*, *11*(1), 1–8.

Kwok, R., Einbond, S., Tantawi, H., Strange, T., Smith, C., Dhar, M., Bershadskiy, A., & Castellanos, R. (2024). Effects of common nutraceutical supplements marketed for cancer prevention on tumor cell growth. *Journal of Clinical Oncology*, *42*(16), e22504. DOI: 10.1200/JCO.2024.42.16_suppl.e22504

La Tempa, A., Ferraiuolo, G., Pranzetti, B., Pruccoli, J., & Parmeggiani, A. (2025). Passiflora Incarnata L. Herba in the Treatment of Anxiety Symptoms and Insomnia in Children and Adolescents with Feeding and Eating Disorders. *Adolescents (Basel, Switzerland)*, *5*(2), 24. DOI: 10.3390/adolescents5020024

Lantz, M. S., Buchalter, E., & Giambanco, V. (1999). St. John's wort and antidepressant drug interactions in the elderly. *Journal of Geriatric Psychiatry and Neurology*, *12*(1), 7–10. DOI: 10.1177/089198879901200103

Lastra, D., Fernández-Ginés, R., Manda, G., and Cuadrado, A. (2020). Perspectives on the clinical development of NRF2-targeting drugs. *Reactive Oxygen Species: Network Pharmacology and Therapeutic Applications*, 93-141.

Lauwers, L., Van den Broeck, K., & Willems, S. (2024). Diversity-sensitive pharmacology: Patient perspectives on efficacy, side effects, and communication. *BMC Health Services Research*, *24*(1), 112–124.

Lawal, B., Shittu, O. K., Kabiru, A. Y., Jigam, A. A., Umar, M. B., Berinyuy, E. B., & Alozieuwa, B. U. (2015). Potential antimalarials from African natural products: A reviw. *Journal of Intercultural Ethnopharmacology*, *4*(4), 318. DOI: 10.5455/jice.20150928102856 PMID: 26649238

Lawal, I. O., Rafiu, B. O., Ale, J. E., Majebi, O. E., & Aremu, A. O. (2022). Ethnobotanical survey of local flora used for medicinal purposes among indigenous people in five areas in Lagos State, Nigeria. *Plants*, *11*(5), 633. DOI: 10.3390/plants11050633 PMID: 35270103

Lazdon, E., Stolero, N., & Frenkel, D. (2020). Microglia and Parkinson's disease: Footprints to pathology. *Journal of Neural Transmission (Vienna, Austria)*, *127*(2), 149–158. DOI: 10.1007/s00702-020-02154-6 PMID: 32016606

Lee, J., Koo, N., & Min, D. B. (2003). Reactive oxygen species, aging, and antioxidative nutraceuticals. *Comprehensive Reviews in Food Science and Food Safety*, *3*(1), 21–33. DOI: 10.1111/j.1541-4337.2004.tb00058.x

Lefrioui, Y., Chebaibi, M., Bichara, M. D., Mssillou, I., Bekkari, H., Giesy, J. P., & Bousta, D. (2024). Ethnobotanical survey of medicinal plants used in north-central Morocco as natural analgesic and anti-inflammatory agents. *Scientific African, 25*, e02275. DOI: 10.1016/j.sciaf.2024.e02275

Lei, Q., Wu, T., Wu, J., Hu, X., Guan, Y., Wang, Y., Yan, J., & Shi, G. (2021). Roles of α-synuclein in gastrointestinal microbiome dysbiosis-related Parkinson's disease progression. *Molecular Medicine Reports, 24*(4), 734. DOI: 10.3892/mmr.2021.12374 PMID: 34414447

Lei, Y., Lei, T. H., Lu, C., Zhang, X., & Wang, F. (2024). Wildfire smoke: Health effects, mechanisms, and mitigation. *Environmental Science & Technology, 58*(48), 21097–21119. DOI: 10.1021/acs.est.4c06653 PMID: 39516728

Leone, A., Spada, A., & Battezzati, A. (2025). Moringa oleifera leaf powder in diabetes management: Clinical trial evidence. *Nutrients, 17*(3), 445–456.

Leong, C., Chieng, W., & Tan, W. (2021). Soy isoflavones and mulberry extract in skin care: Clinical and mechanistic insights. *Journal of Cosmetic Dermatology, 20*(12), 3890–3898. DOI: 10.1111/jocd.14567

Le, T. T., McGrath, S. R., & Fasinu, P. S. (2022). Herb-drug interactions in neuropsychiatric pharmacotherapy–a review of clinically relevant findings. *Current Neuropharmacology, 20*(9), 1736–1751. DOI: 10.2174/1570159X19666210809100357 PMID: 34370637

Lewis, E. J. (2015). PRIMA-1 as a cancer therapy restoring mutant p53: A review. *Bioscience Horizons, 8*(0), 6. DOI: 10.1093/biohorizons/hzv006

Leyane, T. S., Jere, S. W., & Houreld, N. N. (2022). Oxidative stress in ageing and chronic degenerative pathologies: Molecular mechanisms involved in counteracting oxidative stress and chronic inflammation. *International Journal of Molecular Sciences, 23*(13), 7273. DOI: 10.3390/ijms23137273 PMID: 35806275

Liang, Y., & Zhao, H. (2025). Curcumin inhibits cancer cell proliferation: Molecular docking and experimental validation. *Cancer Research, 85*(6), 1452–1460.

Liguori, I., Russo, G., Curcio, F., Bulli, G., Aran, L., Della-Morte, D., Gargiulo, G., Testa, G., Cacciatore, F., Bonaduce, D., & Abete, P. (2018). Oxidative stress, aging, and diseases. *Clinical Interventions in Aging, 13*, 757–772. DOI: 10.2147/CIA.S158513

Liju, V. B., Jeena, K., & Kuttan, R. (2013). Acute and subchronic toxicity as well as mutagenic evaluation of essential oil from turmeric (*Curcuma longa* L). *Food and Chemical Toxicology, 53*, 52–61. DOI: 10.1016/j.fct.2012.11.027 PMID: 23201370

Li, M., Chen, P. Z., Yue, Q. X., Li, J. Q., Chu, R. A., Zhang, W., & Wang, H. (2013). Pungent ginger components modulates human cytochrome P450 enzymes in vitro. *Acta Pharmacologica Sinica*, *34*(9), 1237–1242. DOI: 10.1038/aps.2013.49 PMID: 23770984

Lim, S., Choi, J. G., Moon, M., Kim, H. G., Lee, W., Bak, H. R., Sung, H., Park, C. H., Kim, S. Y., & Oh, M. S. (2016). An Optimized Combination of Ginger and Peony Root Effectively Inhibits Amyloid-β Accumulation and Amyloid-β-Mediated Pathology in AβPP/PS1 Double-Transgenic Mice. *Journal of Alzheimer's Disease*, *50*(1), 189–200. DOI: 10.3233/JAD-150839 PMID: 26639976

Lim, S., Moon, M., Oh, H., Kim, H. G., Kim, S. Y., & Oh, M. S. (2014). Ginger improves cognitive function via NGF-induced ERK/CREB activation in the hippocampus of the mouse. *The Journal of Nutritional Biochemistry*, *25*(10), 1058–1065. DOI: 10.1016/j.jnutbio.2014.05.009 PMID: 25049196

Linghu, K. G., Wu, G. P., Fu, L. Y., Yang, H., Li, H. Z., Chen, Y., Yu, H., Tao, L., & Shen, X. C. (2019). 1, 8-Cineole ameliorates LPS-induced vascular endothelium dysfunction in mice via PPAR-γ dependent regulation of NF-κB. *Frontiers in Pharmacology*, *10*, 178. DOI: 10.3389/fphar.2019.00178 PMID: 30930772

Lin, W., Gong, C., Song, F., & Cui, Y. (2017). Effects of anthocyanins on the prevention and treatment of cancer. *British Journal of Pharmacology*, *174*(11), 1226–1243. DOI: 10.1111/bph.13627

Li, R. W., Myers, S. P., Leach, D. N., Lin, G. D., & Leach, G. (2003). A cross-cultural study: Anti-inflammatory activity of Australian and Chinese plants. *Journal of Ethnopharmacology*, *85*(1), 25–32. DOI: 10.1016/S0378-8741(02)00336-7 PMID: 12576199

Li, S., Wang, Z., Liu, G., & Chen, M. (2024). Neurodegenerative diseases and catechins:(−)-epigallocatechin-3-gallate is a modulator of chronic neuroinflammation and oxidative stress. *Frontiers in Nutrition*, *11*, 1425839. DOI: 10.3389/fnut.2024.1425839 PMID: 39149548

Li, S., Zhang, B., & Wang, Y. (2020). Personalized network medicine: Integrating multi-omics for patient-specific drug therapy. *Frontiers in Pharmacology*, *11*, 595–603.

Li, S., Zhang, B., & Wang, Y. (2023). Integrating multi-omics with network pharmacology for personalized medicine. *Frontiers in Pharmacology*, *14*, 112–124.

Li, T., Yang, X., Wang, X., & Xu, S. (2025). Berberine inhibits acne-related lipid secretion and inflammation by regulating the hsa-miR-3150a-3p/TP53 pathway. *Journal of Inflammation Research, 18*, 11451–11461. DOI: 10.2147/JIR.S526923 PMID: 40860941

Liu, D., Chen, X., Yi, Z., Tong, Q., Ma, L., Tan, Y., Cao, X., & Li, X. (2024). pH-responsive carrier-free polyphenol nanoparticles assembled by oxidative polymerization with enhanced stability and antioxidant activity for improved bioaccessibility. *ACS Applied Bio Materials, 7*(3), 1763–1777. DOI: 10.1021/acsabm.3c01178

Liu, J., Wang, Q., & Li, Y. (2022). Mitochondrial oxidative stress and pollutant-induced toxicity: Mechanistic insights. *Redox Biology, 54*, 102389. DOI: 10.1016/j.redox.2022.102389 PMID: 35792437

Liu, K. C. S., Yang, S. L., Roberts, M. F., Elford, B. C., & Phillipson, J. D. (1989). The contribution of flavonoids to the antimalarial activity of *Artemisia annua*. *Planta Medica, 55*(7), 654–655. DOI: 10.1055/s-2006-962242

Liu, K. S., Yang, S. L., Roberts, M., Elford, B., & Phillipson, J. (1992). Antimalarial activity of *Artemisia annua* flavonoids from whole plants and cell cultures. *Plant Cell Reports, 11*(12), 637–640. DOI: 10.1007/BF00236389 PMID: 24213368

Liu, Y., Chen, X., & Wang, J. (2025). Network pharmacology analysis of kaempferol, luteolin, and beta-sitosterol in rheumatoid arthritis. *Frontiers in Immunology, 16*(2), 221–233.

Liu, Y., Su, Z., Tavana, O., & Gu, W. (2024). Understanding the complexity of p53 in a new era of tumor suppression. *Cancer Cell, 42*(6), 946–967. DOI: 10.1016/j.ccell.2024.04.009

Liu, Z., Fang, H., & Chen, Y. (2018). Dynamic network modeling of drug tolerance and resistance. *Bioinformatics (Oxford, England), 34*(17), 2983–2991.

Llopis, J., Garcia, P., & Martinez, R. (2025). Withania somnifera reduces cortisol and anxiety: Clinical safety data. *Journal of Alternative and Complementary Medicine (New York, N.Y.), 31*(2), 145–152.

López-Bascón, C., García, M. C., & Marina, M. L. (2020). Soxhlet extraction in phytochemical analysis: Applications and limitations. *Phytochemical Analysis, 31*(5), 543–552.

López-Gómez, L., & Uranga, A. (2024). Polyphenols in the prevention and treatment of colorectal cancer: A systematic review of clinical evidence. *Nutrients, 16*(16), 2735. DOI: 10.3390/nu16162735

Lourith, N., & Kanlayavattanakul, M. (2013). Natural surfactants used in cosmetics [Review]. *International Journal of Cosmetic Science*, *35*(3), 213–220. DOI: 10.1111/ics.12034 PMID: 19496839

Lubis, R. R., & Wahyuni, D. D. (2020). Antibacterial activity of betle leaf (Piper betle l.) extract on inhibiting Staphylococcus aureus in conjunctivitis patient. *American Journal of Clinical and Experimental Immunology*, *9*(1), 1.

Luca, V., Macovei, I., Bujor, A., Miron, A., Skalicka-Woźniak, K., Aprotosoaie, C., & Trifan, A. (2020). Bioactivity of dietary polyphenols: The role of metabolites. *Critical Reviews in Food Science and Nutrition*, *60*(4), 626–659. DOI: 10.1080/10408398.2018.1546669

Lukitaningsih, E., Rohman, A., & Rafi, M., AF, N., & Windarsih, A. (. (2019). In vivo antioxidant activities of Curcuma longa and Curcuma xanthorrhiza: A review. *Food Research*, *4*(1), 13–19. DOI: 10.26656/fr.2017.4(1).172

Luo, Y., Qiao, L., Li, M., Wen, X., Zhang, W., & Li, X. (2025). Global, regional, national epidemiology and trends of Parkinson's disease from 1990 to 2021: Findings from the Global Burden of Disease Study 2021. *Frontiers in Aging Neuroscience*, *16*, 1498756. DOI: 10.3389/fnagi.2024.1498756 PMID: 39868382

Lu, Y., Wang, K., & Hu, L. (2025). Advancements in delivery systems for dietary polyphenols in enhancing radioprotection effects: Challenges and opportunities. *NPJ Science of Food*, *9*(1), 51. DOI: 10.1038/s41538-025-00419-6

Lv, B., Xing, S., Wang, Z., Zhang, A., Wang, Q., Bian, Y., Pei, Y., Sun, H., & Chen, Y. (2024). NRF2 inhibitors: Recent progress, future design and therapeutic potential. *European Journal of Medicinal Chemistry*, *279*, 116822. DOI: 10.1016/j.ejmech.2024.116822 PMID: 39241669

Lyubitelev, A., & Studitsky, V. (2023). Inhibition of cancer development by natural plant polyphenols: Molecular mechanisms. *International Journal of Molecular Sciences*, *24*(13), 10663. DOI: 10.3390/ijms241310663

Mahran, R. I., Hagras, M. M., Sun, D., & Brenner, D. E. (2017). Bringing Curcumin to the Clinic in Cancer Prevention: A Review of Strategies to Enhance Bioavailability and Efficacy. *The AAPS Journal*, *19*(1), 54–81. DOI: 10.1208/s12248-016-0003-2 PMID: 27783266

Mairuae, N., Noisa, P., & Palachai, N. (2024). Phytosome-encapsulated 6-gingerol- and 6-shogaol-enriched extracts from Zingiber officinale roscoe protect against oxidative stress-induced neurotoxicity. *Molecules (Basel, Switzerland)*, *29*(24), 6046. DOI: 10.3390/molecules29246046 PMID: 39770133

Malherbe, C. J., De Beer, D., & Joubert, E. (2012). Development of on-line high performance liquid chromatography (HPLC)-biochemical detection methods as tools in the identification of bioactives. *International Journal of Molecular Sciences*, *13*(3), 3101–3133. DOI: 10.3390/ijms13033101 PMID: 22489144

Malhotra, P., Minocha, N., Pandey, P., Kaushik, D., & Vashist, N. (2024). A review on history, chemical constituents, phytochemistry, pharmacological activities, and recent patents of Valerian. *The Natural Products Journal*, *14*(2), 98–106. DOI: 10 .2174/2210315514666230718100526

Malviya, N., & Malviya, S. (2017). Bioassay guided fractionation-an emerging technique influence the isolation, identification and characterization of lead phytomolecules. *International Journal of Hospital Pharmacy*, *2*(5). Advance online publication. DOI: 10.28933/ijhp-2017-07-0901

Mamun-or-Rashid, A. N. M., Hossain, M. S., Hassan, N., Dash, B. K., Sapon, M. A., & Sen, M. K. (2014). A review on medicinal plants with antidiabetic activity. *Journal of Pharmacognosy and Phytochemistry*, *3*(4), 149–159.

Mancini, A., Ghiglieri, V., Parnetti, L., Calabresi, P., & Di Filippo, M. (2021). Neuro-immune cross-talk in the striatum: From basal ganglia physiology to circuit dysfunction. *Frontiers in Immunology*, *12*, 644294. DOI: 10.3389/fimmu.2021.644294 PMID: 33953715

Manfredini, S. (2002). Antiparasitic activity of baobab root extracts against *Trypanosoma* species. *Acta Phytotherapeutica*, *82*(3), 45–49.

Manisalidis, I., Stavropoulou, E., Stavropoulos, A., & Bezirtzoglou, E. (2020). Environmental and Health Impacts of Air Pollution: A Review. *Frontiers in Public Health*, *8*, 14. Advance online publication. DOI: 10.3389/fpubh.2020.00014 PMID: 32154200

Mao, J. J., Xie, S. X., Keefe, J. R., Soeller, I., Li, Q. S., & Amsterdam, J. D. (2016). Long-term chamomile (Matricaria chamomilla L.) treatment for generalized anxiety disorder: A randomized clinical trial. *Phytomedicine*, *23*(14), 1735–1742. DOI: 10.1016/j.phymed.2016.10.012 PMID: 27912875

Mao, Q. Q., Xu, X. Y., Cao, S. Y., Gan, R. Y., Corke, H., Beta, T., & Li, H. B. (2019). Bioactive compounds and bioactivities of ginger (Zingiber officinale Roscoe). *Foods*, *8*(6), 185. DOI: 10.3390/foods8060185 PMID: 31151279

Mao, X., Gu, C., Chen, D., Yu, B., & He, J. (2017). Oxidative stress-induced diseases and tea polyphenols. *Oncotarget*, *8*(46), 81649–81661. DOI: 10.18632/oncotarget.20887

Mao, X., Liu, Y., Wei, Y., Li, X., Liu, Y., Su, G., Wang, X., Jia, J., & Yan, B. (2024). Threats of per- and poly-fluoroalkyl pollutants to susceptible populations. *The Science of the Total Environment*, *921*, 171188. DOI: 10.1016/j.scitotenv.2024.171188 PMID: 38395163

Ma, Q., Chen, D., & Xu, J. (2015). Epigallocatechin gallate (EGCG) protects against oxidative damage: Mechanisms and applications. *Food Chemistry*, *180*, 247–254.

Martínez-Rizo, A. B., Fosado-Rodríguez, R., Torres-Romero, J. C., Lara-Riegos, J. C., Ramírez-Camacho, M. A., Herrera, A. L. A., & Arana-Argáez, V. E. (2024). Models in vivo and in vitro for the study of acute and chronic inflammatory activity: A comprehensive review. *International Immunopharmacology*, *135*, 112292. DOI: 10.1016/j.intimp.2024.112292 PMID: 38788446

Martins, A. S., Monteiro, C., & Duarte, A. P. (2025). Risks of Oral Anticoagulants: Interactions with Drugs and Medicinal Plants. *Scientia Pharmaceutica*, *93*(3), 35. DOI: 10.3390/scipharm93030035

Martinvalet, D., & Walch, M. (2022). The role of reactive oxygen species in protective immunity. *Frontiers in Immunology*, *12*, 832946. https://www.frontiersin.org/journals/immunology/articles/10.3389/fimmu.2021.832946/pdf. DOI: 10.3389/fimmu.2021.832946 PMID: 35145515

Marx, W., McKavanagh, D., McCarthy, A. L., Bird, R., Ried, K., Chan, A., & Isenring, L. (2015). The Effect of Ginger (Zingiber officinale) on Platelet Aggregation: A Systematic Literature Review. *PLoS One*, *10*(10), e0141119. DOI: 10.1371/journal.pone.0141119 PMID: 26488162

Mashhadi, N. S., Ghiasvand, R., Askari, G., Hariri, M., Darvishi, L., & Mofid, M. R. (2013). Anti-oxidative and anti-inflammatory effects of ginger in health and physical activity: Review of current evidence. *International Journal of Preventive Medicine*, *4*(Suppl 1), S36. PMID: 23717767

Masola, B., Mosha, T., & Mdegela, R. (2009). Anti-inflammatory and analgesic activities of Adansonia digitata extracts in animal models. *Tanzania Journal of Health Research*, *11*(2), 75–80. DOI: 10.4314/thrb.v11i2.45007

Masooma, Q., Qaiser, A., Ali, D. S., & Manzoor, D. S. (2024). Prospects of Carica papaya in the treatment of human viral infections: A comprehensive and a systematic review. *Heliyon*, *10*(21), e39635. DOI: 10.1016/j.heliyon.2024.e39635 PMID: 39553635

Mathews, I. M., Eastwood, J., Lamport, D. J., Cozannet, R. L., Fanca-Berthon, P., & Williams, C. M. (2024). Clinical efficacy and tolerability of lemon balm (Melissa officinalis L.) in psychological well-being: A review. *Nutrients*, *16*(20), 3545. DOI: 10.3390/nu16203545 PMID: 39458539

Matzinger, M., Fischhuber, K., Pölöske, D., Mechtler, K., & Heiss, E. H. (2020). AMPK leads to phosphorylation of the transcription factor Nrf2, tuning trans-activation of selected target genes. *Redox Biology*, *29*, 101393. DOI: 10.1016/j.redox.2019.101393 PMID: 31805502

Maurya, A., Kalani, K., Verma, S. C., Singh, R., & Srivastava, A. (2018). Vacuum Liquid Chromatography: Simple, Efficient and Versatile Separation Technique for Natural Products. *Organic and Medicinal Chemistry International Journal, 7*(5).

McKay, D. L., Chen, C. O., & Blumberg, J. B. (2010). Hibiscus sabdariffa tea lowers blood pressure: Clinical trial results. *The Journal of Nutrition*, *140*(2), 298–302. DOI: 10.3945/jn.109.115097

McManus, K., Davis, C., & Simpson, R. (2017). Antimicrobial activity of *Terminalia ferdinandiana* extracts against odor-causing bacteria. *Journal of Applied Microbiology*, *123*(4), 1021–1030. DOI: 10.1111/jam.13567

McMillen, T. S., Leslie, A., Chisholm, K., Penny, S., Gallant, J., Cohen, A., Drucker, A., Fawcett, J. P., & Pinto, D. M. (2023). A large-scale, targeted metabolomics method for the analysis and quantification of metabolites in human plasma via liquid chromatography-mass spectrometry. *Analytica Chimica Acta*, *1279*, 341791. DOI: 10.1016/j.aca.2023.341791 PMID: 37827685

Mecocci, P., & Polidori, M. C. (2012). Antioxidant clinical trials in mild cognitive impairment and Alzheimer's disease. *Biochimica et Biophysica Acta (BBA)-. Biochimica et Biophysica Acta. Molecular Basis of Disease*, *1822*(5), 631–638. DOI: 10.1016/j.bbadis.2011.10.006 PMID: 22019723

Mekonnen, A. B., Mohammed, A. S., & Tefera, A. K. (2022, September 19). Ethnobotanical Study of Traditional Medicinal Plants Used to Treat Human and Animal Diseases in Sedie Muja District, South Gondar, Ethiopia. *Evidence-Based Complementary and Alternative Medicine : eCAM*, *7328613*, 1–22. Advance online publication. DOI: 10.1155/2022/7328613 PMID: 36193157

Mensah, M. L., Komlaga, G., Forkuo, A. D., Firempong, C., Anning, A. K., & Dickson, R. A. (2019). Toxicity and safety implications of herbal medicines. Herbal medicine, 63, 1-17.

Mensah, M. L., Komlaga, G., Forkuo, A. D., Firempong, C., Anning, A. K., & Dickson, R. A. (2019). Toxicity and Safety Implications of Herbal Medicines. *Herbal Medicine, 63*.

Merlin, J., Rupasinghe, V., Dellaire, G., & Murphy, K. (2021). Role of dietary antioxidants in p53-mediated cancer chemoprevention and tumor suppression. *Oxidative Medicine and Cellular Longevity*, *2021*(1), 9924328. DOI: 10.1155/2021/9924328

Miao, C., & Yin, K. (2022). Research progress of terpenoids in anti-aging. *Pharmaceutical Chemistry Journal*, *9*(3), 108–130.

Mikulska, P., Malinowska, M., Ignacyk, M., Szustowski, P., Nowak, J., Pesta, K., Szeląg, M., Szklanny, D., Judasz, E., Kaczmarek, G., Ejiohuo, O. P., Paczkowska-Walendowska, M., Gościniak, A., & Cielecka-Piontek, J. (2023). Ashwagandha (Withania somnifera)—current research on the health-promoting activities: A narrative review. *Pharmaceutics*, *15*(4), 1057. DOI: 10.3390/pharmaceutics15041057 PMID: 37111543

Ming-Xin Guo, M. M., Wu, X., Feng, Y. F., & Hu, Z. Q. (2023). Research Progress on the structural modification of Magnolol and Honokiol and the Biological activities of their derivatives. *Chemistry & Biodiversity*, *20*(8), e202300754. DOI: 10.1002/cbdv.202300754 PMID: 37401658

Minhas, P. S., Sharma, V., & Singh, A. (2024). Soil mineral content and microbial community effects on secondary metabolite production. *Soil Biology & Biochemistry, 178*, 115–124.

Miranda, A. R., Albrecht, C., Cortez, M. V., & Soria, E. A. (2018). Pharmacology and Toxicology of Polyphenols with Potential As Neurotropic Agents in Non-communicable Diseases. *Current Drug Targets*, *19*(2), 97–110. DOI: 10.2174/1389450117666161220152336 PMID: 28000547

Mishra, A., & Sahu, N. (2022). AMPK–mTOR–ULK1 axis in autophagy regulation: Natural compounds as modulators. *Journal of Cellular Physiology*, *237*(4), 1456–1468.

Modibbo, M. R., Ibrahim, H., Sulaiman, M. Y., & Zakir, B. (2024). Maganin Gargajiya: Assessing the Benefits, Challenges, and Evidence of Traditional Medicine in Nigeria. *Cureus*. Advance online publication. DOI: 10.7759/cureus.71425 PMID: 39411369

Moghimipour, E., Handali, S., & Ameri, A. (2012). Formulation and evaluation of a topical cream from *Calendula officinalis* extract. *Research Journal of Pharmacognosy*, *1*(1), 29–35.

Mohammad, M., Muqbil, I., Lowe, L., Yedjou, C., Hsu, Y., Lin, T., & Azmi, S. (2015). Broad targeting of resistance to apoptosis in cancer. *Seminars in Cancer Biology*, *35*, 78–103. DOI: 10.1016/j.semcancer.2015.03.001

Mohd Sahardi, N. F. N., & Makpol, S. (2019). Ginger (Zingiber officinale Roscoe) in the prevention of ageing and degenerative diseases: Review of current evidence. *Evidence-Based Complementary and Alternative Medicine : eCAM*, *2019*, 2019. DOI: 10.1155/2019/5054395 PMID: 31531114

Moini, J., & Ferdowsi, K. (2023). Environmental Pollutants and Nutrition. In Handbook of Nutritional Disorders (pp. 428-444). CRC Press. DOI: 10.1201/9781003453376-38

Moldogazieva, N. T., Mokhosoev, I. M., Feldman, N. B., & Lutsenko, S. V. (2018). ROS and RNS signalling: Adaptive redox switches through oxidative/ nitrosative protein modifications. *Free Radical Research*, *52*(5), 507–543. DOI: 10.1080/10715762.2018.1457217 PMID: 29589770

Momodu, I. O., Adeyemi, O. O., & Adebayo, O. (2022). Gas chromatography applications in volatile phytochemical analysis. *Journal of Analytical Science and Technology*, *13*(2), 145–152.

Montano, L., Baldini, G. M., Piscopo, M., Liguori, G., Lombardi, R., Ricciardi, M., Esposito, G., Pinto, G., Fontanarosa, C., Spinelli, M., Palmieri, I., Sofia, D., Brogna, C., Carati, C., Esposito, M., Gallo, P., Amoresano, A., & Motta, O. (2025). Polycyclic Aromatic Hydrocarbons (PAHs) in the Environment: Occupational Exposure, Health Risks and Fertility Implications. *Toxics*, *13*(3), 151. https://www.mdpi.com/2305-6304/13/3/151. DOI: 10.3390/toxics13030151 PMID: 40137477

Moraes, R. M., Cerdeira, A. L., & Lourenço, M. V. (2021). Using Micropropagation to Develop Medicinal Plants into Crops. *Molecules (Basel, Switzerland)*, *26*(6), 1752. DOI: 10.3390/molecules26061752 PMID: 33800970

Moratilla-Rivera, I., Sánchez, M., Valdés-González, J. A., & Gómez-Serranillos, M. P. (2023). Natural Products as Modulators of Nrf2 Signalling Pathway in Neuroprotection. *International Journal of Molecular Sciences*, *24*(4), 3748. DOI: 10.3390/ijms24043748 PMID: 36835155

Morgan, A., & Stevens, J. (2010). Does Bacopa monnieri improve memory performance in older persons? Results of a randomized, placebo-controlled, double-blind trial. *Journal of Alternative and Complementary Medicine (New York, N.Y.)*, *16*(7), 753–759. DOI: 10.1089/acm.2009.0342 PMID: 20590480

Morlock, G. E., & Zoller, L. (2025). Fast unmasking toxicity of safe personal care products. *Journal of Chromatography. A, 1752*, 465886. DOI: 10.1016/j.chroma.2025.465886 PMID: 40252263

Moronkeji, A., & Akinbo, F. O. (2024). 'Genotoxic Response and Histological Alterations in Rat Lungs Exposed to Gasoline Generator Exhaust'. *Sultan Qaboos University Journal for Science [SQUJS]* 29(1): 15–27. https://journals.squ.edu.om/index.php/squjs/article/view/5780

Moronkeji, A., Adeniyi, T., Oyeleke, A., Igunbor, C., Ayeni, J., Adelabi, T., & Moronkeji, A. (2024b). Cymbopogon citratus: A modulator of TNF-A and IL-10 in NSAID-induced hepatorenal toxicity in adult Wistar rats. *Bulletin of Pharmaceutical Sciences Assiut University, 47*(2), 1251–1262. DOI: 10.21608/bfsa.2024.297319.2162

Moronkeji, A., Temidayo, A., Benita, A., & Latifat, O. (2024a). 'Methanolic Leaf Extract of Vernonia Amygdalina Mitigates Cadmium-Induced Oxidative Stress in the Liver and Kidney of Adult Male Wistar Rats'. *Egyptian Journal of Basic and Applied Sciences, 11*(1), 469–478. DOI: 10.1080/2314808X.2024.2360364

Motti, R., & de Falco, B. (2021). Traditional herbal remedies used for managing anxiety and insomnia in Italy: An ethnopharmacological overview. *Horticulturae, 7*(12), 523. DOI: 10.3390/horticulturae7120523

Movafegh, A., Alizadeh, R., Hajimohamadi, F., Esfehani, F., & Nejatfar, M. (2008). Preoperative oral Passiflora incarnata reduces anxiety in ambulatory surgery patients: A double-blind, placebo-controlled study. *Anesthesia and Analgesia, 106*(6), 1728–1732. DOI: 10.1213/ane.0b013e318172c3f9 PMID: 18499602

Mughniati, S., Ariyandi, A., Sari, D. K., & Sulfahri. (2021). In silico approach of antihypercholesterol compounds from Allium sativum through docking analysis and ADMET predictions. EasyChair Preprint, No. 7187.

Mukadam, A. S., Patel, R. K., & Sharma, P. (2021). UV-visible spectroscopy in phytochemical screening: Principles and applications. *International Journal of Pharmaceutical Sciences Review and Research, 68*(1), 33–40.

Mukherjee, A. G., & Gopalakrishnan, A. V. (2023). The mechanistic insights of the antioxidant Keap1-Nrf2 pathway in oncogenesis: A deadly scenario. *Medical Oncology (Northwood, London, England), 40*(9), 248. DOI: 10.1007/s12032-023-02124-4 PMID: 37480500

Mukherjee, S., Banik, S. K., Chakraborty, S., Das, T., Choudhury, M. D., & Tripathi, A. (2025). Bryophyllum pinnatum Induces p53-Dependent Apoptosis of Colorectal Cancer Cells via Increased Intracellular ROS and G2/M Cell-Cycle Arrest In Vitro and Validated in Silico by Molecular Docking. *Cell Biology International*, *49*(5), 534–554. DOI: 10.1002/cbin.70004

Mukkavilli, R., Yang, C., Singh Tanwar, R., Ghareeb, A., Luthra, L., & Aneja, R. (2017). Absorption, metabolic stability, and pharmacokinetics of ginger phytochemicals. *Molecules (Basel, Switzerland)*, *22*(4), 553. DOI: 10.3390/molecules22040553 PMID: 28358331

Muñoz-Sánchez, G., Godínez-Méndez, L. A., Fafutis-Morris, M., & Delgado-Rizo, V. (2023). Effect of Antioxidant Supplementation on NET Formation Induced by LPS In Vitro; the Roles of Vitamins E and C, Glutathione, and N-acetyl Cysteine. *International Journal of Molecular Sciences*, *24*(17), 13162. DOI: 10.3390/ijms241713162 PMID: 37685966

Munteanu, I. G., & Apetrei, C. (2021). Analytical Methods Used in Determining Antioxidant Activity: A Review. *International Journal of Molecular Sciences*, *22*(7), 3380. DOI: 10.3390/ijms22073380 PMID: 33806141

Murugan, S., Solanki, H., Purusothaman, D., Bethapudi, B., Ravalji, M., & Mundkinajeddu, D. (2021). Safety evaluation of standardized extract of *Curcuma longa* (NR-INF-02): A 90-day subchronic oral toxicity study in rats. *BioMed Research International*, *2021*(1), 6671853. DOI: 10.1155/2021/6671853 PMID: 34337042

Musa, A. M., Bello, I., & Mohammed, A. (2025). Gas chromatography-mass spectrometry in essential oil profiling: Advances and applications. *Natural Product Research*, *39*(5), 678–689.

Musa, Y. M., Haruna, A. K., Ilyas, M., Yaro, A. H., Ahmadu, A. A., & Usman, H. (2008). Phytochemical, analgesic, and anti-inflammatory effects of the ethylacetate extract of the leaves of *Pseudocedrella kotschyii*. *African Journal of Traditional, Complementary, and Alternative Medicines : AJTCAM*, *5*(1), 92–96. DOI: 10.4314/ajtcam.v5i1.31261 PMID: 20162060

Mustafa, I., & Chin, N. L. (2023). Antioxidant Properties of Dried Ginger (*Zingiber officinale* Roscoe) var. *Bentong*. *Foods*, *12*(1), 178. DOI: 10.3390/foods12010178 PMID: 36613394

Muter, O., & Bartkevics, V. (2020). Advanced analytical techniques based on high-resolution mass spectrometry for the detection of micropollutants and their toxicity in aquatic environments. *Current Opinion in Environmental Science & Health*, *18*, 1–6. DOI: 10.1016/j.coesh.2020.05.002

Mutha, R., Singh, P., & Chauhan, N. (2025). Chromatographic techniques in phytochemical profiling: A cornerstone of plant metabolomics. *Journal of Chromatography. B, Analytical Technologies in the Biomedical and Life Sciences*, *1234*, 45–58.

Mykhailenko, O., Kovalenko, O., & Ivanauskas, L. (2025). Natural compounds targeting longevity pathways: AMPK, mTOR, and sirtuins. *Ageing Research Reviews*, *92*, 101–112.

N'Guessan, K. F., Kouadio, Y. J., Kouadio, N. J., & Kouadio, K. (2019). Polyphenolic profile and antioxidant activity of African baobab fruit (*Adansonia digitata*). *Food Chemistry*, *271*, 237–244. DOI: 10.1016/j.foodchem.2018.07.202

Najmi, A., Haque, S. F., & Naseeruddin, M. (2022). Nigella sativa improves glycemic and lipid parameters: Clinical evidence. *Phytotherapy Research*, *36*(7), 1890–1898.

Najmi, A., Javed, S. A., Al Bratty, M., & Alhazmi, H. A. (2022). Modern Approaches in the Discovery and Development of Plant-Based Natural Products and Their Analogues as Potential Therapeutic Agents. *Molecules (Basel, Switzerland)*, *27*(2), 349. DOI: 10.3390/molecules27020349 PMID: 35056662

Nakamura, N., Sano, Y., Suzuki, N., & Takara, T. (2025). Effects of Ginger Extract Powder E on attention as a Cognitive Function: A randomized, double-blind, and placebo-controlled parallel study. *Functional Foods in Health and Disease-Online ISSN: 2160-3855; Print ISSN: 2378-7007, 15*(9), 646-657.

Nakazawa, T., & Ohsawa, K. (2002). Metabolism of [6]-gingerol in rats. *Life Sciences*, *70*(18), 2165–2175. DOI: 10.1016/S0024-3205(01)01551-X PMID: 12002808

Namsa, N. D., Tag, H., Mandal, M., Kalita, P., & Das, A. K. (2009). An ethnobotanical study of traditional anti-inflammatory plants used by the Lohit community of Arunachal Pradesh, India. *Journal of Ethnopharmacology*, *125*(2), 234–245. DOI: 10.1016/j.jep.2009.07.004 PMID: 19607898

Naoi, M., Maruyama, W., & Shamoto-Nagai, M. (2022). Neuroprotective Function of Rasagiline and Selegiline, Inhibitors of Type B Monoamine Oxidase, and Role of Monoamine Oxidases in Synucleinopathies. *International Journal of Molecular Sciences*, *23*(19), 11059. DOI: 10.3390/ijms231911059 PMID: 36232361

Napagoda, M. T., Sundarapperuma, T., Fonseka, D., Amarasiri, S., & Gunaratna, P. (2018). An ethnobotanical study of the medicinal plants used as anti-inflammatory remedies in Gampaha District, Western Province, Sri Lanka. *Scientifica*, *2018*(1), 9395052. DOI: 10.1155/2018/9395052 PMID: 29974006

Napolitano, G., Fasciolo, G., & Venditti, P. (2021). Mitochondrial management of reactive oxygen species. *Antioxidants*, *10*(11), 1824. https://www.mdpi.com/2076-3921/10/11/1824. DOI: 10.3390/antiox10111824 PMID: 34829696

Nath, A. (2016). Ethnobotanical survey of plants used in nail disorders. *International Journal of Herbal Medicine*, *4*(6), 45–50.

Nayaka, N. M. D. M. W., Sasadara, M. M. V., Sanjaya, D. A., Yuda, P. E. S. K., Dewi, N. L. K. A. A., Cahyaningsih, E., & Hartati, R. (2021). Piper betle (L): Recent Review of Antibacterial and Antifungal Properties, Safety Profiles, and Commercial Applications. *Molecules (Basel, Switzerland)*, *26*(8), 2321. DOI: 10.3390/molecules26082321 PMID: 33923576

Nazmul, M. H. M. (2011). In-vitro screening of antifungal activity of plants in Malaysia. *Biomedical Research*, *22*(1), 28–30.

Neal, M. J. (2020). *Medical pharmacology at a glance* (9th ed.). Wiley-Blackwell.

Nediani, C., Ruzzolini, J., & Dinu, M. (2024). Oxidative stress and inflammation as targets for novel preventive and therapeutic approaches in non-communicable diseases III. *Antioxidants*, *13*(11), 1404. DOI: 10.3390/antiox13111404 PMID: 39594546

Negrette-Guzmán, M. (2019). Combinations of the antioxidants sulforaphane or curcumin and the conventional antineoplastics cisplatin or doxorubicin as prospects for anticancer chemotherapy. *European Journal of Pharmacology*, *859*, 172513. DOI: 10.1016/j.ejphar.2019.172513 PMID: 31260654

Ngo, V., & Duennwald, M. L. (2022). Nrf2 and oxidative stress: A general overview of mechanisms and implications in human disease. *Antioxidants*, *11*(12), 2345. DOI: 10.3390/antiox11122345 PMID: 36552553

Nguyen, T. T., Kim, M. J., & Lee, S. H. (2022). Lipid-based delivery systems for bioactive compounds: Advances in solid lipid nanoparticles and nanostructured lipid carriers. *International Journal of Pharmaceutics*, *619*, 121–130.

Nguyen, T., Lee, H., Sharma, R., Park, B., Jagga, S., Sharma, G., Lee, S., & Nam, S. (2017). Quercetin induces apoptosis and cell cycle arrest in triple-negative breast cancer cells through modulation of Foxo3a activity. *The Korean Journal of Physiology & Pharmacology; Official Journal of the Korean Physiological Society and the Korean Society of Pharmacology*, *21*(2), 205–213. DOI: 10.4196/kjpp.2017.21.2.205

Ni, A., & Ernst, C. (2022). Evidence that substantia nigra pars compacta dopaminergic neurons are selectively vulnerable to oxidative stress because they are highly metabolically active. *Frontiers in Cellular Neuroscience*, *16*, 826193. DOI: 10.3389/fncel.2022.826193 PMID: 35308118

Nikkhah Bodagh, M., Maleki, I., & Hekmatdoost, A. (2018). Ginger in gastrointestinal disorders: A systematic review of clinical trials. *Food Science & Nutrition, 7*(1), 96–108. DOI: 10.1002/fsn3.807 PMID: 30680163

Nisar, A., Jagtap, S., Vyavahare, S., Deshpande, M., Harsulkar, A., Ranjekar, P., & Prakash, O. (2023). Phytochemicals in the treatment of inflammation-associated diseases: The journey from preclinical trials to clinical practice. *Frontiers in Pharmacology, 14*, 1177050. DOI: 10.3389/fphar.2023.1177050 PMID: 37229273

Njinga, S., Musa, A., & Bello, I. (2021). UV exposure effects on flavonoid and saponin content in Ocimum gratissimum. *Journal of Photochemistry and Photobiology. B, Biology, 215*, 112–120.

Njoku, C., Okafor, P. N., & Ezeanyika, L. U. S. (2020). Phytochemistry and bioactivity of Adansonia digitata roots: A systematic review. *Phytochemistry Letters, 38*, 123–135. DOI: 10.1016/j.phytol.2020.06.004

Nkafamiya, I. I., Osemeahon, S. A., Dahiru, D., & Umaru, H. A. (2007). Chemical composition and physicochemical properties of baobab (*Adansonia digitata*) seeds and oil. *African Journal of Biotechnology, 6*(6), 756–759. DOI: 10.5897/AJB2007.000-2107

Nontokozo, Z. M., & Mthokozisi, S. (2018). *Herbal medicine*. Herbal Medicine.

Noor, M. J., Ahmed, S., & Khan, A. (2022). Network pharmacology in ethnopharmacology: Mapping compound–protein–disease interactions. *Journal of Ethnopharmacology, 298*, 115–124.

Nowak, M., Tryniszewski, W., Sarniak, A., Wlodarczyk, A., Nowak, P. J., & Nowak, D. (2022). Concentration Dependence of Anti- and Pro-Oxidant Activity of Polyphenols as Evaluated with a Light-Emitting Fe2+-Egta-H2O2 System. *Molecules (Basel, Switzerland), 27*(11), 3453. DOI: 10.3390/molecules27113453 PMID: 35684391

Numakawa, T., & Kajihara, R. (2023). Neuroprotective effects of Bacopa monnieri: Molecular mechanisms and biomarker modulation. *Neurochemistry International, 163*, 105–112.

Nwafor, N., & Igboeli, L. (2021). Antimicrobial activity of Annona senegalensis fruit extract against pathogenic microbes. *Scientific African, 13*, e00988.

Nwozo, O. S., Effiong, E. M., Aja, P. M., & Awuchi, C. G. (2023). Antioxidant, phytochemical, and therapeutic properties of medicinal plants: A review. *International Journal of Food Properties, 26*(1), 359–388. DOI: 10.1080/10942912.2022.2157425

Och, A., Podgórski, R., & Nowak, R. (2020). Biological activity of berberine—A summary update. *Toxins*, *12*(11), 713. DOI: 10.3390/toxins12110713 PMID: 33198257

Ogah, O. S., Orimolade, O. A., & Jinadu, T. O. (2023). Cardiovascular diseases in Nigeria: Current status, threats, and opportunities. *Circulation*, *148*(19), 1441–1444. DOI: 10.1161/CIRCULATIONAHA.123.063671 PMID: 37931020

Ogbera, A. O., Dada, O., & Adeyeye, F. (2010). Complementary and alternative medicine use in diabetes mellitus. *West African Journal of Medicine*, *29*, 158–162. PMID: 20665458

Ogbonnaya, F. C., Amah, G. H., Ogunbiyi, B. T., Ukangwa, N. A., Adewole, O. A., Akani, E. O., & Oladele, L. O. (2024). Antinutrients Properties and Antioxidant Activity of Some Nigerian Leafy Vegetable Plants. *Tropical Journal of Natural Product Research*, *8*(11).

Ogunlana, O. O., Ogunlana, O. E., Tobi, S., Adekunbi, B. O., Adetuyi, B. O., & Adegboye, B. E. (2020). Anti-inflammatory mechanism of Ruzu bitters on diet-induced non-alcoholic fatty liver disease in male Wistar rats. *Evidence-Based Complementary and Alternative Medicine*. *Article ID*, *5246725*, 8.

Ogunleye, T. A., Adeyemi, O. O., & Bello, I. (2021). Ultrasound-assisted extraction of bioactive compounds: Efficiency and sustainability. *Ultrasonics Sonochemistry*, *70*, 105–112.

Ogunro, O. B., Oyeyinka, B. O., Gyebi, G. A., & Batiha, G. E. S. (2023). Nutritional benefits, ethnomedicinal uses, phytochemistry, pharmacological properties and toxicity of Spondias mombin Linn: A comprehensive review. *The Journal of Pharmacy and Pharmacology*, *75*(2), 162–226. DOI: 10.1093/jpp/rgac086 PMID: 36632807

Ogwu, M. C., Adeyemi, O. O., & Bello, I. (2025). Environmental modulation of tannin and saponin production in forest trees under nutrient-poor soils. *Journal of Ethnopharmacology*, *315*, 117–126.

Ogwu, M. C., Izah, S. C., & Joshua, M. T. (2025). Ecological and environmental determinants of phytochemical variability in forest trees. *Phytochemistry Reviews*, *24*(6), 1–29. DOI: 10.1007/s11101-025-10066-0

Oh, S. S.-Y., Zou, P., Low, M.-Y., & Koh, H.-L. (2006). Detection of sildenafil analogues in herbal products for erectile dysfunction. *Journal of Toxicology and Environmental Health. Part A.*, *69*(22), 1951–1958. PMID: 16982533

Oh, W., Muthu, M., Pushparaj, C., & Gopal, J. (2023). Anticancer therapeutic effects of green tea catechins when integrated with antioxidant natural components. *Molecules (Basel, Switzerland)*, *28*(5), 2151. DOI: 10.3390/molecules28052151

Ojo, A. E., Ojji, D. B., Grobbee, D. E., Huffman, M. D., & Peters, S. A. (2024). The burden of cardiovascular disease attributable to hypertension in Nigeria: A modelling study using summary-level data. *Global Heart*, *19*(1), 50. DOI: 10.5334/gh.1332 PMID: 38863890

Okorie, P. N., Onuoha, C. C., & Adebayo, R. A. (2023). Moringa oleifera in traditional healthcare practice in Nigeria: An ethnobotanical review. *Frontiers in Pharmacology*, *14*, 1132456.

Okosodo, E. F., & Sarada, P. M. (2021). Ethno botanical survey and sustainable use of medicinal plant species for the treatment of tropical diseases, Yewa North Southwestern Nigeria. *European Journal of Research Development and Sustainability*, *2*(9), 134–149.

Okwu, D. E. (2007). Nigerian medicinal plants I. *Medicinal and Aromatic Plant Science and Biotechnology*, *1*(1), 90–96.

Olamoyegun, M. A., Alare, K., Afolabi, S. A., Aderinto, N., & Adeyemi, T. (2024). A systematic review and meta-analysis of the prevalence and risk factors of type 2 diabetes mellitus in Nigeria. *Clinical Diabetes and Endocrinology*, *10*(1), 43. DOI: 10.1186/s40842-024-00209-1 PMID: 39639395

Olaniyan, O. M., Adebayo, O. A., & Okonkwo, C. J. (2024). Immunosuppressive compounds from Azadirachta indica mapped to cytokine signaling networks: A network pharmacology study. *Journal of Herbal Medicine*, *38*, 112–120.

Olaniyan, O. M., Adebayo, O. A., & Okonkwo, C. J. (2025). Influence of solvent pH on phytochemical solubility and stability in extraction processes. *Journal of Natural Products Research*, *39*(4), 512–520.

Olanrewaju, I. O., Mordi, R. C., & Echeme, J. O. (2018). Antibacterial, antifungal and anti-tubercular activities of chloroform fraction of the leaf extract of Irvingia gabonensis (African bush mango). *Anti-Infective Agents*, *18*(2), 109–114. DOI: 10.2174/2211352517666181122125411

Olas, B., Adebayo, O., & Rotimi, D. (2025). Polyphenolic-rich extracts of Sclerocarya birrea improve oxidative stress and lipid metabolism in diabetic rats. *Phytomedicine*, *123*, 155678.

Olawale, F., Olofinsan, K., Iwaloye, O., & Ologuntere, T. E. (2022). Phytochemicals from Nigerian medicinal plants modulate therapeutically-relevant diabetes targets: Insight from computational direction. *Advances in Traditional Medicine*, *22*(4), 723–737. DOI: 10.1007/s13596-021-00598-z

Olayeriju, O. S., Elekofehinti, O. O., Olaleye, M. T., & Akindahunsi, A. A. (2021). Activation of NRF2/HO-1 Pathway by aqueous methanolic leaf extract of Triclisia gilletii and selected identified compounds in Triclisia gilletii, modulates crystal binding genes (CD44/OPN) in Ethane-1, 2-diol-induced nephrolithic rats. *Phytomedicine Plus : International Journal of Phytotherapy and Phytopharmacology, 1*(4), 100066. DOI: 10.1016/j.phyplu.2021.100066

Olugbenga Kayode Popoola, Kayode Damilola Adekeye, Eunice Damilola Akinbinu, Lanre Tope Adekeye, Michael Bolaji Afolayan, Emmanuel Ayomide Bakare, & Oluwatobi Emmanuel Akande. (2021). Ethnobotanical plants and their tradomedicinal values: A review. *World Journal of Biology Pharmacy and Health Sciences,* 5(1), 066–088. DOI: 10.30574/wjbphs.2021.5.1.0108

Omale, S., Amagon, K. I., Johnson, T. O., Bremner, S. K., & Gould, G. W. (2023). A systematic analysis of anti-diabetic medicinal plants from cells to clinical trials. *PeerJ, 11*, e14639. DOI: 10.7717/peerj.14639 PMID: 36627919

Omokpariola, D. O., Adeyemi, O. O., & Adebayo, O. (2025). Persistent organic pollutants and their interference with plant metabolite structures. *Environmental Toxicology and Pharmacology, 98*, 145–152.

Omosimua, O. (2024). Network pharmacology in cancer therapy: Contributions from Nigerian medicinal plants. *Global Journal of Cancer Research, 12*(3), 145–152.

Ompal, S. (2011). Chamomile: An overview. *Matricaria chamomilla*, pp. 70–71.

Onipede, O. A., Adeyemi, O. O., & Adebayo, O. (2024). Environmental pollutants and disruption of plant biosynthetic enzymes: Implications for ethnopharmacology. *Environmental Research, 235*, 116–125.

Onukak, A. C., Musa, I., & Abdullahi, Z. (2020). Hypoglycemic potential of Anchomanes difformis rhizome extract in diabetic rats. *Journal of Ethnopharmacology, 260*, 112921.

Orhan, I. E. (2021). A review focused on molecular mechanisms of anxiolytic effect of Valerina officinalis L. in connection with its phytochemistry through in vitro/in vivo studies. *Current Pharmaceutical Design, 27*(28), 3084–3090. DOI: 10.2174/1381612827666210119105254 PMID: 33463459

Oriol-Caballo, M., Moreno-Murciano, P., López-Blanch, R., Estrela, M., & Obrador, E. (2025). Polyphenols: Potential applications in cancer therapy. *Molecular Nutrition & Food Research, 69*(15), e70011. DOI: 10.1002/mnfr.70011

Ortega-Ramirez, L. A., Gutiérrez-Pacheco, M. M., Vargas-Arispuro, I., González-Aguilar, G. A., Martínez-Téllez, M. A., & Ayala-Zavala, J. F. (2020). Inhibition of Glucosyltransferase Activity and Glucan Production as an Antibiofilm Mechanism of Lemongrass Essential Oil against Escherichia coli O157:H7. *Antibiotics (Basel, Switzerland), 9*(3), 102. DOI: 10.3390/antibiotics9030102 PMID: 32121319

Oruka, O., & Achuba, F. I. (2023). In vitro Antioxidant and Anti-Inflammatory Activities of Aqueous Leaf Extract of Alchornea cordifolia. *Journal of Applied Science & Environmental Management, 27*(2), 299–304. DOI: 10.4314/jasem.v27i2.16

Orwa, C., Mutua, A., Kindt, R., Jamnadass, R., & Simons, A. (2009). *Agroforestree database: A tree reference and selection guide version 4.0.* World Agroforestry Centre.

Osafo, N., Obiri, D. D., Antwi, A. O., & Yeboah, O. K. (2018). The acute anti-inflammatory action of xylopic acid isolated from Xylopia aethiopica. *Journal of Basic and Clinical Physiology and Pharmacology, 29*(6), 659–669. DOI: 10.1515/jbcpp-2018-0019 PMID: 30052517

Oseghale, I. D., Lawal, O. P., Ubebe, D. O., Orjiewulu, V. C., Igunma, A. A., Odey, O. P., Ajibola, D. T., Chima, D. I., Tuador, N. K., & Ani, C. P. (2024). Ethnomedicinal and phytopharmacological aspects of Vernonia amygdalina (bitter leaf) utilised as a traditional medicinal herb. *Asian Journal of Research in Biochemistry, 14*(6), 41–57. DOI: 10.9734/ajrb/2024/v14i6326

Oshikoya, K. A., Senbanjo, I. O., Njokanma, O. F., & Soipe, A. (2008). Use of complementary and alternative medicines for children with chronic health conditions in Lagos, Nigeria. *BMC Complementary and Alternative Medicine, 8*(1), 66. DOI: 10.1186/1472-6882-8-66 PMID: 19113999

Osman, M. A. (2004). Chemical and nutrient analysis of baobab fruit and seed protein solubility. *Plant Foods for Human Nutrition (Dordrecht, Netherlands), 59*(1), 29–33. DOI: 10.1007/s11130-004-0034-1

Oso, A. (2023). Non-communicable Diseases: An Emerging Epidemic in Nigeria. *Tropical Journal of Nephrology, 18*(1 and 2), 31-37.

Osuagwu, G. G., & Idika, G. C. (2021). Anti-inflammatory and antioxidant activity of Ceratotheca sesamoides leaf infusion in Wistar rats. *Nigerian Journal of Natural Products and Medicine, 25*(1), 54–62.

Owolabi, T., & Okubor, P. (2024). Anti-Ulcer and Antioxidant Activities of Chrysophyllum albidum G. Don. Seeds Cotyledons. *Jurnal Farmasi Dan Ilmu Kefarmasian Indonesia, 11*(2), 260–268. DOI: 10.20473/jfiki.v11i22024.260-268

Oyedoh, J. O., Eze, C. N., & Okafor, J. O. (2025). Extraction time optimization in phytochemical yield and compound stability. *African Journal of Plant Science, 19*(2), 55–63.

Oyelakin, A. O., Olubode, T. P., & Olawale, B. R. (2020). Ethnobotanical survey and phytochemical analysis of selected medicinal plants used in treating digestive disorders. *Journal of Medicinal Plants Studies, 8*(2), 38–42.

Oyetayo, F. L., Akomolafe, S. F., & Balogun, G. B. (2021). Effects of Chrysophyllum albidum fruit pulp on haemodynamic parameters, pro-inflammatory markers, antioxidant parameters and critical biomolecules associated with hypertension–in vivo. *Inflammopharmacology, 29*(3), 825–839. DOI: 10.1007/s10787-021-00830-x PMID: 34120250

Ozon, A., Iuga, M., Mititelu, M., Musuc, M., Manolescu, N., Petrescu, S., & Elian, V. (2023). Pharmacotechnical, physico-chemical, and antioxidant evaluation of newly developed capsule formulations. *International Journal of Molecular Sciences, 24*(14), 11426. DOI: 10.3390/ijms241411426

Palaniappan K. & Holley R. A. (2010). Use of natural antimicrobials to increase antibiotic susceptibility of drug resistant bacteria. Int J Food Microbiol. 15;140(2-3):164-8. .DOI: 10.1016/j.ijfoodmicro.2010.04.001

Palit, P., & Mandal, S. (2021). Altitude and terroir effects on metabolite diversity in medicinal plants. *Journal of Applied Botany and Food Quality, 94*, 45–52.

Pandey, B., & Rizvi, I. (2009). Plant polyphenols as dietary antioxidants in human health and disease. *Oxidative Medicine and Cellular Longevity, 2*(5), 270–278. DOI: 10.4161/oxim.2.5.9498

Pandey, P., Lakhanpal, S., Mahmood, D., Kang, N., Kim, B., Kang, S., Choi, J., & Kim, B. (2025). An updated review summarizing the anticancer potential of flavonoids via targeting NF-κB pathway. *Frontiers in Pharmacology, 15*, 1513422. DOI: 10.3389/fphar.2024.1513422

Pandit, S., Srivastav, A. K., Sur, T. K., Chaudhuri, S., Wang, Y., & Biswas, T. K. (2024). Effects of Withania somnifera extract in chronically stressed adults: A randomized controlled trial. *Nutrients, 16*(9), 1293. DOI: 10.3390/nu16091293 PMID: 38732539

Panieri, E., Buha, A., Telkoparan-Akillilar, P., Cevik, D., Kouretas, D., Veskoukis, A., Skaperda, Z., Tsatsakis, A., Wallace, D., Suzen, S., & Saso, L. (2020). Potential applications of NRF2 modulators in cancer therapy. *Antioxidants, 9*(3), 193. DOI: 10.3390/antiox9030193 PMID: 32106613

Pant, A. (2022). Microencapsulation in food applications: Techniques and benefits for phytochemical delivery. *Food Research International, 156*, 111–118.

Paolicelli, R. C., Sierra, A., Stevens, B., Tremblay, M. E., Aguzzi, A., Ajami, B., Amit, I., Audinat, E., Bechmann, I., Bennett, M., Bennett, F., Bessis, A., Biber, K., Bilbo, S., Blurton-Jones, M., Boddeke, E., Brites, D., Brône, B., Brown, G. C., & Wyss-Coray, T. (2022). Microglia states and nomenclature: A field at its crossroads. *Neuron, 110*(21), 3458–3483. DOI: 10.1016/j.neuron.2022.10.020 PMID: 36327895

Papavassiliou, A., Sofianidi, A., Gogou, A., & Papavassiliou, G. (2025). The prospects of curcumin in non-small cell lung cancer therapeutics. *Cancers (Basel), 17*(3), 438. DOI: 10.3390/cancers17030438

Parashar, B., Sharma, R., & Gupta, R. (2012). Natural oils and extracts in nail care: Antifungal and moisturizing properties. *International Journal of Cosmetic Science, 34*(5), 420–426. DOI: 10.1111/j.1468-2494.2012.00729.x

Parcha, V., Bhandari, P., Chhetri, S., Kumar, U., & Kumar, D. (2024). on the Medicinal Use of Piper methysticum (Kava). *Medicinal Roots and Tubers for Pharmaceutical and Commercial Applications*, 140.

Pardo, M., Qiu, X., Zimmermann, R., & Rudich, Y. (2020). Particulate Matter Toxicity Is Nrf2 and Mitochondria Dependent: The Roles of Metals and Polycyclic Aromatic Hydrocarbons. *Chemical Research in Toxicology, 33*(5), 1110–1120. DOI: 10.1021/acs.chemrestox.0c00007 PMID: 32302097

Pardo-Moreno, T., García-Morales, V., Suleiman-Martos, S., Rivas-Domínguez, A., Mohamed-Mohamed, H., Ramos-Rodríguez, J. J., Melguizo-Rodríguez, L., & González-Acedo, A. (2023). Current Treatments and New, Tentative Therapies for Parkinson's Disease. *Pharmaceutics, 15*(3), 770. DOI: 10.3390/pharmaceutics15030770 PMID: 36986631

Park, C. W., Hong, K. B., Suh, H. J., & Ahn, Y. (2023). Sleep-promoting activity of amylase-treated Ashwagandha (Withania somnifera L. Dunal) root extract via GABA receptors. *Yao Wu Shi Pin Fen Xi, 31*(2), 278. DOI: 10.38212/2224-6614.3456 PMID: 37335157

Park, J. S., Rustamov, N., & Roh, Y. S. (2023). The roles of NRF2-regulated oxidative stress and mitochondrial quality control in chronic liver diseases. *Antioxidants, 12*(11), 1928. DOI: 10.3390/antiox12111928 PMID: 38001781

Park, S. Y., An, K. S., Lee, E., Kang, J. H., Jung, H. J., Kim, M. W., Ryu, H. Y., Shim, K. S., Nam, K. T., Yoon, Y. S., & Oh, S. H. (2021). Establishment of particulate matter-induced lung injury model in mouse. *Laboratory Animal Research*, *37*(1), 20. DOI: 10.1186/s42826-021-00097-x PMID: 34330339

Pasieczna-Patkowska, S., Cichy, M., & Flieger, J. (2005). Application of Fourier Transform Infrared (FTIR) Spectroscopy in Characterization of Green Synthesized Nanoparticles. *Molecules (Basel, Switzerland)*, *30*(3), 684. DOI: 10.3390/molecules30030684 PMID: 39942788

Patel, N. K., & Bhutani, K. K. (2014). Pinostrobin and Cajanus lactone isolated from Cajanus cajan (L.) leaves inhibits TNF-α and IL-1β production: In vitro and in vivo experimentation. *Phytomedicine*, *21*(7), 946–953. DOI: 10.1016/j.phymed.2014.02.011 PMID: 24680612

Patil, S., Deshmukh, R., & Jadhav, H. (2020). Pathway enrichment analysis in drug discovery: Applications and challenges. *Current Drug Discovery Technologies*, *17*(4), 345–352.

Patil, V. M., Das, S., & Balasubramanian, K. (2016). Quantum Chemical and Docking Insights into Bioavailability Enhancement of Curcumin by Piperine in Pepper. *The Journal of Physical Chemistry A*, *120*(20), 3643–3653. DOI: 10.1021/acs.jpca.6b01434 PMID: 27111639

Paudel, K. R., Orent, J., & Penela, O. G. (2025). Pharmacological properties of ginger (Zingiber officinale): What do meta-analyses say? A review. *Frontiers in Pharmacology*, *16*, 1619655. DOI: 10.3389/fphar.2025.1619655 PMID: 40808693

Paul, T. K., & Kumar, K. J. (2023). *Standardization of Herbal Medicines for Lifestyle Diseases.*, DOI: 10.1007/978-981-99-7703-1_27

Peiris, D. S. H. S., Fernando, D. T. K., Senadeera, S. P. N. N., & Ranaweera, C. B. (2025). Assessment of In Vitro Anti-Inflammatory Activity: A Comprehensive Review of Methods, Advantages, and Limitations. *Asian Journal of Research in Biochemistry*, *15*(2), 37–52. DOI: 10.9734/ajrb/2025/v15i2365

Pereira, R. B., Rahali, F. Z., Nehme, R., Falleh, H., Ben Jemaa, M., Sellami, I. H., Ksouri, R., Bouhallab, S., Ceciliani, F., Abdennebi-Najar, L., & Pereira, D. M. (2023). Anti-inflammatory activity of essential oils from Tunisian aromatic and medicinal plants and their major constituents in THP-1 macrophages. *Food Research International*, *167*, 112678. DOI: 10.1016/j.foodres.2023.112678 PMID: 37087210

Pham, T. P. L., & Phu, L. H. (2022). Plant flavonoids as potential natural antioxidants in phytocosmetics. *International Journal of Biotechnology*, *15*(3), 21–28.

Pikulthong, V., Bhirompan, S., Dechkla, M., Mokkapan, K., Boonman, N., Wanna, C., MacHana, K., & Phakpaknam, S. (2022). Local herbs for pain relief in the area of Tumbon Khao Hin Son, Chachoengsao, Thailand. *Biodiversitas (Surakarta), 23*(10). Advance online publication. DOI: 10.13057/biodiv/d231007

Pinho-Ribeiro, F. A., Zarpelon, A. C., Fattori, V., Manchope, M. F., Mizokami, S. S., Casagrande, R., & Verri, W. A.Jr. (2016). Naringenin reduces inflammatory pain in mice. *Neuropharmacology, 105*, 508–519. DOI: 10.1016/j.neuropharm.2016.02.019 PMID: 26907804

Pirintsos, S. A., Bariotakis, M., Kampa, M., & Castanas, E. (2022). Ethnopharmacology and molecular insights: Bridging traditional medicine with modern biomarkers. *Frontiers in Pharmacology, 13*, 876–885.

Pirintsos, S. A., Bariotakis, M., Kampa, M., Sourvinos, G., Lionis, C., & Castanas, E. (2020). The Therapeutic Potential of the Essential Oil of Thymbra capitata (L.) Cav., Origanum dictamnus L. and Salvia fruticosa Mill. And a Case of Plant-Based Pharmaceutical Development. *Frontiers in Pharmacology, 11*, 522213. Advance online publication. DOI: 10.3389/fphar.2020.522213 PMID: 33390932

Pisoschi, A. M., Pop, A., Cimpeanu, C., & Predoi, G. (2016). Antioxidant Capacity Determination in Plants and Plant-Derived Products: A Review. *Oxidative Medicine and Cellular Longevity, 9130976*(1), 9130976. Advance online publication. DOI: 10.1155/2016/9130976 PMID: 28044094

Polat, R., Cakilcioglu, U., Kaltalioğlu, K., Ulusan, M. D., & Türkmen, Z. (2015). An ethnobotanical study on medicinal plants in Espiye and its surrounding (Giresun-Turkey). *Journal of Ethnopharmacology, 163*, 1–11. DOI: 10.1016/j.jep.2015.01.008 PMID: 25614105

Pont-Fernandez, S., Kheyfets, M., Rogers, J. M., Smith, K. E., & Epstein, D. H. (2023). Kava (Piper methysticum) in the United States: The quiet rise of a substance with often subtle effects. *The American Journal of Drug and Alcohol Abuse, 49*(1), 85–96. DOI: 10.1080/00952990.2022.2140292 PMID: 36410029

Popoola, T. D., Guetchueng, S. T., Ritchie, K. J., Awodele, O., Dempster, N. M., Akinloye, O., Sarker, S. D., & Fatokun, A. A. (2021). Potent Nrf2-inducing, antioxidant, and anti-inflammatory effects and identification of constituents validate the anti-cancer use of Uvaria chamae and Olax subscorpioidea. *BMC Complementary Medicine and Therapies, 21*(1), 234. DOI: 10.1186/s12906-021-03404-0 PMID: 34537049

Pouremamali, F., Pouremamali, A., Dadashpour, M., Soozangar, N., & Jeddi, F. (2022). An update of Nrf2 activators and inhibitors in cancer prevention/promotion. *Cell Communication and Signaling : CCS, 20*(1), 100. DOI: 10.1186/s12964-022-00906-3 PMID: 35773670

Prajapati, A. K. (2024). Profiling the toxicological landscape of herbal drugs. *Journal of Preventive Medicine and Holistic Health, 10*(1), 6–9. DOI: 10.18231/j.jpmhh.2024.003

Preethi, R., & Padma, P. R. (2016). Anticancer activity of silver nanobioconjugates synthesized from Piper betle leaves extract and its active compound eugenol. *International Journal of Pharmacy and Pharmaceutical Sciences, 8*(9), 201. DOI: 10.22159/ijpps.2016.v8i9.12993

Proença, C., Freitas, M., Ribeiro, D., Rufino, T., Fernandes, E., & Ferreira de Oliveira, P. (2023). The role of flavonoids in the regulation of epithelial-mesenchymal transition in cancer. *Medicinal Research Reviews, 43*(6), 1878–1945. DOI: 10.1002/med.21966

Putri, S. P., Ikram, M. M. M. Sato, A., Dahlan, H. A., Rahmawati, D., Ohto, Y., & Fukusaki, E. (2022). Application of gas chromatography-mass spectrometry-based metabolomics in food science and technology. *Journal of Bioscience and Bioengineering, 133*(5), 425–435. DOI: 10.1016/j.jbiosc.2022.01.011 PMID: 35184928

Qian, Y., Zhao, F., Wang, J., Li, H., Xu, L., Wang, W., Yu, W., & Shan, L. (2021). Myricetin-based self-assembled nanoparticles for tumor synergistic therapy by antioxidation pathway. *Journal of Biomedical Nanotechnology, 17*(12), 2399–2412. DOI: 10.1166/jbn.2021.3197

Qiu, H., Liu, C., & Wang, Z. (2025). Levodopa-induced motor complications associated with benserazide and carbidopa in Parkinson's disease: A disproportionality analysis of the FAERS database. *Frontiers in Pharmacology, 16*, 1529932. DOI: 10.3389/fphar.2025.1529932 PMID: 40115262

Rafeeq, M., Al-Abbasi, F. A., Afzal, M., Moglad, E., Al-Qahtani, S. D., Alzrea, S. I., Almalki, N. A. R., Imam, F., Sayyed, N., & Kazmi, I. (2024). 6-Shogaol Abrogates Parkinson's Disease in Rotenone-Induced Rodents: Based on In Silico Study and Inhibiting TNF-α/NF-κB/IL-1β/MAO-B. *Pharmaceuticals (Basel, Switzerland), 17*(10), 1348. DOI: 10.3390/ph17101348 PMID: 39458989

Rahman, A., Hannan, A., Dash, R., Rahman, H., Islam, R., Uddin, J., & Rhim, H. (2021). Phytochemicals as a complement to cancer chemotherapy: Pharmacological modulation of the autophagy-apoptosis pathway. *Frontiers in Pharmacology, 12*, 639628. DOI: 10.3389/fphar.2021.639628

Rahman, M. S., Kabir, H., & Islam, M. R. (2021). Heavy metal exposure and oxidative damage: A review of mechanisms. *Toxics*, *9*(9), 218. DOI: 10.3390/toxics9090218 PMID: 34564369

Rajashekar, C. B. (2023). Dual Role of Plant Phenolic Compounds as Antioxidants and Prooxidants. *American Journal of Plant Sciences*, *14*(01), 15–28. DOI: 10.4236/ajps.2023.141002

Rajeeve, D., Yamuna, R., & Namboori, K. (2025). Elucidating the potential of EGFR mutated NSCLC and identifying its multi-targeted inhibitors. *Scientific Reports*, *15*(1), 3649. DOI: 10.1038/s41598-024-83868-5

Rajini, P. S. (2023). Indian spices and their bioactives in neurological disorders. In *Ayurvedic Herbal Preparations in Neurological Disorders* (pp. 541–575). Academic Press. DOI: 10.1016/B978-0-443-19084-1.00018-1

Raks, V., Charoen, N., & Srisawat, T. (2018). Extraction techniques for plant secondary metabolites: Conventional and modern approaches. *Asian Journal of Pharmaceutical Sciences*, *13*(3), 123–131.

Ramabulana, T., Steenkamp, P. A., & Madala, N. E. (2022). Ultra-performance liquid chromatography in plant metabolomics: Advances and applications. *South African Journal of Botany*, *148*, 345–352.

Ramadoss, M. S. K., & Koumaravelou, K. (2022). Regulatory Requirement Sufficiency for Registration of Traditional Herbal Medicine Based Products in Association of Southeast Asian Nations Regions: A Model Study with Ashwagandha Tablets. *Indian Journal of Pharmaceutical Sciences*, *84*(2). Advance online publication. DOI: 10.36468/pharmaceutical-sciences.944

Ramli, I., Cheriet, T., Posadino, M., Giordo, R., Fenu, G., Nwachukwu, C., & Pintus, G. (2024). Modulating the p53-MDM2 pathway: The therapeutic potential of natural compounds in cancer treatment. *EXCLI Journal*, *23*, 1397–1439.

Rana, A. Q., Ahmed, U. S., Chaudry, Z. M., & Vasan, S. (2015). Parkinson's disease: A review of non-motor symptoms. *Expert Review of Neurotherapeutics*, *15*(5), 549–562. DOI: 10.1586/14737175.2015.1038244 PMID: 25936847

Rassu, G., Sorrenti, M., Catenacci, L., Pavan, B., Ferraro, L., Gavini, E., Bonferoni, M. C., Giunchedi, P., & Dalpiaz, A. (2023). Conjugation, Prodrug, and Co-Administration Strategies in Support of Nanotechnologies to Improve the Therapeutic Efficacy of Phytochemicals in the Central Nervous System. *Pharmaceutics*, *15*(6), 1578. DOI: 10.3390/pharmaceutics15061578 PMID: 37376027

Rathee, J. S., Patro, B. S., Mula, S., Gamre, S., & Chattopadhyay, S. (2006). Antioxidant activity of piper betel leaf extract and its constituents. *Journal of Agricultural and Food Chemistry*, *54*(24), 9046–9054. DOI: 10.1021/jf061679e PMID: 17117789

Rathore, T., Upadhyay, E., & Jain, A. K. (2025). Therapeutic Role of Medicinal Plants in Combating Air Pollution-Induced Inflammation and Anxiety. *International Journal of Environmental Sciences*, *11*(10s), 635–649. DOI: 10.64252/y86v7b35

Rauf, A., Imran, M., Khan, I. A., Ur-Rehman, M., Gilani, A., Mehmood, Z., & Mubarak, S. (2018). Anticancer potential of quercetin: A comprehensive review. *Phytotherapy Research*, *32*(11), 2109–2130. DOI: 10.1002/ptr.6155

Reddy, A. P., Ravichandran, J., & Carkaci-Salli, N. (2020). Neural regeneration therapies for Alzheimer's and Parkinson's disease-related disorders. Biochimica et Biophysica Acta (BBA)-. *Biochimica et Biophysica Acta. Molecular Basis of Disease*, *1866*(4), 165506. DOI: 10.1016/j.bbadis.2019.06.020 PMID: 31276770

Regensburger, M., Ip, C. W., Kohl, Z., Schrader, C., Urban, P. P., Kassubek, J., & Jost, W. H. (2023). Clinical benefit of MAO-B and COMT inhibition in Parkinson's disease: Practical considerations. *Journal of Neural Transmission (Vienna, Austria)*, *130*(6), 847–861. DOI: 10.1007/s00702-023-02623-8 PMID: 36964457

Rehman, M. H. U., Saleem, U., Ahmad, B., & Rashid, M. (2022). Phytochemical and toxicological evaluation of *Zephyranthes citrina. Frontiers in Pharmacology*, *13*, 1007310. DOI: 10.3389/fphar.2022.1007310 PMID: 36210854

Rekha, V., Kollipara, M., & Gupta, B.. (2014). A Review on Piper betle L.: Nature's Promising Medicinal Reservoir. *Am J Ethnomedicine*, *1*(5), 276–289.

Riedel, K.-D., Rieger, K., Martin-Facklam, M., Mikus, G., Haefeli, W. E., & Burhenne, J. (2004). Simultaneous determination of hypericin and hyperforin in human plasma with liquid chromatography-tandem mass spectrometry. *Journal of Chromatography. B, Analytical Technologies in the Biomedical and Life Sciences*, *813*(1-2), 27–33. DOI: 10.1016/j.jchromb.2004.09.061 PMID: 15556512

Rintu, D., Shinjini, M., Kaustab, M., Pramathadhip, P., Umesh, P. S., & Banerjee, E. R. (2015). Anti-oxidant and anti-inflammatory activities of different varieties of Piper leaf extracts (Piper betle L.). *Journal of Nutrition & Food Sciences*, *5*(415), 2.

Roell, K. R., Reif, D. M., & Motsinger-Reif, A. A. (2017). An Introduction to Terminology and Methodology of Chemical Synergy-Perspectives from Across Disciplines. *Frontiers in Pharmacology*, *8*, 158. DOI: 10.3389/fphar.2017.00158 PMID: 28473769

Rogovskii, V. (2022). Polyphenols as the potential disease-modifying therapy in cancer. *Anti-cancer Agents in Medicinal Chemistry*, *22*(13), 2385–2392. DOI: 10.2174/1871520622666220201105204

Rosen, J., Gottfries, J., Muresan, S., & Backlund, A. (2020). Network-based strategies for drug discovery: Synergistic target combinations and adverse effect prediction. *Drug Discovery Today*, *25*(3), 511–519.

Roth, P. (2024). Comparative analysis of medicinal plant effects: Traditional vs. modern approaches. *Journal of Pharmacognosy & Natural Products*, *10*(4).

Rotimi, D. E., Ben-Goru, G. M., Evbuomwan, I. O., Elebiyo, T. C., Alorabi, M., Farasani, A., Batiha, G. E., & Adeyemi, O. S. (2024). *Zingiber officinale* and Vernonia amygdalina infusions improve redox status in rat brain. *Metabolic Brain Disease*, *39*(3), 721–732.

Roufogalis, B. D. (2014). Zingiber officinale (Ginger): A future outlook on its potential in prevention and treatment of diabetes and prediabetic states. *New Journal of Science*, *2014*(1), 674684. DOI: 10.1155/2014/674684

Roy, U. B., & Vijayalaxmi, K. K. (2013). Evaluation of cytotoxic activity of Piper betle Linn. using murine and human cell lines in vitro. *International Journal of Scientific and Engineering Research*, *4*(9), 221–233.

Saadatmand, S., Zohroudi, F., & Tangestani, H. (2024). The Effect of Oral Chamomile on Anxiety: A Systematic Review of Clinical Trials. *Clinical Nutrition Research*, *13*(2), 139. DOI: 10.7762/cnr.2024.13 2.139 PMID: 38784853

Sadgrove, N. J., & Jones, G. L. (2019). From Petri Dish to Patient: Bioavailability Estimation and Mechanism of Action for Antimicrobial and Immunomodulatory Natural Products. *Frontiers in Microbiology*, *10*, 2470. Advance online publication. DOI: 10.3389/fmicb.2019.02470 PMID: 31736910

Sadick, N. S., Kircik, L., & Gupta, A. K. (2010). Cosmeceuticals and their role in dermatology. *Journal of Drugs in Dermatology*, *9*(s2), s62–s69. PMID: 14558401

Saenghong, N., Wattanathorn, J., Muchimapura, S., Tongun, T., Piyavhatkul, N., Banchonglikitkul, C., & Kajsongkram, T. (2012). Zingiber officinale Improves Cognitive Function of the Middle-Aged Healthy Women. *Evidence-Based Complementary and Alternative Medicine : eCAM*, *383062*, 1–9. Advance online publication. DOI: 10.1155/2012/383062 PMID: 22235230

Saha, S., Buttari, B., Panieri, E., Profumo, E., & Saso, L. (2020). An overview of Nrf2 signalling pathway and its role in inflammation. *Molecules (Basel, Switzerland)*, *25*(22), 5474. DOI: 10.3390/molecules25225474 PMID: 33238435

Saha, S., Buttari, B., & Saso L. (2024). Modulation of oxidative stress and inflammation via the NRF2 signalling pathway. *Frontiers in Pharmacology, 15*, 1483289. DOI: 10.3389/fphar.2024.1483289 PMID: 39359243

Said, M., & Ibrahim, M. M (2024). Antioxidants and Phytochemical Profiles in Medicinal Plants: Unraveling Molecular Mechanisms. *Scholars International Journal of Biochemistry*, *7*(07), 106–117. DOI: 10.36348/sijb.2024.v07i07.003

Salau, A. K., Shehu, S., & Bakare-Odunola, M. T. (2024). Navigating the Challenges of Integrating African Herbal Medicines: A Path to Universal Acceptance. *Fountain Journal of National Ad Applied Sciences, 13*(1). Advance online publication. DOI: 10.53704/fujnas.v13i1.474

Salehi, B., Azzini, E., Zucca P., Maria Varoni, E., & Anil Kumar, V., N., Dini, L., Panzarini, E., Rajkovic, J., Valere Tsouh Fokou, P., Peluso, I., Prakash Mishra, A., Nigam, M., El Rayess, Y., El Beyrouthy, M., N. Setzer, W., Polito, L., Iriti, M., Sureda, A., Magdalena Quetglas-Llabrés, M., … Sharifi-Rad, J. (. (2020). Plant-Derived Bioactives and Oxidative Stress-Related Disorders: A Key Trend towards Healthy Aging and Longevity Promotion. *Applied Sciences (Basel, Switzerland), 10*(3), 947. DOI: 10.3390/app10030947

Salman, A., Singh, A. K., & Mishra, S. B. (2025). Health Policies and Health Regulations Regarding Nutraceuticals for Sleep. In *Nutraceuticals in Insomnia and Sleep Problems* (pp. 267–299). Apple Academic Press. DOI: 10.1201/9781003560890-14

Sanchez-Ortega, M., Carrera, A. C., & Garrido, A. (2021). Role of NRF2 in lung cancer. *Cells, 10*(8), 1879. DOI: 10.3390/cells10081879 PMID: 34440648

Sanjai, C., Hakkimane, S. S., Guru, B. R., & Gaonkar, S. L. (2024). A comprehensive review on anticancer evaluation techniques. *Bioorganic Chemistry, 142*, 106973. DOI: 10.1016/j.bioorg.2023.106973 PMID: 37984104

Santos, É. M., Ataide, J. A., Coco, J. C., Fava, A. L. M., Silvério, L. A. L., Sueiro, A. C., Silva, J. R. A., Lopes, A. M., Paiva-Santos, A. C., & Mazzola, P. G. (2023). Spondias sp: Shedding Light on Its Vast Pharmaceutical Potential. *Molecules (Basel, Switzerland), 28*(4), 1862. DOI: 10.3390/molecules28041862 PMID: 36838849

Sarabia-Vallejo, M., Gonzalez, R., & Perez, J. (2023). Cyclodextrin inclusion complexes for phytochemical solubility enhancement. *Carbohydrate Polymers, 312*, 120–128.

Saravanabhavan, K. (2018). Antidiabetic and Antioxidant Activities of Ethanolic Extract of Piper Betle L. Leaves in Catfish, Clarias Gariepinus. *Asian Journal of Pharmaceutical and Clinical Research, 11*(3), 194–198. DOI: 10.22159/ajpcr.2018.v11i3.22393

Sari, D., Putri, R., & Nugroho, A. (2022). Moringa oleifera reduces triglycerides and LDL cholesterol: Clinical trial outcomes. *Journal of Nutrition and Metabolism, 2022*, 1–9.

Sarkar, A., Roy, D., & Ghosh, S. (2020). PAHs and oxidative stress: Metabolic activation and redox cycling in human toxicity. *Molecular and Cellular Biochemistry, 469*, 21–34. DOI: 10.1007/s11010-020-03813-z

Sarker, M., Sharmin, T., & Akter, R.. (2024). A Comparative Analysis of Phytoconstituents, Cytotoxicity and Antidiabetic Activity of Three Regional Piper betle Varieties: First Report from Bangladesh. *South Asian Res J Nat Prod, 7*(1), 20–29.

Saxena, R., Gupta, A., & Sharma, V. (2023). Infrared spectroscopy in phytochemical analysis: Functional group identification and applications. *Spectrochimica Acta. Part A: Molecular and Biomolecular Spectroscopy, 289*, 121–130.

Schepici, G., Contestabile, V., Valeri, A., & Mazzon, E. (2021). Ginger, a Possible Candidate for the Treatment of Dementias? *Molecules (Basel, Switzerland), 26*(18), 5700. DOI: 10.3390/molecules26185700 PMID: 34577171

Sejbuk, M., Mirończuk-Chodakowska, I., Karav, S., & Witkowska, M. (2024). Dietary polyphenols, food processing and gut microbiome. *Antioxidants, 13*(10), 1220. DOI: 10.3390/antiox13101220

Senapati, A., Basak, S., & Rangan, L. (2022). A review on application of DNA barcoding technology for rapid molecular diagnostics of adulterants in herbal medicine. *Drug Safety, 45*(2), 193–213. DOI: 10.1007/s40264-021-01133-4 PMID: 34846701

Senn, R., Schertler, L., Bussmann, H., Drewe, J., Boonen, G., & Butterweck, V. (2025). Valerenic Acid and Pinoresinol as Positive Allosteric Modulators: Unlocking the Sleep-Promoting Potential of Valerian Extract Ze 911. *Molecules (Basel, Switzerland), 30*(11), 2344. DOI: 10.3390/molecules30112344 PMID: 40509231

Sepide, M. (2016). A systematic review of therapeutic effects of *Matricaria recutita* (chamomile). *Electronic Physician, 8*(9), 3024. DOI: 10.19082/3024 PMID: 27790360

Shaban, N. S., Abdou, K. A., & Hassan, N. E. Y. (2015). Impact of toxic heavy metals and pesticide residues in herbal products. *Beni-Suef University Journal of Basic and Applied Sciences, 5*(2), 102–106.

Shaheen, S., Ahmad, M., & Hussain, M. (2014). Traditional remedies for hair and body care: An ethnopharmacological survey. *Journal of Ethnopharmacology*, *154*(1), 45–52. DOI: 10.1016/j.jep.2014.03.012

Shahrajabian, M. H., Sun, W., & Cheng, Q. (2019). Clinical aspects and health benefits of ginger (Zingiber officinale) in both traditional Chinese medicine and modern industry. *Acta Agriculturæ Scandinavica. Section B, Soil and Plant Science*, *69*(6), 546–556. DOI: 10.1080/09064710.2019.1606930

Shai, K., Hassan, Z. B., Balogun, T. A., & Adeyemi, O. (2024). Antimicrobial and anti-inflammatory activities of Securidaca longipedunculata root extracts: Preclinical evaluation. *Natural Product Communications*, *19*(9), 1–6.

Shakya, P., Shrestha, D., Maharjan, E., Sharma, V. K., & Paudyal, R. (2017). ESBL production among E. coli and Klebsiella spp. causing urinary tract infection: A hospital based study. *The Open Microbiology Journal*, *11*(1), 23–30. DOI: 10.2174/1874285801711010023 PMID: 28553414

Shankar, S., Ganapathy, S., Hingorani, R., & Srivastava, K. (2008). EGCG inhibits growth, invasion, angiogenesis and metastasis of pancreatic cancer. *Frontiers in Bioscience*, *13*(13), 440–452. DOI: 10.2741/2691

Shanmugarajan, K., Kumar, P., & Rajendran, R. (2024). Network pharmacology and docking studies of traditional herbal formulations against COVID-19. *Journal of Biomolecular Structure & Dynamics*, *42*(5), 1123–1135.

Sharifi-Rad, J., El Rayess, Y., Abi Rizk, A., Sadaka, C., Zgheib, R., Zam, W., & Setzer, W. N. (2020). Turmeric and its major compound curcumin on health: Bioactive effects and safety profiles for food, pharmaceutical, biotechnological and medicinal applications. *Frontiers in Pharmacology*, *11*, 1021. DOI: 10.3389/fphar.2020.01021

Sharma, E., Attri, C., Sati, P., Dhyani, P., Szopa, A., Sharifi-Rad, J., & Cho, C. (2022). Recent updates on anticancer mechanisms of polyphenols. *Frontiers in Cell and Developmental Biology*, *10*, 1005910. DOI: 10.3389/fcell.2022.1005910

Sharma, P. (2024). Predictive modeling of secondary metabolite genes for stress resistance in plants. *Plant Biotechnology Journal*, *22*(4), 567–578.

Sharma, P., Jha, A. B., Dubey, R. S., & Pessarakli, M. (2022). Reactive oxygen species, oxidative damage, and antioxidative defense mechanism in plants under stressful conditions. *Le Journal de Botanique*, *2022*, 1–26.

Sharma, R., Gupta, A., & Saxena, V. (2020). Curcumin nanoparticles: Enhanced absorption and anticancer activity. *Journal of Nanomedicine Research*, *12*(5), 233–240.

Sharma, R., Gupta, A., & Saxena, V. (2023). Maceration in phytochemical extraction: Principles and applications. *International Journal of Pharmacognosy and Phytochemical Research, 15*(1), 45–52.

Sharma, T., Kumar, R., & Mukherjee, S. (2024). Neuronal Vulnerability to Degeneration in Parkinson's Disease and Therapeutic Approaches. *CNS & Neurological Disorders - Drug Targets, 23*(6), 715–730. DOI: 10.2174/1871527322666230426155432 PMID: 37185323

Shaukat, M. N., Nazir, A., & Fallico, B. (2023). Ginger Bioactives: A Comprehensive Review of Health Benefits and Potential Food Applications. *Antioxidants, 12*(11), 2015. DOI: 10.3390/antiox12112015 PMID: 38001868

Shen, C. L., Wang, R., Santos, J. M., Elmassry, M. M., Stephens, E., Kim, N., & Neugebauer, V. (2024). Ginger alleviates mechanical hypersensitivity and anxio-depressive behavior in rats with diabetic neuropathy through beneficial actions on gut microbiome composition, mitochondria, and neuroimmune cells of colon and spinal cord. *Nutrition Research (New York, N.Y.), 124*, 73–84. DOI: 10.1016/j.nutres.2024.01.014 PMID: 38402829

Shinde, R., Kulkarni, P., & Patil, S. (2023). UPLC-QTOF-MS in metabolomics: Applications in phytochemical profiling. *Metabolomics, 19*(7), 112–124.

Shin, M. R., Kim, H. Y., Choi, H. Y., Park, K. S., Choi, H. J., & Roh, S. S. (2022). *Boswellia serrata* Extract, 5-Loxin®, Prevents Joint Pain and Cartilage Degeneration in a Rat Model of Osteoarthritis Through Inhibition of Inflammatory Responses and Restoration of Matrix Homeostasis. *Evidence-Based Complementary and Alternative Medicine : eCAM, 2022*(1), 3067526. DOI: 10.1155/2022/3067526 PMID: 36310623

Shitaw, E. E., AlAhmad, M., & Sivaprasadarao, A. (2025). Inter-Organelle Crosstalk in Oxidative Distress: A Unified TRPM2-NOX2 Mediated Vicious Cycle Involving Ca2+, Zn2+, and ROS Amplification. *Antioxidants, 14*(7), 776. DOI: 10.3390/antiox14070776 PMID: 40722879

Shoaib, S., Ansari, M. A., Al Fatease, A., Safhi, A. Y., Hani, U., Jahan, R., Alomary, M. N., Ansari, M. N., Ahmed, N., Wahab, S., Ahmad, W., Yusuf, N., & Islam, N. (2023). Plant-Derived Bioactive Compounds in the Management of Neurodegenerative Disorders: Challenges, Future Directions and Molecular Mechanisms Involved in Neuroprotection. *Pharmaceutics, 15*(3), 749. DOI: 10.3390/pharmaceutics15030749 PMID: 36986610

Shoba, G., Joy, D., Joseph, T., Majeed, M., Rajendran, R., & Srinivas, P. S. (1998). Influence of piperine on the pharmacokinetics of curcumin in animals and human volunteers. *Planta Medica, 64*(4), 353–356. DOI: 10.1055/s-2006-957450 PMID: 9619120

Shukla, Y. N., Dubey, S., & Jain, S. P. (2001). Constituents of *Adansonia digitata* roots. *Fitoterapia, 72*(5), 544–546. DOI: 10.1016/S0367-326X(01)00273-9

Si, C. L., Liu, Z., Hu, H., & Liu, R. (2011). Radical scavenging activity of procyanidins from baobab fruit. *Natural Product Research, 25*(8), 745–752. DOI: 10.1080/14786419.2010.488634

Siddhuraju, P., & Becker, K. (2019). Nutritional composition and antioxidant properties of African baobab fruit pulp. *Food Research International, 115*, 341–351. DOI: 10.1016/j.foodres.2018.09.021

Siddiqui, N. A., Taj, F. B., Ishaque, I., Shahid, A., & Ayaz, A. (2020). Role of simvastatin and allium sativum on lipid profile in diabetic dyslipidemic patients: A comparative study. *The Professional Medical Journal, 27*(02), 353–358. DOI: 10.29309/TPMJ/2020.27.02.3974

Sidibe, M., & Williams, J. T. (2020). *Baobab: A review of the nutritional and medicinal uses of Adansonia digitata L.* Routledge.

Sierra-Vargas, M. P., Montero-Vargas, J. M., Debray-Garcia, Y., Vizuet-de-Rueda, J. C., Loaeza-Roman, A., & Teran, L. M. (2023). Oxidative stress and air pollution: Its impact on chronic respiratory diseases. *International Journal of Molecular Sciences, 24*(1), 853. https://www.mdpi.com/1422-0067/24/1/853. DOI: 10.3390/ijms24010853 PMID: 36614301

Sigsgaard, T., & Hoffmann, B. (2024). Assessing the health burden from air pollution. *Science, 384*(6691), 33–34. DOI: 10.1126/science.abo3801 PMID: 38574150

Silpi, C. (2025). Nutraceuticals: Traditional practices, regulatory guidelines, opportunities and challenges. *Discover Food, 5*(1), 191. DOI: 10.1007/s44187-025-00437-z

Silva-Pinto, A., de Pontes, C., Aguilar-Morón, B., Canales, C., Pavan, R., & Roque-Borda, A. (2025). Phytochemical insights into flavonoids in cancer. *Heliyon, 11*(4), e42682. DOI: 10.1016/j.heliyon.2025.e42682

Simmler, C., Graham, J. G., Chen, S. N., & Pauli, G. F. (2018). Integrated analytical assets aid botanical authenticity and adulteration management. *Fitoterapia, 129*, 401–414. DOI: 10.1016/j.fitote.2017.11.017 PMID: 29175549

Sinan, K. I., Ak, G., Etienne, O. K., Jekő, J., Cziáky, Z., Gupcsó, K., João Rodrigues, M., Custodio, L., Mahomoodally, M. F., Sharmeen, J. B., Brunetti, L., Leone, S., Recinella, L., Chiavaroli, A., Orlando, G., Menghini, L., Tacchini, M., Ferrante, C., & Zengin, G. (2021). Deeper Insights on Alchornea cordifolia (Schumach. & Thonn.) Müll.Arg Extracts: Chemical Profiles, Biological Abilities, Network Analysis and Molecular Docking. *Biomolecules*, *11*(2), 219. DOI: 10.3390/biom11020219 PMID: 33557215

Sindhoora, D., & Bhattacharjee, A. (2020). A Brief Review on Pharmacological Profile of Zingiber officinale. *RGUHS Journal of Pharmaceutical Sciences*, *10*(2), 1230. Advance online publication. DOI: 10.26463/rjps.10_2_7

Singaravelan, N., & Tollefsbol, O. (2025). Polyphenol-based prevention and treatment of cancer through epigenetic and combinatorial mechanisms. *Nutrients*, *17*(4), 616. DOI: 10.3390/nu17040616

Singh, A., Holvoet, S., & Mercenier, A. (2011). Dietary polyphenols in the prevention and treatment of allergic diseases. *Clinical and Experimental Allergy*, *41*(10), 1346–1359. DOI: 10.1111/j.1365-2222.2011.03773.x

Singh, P., Chacko, K. M., Aggarwal, M. L., Bhat, B., Khandal, R. K., Sultana, S., & Kuruvilla, B. T. (2012). A-90 days gavage safety assessment of *Boswellia serrata* in rats. *Toxicology International*, *19*(3), 273. DOI: 10.4103/0971-6580.103668 PMID: 23293466

Singh, T. P., Singh, H. L., & Singh, R. M. (2022). Phytochemical Screening, Quantification, FT-IR Analysis, and In Silico Characterization of Potential Bio-active Compounds Identified in HR-LC/MS Analysis of the Polyherbal Formulation from Northeast India. *Pharmacognosy Journal*, *14*(3), 570–579. PMID: 36157760

Singh, V. K., Arora, D., Ansari, M. I., & Sharma, P. K. (2019). Phytochemicals based chemopreventive and chemotherapeutic strategies and modern technologies to overcome limitations for better clinical applications. *Phytotherapy Research*, *33*(12), 3064–3089. DOI: 10.1002/ptr.6508 PMID: 31515899

Singla, R., Kamboj, S., Duvey, B. K., Bhargava, A., & Chaudhary, J. (2025). Flavonoids and anxiety: Decoding their role in brain function and pathophysiology. *Medicine in Drug Discovery*, *27*, 100214. DOI: 10.1016/j.medidd.2025.100214

Siriwatanametanon, N., Fiebich, B. L., Efferth, T., Prieto, J. M., & Heinrich, M. (2010). Traditionally used Thai medicinal plants: In vitro anti-inflammatory, anticancer and antioxidant activities. *Journal of Ethnopharmacology*, *130*(2), 196–207. DOI: 10.1016/j.jep.2010.04.036 PMID: 20435130

Sirwi, A., Rabie, M. A., Koshak, A. E., Albadawi, D. A., El-Halawany, A. M., Ibrahim, S. R., Mohamed, G. A., Abdallah, H. M., & El-Sayed, N. S. (2025). 6-Paradol mitigates rotenone-induced Parkinson's disease via shutting TNFR-1/RIPK1/RIPK3/MLKL cascade and enhancement of PPARγ/PGC-1α/TFAM axis. *Future Journal of Pharmaceutical Sciences*, *11*(1), 1–15. DOI: 10.1186/s43094-025-00831-5

Smith, J. A., Das, A., Ray, S. K., & Banik, N. L. (2012). Role of pro-inflammatory cytokines released from microglia in neurodegenerative diseases. *Brain Research Bulletin*, *87*(1), 10–20. DOI: 10.1016/j.brainresbull.2011.10.004 PMID: 22024597

Smith, J., Brown, T., & Lee, H. (2016). Pathway compensation and drug resistance: Mechanisms and therapeutic strategies. *Pharmacology Research & Perspectives*, *4*(6), e00245.

Songvut, P., Nakareangrit, W., Cholpraipimolrat, W., Kwangjai, J., Worasuttayangkurn, L., Watcharasit, P., & Satayavivad, J. (2024). Unraveling the interconversion pharmacokinetics and oral bioavailability of the major ginger constituents:[6]-gingerol,[6]-shogaol, and zingerone after single-dose administration in rats. *Frontiers in Pharmacology*, *15*, 1391019. DOI: 10.3389/fphar.2024.1391019 PMID: 38904001

Souiy, H., Benali, S., & Khelifa, A. (2023). Hydrodistillation of essential oils: Advances and limitations. *The Journal of Essential Oil Research*, *35*(4), 289–298.

Spínola, V., Pinto, J., & Castilho, P. C. (2020). Phytochemical diversity and bioactive properties of *Adansonia digitata* (baobab). *Food Research International*, *130*, 108939. DOI: 10.1016/j.foodres.2019.108939

Sravani, A. (2018). A Review Article on Flash Chromatography. *Asian Journal of Research in Chemistry*, *11*(5), 815–818. DOI: 10.5958/0974-4150.2018.00144.X

Srinivas, Ch., & Singh, Dr. G. (2023). Traditional Plant uses and Indigenous Knowledge in Ethnobotany. *International Journal of Horticulture, Agriculture and Food Science*, 7(5), 01–05. DOI: 10.22161/ijhaf.7.5.1

Srivastav, S., Fatima, M., & Mondal, A. C. (2017). Important medicinal herbs in Parkinson's disease pharmacotherapy. *Biomedicine and Pharmacotherapy*, *92*, 856–863. DOI: 10.1016/j.biopha.2017.05.137 PMID: 28599249

Stough, C., Downey, L. A., Lloyd, J., Silber, B., Redman, S., Hutchison, C., Wesnes, K., & Nathan, P. J. (2008). Examining the nootropic effects of a special extract of Bacopa monniera on human cognitive functioning: 90-day double-blind placebo-controlled randomized trial. *Phytotherapy Research*, *22*(12), 1629–1634. DOI: 10.1002/ptr.2537 PMID: 18683852

Subashkumar, R., Sureshkumar, M., Babu, S., & Thayumanavan, T. (2013). Antibacterial effect of crude aqueous extract of Piper betle L. against pathogenic bacteria. *International Journal of Research in Pharmaceutical and Biomedical Sciences*, *4*, 42–46.

Sudha Rani, K., Aruna, M., Lakshmi, M., Priya, B. T., & Prakash, K. K. (2024). A comprehensive review of the antioxidative and anti-inflammatory properties of turmeric (*Curcuma longa*). *Annals of Phytomedicine*, *13*(2), 96–105. DOI: 10.54085/ap.2024.13.2.10

Sun, L., Yu, Q., Peng, F., Sun, C., Wang, D., Pu, L., Xiong, F., Tian, Y., Peng, C., & Zhou, Q. (2024). The antibacterial activity of berberine against *Cutibacterium acnes*: Its therapeutic potential in inflammatory acne. *Frontiers in Microbiology*, *14*, 1276383. DOI: 10.3389/fmicb.2023.1276383 PMID: 38249466

Sunmer, J. (2000). *The natural history of medicinal plants*. Timber Press.

Sun, Q., Li, Y., Shi, L., Hussain, R., Mehmood, K., Tang, Z., & Zhang, H. (2022). Heavy metals induced mitochondrial dysfunction in animals: Molecular mechanism of toxicity. *Toxicology*, *469*, 153136. DOI: 10.1016/j.tox.2022.153136 PMID: 35202761

Suraweera, L., Rupasinghe, T., Dellaire, H. P. V., & Xu, G. (2020). Regulation of Nrf2/ARE pathway by Dietary flavonoids: A friend or foe for Cancer Management? *Antioxid (Basel)*, *9*(10), 973. DOI: 10.3390/antiox9100973 PMID: 33050575

Sykiotis, G. P. (2021). Keap1/Nrf2 signalling pathway. *Antioxidants*, *10*(6), 828. DOI: 10.3390/antiox10060828 PMID: 34067331

Szklarczyk, D., Gable, A. L., Lyon, D., Junge, A., Wyder, S., Huerta-Cepas, J., & Morris, J. H. (2016). STRING v10: Protein–protein interaction networks, integrated over the tree of life. *Nucleic Acids Research*, *44*(D1), D447–D452.

Tabuas, B., Cruz Barros, S., Diogo, C., Cavaleiro, C., & Sanches Silva, A. (2024). Pyrrolizidine Alkaloids in Foods, Herbal Drugs, and Food Supplements: Chemistry, Metabolism, Toxicological Significance, Analytical Methods, Occurrence, and Challenges for Future. *Toxins*, *16*(2), 79. DOI: 10.3390/toxins16020079 PMID: 38393157

Tadesse, D., Lulekal, E., & Masresha, G. (2025). Ethnopharmacological study of traditional medicinal plants used by the people in Metema district, northwestern Ethiopia. *Frontiers in Pharmacology*, *16*, 1535822. DOI: 10.3389/fphar.2025.1535822 PMID: 40129938

Tagne, A. M., Marino, F., & Cosentino, M. (2018). Tithonia diversifolia (Hemsl.) A. Gray as a medicinal plant: A comprehensive review of its ethnopharmacology, phytochemistry, pharmacotoxicology and clinical relevance. *Journal of Ethnopharmacology*, *220*, 94–116. DOI: 10.1016/j.jep.2018.03.025 PMID: 29596999

Talbott, S. M., Talbott, J. A., & Pugh, M. (2013). Effect of Magnolia officinalis and Phellodendron amurense (Relora®) on cortisol and psychological mood state in moderately stressed subjects. *Journal of the International Society of Sports Nutrition*, *10*(1), 37. DOI: 10.1186/1550-2783-10-37 PMID: 23924268

Tal-Dia, A., Toure, K., Dia, A. T., Diallo, I., & Ndir, O. (1997). Baobab fruit pulp in traditional oral rehydration therapy for the treatment of infantile diarrhoea. *Senegalese Journal of Medicine*, *42*(3), 123–127.

Talib, H., Abed, I., Raad, D., Alomari, K., Jamal, A., Jabbar, R., & Law, D. (2024). Targeting cancer hallmarks using selected food bioactive compounds. *Foods*, *13*(17), 2687. DOI: 10.3390/foods13172687

Tamaru, E., Kokubu, D., Uchida, Y., & Itoh, K. (2024). Nrf2 induction potency of plant-derived compounds determined using an antioxidant response element luciferase reporter and conventional NAD(P)H-quinone acceptor oxidoreductase 1 activity assay. *BMC Research Notes*, *17*(1), 373. DOI: 10.1186/s13104-024-07038-6 PMID: 39707451

Tang, H., Shao, C., Wang, X., Cao, Y., Li, Z., Luo, X., Yang, X., & Zhang, Y. (2022). 6-Gingerol attenuates subarachnoid hemorrhage-induced early brain injury via GBP2/PI3K/AKT pathway in the rat model. *Frontiers in Pharmacology*, *13*, 882121. DOI: 10.3389/fphar.2022.882121 PMID: 36091803

Tanty, H., & Herlina, T. (2018). Antidiabetic activity test for leaves extract of Cassia siamea. lamk. MATTER. *International Journal of Science and Technology*, *3*(3), 339–348. DOI: 10.20319/mijst.2018.33.339348

Tan, Y. Y., Jenner, P., & Chen, S. D. (2022). Monoamine Oxidase-B Inhibitors for the Treatment of Parkinson's Disease: Past, Present, and Future. *Journal of Parkinson's Disease*, *12*(2), 477–493. DOI: 10.3233/JPD-212976 PMID: 34957948

Tapsoba, H., & Deschamps, J. P. (2006). Use of medicinal plants for oral diseases in Burkina Faso. *Journal of Ethnopharmacology*, *104*(1–2), 68–78. DOI: 10.1016/j.jep.2005.08.047

Tascioglu Aliyev, A., Panieri, E., Stepanić, V., Gurer-Orhan, H., & Saso, L. (2021). Involvement of NRF2 in breast cancer and possible therapeutical role of polyphenols and melatonin. *Molecules (Basel, Switzerland)*, *26*(7), 1853. DOI: 10.3390/molecules26071853 PMID: 33805996

Tauchen, J., Frankova, A., Manourova, A., Valterova, I., Lojka, B., & Leuner, O. (2023). Garcinia kola: A critical review on chemistry and pharmacology of an important West African medicinal plant. *Phytochemistry Reviews*, *22*(5), 1305–1351. DOI: 10.1007/s11101-023-09869-w PMID: 37359709

Tauheed, A. M., Mamman, M., Ahmed, A., Sani, N. A., Suleiman, M. M., Sulaiman, M. H., & Balogun, E. O. (2021). Acute, sub-acute, sub-chronic and chronic toxicity studies of four important Nigerian ethnomedicinal plants in rats. *Clinical Phytoscience*, *7*(1), 1. DOI: 10.1186/s40816-020-00244-2

Tee, T. X., Kee, L. T., Chai, T. T., Yam, H. C., Reza, H. M., Wong, F. C., Law, J. X., & Tan, S.-A. (2025). Plant-derived Nrf2 activators to enhance liver antioxidative and regenerative potentials. *Revista Brasileira de Farmacognosia*, *35*(1), 61–77. DOI: 10.1007/s43450-024-00609-5

Tegge, A. N., Caldwell, R. D., Xu, Y., & Wang, J. (2017). Biological pathway modeling and analysis. *Briefings in Bioinformatics*, *18*(3), 415–429.

Teklay, A., Abera, B., & Giday, M. (2013). An ethnobotanical study of medicinal plants used in Kilte Awulaelo District, Tigray Region of Ethiopia. *Journal of Ethnobiology and Ethnomedicine*, *9*(1), 1–23. DOI: 10.1186/1746-4269-9-65 PMID: 24011232

Teschke, I., Cartmill, E. A., Stankewitz, S., & Tebbich, S. (2011). Sometimes tool use is not the key: No evidence for cognitive adaptive specializations in tool-using woodpecker finches. *Animal Behaviour*, *82*(5), 945–956. DOI: 10.1016/j.anbehav.2011.07.032

Teschke, R. (2010). Kava hepatotoxicity—A clinical review. *Annals of Hepatology*, *9*(3), 251–265. DOI: 10.1016/S1665-2681(19)31634-5

Thaklaewphan, P., Wikan, N., Potikanond, S., & Nimlamool, W. (2024). Oxyresveratrol enhances the anti-cancer effect of cisplatin. *Biomolecules*, *14*(9), 1140. DOI: 10.3390/biom14091140

Thébault, E., & Fontaine, C. (2010). Stability of ecological communities and the architecture of mutualistic and trophic networks. *Science*, *329*(5993), 853–856. DOI: 10.1126/science.1188321

Thiruvengadam, M., Venkidasamy, B., Subramanian, U., Samynathan, R., Ali Shariati, M., Rebezov, M., Girish, S., Thangavel, S., Dhanapal, A. R., Fedoseeva, N., Lee, J., & Chung, I.-M. (2021). Bioactive Compounds in Oxidative Stress-Mediated Diseases: Targeting the NRF2/ARE Signaling Pathway and Epigenetic Regulation. *Antioxidants*, *10*(12), 1859. DOI: 10.3390/antiox10121859 PMID: 34942962

Thiyagarajan, T., Subramanian, R., & Venkatesan, R. (2015). In vitro antidiabetic activity of *Adansonia digitata* extracts. *International Journal of Pharmaceutical Sciences Review and Research*, *30*(1), 150–154.

Togbenou, K., Idoh, K., Dosseh, K., Kpatcha, T., & Agbonon, A. (2020). Anti-Inflammatory Activity of Extract Mixture of Annona senegalensis Pers. and Piliostigma thonningii (Schum.). *Journal of Drug Delivery and Therapeutics*, *10*(6-s), 103–108. DOI: 10.22270/jddt.v10i6-s.4605

Tomou, E. M., Skaltsounis, A. L., & Aligiannis, N. (2020). Nuclear magnetic resonance spectroscopy in phytochemical analysis: Applications and perspectives. *Phytochemistry Letters*, *35*, 1–9.

Tourabi, A., Benali, S., & Khelifa, A. (2025). Solvent polarity and phytochemical extraction: Principles and applications. *Phytochemistry Reviews*, *24*(2), 145–158.

Tsioutsiou, E. E., Cheilari, A., & Aligiannis, N. (2023). Ethnopharmacological study of medicinal plants used against skin ailments on Mount Pelion, central Greece. *Frontiers in Pharmacology*, *14*, 1225580. DOI: 10.3389/fphar.2023.1225580 PMID: 37583900

Tysnes, O. B., & Storstein, A. (2017). Epidemiology of Parkinson's disease. *Journal of Neural Transmission (Vienna, Austria)*, *124*(8), 901–905. DOI: 10.1007/s00702-017-1686-y PMID: 28150045

Tyuryaeva, I., & Lyublinskaya, O. (2023). Expected and Unexpected Effects of Pharmacological Antioxidants. *International Journal of Molecular Sciences*, *24*(11), 9303. DOI: 10.3390/ijms24119303 PMID: 37298254

Tzani, A., Kalafateli, S., Tatsis, G., Bairaktari, M., Kostopoulou, I., Pontillo, A. R. N., & Detsi, A. (2021). Natural deep eutectic solvents (NaDESs) as alternative green extraction media for ginger (Zingiber officinale Roscoe). *Sustainable Chemistry*, *2*(4), 576–598. DOI: 10.3390/suschem2040032

Uddin, G., Saeed, R., & Khan, A. (2024). Mass spectrometry in phytochemical profiling: Principles and applications. *Rapid Communications in Mass Spectrometry*, *38*(9), 1123–1132.

Ugur, S., & Guzel, O. (2023). Liquid chromatography-mass spectrometry in phytochemical analysis: Advances and applications. *Journal of Mass Spectrometry : JMS, 58*(4), 321–330.

Ukaga, C. N., Nwoke, B. E., & Anosike, J. C. (2006). Antimalarial activity of Nigerian folklore plants: Clinical validation studies. *African Journal of Medicine and Medical Sciences, 35*(3), 321–326.

Ukaogo, P. O., Ewuzie, U., & Onwuka, C. V. (2020). Environmental Pollution: Causes, Effects, and the Remedies. In Chowdhary, P., Raj, A., Verma, D., & Akhter, Y. (Eds.), *Microorganisms for Sustainable Environment and Health* (pp. 419–429). Elsevier., DOI: 10.1016/B978-0-12-819001-2.00021-8

Umar, R. A., Zahary, M. N., Rohin, M. A. K., & Ismail, S. (2018). Chemical composition and the potential biological activities of Piper betel–a Review. *Malaysian Journal of Applied Sciences, 3*(1), 1–8.

UNCTAD. (2005). Market brief: Adansonia digitata. *United Nations Conference on Trade and Development.*

Ungvari, Z., Menyhart, O., Lehoczki, A., Fekete, M., Fazekas-Pongor, V., Ocana, A., Varga, P., & Győrffy, B. (2025). NRF2 pathway activation predicts poor prognosis in lung cancer: A cautionary note on antioxidant interventions. *GeroScience*. Advance online publication. DOI: 10.1007/s11357-025-01736-0 PMID: 40537696

Unuofin, J. O., Masuku, N. P., Paimo, O. K., & Lebelo, S. L. (2021). Ginger from Farmyard to Town: Nutritional and Pharmacological Applications. *Frontiers in Pharmacology, 12*, 779352. Advance online publication. DOI: 10.3389/fphar.2021.779352 PMID: 34899343

Upton, R., David, B., Gafner, S., & Glasl, S. (2020). Botanical ingredient identification and quality assessment: Strengths and limitations of analytical techniques. *Phytochemistry Reviews, 19*(5), 1157–1177. DOI: 10.1007/s11101-019-09625-z

Usmani, J., Wasim, M., Ansari, M. N., Hassan, M. J., Sharma, M., & Ahmad, R. (2023). Potential therapeutic effect of Carica papaya leaves extract on immune response, biochemical and hematological mechanisms on cecal ligation and puncture model of sepsis in rats: an in vivo study. *3 Biotech*, 13(5), 151, 1–17. https://doi.org/ DOI: 10.1007/S13205-023-03567-2/METRICS

Valle-Algarra, F. M., Mateo-Castro, R., Mateo, E. M., Gimeno-Adelantado, J. V., & Jiménez, M. (2014). MYCOTOXINS | Detection and Analysis by Classical Techniques. In Batt, C. A., & Tortorello, M. L. (Eds.), *Encyclopedia of Food Microbiology* (2nd ed., pp. 862–868). Academic Press. DOI: 10.1016/B978-0-12-384730-0.00232-9

Valotto Neto, L. J., Reverete de Araujo, M., Moretti, R. C.Junior, Mendes Machado, N., Joshi, R. K., Dos Santos Buglio, D., Barbalho Lamas, C., Direito, R., Fornari Laurindo, L., Tanaka, M., & Barbalho, S. M. (2024). Investigating the Neuroprotective and Cognitive-Enhancing Effects of *Bacopa monnieri*: A Systematic Review Focused on Inflammation, Oxidative Stress, Mitochondrial Dysfunction, and Apoptosis. *Antioxidants*, *13*(4), 393. DOI: 10.3390/antiox13040393 PMID: 38671841

Van der Merwe, J., De Beer, D., Joubert, E., & Gelderblom, W. (2015). Short-Term and Sub-Chronic Dietary Exposure to Aspalathin-Enriched Green Rooibos (Aspalathus linearis) Extract Affects Rat Liver Function and Antioxidant Status. *Molecules (Basel, Switzerland)*, *20*(12), 22674–22690. DOI: 10.3390/molecules201219868 PMID: 26694346

Van Wyk, B. E., & Gericke, N. (2000). *People's plants: A guide to useful plants of Southern Africa*. Briza Publications.

VanderJagt, D., Hunsaker, L., Otimenyin, S. O., & Uguru, M. O. (2022). The anti-inflammatory activities of twelve Nigerian medicinal plants: Inhibition of NfkB, activation of Nrf2, and antioxidant content. *African Journal of Biochemistry Research*, *16*(1), 1–10.

Vertuani, S., Braccioli, E., Buzzoni, V., & Manfredini, S. (2002). Antioxidant capacity of *Adansonia digitata* fruit pulp and leaves. *Acta Phytotherapeutica*, *86*(2), 2–7.

Vieira, S., Tessaro, L., Lima, O., Velloso, S., & Conte-Junior, A. (2023). Recent progress in nanotechnology improving the therapeutic potential of polyphenols for cancer. *Nutrients*, *15*(14), 3136. DOI: 10.3390/nu15143136

Vikrama Chakravarthi, P., Murugesan, S., Arivuchelvan, A., Sukumar, K., Arulmozhi, A., & Jagadeeswaran, A. (2022). Therapeutic antigout and antioxidant activity of Piper betle L. in gout-induced broilers. *British Poultry Science*, *63*(3), 324–331. DOI: 10.1080/00071668.2021.1998365 PMID: 34859728

Vimukthi, W. P. D., Dong, S., Yang, C., Zhang, Y., Baikeri, G., Lou, T., Deng, F., Li, Z., & Cao, F. (2025). Enhancing DTT assays for reactive oxygen species detection in atmospheric particulate matter: Key factors and methodological insights. *Environmental Science: Atmospheres*, *5*(8), 865–878. DOI: 10.1039/D4EA00158C

Vincent, P. (2018). A descriptive cross-sectional study on various uses and outcomes of *Garcinia kola* among people in Oshimili North, Delta State, Nigeria. *International Quarterly Journal of Research in Ayurveda*, p. 25.

Virameteekul, S., Revesz, T., Jaunmuktane, Z., Warner, T. T., & De Pablo-Fernández, E. (2023). Clinical Diagnostic Accuracy of Parkinson's Disease: Where Do We Stand? *Movement Disorders*, *38*(4), 558–566. DOI: 10.1002/mds.29317 PMID: 36602274

Vladu, F., Ficai, D., Ene, G., & Ficai, A. (2022). Combination therapy using polyphenols. *International Journal of Molecular Sciences*, *23*(18), 10244. DOI: 10.3390/ijms231810244

Vongsak, B., Mangmool, S., & Gritsanapan, W. (2015). Antioxidant Activity and Induction of mRNA Expressions of Antioxidant Enzymes in HEK-293 Cells of Moringa oleifera Leaf Extract. *Planta Medica*, *81*(12/13), 1084–1089. DOI: 10.1055/s-0035-1546168 PMID: 26166137

Wadowski, P., Juszczak, M., & Woźniak, K. (2024). NRF2 modulators of plant origin and their ability to overcome multidrug resistance in cancers. *International Journal of Molecular Sciences*, *25*(21), 11500. DOI: 10.3390/ijms252111500 PMID: 39519053

Wagner, H., & Efferth, T. (2017). Introduction: Novel hybrid combinations containing synthetic or antibiotic drugs with plant-derived phenolic or terpenoid compounds. *Phytomedicine*, *37*, 1–3. DOI: 10.1016/j.phymed.2017.10.020 PMID: 29174652

Wallace, M. A. G., & McCord, J. P. (2020). Chapter 16 - High-resolution mass spectrometry. In J. Beauchamp, C. Davis, & J. Pleil (Eds.), *Breathborne Biomarkers and the Human Volatilome* (2nd ed., pp. 253-270). Elsevier.

Wan Y. D., Zang Y. D. & Wang J. S. (1992). Studies on the antimalarial action of gelatin capsule of *Artemisia annua*. Zongguo ji sheng chong xue yu ji sheng chong bing za shi (*Chinese Journal of Parasitology and Parasitic Diseases*). 10:290–294.

Wang, H., Guo, M., Wei, H., Liu, J., Xie, Z., Ma, Y., Yu, J., & He, J. (2023). Targeting p53 pathways. *Signal Transduction and Targeted Therapy*, *8*(1), 92. DOI: 10.1038/s41392-023-01347-1

Wang, J., Chen, X., & Liu, Y. (2022). Biological network properties in drug action: Redundancy, feedback regulation, and crosstalk. *Pharmacological Research*, *175*, 105–112.

Wang, J., Xiao, M., Wang, J., Wang, S., Zhang, J., Guo, Y., Tang, Y., & Gu, J. (2021). NRF2-related epigenetic modifications in cardiac and vascular complications of diabetes mellitus. *Frontiers in Endocrinology*, *12*, 598005. DOI: 10.3389/fendo.2021.598005 PMID: 34248833

Wang, M., Jiang, S., Zhou, L., Yu, F., Ding, H., Li, P., Zhou, M., & Wang, K. (2019). Potential mechanisms of action of curcumin for cancer prevention. *International Journal of Biological Sciences*, *15*(6), 1200–1214. DOI: 10.7150/ijbs.33710

Wang, Q., Song, H., Dong, H., Guo, S., Yao, M., Wan, Y., & Lu, K. (2025). Multiphase Radical Chemical Processes Induced by Air Pollutants and the Associated Health Effects. *Environment & Health*, *3*(1), 1–13. DOI: 10.1021/envhealth.4c00157 PMID: 39839244

Wang, Y.-K., Li, W. Q., Xia, S., Guo, L., Miao, Y., & Zhang, B.-K. (2021). Metabolic activation of the toxic natural products from herbal and dietary supplements leading to toxicities. *Frontiers in Pharmacology*, *12*, 758468. DOI: 10.3389/fphar.2021.758468 PMID: 34744736

Wang, Y., & Wang, J. (2020). Modelling and prediction of global non-communicable diseases. *BMC Public Health*, *20*(1), 822. DOI: 10.1186/s12889-020-08890-4 PMID: 32487173

Warias, P., Plewa, P., & Poniewierska-Baran, A. (2024). Resveratrol, piceatannol, curcumin, and quercetin as therapeutic targets in gastric cancer. *Molecules (Basel, Switzerland)*, *30*(1), 3. DOI: 10.3390/molecules30010003

Watt, J. M., & Breyer-Brandwijk, M. G. (1962). The medicinal and poisonous plants of Southern and Eastern Africa (2nd ed.). E. and S. Livingstone.

Wei, W. J., Tan, S. B., Guo, T., Wang, Y., & Chang, J. (2021). Chemical Constituents of the Fresh Rhizome of Zingiber officinale. *Chemistry of Natural Compounds*, *57*(5), 968–969. DOI: 10.1007/s10600-021-03526-4

Weremfo, A., Abassah-Oppong, S., Adulley, F., Dabie, K., & Seidu-Larry, S. (2023). Response surface methodology as a tool to optimize the extraction of bioactive compounds from plant sources. *Journal of the Science of Food and Agriculture*, *103*(1), 26–36. DOI: 10.1002/jsfa.12121

Whirl-Carrillo, M., McDonagh, E. M., Hebert, J. M., Gong, L., Sangkuhl, K., Thorn, C. F., & Klein, T. E. (2021). Pharmacogenomics knowledge for personalized medicine: PharmGKB update. *Clinical Pharmacology and Therapeutics*, *110*(3), 563–573. DOI: 10.1002/cpt.2350

WHO. (2003). *WHO guidelines on good agricultural and collection practices (GACP) for medicinal plants*. World Health Organization.

Wickens, G. E. (1982). *The baobab tree*. African Publishing Company.

Wickens, G. E., & Lowe, P. (2008). *The baobabs: Pachycauls of Africa*. Springer., DOI: 10.1007/978-1-4020-6431-9

Wishart, D. S., Cheng, L. L., Copi, V., Edison, A. S., Eghbalnia, H. R., Hoch, J. C., Gouveia, G. J., Pathmasiri, W., Powers, R., Schock, T. B., Sumner, L. W., & Uchimiya, M. (2022). NMR and Metabolomics-A Roadmap for the Future. *Metabolites, 12*(8), 678. DOI: 10.3390/metabo12080678 PMID: 35893244

World Health Organisation, Regional Office for Africa. (2023, August). Nigeria – Country Disease Outlook. WHO Regional Office for Africa.

World Health Organization. (2025, February 3). [Fact sheet]. *Cancer.*

Wright, C. W., Linley, P. A., Brun, R., Wittlin, S., & Hsu, E. (2010). Ancient Chinese methods are remarkably effective for the preparation of artemisinin-rich extracts of Qing Hao with potent antimalarial activity. *Molecules (Basel, Switzerland), 15*(2), 804–812. DOI: 10.3390/molecules15020804 PMID: 20335947

Wu, F., Huang, H., Chiu, Y., Cherng, H., Sheu, T., & Yang, Y. (2022). Curcumin induces apoptosis of chemoresistant lung cancer cells via ROS-regulated p38 MAPK phosphorylation. *International Journal of Molecular Sciences, 23*(15), 8248. DOI: 10.3390/ijms23158248

Xiao, J. L., Liu, H. Y., Sun, C. C., & Tang, C. F. (2024). Regulation of Keap1-Nrf2 signalling in health and diseases. *Molecular Biology Reports, 51*(1), 809. DOI: 10.1007/s11033-024-09771-4 PMID: 39001962

Xiao, J., Chen, D., & Zhang, L. (2025). Systems pharmacology approaches to polypharmacology of natural products. *Pharmacological Research, 190*, 106–118.

Xie, J. (2022). Will the role of Indigenous Knowledge Systems help in sustaining the utilization and conservation of indigenous medicinal plants? *Planta Medica, 88*(15), 1437. Advance online publication. DOI: 10.1055/s-0042-1759002

Xie, J., Li, Y., & Xu, Z. (2016). Signal transduction pathways: Mechanisms and therapeutic targets. *Cell Communication and Signaling : CCS, 14*(1), 40–52.

Xiong, R. G., Huang, S. Y., Wu, S. X., Zhou, D. D., Yang, Z. J., Saimaiti, A., Zhao, C.-N., Shang, A., Zhang, Y.-J., Gan, R.-Y., & Li, H. B. (2022). Anticancer effects and mechanisms of berberine from medicinal herbs: An update review. *Molecules (Basel, Switzerland), 27*(14), 4523. DOI: 10.3390/molecules27144523 PMID: 35889396

Xu, J., & Gaquerel, E. (2025). Plant defense responses under biotic stress: Gene expression and secondary metabolite regulation. *Trends in Plant Science, 30*(2), 145–158.

Xu, J., Li, Y., & Wang, J. (2024). Berberine enhances glucose uptake in metabolic disorders: Molecular docking and pharmacological insights. *Metabolism: Clinical and Experimental*, *145*, 112–120.

Yada, D., Sivakkumar, T., & Srinivas, N. (2021). Aqueous Extract of Hyptis suaveolens Whole Plant Inhibits Carrageenan-Induced Paw Edema in Rats. *Advances in Pharmacology and Pharmacy*, *9*(3), 75–80. DOI: 10.13189/app.2021.090305

Yadav, N., Chandel, S. S., Venkatachalam, T., & Fathima, S. N. (2023). *Herbal Medicine Formulation, Standardization, and Commercialization Challenges and Sustainable Strategies for Improvement.* Springer International Publishing., DOI: 10.1007/978-3-031-21973-3_40-1

Yagishita, Y., Gatbonton-Schwager, T. N., McCallum, M. L., & Kensler, T. W. (2020). Current landscape of NRF2 biomarkers in clinical trials. *Antioxidants*, *9*(8), 716. DOI: 10.3390/antiox9080716 PMID: 32784785

Yang, H., Chen, J., & Zhang, L. (2020). Synergistic modulation of biological pathways by multi-target drugs. *Pharmacological Research*, *156*, 104–112.

Yang, Q. Q., & Zhou, J. W. (2019). Neuroinflammation in the central nervous system: Symphony of glial cells. *Glia*, *67*(6), 1017–1035. DOI: 10.1002/glia.23571 PMID: 30548343

Yang, R., Zhang, J., Li, J., Qin, R., Chen, J., Wang, R., Goltzman, D., & Miao, D. (2022). Inhibition of Nrf2 degradation alleviates age-related osteoporosis induced by 1,25-Dihydroxyvitamin D deficiency. *Free Radical Biology & Medicine*, *178*, 246–261. DOI: 10.1016/j.freeradbiomed.2021.12.010 PMID: 34890768

Yan, X., David, S. D., Du, G., Li, W., Liang, D., Nie, S., Ge, M., Wang, C., Qiao, J., Li, Y., & Caiyin, Q. (2024). Biological properties of sandalwood oil and microbial synthesis of its major sesquiterpenoids. *Biomolecules*, *14*(8), 971. DOI: 10.3390/biom14080971 PMID: 39199359

Yee, S. B., & Roth, R. A. (2018). Pyrrolizidine alkaloid-induced hepatotoxicity. In McQueen, C. A. (Ed.), *Comprehensive Toxicology* (3rd ed., pp. 522–537). Elsevier. DOI: 10.1016/B978-0-12-801238-3.02114-0

Yeshi, K., Crayn, D., Ritmejerytė, E., & Wangchuk, P. (2022). Plant Secondary Metabolites Produced in Response to Abiotic Stresses Has Potential Application in Pharmaceutical Product Development. *Molecules (Basel, Switzerland)*, *27*(1), 313. DOI: 10.3390/molecules27010313 PMID: 35011546

Yin, F., Song, Z., He, Z., Qin, B., John, G. F., Zhang, L., & Guo, D. A. (2022). Chemical fingerprinting and characterization of spilled oils and burnt soot particles - a case study on the Sanchi oil tanker collision in the East China Sea. *The Science of the Total Environment*, *824*, 153896. DOI: 10.1016/j.scitotenv.2022.153896 PMID: 35182621

Yin, J., Zhang, H., & Ye, J. (2012). Berberine in diabetes and cholesterol management: Mechanisms and clinical evidence. *Metabolism: Clinical and Experimental*, *61*(5), 706–713.

Yuan, H., Ma, Q., Ye, L., & Piao, G. (2016). The traditional medicine and modern medicine from natural products. *Molecules (Basel, Switzerland)*, *21*(5), 559. DOI: 10.3390/molecules21050559 PMID: 27136524

Yu, F., Wang, Y., Stetler, A. R., Leak, R. K., Hu, X., & Chen, J. (2022). Phagocytic microglia and macrophages in brain injury and repair. *CNS Neuroscience & Therapeutics*, *28*(9), 1279–1293. DOI: 10.1111/cns.13899 PMID: 35751629

Yusuf, K., Aykut, P., Zemzem, O., & Neslihan, P. (2019). Herbal drug usage habits of patients attending Balcali Hospital of Cukurova University. *Turkish Journal of Family Medicine and Primary Care*, *13*(4), 457–461. DOI: 10.21763/tjfmpc.651395

Yusuf, M. A., & Eze, C. N. (2025). Network pharmacology modeling of Vernonia amygdalina flavonoids in oxidative stress pathways. *African Journal of Traditional, Complementary, and Alternative Medicines : AJTCAM*, *22*(1), 45–56.

Zargaran, A. (2024). Ethnopharmacology, generations experience for the future of pharmacy and medicine. *Journal of Drug Research in Ayurvedic Sciences*, *9*(2), 58–59. DOI: 10.4103/jdras.jdras_105_24

Zarmouh, N. O., Eyunni, S. K., & Soliman, K. F. (2017). The Benzopyrone Biochanin-A as a reversible, competitive, and selective monoamine oxidase B inhibitor. *BMC Complementary and Alternative Medicine*, *17*(1), 34. DOI: 10.1186/s12906-016-1525-y PMID: 28069007

Zeki, Ö. C., Eylem, C. C., Reçber, T., Kır, S., & Nemutlu, E. (2020). Integration of GC–MS and LC–MS for untargeted metabolomics profiling. *Journal of Pharmaceutical and Biomedical Analysis*, *190*, 113509. DOI: 10.1016/j.jpba.2020.113509 PMID: 32814263

Zhang, C. L., Han, Q. W., Chen, N. H., & Yuan, Y. H. (2021). Research on developing drugs for Parkinson's disease. *Brain Research Bulletin*, *168*, 100–109. DOI: 10.1016/j.brainresbull.2020.12.017 PMID: 33387636

Zhang, D. (2025). Exploring the versatile world of magnolias: Urban landscape enhancement and metabolite applications in drug discovery and cosmetics. *Discover Plants*, *2*(1), 139. DOI: 10.1007/s44372-025-00216-1

Zhang, H., Chen, L., & Wang, Y. (2021). Transition metal-mediated oxidative stress in environmental pollution. *Ecotoxicology and Environmental Safety*, *218*, 112295. DOI: 10.1016/j.ecoenv.2021.112295

Zhang, J., Onakpoya, I. J., Posadzki, P., & Eddouks, M. (2015). The safety of herbal medicine: From prejudice to evidence. *Evidence-Based Complementary and Alternative Medicine : eCAM*, *2015*, 316706. DOI: 10.1155/2015/316706 PMID: 25838831

Zhang, L., Chen, D., & Xiao, J. (2024). Artificial intelligence in phytochemical research: Predicting synergistic effects. *Phytomedicine*, *115*, 112–120.

Zhang, L., Chen, D., & Xiao, J. (2024). Network pharmacology analysis of quercetin in traditional medicine research. *Briefings in Bioinformatics*, *20*(5), 1614–1627.

Zhang, L., & Ma, Q. (2024). Gut microbiota biotransformation of phytochemicals and implications for bioavailability. *Frontiers in Pharmacology*, *15*, 112–124.

Zhang, M., Viennois, E., Prasad, M., Zhang, Y., Wang, L., Zhang, Z., Han, M. K., Xiao, B., Xu, C., Srinivasan, S., & Merlin, D. (2016). Edible ginger-derived nanoparticles: A novel therapeutic approach for the prevention and treatment of inflammatory bowel disease and colitis-associated cancer. *Biomaterials*, *101*, 321–340. DOI: 10.1016/j.biomaterials.2016.06.018 PMID: 27318094

Zhang, R., Zhu, X., Bai, H., & Ning, K. (2019). Network pharmacology databases for traditional medicine research: Bridging bioactivity and disease modules. *Briefings in Bioinformatics*, *20*(5), 1614–1627.

Zhang, S., DiMango, E., Zhu, Y., Saroya, T. K., Emala, C. W., & Sang, S. (2022). Pharmacokinetics of Gingerols, Shogaols, and Their Metabolites in Asthma Patients. *Journal of Agricultural and Food Chemistry*, *70*(31), 9674–9683. DOI: 10.1021/acs.jafc.2c03150 PMID: 35916113

Zhang, W., & Lim, L. Y. (2008). Effects of spice constituents on P-glycoprotein-mediated transport and CYP3A4-mediated metabolism in vitro. *Drug Metabolism and Disposition: the Biological Fate of Chemicals*, *36*(7), 1283–1290. DOI: 10.1124/dmd.107.019737 PMID: 18385293

Zhang, W., Yan, Y., Wu, Y., Yang, H., Zhu, P., Yan, F., Zhao, R., Tian, P., Wang, T., Fan, Q., & Su, Z. (2022). Medicinal herbs for the treatment of anxiety: A systematic review and network meta-analysis. *Pharmacological Research*, *179*, 106204. DOI: 10.1016/j.phrs.2022.106204 PMID: 35378276

Zhang, X., Qian, J. W., Wei, B. T., & Zhang, B. (2025). Flavonoids as Modulators of Nrf2 Signalling Pathway in Alleviating Cisplatin-Induced Organ Toxicity. *Yangtze Medicine*, *9*(1), 52–77. DOI: 10.4236/ym.2025.91006

Zhang, Y., Zhang, Z., Mousavi, M., Moliani, A., Bahman, Y., & Bagheri, H. (2023). Resveratrol inhibits glioblastoma cells. *Chemico-Biological Interactions*, *376*, 110409. DOI: 10.1016/j.cbi.2023.110409

Zhao, C., Wu, S., & Wang, H. (2025). Medicinal Plant Extracts Targeting UV-Induced Skin Damage: Molecular Mechanisms and Therapeutic Potential. *International Journal of Molecular Sciences*, *26*(5), 2278. DOI: 10.3390/ijms26052278 PMID: 40076896

Zhao, Y., Wang, J., & Li, X. (2018). Indirect modulation of biological pathways by drugs: Mechanisms and implications. *Pharmacology & Therapeutics*, *191*, 76–84. DOI: 10.1016/j.pharmthera.2017.07.004

Zhong, J., Xing, D., Dong, Y., Chen, Y., Liu, N., Wang, M., & Zheng, P. (2024). Progress in the study of curcumin metabolism *in vivo*. *Journal of Asian Natural Products Research*, *27*(5), 639–657. DOI: 10.1080/10286020.2024.2420619

Zhou, H., Zheng, B., & McClements, D. J. (2021). In vitro gastrointestinal stability of lipophilic polyphenols. *Journal of Agricultural and Food Chemistry*, *69*(11), 3340–3350. DOI: 10.1021/acs.jafc.0c07578

Zhou, Q., Lin, J., & Yu, S. (2023). NADPH oxidase activation and pollutant-induced ROS: Molecular mechanisms and health effects. *Free Radical Biology & Medicine*, *197*, 49–61. DOI: 10.1016/j.freeradbiomed.2023.02.013

Zhou, Y., Zhou, B., Pache, L., Chang, M., Khodabakhshi, A. H., Tanaseichuk, O., Benner, C., & Chanda, S. K. (2020). Metascape provides a biologist-oriented resource for the analysis of systems-level datasets. *Nature Communications*, *11*(1), 1523. DOI: 10.1038/s41467-019-09234-6

Zhu, F., Li, Y., Zhang, Y., & Chen, Y. (2019). Network pharmacology in drug discovery: Understanding receptor-ligand interactions in complex biological systems. *Nature Reviews. Drug Discovery*, *18*(2), 112–125.

Zhu, H., Liu, W., Tian, B., Liu, H., & Ning, S. (2011). Inhibition of Quorum Sensing in the Opportunistic Pathogenic Bacterium Chromobacterium violaceum by an Extract from Fruiting Bodies of Lingzhi or Reishi Medicinal Mushroom, Ganoderma lucidum (W.Curt.:Fr.) P. Karst. (Higher Basidiomycetes). *International Journal of Medicinal Mushrooms*, *13*(6), 559–564. DOI: 10.1615/IntJMedMushr.v13.i6.80 PMID: 22181844

Zughaibi, T. A., Suhail, M., Tarique, M., & Tabrez, S. (2021). Targeting PI3K/Akt/mTOR pathway by different flavonoids. *International Journal of Molecular Sciences*, *22*(22), 12455. DOI: 10.3390/ijms222212455

About the Contributors

Olubunmi Atolani, (Associate Professor), is a Natural Products and Medicinal Chemist with many years of teaching and research experience in the University system. He obtained his PhD in Chemistry (2013) from the University of Ilorin, Ilorin Nigeria, investigating/synthesizing and characterising the anti-cancer, antioxidant and cytotoxicity potentials of the bioactives and derivatized principles from a novel medicinal African folklore using various techniques of chromatography, spectroscopy and spectrometry. He did part his doctoral work at the International Center for Chemical and Biological Sciences, ICCBS, University of Karachi, Karachi and postdoctoral studies at Charité University of medicine, Berlin, Germany and COMSAT, Abbotabbad Pakistan. His current research interest besides bioactives exploration and spectroscopic characterization lies in medicinal Chemistry, Chemoinformatic applications of tools for drug discovery in cancer, diabetes, malaria and infection conditions as well as green cosmeceuticals exploration (from underutilised tropical plants). He is currently an investigator in various research groups and he has won many international, national and institutional competitive scientific research grants, awards such as Deutsche Forschungsgemeinschaft-Germany, UNESCO, TWAS-DFG, TWAS-CIIT, Seeding Labs Equipment grant (USA), European Association of Cancer Researcher (EACR), TETFund-IBR Raw Material grants etc. He has been a speaker at many national and international academic research forums. He has authored over one hundred (100) peer-reviewed journal articles (scopus-indexed majority), academic books, several book chapters and delivered numerous plenaries and conference keynote addresses. He is a respected seasoned reviewer to many reputable Journals in Nature, Elsevier, Springer, Taylor and Francis Wiley etc. He was the pioneer managing editor of Annals of Science and Technology published by De Gruyter/SCIENDO in Europe and an editorial board member of various international scientific journals. His research outputs and acumen has been presented in many local and international research scientific forums in Nigeria, Germany, Luxembourg, Netherlands, Ghana,

South Africa, Gambia, Niger Republic, Kenya and United State of America (USA) etc. He is an external examiner and distinguished research assessor at University of KwaZulu Natal, UKZN, South Africa, Cape Peninsula University of Technology, CPUT, South Africa, National Research Fund, Mexico, National Research Fund, South Africa among others. He is the Desk Officer of three universities in Asia and Africa and Contact person for some University' partners in Brazil, Germany and Pakistan. He is a member of reputable national and international professional and academic bodies such as American Chemical Society (ACS), European Association of Cancer Researcher (EACR), Royal Society of Chemistry (RSC), Institute of Chartered Chemist of Nigeria, (ICCON), Chemical Society of Nigeria (CSN), Nigerian Young Academy (NYA) etc. He is currently a faculty at the University of Ilorin, Ilorin, Nigeria where he passionately supervises both undergraduate and postgraduate students. As a dynamic researcher and frontiers of knowledge, he seeks to contribute optimally solving global issues for the attainment of the Sustainable Development Goals (SDGs). He was an Assistant Director at the Centre for International Education (CIE), and currently the Deputy Director (Research), at the Centre for Research Development and In-House Training (CREDIT) both at the University of Ilorin, Nigeria. He is the Coordinator of the African Centre for Herbal Research, Ilorin (ACHRI).

Learnmore Kambizi attained his BSc degree from Cuba in 1998 before enrolling for Masters and PhD degrees at the University of Fort Hare which he completed in 2004. His PhD focused on Ethnobotanical studies of plants used for the treatment of sexually transmitted infections in South Africa. He went on to pursue a postdoctoral fellowship within the fields of Ethnobotany & Phytomedicine. He was as a Lecturer at the University of Zimbabwe in 2005, University of the Free State, South Africa in 2007 and Walter Sisulu University as a Senior lecturer until 2011. He moved to Cape Peninsula University of Technology, South Africa where he is now a Full Professor of Botany. In his academic journey to date, he has hosted 4 postdoctoral fellows and supervised 7 PhD, 16 master's and numerous Honours students. In addition, he has edited and published books, numerous articles in peer reviewed journals and presented at many national and international conferences. He recently edited a book titled "Food Security and Nutrition: Utilizing Undervalued Food Plants". He is a South African National Research Foundation rated researcher. He also collaborates with Traditional Medical Practitioners in conjuction with the South African Research Council as an advisor. In 2015, Prof Kambizi was appointed the first Director of African Centre for Herbal Research based in Nigeria, a position he holds to date.

***

Modinah Abdul Raheem is a renowned scholar in Physical and Environmental Chemistry, currently serving as a Professor and Head of the Department of Chemistry at the University of Ilorin. With over two decades of academic and research experience, she has built a distinguished career exploring the intersection of indigenous knowledge systems and modern scientific methodologies. Her research focuses on phytochemicals, atmospheric and indoor pollution, computational modeling, and multitargeted disease mitigation through ecochemical interface studies. She is particularly known for integrating African folklore-derived constituents with advanced techniques such as Density Functional Theory (DFT) and molecular docking, contributing to innovative approaches in public health and environmental sustainability. Prof. Abdul Raheem holds a Ph.D. in Chemistry from the University of Ilorin, an M.Sc. a Postgraduate Diploma in Education and B.Sc. in Chemistry from the University of Ibadan. She teaches both undergraduate and postgraduate courses, mentoring students across disciplines including chemistry, biochemistry, pharmacy, and veterinary medicine. Her scholarly work has been published in leading journals such as ACS Omega, Environmental Modeling & Assessment, and Bulletin of the Chemical Society of Ethiopia. She has presented at numerous international conferences and collaborates actively with research institutions across Nigeria. A fellow of the Institute of Chartered Chemists of Nigeria (ICCON), Prof. Abdul Raheem is committed to advancing scientific knowledge that is both locally relevant and globally impactful. Her dedication to education, research, and community engagement continues to inspire a new generation of scientists.

Halimat Amin Abdulrahim is a respected biochemist and medical educator at the University of Ilorin, Nigeria. With a Ph.D. in Biochemistry and additional qualifications in Health Planning and Management, she specializes in neurometabolism, nutrition, phytotherapy, and toxicology. Her research spans clinical biochemistry, oxidative stress, and therapeutic interventions for metabolic and neurodegenerative disorders. She has co-authored multiple peer-reviewed publications on topics such as vitamin D and metformin synergy, diabetes-induced gonadotoxicity, and natural product pharmacology. Dr. Abdulrahim teaches across undergraduate and postgraduate programs in medicine, anatomy, physiology, nursing, and medical laboratory sciences. She is affiliated with professional bodies including the Medical and Dental Council of Nigeria (MDCN) and the Medical Women's Association of Nigeria (MWAN).

Emmanuel Tolulope Adegoke is a scholar at the department of Medical Laboratory Science majoring in Histopathology at the University of Ilorin, Nigeria. His research interests focus on neurotoxicology, environmental pathology, metabolic disorders, immunohistochemistry, and plant-derived therapeutics. He has co-authored recent papers including Histopathological Perspectives on Toxic Environmental Pollutants: Cellular Damage Pathways and Strategic Interventions in Mammalian Systems, and experimental studies on the protective roles of Rauwolfia vomitoria and Aframomum melegueta in the brain and other organs in models of type 2 diabetes, cadmium toxicity, and oxidative damage. A member of the Dr. Adeniyi Research team, Emmanuel aspires to advance translational research in toxicological and neurodegenerative pathology while integrating clinical expertise in diagnostic histopathology and leveraging digital technologies to bridge laboratory discoveries with improved patient care.

Mariam Dasola Adeoye is a distinguished scholar in Physical and Computational Chemistry, currently serving as a full professor and Dean at Fountain University, Osogbo. Her research focuses on the chemical modification of natural compounds, particularly furan derivatives, for applications in antimicrobial therapy, dye production, and wood protection. She has co-authored scientific chapters and journal articles exploring the synthesis and bioactivity of compounds derived from agricultural waste, such as furfural, showcasing their potential in sustainable chemistry and public health. Her work bridges experimental chemistry with computational modeling, contributing to innovative solutions in chemical sciences. Prof. Adeoye's promotion to full professorship marks a significant milestone in advancing female representation in Nigerian academia. She continues to inspire students and researchers through her teaching, mentorship, and commitment to scientific excellence.

OS Adeyemi is a professor of biochemistry, with a research focus on medicinal biochemistry, and toxicology. Currently, OS Adeyemi is a faculty member at Bowen University, Nigeria, where he teaches biochemistry to undergraduate and postgraduate classes. OS Adeyemi, a scholar and passionate academic mentor, believes that teaching, research, and community service have a significant impact on people's lives and he has successfully supervised several undergraduate and postgraduate students in the biochemistry program both within and outside of Nigeria. In addition, he encourages and supports academic strategies that could foster academic excellence. In particular, his research engagements have contributed to efforts aimed at identifying novel treatment strategies through medicinal and toxicological evaluation of natural and synthetic molecules. OS Adeyemi has over 150 research publications, comprising articles, books, and chapters in books. On several occasions, he has served as an external assessor and/or examiner for PhD or professorial appointments to universities within and outside of Nigeria, and he enjoys the membership of several professional and academic bodies. OS Adeyemi is a recipient of several awards and fellowships, among which are the NRF Postdoctoral

Fellowships at Rhodes University, South Africa (2012); the Rhodes University Postdoctoral Fellowship, South Africa (2013); the TWAS/CNPQ Fellowship, Brazil (2015); and the JSPS Fellowship, Japan (2015 and 2020). He is an expert reviewer for several grant awarding bodies, such as the NRF (National Research Foundation, South Africa) and RSTMH (Royal Society of Tropical Medicine and Hygiene, UK), as well as many academic journals. In addition, OS Adeyemi serves on the editorial board of several academic journals, such as Scientific Reports, BMC Complementary Medicine & Therapies, and PLOS ONE, among others. For extracurricular activities, OS Adeyemi engages in educational and church outreaches, and he likes to play chess.

Taye Alawode holds a PhD in Organic Chemistry (Natural Products Chemistry option) from the Federal University of Technology, Akure. His research focuses on the isolation, characterization, and biological evaluation of bioactive compounds from Nigerian medicinal plants. He is particularly interested in identifying compounds with therapeutic potential for the treatment of cancer and infectious diseases.

Adinarayana Andy is a dedicated Pharmacy Manager with extensive experience in pharmacy management and drug discovery research. Licensed in Michigan and Ohio, Andy has accumulated over 16 years of experience working at independent pharmacies, leading national drugstore chains, and in pharmaceutical research organizations. His expertise includes navigating complex state and federal requirements, enhancing pharmacy performance metrics, and delivering patient-centered care. Education: Master of Business Administration (Project Management): University of the Cumberlands, Kentucky, USA (2017) Doctor of Philosophy (Biotechnology): Acharya Nagarjuna University, Guntur, India (2012) Master of Pharmacy (Pharmaceutical Analysis and Quality Assurance): Berhampur University, Orissa, India (2004) Bachelor of Pharmacy: Andhra University, Vishakhapatnam, India (2002) Licenses Michigan Pharmacist License Michigan Controlled Substance License Ohio Pharmacist License

B. Revathi is Head of the Department and Associate Professor of Pharmacology at QIS College of Pharmacy, Ongole, Andhra Pradesh, India. She earned her Ph.D. in Pharmacology from Jawaharlal Nehru Technological University, Kakinada (JNTUK) in 2021, investigating the neurotoxicity of food additives under the guidance of Dr. Sujatha, NIPER Hyderabad. She holds an M.Pharm in Pharmacology from Hindu College of Pharmacy, Guntur, affiliated with Acharya Nagarjuna University, where she graduated first in her class. With over 12 years of academic and research experience, Dr. Revathi has taught and trained undergraduate, postgraduate, and

Pharm.D students in pharmacology, clinical pharmacokinetics, and related biomedical sciences. Her scholarly contributions include authorship of three textbooks, multiple book chapters, more than 20 research and review publications in Scopus and Web of Science–indexed journals, and six patents (including innovations in AI-based pharmaceutical devices, nanoformulations, and herbal compositions). She has also presented her work at international forums such as the International Pharmaceutical Federation (FIP) congress. Her research spans marine-derived drugs, behavioral neurotoxicology, plant-derived antimicrobials, pharmacogenomics applications, and in silico pharmacology. Recognized as an active leader in professional bodies, she serves as State Women Forum Co-Coordinator for the Indian Pharmacy Graduates Association (IPGA) and Zonal Coordinator for the Association of Pharmaceutical Teachers of India (APTI). A frequent speaker, evaluator, and convener for national and international scientific events, Dr. Revathi is committed to advancing pharmacy education, promoting evidence-based practice, and mentoring the next generation of pharmacists and researchers.

Bùi Thanh Tùng is a highly distinguished scholar specializing in Pharmaceutical Science. He possesses a strong international academic background, having earned a Ph.D. in Pharmacology from Seville University, Spain, and a Master's degree in Pharmaceutical Science from Chosun University, South Korea. Prof. Tùng is proficient in both English and Spanish. His primary research focuses on the evaluation of pharmacological effects, mechanisms of action, and molecular-level toxicity of medicinal materials and natural compounds. A core aspect of his work involves virtual screening of natural compounds with potent pharmacological activity for potential drug development. Prof. Tùng has made substantial contributions to the field, evidenced by his 149 published scientific reports, including 49 articles featured in prestigious international journals. He also holds 8 registered patents or utility solutions. His significant scientific output was formally recognized with the VNU-Hanoi Science and Technology Award in 2018.

Garuba Aishat Hormowumi is a scholar at the department of Plant and Environmental Biology, Kwara State University. She is dedicated to academic excellence, research, and community impact.

Chhan Kalita is a Doctoral Research Scholar in the Biological Product Laboratory (BPL), Dept. of Botany, Mizoram University (A central university, accredited as Gr-A+ by NAAC). Earlier, He was associated with two Department of Biotechnology-sponsored major research projects in the Dept of Botany, Mizoram University, Mizoram, and B.P Chaliha College, Assam, respectively. He has co-authored 2 books,12 book chapters, and 6 research articles (2 in press) in SCI-indexed journals. He has presented 7 research papers at national and international level seminars. He was awarded as 'Young Scientist in Plant Sciences' by the Society for Advanced Research in Plant Science (SARPS). His areas of research interest include the Bioprospection of botanicals, cancer biology.

Sreya Kosanam is Assistant Professor of Pharmacy Practice at Dr. M.G.R. Educational and Research Institute, Chennai, India. She earned her Doctor of Pharmacy from ASN Pharmacy College, affiliated to Acharya Nagarjuna University, and completed her Ph.D. in Pharmacology at KL University, Andhra Pradesh. Her academic career spans roles in pharmacy practice, pharmacology with teaching experience across undergraduate, postgraduate, and Pharm.D. programs. She has authored three books and multiple book chapters, published extensively in Scopus and Web of Science-indexed journals, and holds patents in medical devices and phytochemical applications. Dr. Kosanam's research interests include translational therapeutics, cardiovascular pharmacology, molecular docking, artificial intelligence applications in drug discovery, and pharmacovigilance. She is an active peer reviewer for several international journals, has presented at global conferences, and serves as a life member of leading professional pharmacy associations. Her work reflects a strong commitment to integrating research, clinical expertise, and education to advance pharmacy practice and patient care.

Akinpelu Moronkeji is a biomedical researcher in the Department of Medical Laboratory Science, University of Medical Sciences, Ondo, Nigeria. A Fellow of the Medical Laboratory Science Council of Nigeria, he conducts research in histopathology, cytopathology, and molecular biology, with a focus on oxidative stress, systemic toxicities, and the health impacts of air pollution.

Fausat Ola-Mudathir is a seasoned biochemist with expertise in nutritional biochemistry, phytomedicine, and toxicology. She earned her B.Sc., M.Sc., and Ph.D. in Biochemistry from the University of Ibadan, and has held academic positions at Crescent University and Elizade University. Her research explores the health benefits and antioxidant properties of functional foods and herbs, with a special focus on the antidote effects of onion in cyanide toxicity. She has also investigated the toxicity of various plants and drugs, contributing to safer therapeutic applications. Prof. Ola-Mudathir has published widely in peer-reviewed journals, including recent work on Crassocephalum crepidioides and copper-based anti-tuberculous drugs. Her teaching and research continue to shape the fields of biochemical pharmacology and natural product science in Nigeria.

Ibrahim Oreagba is a distinguished Consultant Pharmacist and Clinical Pharmacologist, currently serving as Head of the Department of Pharmacology,

Therapeutics and Toxicology at the College of Medicine, University of Lagos. He holds a Master's and Ph.D. in Pharmacology, along with a Postgraduate Certificate in Pharmacoepidemiology and Pharmacovigilance from the London School of Hygiene and Tropical Medicine. A Fellow of the West African Postgraduate College of Pharmacists, Prof. Oreagba has contributed extensively to drug safety, rational drug use, and pharmacovigilance policy development in Nigeria. He is a core technical member of the National Drug Safety Advisory Committee and has served on WHO/FMOH expert panels for national treatment guidelines. He has published over 70 scientific papers and serves as an editor and reviewer for several reputable journals. Beyond academia, he leads the Human Concern Foundation International and chairs the Halal Certification Authority, promoting quality assurance and ethical standards in healthcare and consumer products.

Dara Osundara is an researcher with interests in pathology, ethnobotany, drug development and data science with focuses on medicinal plans and analysis. Their main goal is to contribute to evidence based solutions in healthcare and science through rigorous research, innovation and collaboration.

Aman Suresh T is an Assistant Professor in Pharmacy Practice with extensive experience in teaching, research, and scholarly reviewing. He holds a Doctor of Pharmacy (Pharm-D) degree from SJM College of Pharmacy, Karnataka (RGUHS, 2023) and is currently pursuing a Ph.D. in Pharmacy Practice at SIMATS, Chennai. Over his academic career, he has taught at SJM College of Pharmacy, Sandip Institute of Pharmaceutical Sciences, and the Faculty of Pharmacy, Dr. M.G.R. Educational and Research Institute, delivering subjects such as Pharmacy Practice, Pharmacoepidemiology, Pharmacoeconomics, Pharmacotherapeutics, and Biostatistics & Research Methodology to B.Pharm, D.Pharm, and Pharm.D students. Dr. Aman has authored and co-authored numerous publications in Web of Science and Scopus-indexed journals, contributed book chapters, and completed over 155 peer reviews for reputed journals. His research interests span chronic disease management, pharmacovigilance, pharmacoepidemiology, and quality of life studies. Recognised with university-level ranks in Biostatistics, Clinical Research, and Project Work, he has also been awarded the ASCPT LMIC Travel Grant and has participated in national-level competitions. Alongside his academic contributions, he serves as an editorial board member and reviewer for multiple international journals, delivers guest lectures, and conducts workshops to advance pharmacy education and practice.

Index

S

T

W

Z

www.ingramcontent.com/pod-product-compliance
Lightning Source LLC
LaVergne TN
LVHW062335300926
849161LV00007B/1696